SALEM HEALTH
NUTRITION

SALEM HEALTH
NUTRITION

First Edition WITHDRAWN

Volume 1
Food Groups
Beverages
Herbs & Spices
Fats & Oils
USDA Information

Executive Editor

Sharon Richman, MSPT
EBSCO Information Services, Inc.

General Editor

Dawn Ortiz, MS RDN

SALEM PRESS
A Division of EBSCO Information Services, Inc.
IPSWICH, MASSACHUSETTS

GREY HOUSE PUBLISHING

Publisher's Cataloging-In-Publication Data
(Prepared by The Donohue Group, Inc.)

Names: Ortiz, Dawn, editor.
Title: Nutrition / editor, Dawn Ortiz, MS RDN.
Other Titles: Salem health | Salem health (Pasadena, Calif.)
Description: First edition. | Ipswich, Massachusetts : Salem Press, a division of EBSCO Information Services, Inc. ; Amenia, NY : Grey House Publishing, [2016] | Includes bibliographical references and index. | Contents: Volume 1. Food Groups; Beverages; Herbs & Spices; Fats & Oils—Volume 2. Medical Nutrition Therapy for Various Disease States—Volume 3. Dietary Considerations; Nutrition Through the Lifespan; Micronutrients; Appendixes; Index.
Identifiers: ISBN 978-1-68217-135-6 (set) | ISBN 978-1-68217-136-3 (v.1) | ISBN 978-1-68217-137-0 (v.2) | ISBN 978-1-68217-138-7 (v.3)
Subjects: LCSH: Nutrition—Encyclopedias. | Diet therapy—Encyclopedias.
Classification: LCC RA784 .N88 2016 | DDC 613.203—dc23

FIRST PRINTING
PRINTED IN THE UNITED STATES OF AMERICA

PUBLISHER'S NOTE

This is the first edition of *SALEM HEALTH: Nutrition*. It joins the family of Salem Health encyclopedias, including *Magill's Medical Guide, Psychology & Behavioral Health, Addictions & Substance Abuse, Complementary & Alternative Medicine, Infectious Diseases & Conditions, Genetics, Cancer,* and *Adolescent Health & Wellness*. This three-volume set—with 255 entries—covers not only the nutritional value of dozens of foods and food groups, but includes nutritional therapy, how diet affects certain medical conditions, and societal issues such as fad diets and obesity.

Volume 1—Food Groups—covers Fruits, Vegetables, Grains, Protiens, and Dairy—with individual, detailed entries on specific foods, followed by entries on specific Beverages, Herbs & Spices, and Fats & Oils. Following the entries in Volume 1 is nutrition information from the USDA.

Volume 2—Medical Nutrition Therapy for Various Diseases—offers information on how what you eat affects a variety of medical and mental conditions from autism and bipolar disorder to ulcers and uriniary tract infections. You'll read about which foods will help and what to avoid. This volume includes a cancer prevention diet, food addiction, and food allergies.

Volume 3 includes Dietary Considerations, Nutrition Through the Lifespan, and Micronutrients. It covers various diets, eating for your age, and specific information on vitamins and minerals. Volume 3 also includes two appendixes and a detailed index.

ORGANIZATION AND FORMAT

Entries in *Nutrition* range from one to eight pages in length. The text of each entry offers a clear and concise discussion of the topic. Subheads appear frequently, and include What We Know, Nutrients, Medical Nutrition, Research Findings, and Risk Factors.

Each entry includes not only the author's name but the names of those who reviewed the material as well.

RESOURCES AND INDEXES

A complete Table of Contents appears at the beginning of each volume. USDA information appears at the end of volume 1. Appendixes and Index appear at the end of Volume 3.

USDA INFORMATION

This section comprises 70 pages of information from the U.S. Department of Agriculture. A detailed table of contents lists the 33 charts and tables in this section, including the 2015-2020 Dietary Guidelines for Americans, Eating Patterns, Making Healthy Shifts, Average Intakes of Grain, Fats, Sugar, and Sodium, MyPlate food guidelines, several healthy eating patterns, and the new food label.

APPENDIXES

No Nutritional Value But Some Benefits

This section includes items like artificial sweeteners (helps with weight control), chewing gum (reduces tooth decay), and popcorn (increases fiber intake).

Cultural Challenges to Good Nutrition

Read about Food Deserts (urban neighborhoods and rural areas without access to nutritious food), Obesity in both the general population and among Veterans, and Ramadan Fasting (28 days of fasting in observance of Muslim holy days).

INDEX

Subject Index alphabetically lists all the significant people, places and concepts covered in this set.

ACKNOWLEDGMENTS

Salem Press gratefully acknowledges CINAHL Information Systems, who developed this material, and Dawn Ortiz, MS, RDN, editor of this edition, whose introduction to the work follows this Publisher's Note.

EDITOR'S INTRODUCTION

The topic of nutrition is unique in that it affects every single person in the world. We all eat. Every human being on the planet requires nutrition to fuel their body. For years, media, marketing teams, and food and drug manufacturers – from milk farmers to vitamin makers – have been capitalizing on the fact that we all want to be healthy and fit. The barrage of messages to consumers are often confusing and conflicting. There are endless opinions about what it means to follow a healthy diet and how to receive optimal nutrition from food. *Salem Health: Nutrition* is designed to help consumers focus on the source of nutrition information. As a registered dietitian nutritionist (RDN), two of my important goals are 1. help consumers decipher between fad diets and food trends and 2. provide healthy and sick individuals of all ages guidance on how the proper diet can meet their nutritional needs and provide optimum health for their unique medical conditions. In three comprehensive volumes, *Salem Health: Nutrition* meets these goals and more. Remember, you are what you eat!

Following a nutritious diet means eating a variety of delicious, fresh foods, while avoiding processed and fast food options. A good rule of thumb is that if your plate looks like a rainbow of colorful foods, chances are it contains a good variety of protein, grains, vegetables, fruits and dairy. You should avoid following a diet that eliminates food groups or includes an excessive amount of certain "super foods." In addition to what you eat, good nutrition is defined by how much you eat. Healthy eating consists of eating all foods in moderation – no self-deprivation. Focus more on adding healthy foods into your diet, and less on what to avoid. Look at meal time as an opportunity to fuel your body with nutritious goodness, and *Salem Health: Nutrition* as a tool with the information you need to make healthy food choices.

This encyclopedia is conveniently organized into three volumes. Volume 1 analyzes the nutritional value of hundreds of different foods. Each food is categorized according to its appropriate food group – fruits, vegetables, grains, protein, dairy, beverages, herbs/spices and fats/oils. The articles specify nutrient content, dietary intake guidelines and current research findings. You will learn how the simple act of eating your favorite foods is keeping you strong and healthy. Did you know that papaya contains a vitamin that helps build new DNA, or that chicken meat and eggs are rich in energy-producing B complex vitamins? Volume 1 also includes a section of important nutrition material from the United States Department of Agriculture that includes 2015-2020 Dietary Guidelines for Americans, eating patterns, and a variety of healthy eating styles.

Volume 2 focuses on how medical nutrition therapy (MNT) can help treat various disease states, and is a valuable resource for patients, and their families, who are struggling with illness. MNT determines how nutritional status and interventions can impact diseases, such as cancer, diabetes, heart disease and even mental illness. MNT for less severe conditions such as constipation and diarrhea, urinary tract infections and acne is also explored. You will learn how the prevention, progression and treatment of disease may be impacted by the addition or avoidance of certain foods. For example: foods rich in omega-3 fatty acids can reduce the depression and aggressive behavior associated with Alzheimer's disease; complex carbohydrates can stabilize moods swings that often accompany alcohol withdrawal; and soybeans and soy products can reduce high blood pressure.

Volume 3 consists of an assortment of topics associated with a healthy diet, including eating breakfast, avoiding fast food, and getting enough sleep. Furthermore, the nutrition implications associated with the most recent dietary guidelines of MyPlate are compared with the previous MyPyramid model. Volume 3 also includes a section of articles dedicated to the nutrition requirements throughout the lifespan that address how nutritional needs change with age. Coverage includes how best to eat during pregnancy and breastfeeding, how to encourage healthy eating in children, which foods can help reduce menopause symptoms, and how specific food choices can help older adults both mentally and physically. Also in Volume 3 is analysis of micronutrients (vitamins and minerals) by their action in the body, food sources, potential for deficiency/toxicity/medication interaction, and current research. Did you know beans are a good source of vitamin K, or that vitamin B12, required for the formation of RNA and DNA as well as proper function of the nervous system, is only found in foods of animal origin or select fortified foods?

I would like to thank Grey House Publishing and the Salem Press team, for the opportunity to work on this worthwhile project: Kristen Hayes, longtime friend, for referring me; Melissa Rose, for her assistance with all details and her calm, kind demeanor; and Laura Mars, for brainstorming sessions to overcome challenges.

Dawn Ortiz, MS RDN

CONTRIBUTORS

Cherie Marcel, BS

Bruce E. Johansen, Ph.D.

Gina Riley, Ph.D.

Karin Gajewski, RN, BSN

Marylane Wade Koch, RN, MSN

Gilberto Cabrera, MD

Anne Danahy, RDN, MS

Alexia Beauregard, RD, MS, CSP, LD

Carita Caple, RN, BSN, MSHS

Tanja Schub, BS

Suzanne Dixon, MPH, MS, RD

Lydia M. Uribe, PharmD, MLIS

Dianne Haskins, RN, BSN

Suzan E. Jaffe, RN, PhD, ARNP

Leonard Buckley, BS, MD

Eliza Schub, RN, BSN

Sara Richards, MSN, RN

Kathleen Walsh, RN, MSN, CCRN

Margaret White-Guthro, RN, ANP, BC

Penny March, PsyD

Lori Porter, RD, MBA

Christen Miller, RD, LDE

Darlene Strayer, RN, MBA

Teresa-Lynn Spears, RN, BSN, PHN, AE-C

COMPLETE LIST OF CONTENTS

VOLUME 1

Food Groups

Fruits

Vegetables

Grains

Proteins

VOLUME 2

VOLUME 3

Appendix One: No Nutritional Value But Some Benefits

Appendix Two: Cultural Challenges to Good Nutrition

FOOD GROUPS

FRUITS

Acai Berry

WHAT WE KNOW

The dark purple acai berry is the fruit of the acai palm (Euterpe oleracea), which is native to Central and South America. Acai berries grow in clusters of 3–8 berries and have the appearance of oversized blueberries. Unlike the blueberry, the acai berry contains a large seed. With their sweet and slightly tart flavor, acai berries can be eaten raw or made into juices, jellies, syrups, sauces, and many types of commercial beverages. In recent years, the acai berry has been touted as a "super food" with claims that it can fight heart disease, cancer, aging, and arthritis and improve digestion, sleep patterns, sexual performance, and overall health. Scientific support for these claims is lacking. Nutritionally, acai berries are similar to other dark berries in that they contain phytonutrients (i.e., beneficial, plant-derived chemicals) with potent antioxidant and anti-inflammatory properties. Acai berries are also a source of monounsaturated fatty acids (MUFAs) and protein.

NUTRIENTS IN THE ACAI BERRY

Acai berries are a rich source of vitamin A, or retinol, which is a fat-soluble vitamin that is required for vision, maintenance of the surface lining of the eyes and other epithelial tissue, bone growth, immune response, energy regulation, reproduction, embryonic development, and activation of gene expression.

- Acai berry contains calcium, which builds and maintains bones and teeth, regulates muscle contraction, conducts nerve impulses, activates enzymes for energy production and muscle contraction, participates in blood clotting, assists with vitamin B12 absorption, and maintains the structural integrity of intracellular membranes.
- The MUFAs found in acai berry promotes the production of antioxidants and lower triglyceride levels in the blood, reducing the risk for arteriosclerosis (i.e., thickened arteries) and heart disease.

- Acai berry is most noted for its high content of phytochemicals, particularly anthocyanins.
- Anthocyanins are reddish pigments that have high antioxidant, anti-inflammatory, antibiotic, and anti-mutagenic activity. They also promote urinary tract health, protect blood vessels from rupture, and support memory function

RESEARCH FINDINGS

Researchers evaluated the effect of acai berry consumption on risk factors for metabolic syndrome (i.e., cluster of risk factors that raise the risk for heart disease and other health problems, such as diabetes and stroke) in overweight individuals. The results of the uncontrolled pilot study indicated that consuming the fruit pulp of acai berries reduced levels of fasting glucose, fasting insulin, and total cholesterol, suggesting that consumption of acai berries may reduce the risk for metabolic syndrome in overweight individuals. Researchers suggested that further studies are warranted.

SUMMARY

The more consumers know about the physiologic benefits of the acai berry, and share this information with friends and family, the better the chances are for increased acai berry consumption.

The acai berry is a good source of monounsaturated fatty acids (MUFAs), protein, vitamin A, calcium and the phytochemical; anthocyanin. The nutritional benefits of the acai berry include improved function of cells, memory, the urinary tract, and bone growth, while reducing the risk factors associated with developing metabolic syndrome.

—*Cherie Marcel, BS*

REFERENCES

Berry interesting: Acai berry's effect on cancer in question. (2011). CURE: Cancer Updates, 10(3), 56.

Marcason, W. (2009). What is the acai berry and are there health benefits? Journal of the American

Dietetic Association, 109(11), 1968. doi:10.1016/j.jada.2009.09.017

Sego, S. (2009). Alternative meds update. Acai berry. Clinical Advisor for Nurse Practitioners, 12(1), 65-66.

Turcotte, M. (2015, February 18). Acai berry nutrition information. Livestrong.com. Retrieved January 14, 2015, from http://www.livestrong.com/article/111990-acai-berry-nutrition-information/

Udani, J. K., Singh, B. B., Singh, V. J., & Barrett, M. L. (2011). Effects of Acai (Euterpe oleracea Mart.) berry preparation on metabolic parameters in a health overweight population: A pilot study. Nutrition Journal, 10, 45. doi:10.1186/1475-2891-10-45

Wein, D. (2010). Acai berry: Indispensable or superfluous? NSCA's Performance Training Journal, 9(1), 21-22.

REVIEWER(S)

Darlene Strayer, RN, MBA, Cinahl Information Systems, Glendale, CA

Nursing Executive Practice Council, Glendale Adventist Medical Center, Glendale, CA

Apple

WHAT WE KNOW

- The apple, or Malus, is a fruit from the Rosaceae (i.e., rose) family, which includes cherries, peaches, apricots, and plums. Apple origins have been traced to Europe and Asia, but apple trees are now grown worldwide and there are more than 7,000 varieties (e.g., Red and Golden Delicious, Pippins, Granny Smith, Fuji, Braeburn). Apples have red, yellow, green, or red mixed with green skin that covers crisp, white flesh. Apple flavors range from tart to sweet. The apple can be eaten raw, canned, dried, baked in pies and cobblers, and used in jams and sauces. In addition to its culinary value, the apple is a good source of fiber, vitamin C, and many phytonutrients (i.e., protective, plant-derived chemicals). The antihistamine, anti-inflammatory, and antioxidant properties of apple provide many health benefits such as reducing risk for asthma, constipation, diabetes mellitus, type 2 (DM2), heart disease, and cancer (e.g., skin, lung, and colon cancer).

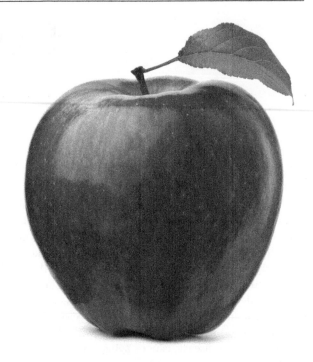

NUTRIENTS IN THE APPLE

- The concentration of nutrients is especially high in the skin of the apple.
- Apple contains many important phytonutrients, including the flavonols; quercetin, kaempferol, and myricetin, which provide strong antioxidant and anti-inflammatory protection and have antihistamine, antimicrobial, anti-diabetic, and anti-carcinogenic (i.e., cancer fighting) properties.
- Phenolic acid (chlorogenic acid) is a plant chemical that exhibits anti-carcinogenic, antimicrobial, and antiviral properties and is believed to inhibit the build-up of low density lipoprotein (LDL) cholesterol (i.e., the "bad" cholesterol).
- The skin of red apples contains anthocyanins, which are reddish color pigments that have high antioxidant and anti-carcinogenic activity, promote urinary tract health, and support memory function.
- Epicatechin is thought to decrease risk for cardiovascular disease (CVD) and hypertension by preventing the oxidation of LDL, enhancing blood vessel relaxation, reducing inflammation, and inhibiting clot formation by simulating blood cell function.
- Apigenin has anti-mutagenic activity and has been shown to reduce the size of prostate tumors

and prevent the development of progestin-induced breast cancer.

- The water-soluble vitamin C in apple neutralizes free radicals, protecting against inflammation and cellular damage. Adequate vitamin C intake is vital for healthy immune system function and is associated with the prevention of heart disease, stroke, and cancer.
- Apple is a good source of dietary fiber, including soluble fiber, which binds with water and slows the digestive process, allowing the body to better manage post-prandial (i.e., after eating) glucose and insulin responses. Fiber also increases the volume of the intestinal contents, which hinders the absorption of cholesterol. The added bulk leads to more regular bowel movements, promoting intestinal health.

RESEARCH FINDINGS

- There is no information in medical literature regarding recommended dosage of apple, adverse effects and contraindications of apple, or interactions of apple with medications.
- There is evidence that the nutrients and phytochemicals found in apple counteract oxidative stress, reduce inflammation, and modulate cellular interactions, which play a protective role against vascular disease and cancer. The prevention of vascular disease is attributed in part to the ability of these nutrients (e.g., epicatechin, chlorogenic acid, and vitamin C) to inhibit blood clotting and lower cholesterol and fat levels. The cancer-preventive properties of the apple lie in the ability of its constituents (e.g., flavonols, anthocyanins, apigenin, and vitamin C) to protect against DNA and cellular damage caused by oxidative stress, modulate carcinogen metabolism, prevent inflammation, induce natural cell death and renewal, and prevent or retard the spread of malignant cells into surrounding tissues. Results of studies indicate that consuming one or more apples a day reduces risk for skin, breast, colon, and lung cancers.
- Evidence indicates that drinking clear apple juice, which does not contain pectin and other important cell wall constituents, is not as effective at lowering cholesterol as eating whole apples. Researchers suggest that the fiber content of whole apples is a necessary component to achieve the cholesterol-lowering effect.
- A 2012 study analyzed the content of arsenic and lead in 15 juices containing apple. Results showed that both arsenic and lead were present in most of the juices analyzed. Although the levels of lead were below the mandated exposure levels in drinking water, 32% of the juices tested had arsenic levels that were close to or exceeded the mandated limit for exposure in drinking water of 10 parts per billion. Researchers suggested that persons who consume apple juice would be better protected if juice was mandated to comply with the same exposure limits that are currently set for drinking water. Additionally, researchers stated that regular testing of juices that contain apple and reporting results would serve to inform consumers of the higher arsenic levels contained in certain types and brands of juice.

SUMMARY

The more consumers know about the physiologic benefits of the apple, and share this information with friends and family, the better the chances are for increased apple consumption.

Apples are a good source of fiber, vitamin C, and many phytonutrients, and the nutritional benefits of apple consumption include reduced risk for asthma, constipation, DM2, heart disease, and cancer.

—*Cherie Marcel, BS*

REFERENCES

Bergmann, H., Triebel, S., Kahle, K., & Richling, E. (2010). The metabolic fate of apple polyphenols in humans. Current Nutrition and Food Science, 6(1), 19-35. doi:10.2174/157340110790909554

Fratianni, F., Coppola, R., & Nazzaro, F. (2011). Phenolic composition and antimicrobial and antiquorum sensing activity of an ethanolic extract of peels from the apple cultivar Annurca. Journal of Medicinal Food, 14(9), 957-963. doi:10.1089/jmf.2010.0170

The George Mateljan Foundation. (n.d.). The world's healthiest foods: Apples. Retrieved February 24, 2015, from http://www.whfoods.com/genpage.php?dbid=15&tname=foodspice

Gerhauser, C. (2008). Cancer chemopreventive potential of apples, apple juice, and apple components. Planta Medica, 74(13), 1608-1624. doi:10.1055/s-0028-1088300

Li, Y., Niu, Y., Sun, Y., Mei, L., Zhang, B., Li, Q., ...
Mei, Q. (2014). An apple oligogalactan potentiates
the growth inhibitory effect of celecoxib on colorec-
talcancer. Nutrition & Cancer, 66(1), 29-37. doi:10.10
80/01635581.2014.847965

Lock, C. (2011). Your child healthy eating. Falling for
apples. Parents, 86(10), 72-82.

Ravn-Haren, G., Dragsted, L. O., Buch-Andersen, T.,
Jensen, E. N., Jensen, R. I., Nemeth-Balogh, M.,
... Bugel, S. (2013). Intake of whole apples or clear
apple juice has contrasting effects on plasma lipids
in healthy volunteers. European Journal of Nutrition,
52(8), 1875-1889. doi:10.1007/s00394-012-0489-z

Tian, H. L., Zhan, P., & Li, K. X. (2010). Analysis of components and study on antioxidant and antimicrobial
activities of oil in apple seeds. International Journal
of Food Sciences and Nutrition, 61(4), 395-403.
doi:10.3109/09637480903535772

Weichselbaum, E., Wyness, L., & Stanner, S. (2010).
Apple polyphenols and cardiovascular disease - a review of the evidence. Nutrition Bulletin, 35(2), 92-
101. doi:10.1111/j.1467-3010.2010.01822.x

Wilson, D., Hooper, C., & Shi, X. (2012). Arsenic and
lead in juice: Apple, citrus, and apple-base. Journal of
Environmental Health, 75(5), 14-20.

REVIEWER(S)

Darlene Strayer, RN, MBA, Cinahl Information Systems,
Glendale, CA

Nursing Executive Practice Council, Glendale Adventist
Medical Center, Glendale, CA

Apricot

WHAT WE KNOW

The apricot, or Prunus armeniaca, is a small stone fruit
from the Rosaceae (i.e., rose) family, along with cherries, peaches, and plums. Its origins are in China over
4,000 years ago, where apricot was believed to enhance
fertility. In the 1700s, Spanish explorers transported
cuttings from apricot trees to the Spanish missions in
California, marking the beginning of California's cultivation of what is now 95% of the apricots grown in the
United States. The soft, peach-like skin of the apricot
is edible and surrounds the sugary sweet and slightly
tart fleshy fruit. Apricots are a delicious culinary treat
when eaten raw, canned, dried, baked into pies and
cobblers, made into jams and sauces, and blended into
drinks. Beyond its value in cuisine, the apricot possesses a wealth of nutrients, including beta carotene
(i.e., the precursor to vitamin A), vitamin C, potassium, lycopene (i.e., a carotenoid responsible for the orange pigmentation), important polyphenolic phytonutrients (i.e., protective plant-derived chemicals), and
fiber. Apricot consumption is associated with reduced
risk of developing macular degeneration and prostate
cancer and with providing antioxidant protection for
the heart. The seed, or kernel (also known as Laetrile
and vitamin B-17) of the apricot contains about 0.5
mg of cyanide, a mitochondrial toxin that can cause
death within minutes to hours of ingestion. In general,
this small amount of cyanide does not pose a threat
to individuals eating the fruit and discarding the kernel. Although controversial, apricot kernels have been
used in certain alternative medicines as a treatment for
cancer. Research is lacking on the benefits of apricot
kernels and their safe administration as a treatment
for cancer.

NUTRIENTS IN THE APRICOT

- Apricots contain important phytonutrients that
  have antioxidant, anti-inflammatory, and anti-
  mutagenic properties, which act to protect deoxyribonucleic acid (DNA) against damage and
  enhance DNA repair.
- The water-soluble vitamin C in apricots neutralizes free radicals, protecting against inflammation
  and cellular damage. Adequate vitamin C intake
  is vital for healthy immune system function and
  is associated with prevention of heart disease,
  stroke, and cancer.
- The beta carotene in apricots is a precursor for
  vitamin A, which provides antioxidant protection
  to the heart and promotes visual health. Results
  of studies show that vitamin A plays a role in preventing age-related macular degeneration.
- Apricots contain potassium, which is an essential element responsible for regulating acid-base
  balance, maintaining fluid balance, supporting
  muscle contraction and cardiac function, contributing to protein synthesis and carbohydrate
  metabolism, and promoting cellular growth and
  transmission of nerve impulses.
- Apricots are an excellent source of dietary fiber,
  which binds and removes toxins from the colon,
  assists in glycemic control, and reduces high cholesterol levels.

- The combination of vitamins A and C, potassium, and polyphenols found in apricots reduces triglycerides and prevents excessive platelet aggregation (i.e., blood clotting).

DIETARY INTAKE GUIDELINES
Excessive intake of apricot kernels may cause cyanide poisoning.

- The lethal cyanide dose is 50–60 apricot kernels
- The Council of Europe and the World Health Organization have established the tolerable daily intake (TDI) of cyanide as follows: 5–9 mcg/lb (12–20 mcg/kg) of body weight
- 1.5–2.5 kernels for a female weighing 140 lb/63.5 kg
- 2–3 kernels for a male weighing 175 lb/79.4 kg
- Other than the potential for cyanide poisoning from excessive kernel ingestion, there is no information in the medical literature about adverse reactions and contraindications of apricot.

RESEARCH FINDINGS
There is evidence that the nutrients and phytochemicals found in apricots counteract oxidative stress, reduce inflammation, and modulate cellular interactions, all of which play a role in protecting against vascular disease and cancer. The prevention of vascular disease is attributed in part to the ability of these phytochemicals (e.g., flavonoids and carotenoids) and nutrients (e.g., vitamin C, vitamin A, and potassium) to limit blood clotting and lower cholesterol levels. The potential chemo-preventive properties of the apricot lie in the ability of its constituents to protect against DNA and cellular damage caused by oxidative stress

Although warnings about the toxicity of apricot kernels due to their cyanide content have prevented apricot use among most healthcare practitioners, some clinicians report their belief in the anti-cancer effects of Laetrile. There are very few recorded cases of death from consuming apricot kernels despite its relatively widespread use as alternative medicine since the 1970s, suggesting that the actual occurrence of cyanide poisoning and death is rare. Results of several studies and many anecdotal accounts supported the medicinal effectiveness of Laetrile extracts for treatment of cancer, bacterial infections (e.g., caused by Staphylococcus aureus or Escherichia coli), and the overgrowth of Candida albicans (i.e, an infectious fungus). Some researchers suggest that more studies be conducted to thoroughly investigate whether or not apricot kernels should be used medicinally and in what quantities and preparations.

SUMMARY
Consumers should be aware of the physiologic benefits of apricot consumption and the risks associated with apricot kernel ingestion. Apricots are a good source of fiber, vitamin C, potassium, beta carotene, lycopene and many important polyphenolic phytonutrients. The nutritional benefits of apricot consumption, include reduced risk of developing macular degeneration and prostate cancer and providing antioxidant protection for the heart. It is also important to note that there is the potential for cyanide poisoning from excessive kernel ingestion.

—*Cherie Marcel, BS*

REFERENCES
Akyildiz, B. N., Kurtoglu, S., Kondolot, M., & Tunç, A. (2010). Cyanide poisoning caused by ingestion of apricot seeds. Annals of Tropical Paediatrics, 30(1), 39-43.

Broihier, K. (2008). Apricot ABC's: Vitamin A, beta-carotene, vitamin C. Environmental Nutrition, 31(5), 8.

Drogoudi, P. D., Vemmos, S., Pantelidis, G., Petri, E., Tzoutzoukou, C., & Karayiannis, I. (2008). Physical characters and antioxidant, sugar, and mineral nutrient contents in fruit from 29 apricot (Prunus armeniaca L.) cultivars and hybrids. Journal of Agricultural and Food Chemistry, 56(22), 10754-10760. doi:10.1021/jf801995x

Krashen, S. (2009). Are apricot kernels toxic? Internet Journal of Health, 9(2), 9.

Latocha, P., Krupa, T., Wolosiak, R., Worobiej, E., & Wilczak, J. (2010). Antioxidant activity and chemical difference in fruit of different Actinidia sp. International Journal of Food Sciences & Nutrition, 61(4), 381-394. doi:10.3109/09637480903517788

Lofshult, D. (2009). The artful apricot. IDEA Fitness Journal, 6(3), 58.

The George Mateljan Foundation. (n.d.). The world's healthiest foods: Apricots. Retrieved February 24, 2015, from http://www.whfoods.com/genpage.php?tname=foodspice&dbid=3

Varga, G. (2010). Are "natural" products really that safe: A case of poisoning in the ER. NENA Outlook, 33(2), 13-15. Retrieved from http://www.whfoods.com/genpage.php?tname=foodspice&dbid=3

Yigit, D., Yigit, N., & Mavi, A. (2009). Antioxidant and antimicrobial activities of bitter and sweet apricot (Prunus armeniaca L.) kernels. Brazilian Journal of Medical and Biological Research, 42(4), 346-352.

Zanteson, L. (2011). Apricot's delicious, healthy appeal. Environmental Nutrition, 34(6), 8.

REVIEWER(S)

Darlene Strayer, RN, MBA, Cinahl Information Systems, Glendale, CA

Nursing Executive Practice Council, Glendale Adventist Medical Center, Glendale, CA

Avocado

WHAT WE KNOW

- The avocado tree, or Persea americana, produces a fruit that is native to Mexico, Central America, and South America, although the avocado is now predominantly grown in California. The meaty, pale green fruit of the avocado grows around a large pit (i.e., the seed) and is surrounded by a thick, dark green skin. The outer skin provides the fruit's protection against disease and insects, reducing the need for using harmful pesticides.
- While avocado is known to be high in fat, approximately 60% of that fat is monounsaturated and 20% is polyunsaturated, leaving only 20% saturated fat. This is valuable because monounsaturated fat protects against heart disease. Avocado is a good source of protein, potassium, magnesium, folate, thiamin, riboflavin, niacin, biotin, pantothenic acid, vitamins E and K, and many phytonutrients (i.e., beneficial plant-derived chemicals). As a result of these nutrients, avocado has been shown to have antioxidant, anti-inflammatory, anti-carcinogenic, anti-thrombotic (i.e., anti-blood clot forming) and anti-hypertensive (i.e., blood pressure lowering) properties. Among the health benefits associated with avocado consumption are prevention of heart disease, cancer (e.g., oral, skin, prostate), diabetes mellitus, type 2 (DM2), obesity, and osteoarthritis (OA).
- Avocado is delicious raw and can be sliced onto salads, spread onto sandwiches, blended into guacamole, or used as a topping on baked potatoes. Because of the smooth texture and fat content, avocado can also be used as a substitute for other fats in some baking recipes.

NUTRIENTS IN THE AVOCADO

- Avocado is rich in nutrients, making it a functional food (i.e., a food that provides health benefits exceeding basic nutrition). Included in these nutrients are the following:
- The monounsaturated fatty acid, oleic acid promotes the production of antioxidants and lowers triglyceride (i.e., main constituent of fat in humans) levels, reducing the risk of atherosclerosis (i.e., thickening of artery walls), heart disease, and cancer.
- Vitamin E protects lipids (i.e. fats) from oxidation, reducing harmful free radicals in the body.
- The fat-soluble vitamin K acts as a coenzyme involved in maintaining normal levels of blood clotting proteins and contributes to bone remodeling.
- The minerals, potassium and magnesium help maintain homeostasis or cell regulation, control blood pressure, promote bone and teeth formation, produce blood cells, and support normal nerve and muscle function.
- Niacin is involved in oxidation-reduction reactions (i.e. transfer of electrons) that derive energy from carbohydrates, lipids, proteins, and alcohol and is integral for the reactions necessary to make new fatty acids and cholesterol.
- Thiamine conducts the flow of nerve and muscle cells and contributes to the function of the nervous system; thiamine contributes to the metabolism or break down of carbohydrates and production of hydrochloric acid, both of which are vital for digestion.
- Pantothenic acid contributes to the metabolism of carbohydrates, proteins, and lipids. It also plays a role in the synthesis of acetylcholine, a neurotransmitter (i.e., transmits nerve impulses) in the central and peripheral nervous systems.
- Folate is essential for the production and maintenance of red blood cells, the metabolism of homocysteine (i.e., an amino acid or broken down protein), and the synthesis of deoxyribonucleic acid (DNA) and ribonucleic acid (RNA), the genetic code for cells.
- Riboflavin activates proteins for respiratory reactions in order to produce energy; plays a role in fatty acid oxidation (i.e., energy production);

contributes to the formation of vitamins B6, B12, and niacin (vitamin B3) and their coenzymes; and is required for conversion of retinol to retinoic acid, which is integral to normal vision.

- Biotin functions as a coenzyme for carboxylases, enzymes required for the metabolism of fatty acids and gluconeogenesis (i.e., the conversion of protein and fat into glucose). It also plays a role in the formation of purines, which are vital elements in DNA and RNA. The health of skin, hair, and nails is also attributed to biotin.
- Glutathione, a tripeptide containing the amino acids, glutamic acid, cysteine, and glycine has powerful antioxidant activity and has been associated with reduced risk of oral and pharyngeal cancer.
- Many valuable phytonutrients (e.g., carotenoids and phytosterols), which exhibit powerful antioxidant, anticoagulant, anti-inflammatory, and anticarcinogenic properties. The phytosterol (i.e., naturally occurring compounds found in plant cell membranes), beta-sitosterol interferes with cholesterol absorption, promoting lower cholesterol levels in the blood.
- Researchers report that consumption of avocado improves the efficiency of conversion of pro-vitamin A carotenoids (i.e., plant pigments responsible for bright red, yellow and orange hues in many fruits and vegetables) to vitamin A within the body because of the lipids contained in avocado.

DIETARY INTAKE GUIDELINES
- While there are no specific guidelines for dietary intake of avocado, it is a significant source of dietary fat. Guidelines for dietary fat intake include the following:
- Reduce risk for CVD, cancer, DM2, and stroke by choosing unsaturated fats (including omega-3 fatty acid) and by limiting total fat intake to 30% or less of daily calories, limiting saturated fat (found in meat, whole milk, cream, butter, and cheese) to less than 10% of daily calories, and consuming less than 200 mg of cholesterol per day.

RESEARCH FINDINGS
- Numerous studies have analyzed the potential efficacy of avocado-soybean unsaponifiables (ASU) for the treatment of OA. ASU are the hydrolyzed (i.e., chemically broken down with water) fraction from avocado and soybean oils, which does not produce soap. ASU has demonstrated anti-inflammatory properties, which appear to prevent joint destruction and possibly promote cartilage repair. While further trials are needed to confirm the significance of these therapeutic actions, researchers suggest that ASU could potentially serve as an alternative nutraceutical treatment (i.e., health benefit from food) for OA.
- Researchers analyzing the wound-healing activity of avocado fruit extract found that the topical application of avocado fruit extract promotes collagen formation in healing wounds, possibly due to its antioxidant and antimicrobial activities, but further study is needed before recommending it for clinical use.
- According to researchers, the results from the National Health Examination Survey (NHANES) 2001-2008 demonstrate a positive correlation between avocado consumption and overall diet quality. Avocado intake was associated with better nutrient intake and a lower risk of developing metabolic syndrome (i.e., cluster of risk factors that raise the risk for heart disease and other health problems, such as diabetes and stroke)
- Avocado oil consumption is similar to olive oil in its liver protecting and lipid lowering effects.

SUMMARY
Becoming more knowledgeable about the physiologic effects of avocado will help increase consumer consumption. While avocado is a high-fat food, it is rich in nutrients, including protein, potassium, magnesium, folate, thiamin, riboflavin, niacin, biotin, pantothenic acid, vitamins E and K, and many phytonutrients. Avocado provides numerous health benefits, including reduced risk of heart disease, DM2, OA, and some cancers.

—*Cherie Marcel, BS*

REFERENCES
Carvajal-Zarrabal, O., Nolasco-Hipolito, C., Aguilar-Uscanga, M. G., Melo, S. G., Hayward-Jones, P. M., & Barradas-Dermitz, D. M. (2014). Effect of dietary intake of avocado oil and olive oil on biochemical markers of liver function in sucrose-fed rats. Biomed Research International, 7pp. doi:10.1155/2014/595479

Carvajal-Zarrabal, O., Nolasco-Hipolito, C., Aguilar-Uscanga, M. G., Melo, S. G., Hayward-Jones, P. M., & Barradas-Dermitz, D. M. (2014). Avocado oil supplementation modifies cardiovascular risk profile markers in a rat model of sucrose-induced metabolic changes. Disease Markers, 386425, 9 pp. doi:10.1155/2014/386425

Chrubasik, J. E., Roufogalis, B. D., & Chrubasik, S. (2007). Evidence of effectiveness of herbal antiinflammatory drugs in the treatment of painful osteoarthritis and chronic low back pain. Phytotherapy Research, 21(7), 675-683. doi:10.1002/ptr.2142

Clayton, J. J. (2007). Nutraceuticals in the management of osteoarthritis. Orthopedics, 30(8), 624-631.

Ding, H., Han, C., Guo, D., Chin, Y., Ding, Y., Kinghorn, A. D., & D'Ambrosio, S. M. (2009). Selective induction of apoptosis of human cancer cell lines by avocado extracts via a ROS-mediated mechanism. Nutrition & Cancer, 61(3), 348-356. doi:10.1080/01635580802567158

Duester, K. C. (2000). Pleasures of the table. Avocados: A look beyond basic nutrition for one of nature's whole foods. Nutrition Today, 35(4), 151-157.

Ernst, E. (2003). Avocado-soybean unsaponifiables (ASU) for osteoarthritis — a systematic review. Clinical Rheumatology, 22(4-5), 285-288. doi:10.1007/s10067-003-0731-4.

Evans, L. Foods for radiant skin. Alive: Canada's Natural Health and Wellness Magazine. Retrieved February 27, 2015, from http://www.alive.com/articles/view/23185/foods_for_radiant_skin

Fulgoni, V. L., Dreher, M., Dreher, M., & Davenport, A. J. (2013). Avocado consumption is associated with better diet quality and nutrient intake, and lower metabolic syndrome risk in US adults: Results from the National Health and Nutrition Examination Survey (NHANES) 2001-2008. Nutrition Journal, 12(1), 6 pp. doi:10.1186/1475-2891-12-1

Gabay, O., Gosset, M., Levy, A., Salvat, C., Sanchez, C., Pigenet, A., & Berenbaum, F. (2008). Stress-induced signaling pathways in hyalin chondrocytes: Inhibition by Avocado-Soybean Unsaponifiables (ASU). Osteoarthritis & Cartilage, 16(3), 373-384. doi:10.1016/j.joca.2007.06.016

The George Mateljan Foundation. (n.d.). The world's healthiest foods: Avocado. Retrieved February 27, 2015, from http://www.whfoods.com/genpage.php?tname=foodspice&dbid=5

Grzanna, M. W., Ownby, S. L., Heinecke, L. F., Au, A. Y., & Frondoza, C. G. (2010). Inhibition of cytokine expression and prostaglandin E2 production in monocyte/macrophage-like cells by avocado/soybean unsaponifiables and chondroitin sulfate. Journal of Complimentary & Integrative Medicine, 7(1), [cover]-16. doi:10.2202/1553-3840.1338

Henrotin, Y. E., Deberg, M. A., Crielaard, J., Piccardi, N., Msika, P., & Sanchez, C. (2006). Avocado/soybean unsaponifiables prevent the inhibitory effect of osteoarthritic subchondral osteoblasts on aggrecan and type II collagen synthesis by chondrocytes. Journal of Rheumatology, 33(8), 1668-1678.

Kopec, R. E., Cooperstone, J. L., Schweiggert, R. M., Young, G. S., Harrison, E. H., Francis, D. M., ... Schwartz, S. J. (2014). Avocado consumption enhances human postprandial provitamin A absorption and conversion from a novel high-carotene tomato sauce and from carrots. The Journal of Nutrition, 144(8), 1158-1166. doi:10.3945/jn.113.187674

Moss, R. (2010). War on cancer. Townsend Letter, 46.

Nayak, B. S., Raju, S. S., & Chalapathi Rao, A. V. (2008). Wound healing activity of Persea americana (avocado) fruit: A preclinical study on rats. Journal of Wound Care, 17(3), 123-126.

Petty, L. (2011). Botanical balms. Alive: Canada's Natural Health and Wellness Magazine, (343), 35-38.

REVIEWER(S)

Darlene Strayer, RN, MBA, Cinahl Information Systems, Glendale, CA

Nursing Executive Practice Council, Glendale Adventist Medical Center, Glendale, CA

Banana

WHAT WE KNOW

Banana is a tropical, fruit-producing plant (Musa sapientum, Musa acuminata, and Musa balbisiana) that belongs to the Musaceae family, along with the lily and the orchid. The creamy banana fruit grows in bunches (also called "hands") and is encased in a tough skin. There are about 1,000 varieties of banana that vary in size, color, and sweetness. The Cavendish variety, which is the common yellow banana accounts for 95% of the international banana trade, although recently the Cavendish banana has become susceptible to a fungus called Panama disease that makes cultivation difficult. Because of this, other sweet banana varieties (e.g., the red banana) are being introduced in the market place. Raw banana is considered delicious to eat and banana is appreciated as a culinary element that adds a sweet flavor and smooth texture to sauces, beverages, and baked goods. The plantain is a firmer and starchier variety banana that can be used as a source of starch in cooking, but it lacks the palatable sweetness of other varieties and is not usually eaten in raw form. The banana contains many nutrients, including vitamins E, C, B1, B2, and B6; magnesium; potassium; fiber; and valuable phytonutrients (i.e., protective plant-derived chemicals), including beta-carotene, the precursor to vitamin A.

NUTRIENTS IN THE BANANA

- Bananas contain important phytochemicals, including carotenoids and flavonoids that exhibit anti-inflammatory, hypolipidemic (i.e., fat lowering), hypoglycemic (i.e., sugar lowering), and antioxidant activity
- The under-ripe banana that appears green or green-tipped in color contains amylase-resistant starch (ARS), which functions much like fiber and is useful in the management of many digestive and metabolic disorders, including the treatment of persistent diarrhea. ARS also protects against mucosal damage associated with indigestion and helps stimulate mucosal resistance in damaged tissue.
- Magnesium and vitamins C, E, and the B vitamins (by combining with manganese) in banana provide antioxidant activity and support the immune and nervous systems.
- The potassium in banana helps eliminate excess sodium from the body.
- Magnesium and potassium help lower blood pressure and reduce risk for coronary artery disease (CAD) and stroke.
- Vitamin B6 stimulates production of serotonin, an enzyme that helps regulate mood.

RESEARCH FINDINGS

- There is evidence that the ARS in the under-ripe green or green-tipped banana provides powerful mucosal protection and treatment for persistent diarrhea. Other benefits of under-ripe banana include lower sugar content and higher fiber, which help burn fat and lower blood glucose levels. Results of

a recent study showed that the methanolic extract of banana seeds is an effective antidiarrheal agent. Researchers also noted that the seed extract exhibited antioxidant and antibacterial activity.

- Researchers recently analyzed the use of flour made from unripe green banana as a gluten-free option for individuals who require a gluten-free diet (e.g., persons with celiac disease). In the study, green banana flour was used to make pasta, which was compared with pasta made from wheat flour. The two pastas showed no significant difference in aroma, flavor, or overall quality, and the pasta made from green banana flour received greater acceptance among study participants than the wheat flour-based pasta. Researchers suggest that the results of this experiment provide support for the use of green banana to develop gluten-free products in order to offer more options to persons following the highly restricted gluten-free diet. Additionally, the use of green banana flour is a good commercial use for green bananas, which are currently considered a sub-product that has low commercial value.
- Researchers studied the effects of consuming 20 g/day for 45 days of green banana flour on the health parameters of overweight women who met metabolic syndrome criteria (e.g., three or more of the following five criteria are met: waist circumference over 40 inches (men) or 35 inches (women), blood pressure over 130/85 mmHg, fasting triglyceride (TG) level over 150 mg/dl, fasting high-density lipoprotein (HDL) cholesterol level less than 40 mg/dl (men) or 50 mg/dl (women) and fasting blood sugar over 100 mg/dl). From study results researchers reported that, while there was no significant change in weight or body composition, the women did experience a decrease in hip circumference and a reduction in systolic blood pressure and fasting glucose levels.

SUMMARY

Consumers should become more knowledgeable about the physiologic benefits of banana consumption. Bananas are rich in nutrients, including vitamins E, C, B1, B2, and B6, magnesium, potassium, fiber, and valuable phytonutrients (e.g., beta-carotene). Bananas provide numerous health benefits, including lowering of blood pressure, reduced risk for CAD and stroke. The under-ripe banana that appears green or green-tipped in color contains ARS, which is useful in the management of many digestive and metabolic disorders, including the treatment of persistent diarrhea.

—*Cherie Marcel, BS*

REFERENCES

Alvarez-Acosta, T., Leon, C., Acosta-Gonzalez, S., Parra-Soto, H., Cluet-Rodriguez, I., Rossel, M. R., ... Colina-Chourio, J. A. (2009). Beneficial role of green plantain [Musa paradisiaca] in the management of persistent diarrhea: A prospective randomized trial. Journal of American College of Nutrition, 28(2), 169-176.

Firpo-Cappiello, R. (2010). Feed what ails you. Prevention, 62(6), 92-97.

Hettiaratchi, U. P., Ekanayake, S., & Welihinda, J. (2011). Chemical compositions and glycemic responses to banana varieties. International Journal of Food Sciences & Nutrition, 62(4), 307-309. doi:10.31 09/09637486.2010.537254

Hossain, M. S., Alam, M. B., Asadujjaman, M., Zahan, R., Islam, M. M., Mazumder, E. H., ... Haque, M. E. (2011). Antidiarrheal, antioxidant and antimicrobial activities of the Musa sapientum seed. Avicenna Journal of Medical Biotechnology, 3(2), 95-105.

Perez-Perez, E. M., Rodriguez-Malaver, A. J., Padilla, N., Medina-Ramirez, G., & Davila, J. (2006). Antioxidant capacity of crude extracts from clones of banana and plane species. Journal of Medicinal Food, 9(4), 517-523.

Rabbani, G. H., Larson, C. P., Islam, R., Saha, U. R., & Kabir, A. (2010). Green banana-supplemented diet in the home management of acute and prolonged diarrhoea in children: A community-based trial in rural Bangladesh. Tropical Medicine & International Health, 15(10), 1132-1139. doi:10.1111/j.1365-3156.2010.02608.x

Raisch, M. (2011). Did you know?. Prevention, 63(5), 86.

Tavares da Silva, S., Araujo Dos Santos, C., Marvila Girondoli, Y., Mello de Azeredo, L., Fernando de Sousa Moraes, L., Keila Viana Gomes Schitini, J., ... Bressan, J. (2014). Women with metabolic syndrome improve antrophometric and biochemical parameters with green banana flour consumption. Nutricion Hospitalaria, 29(5), 1070-1080. doi:10.3305/ nh.2014.29.5.7331

Thakorlal, J., Perera, C. O., Smith, B., Englberger, L., & Lorens, A. (2010). Resistant starch in Micronesian banana cultivars offers health benefits. Pacific Health Dialog, 16(1), 49-59.

Vijayakumar, S., Presannakumar, G., & Vijayalakshmi, N. R. (2008). Antioxidant activity of banana flavonoids. Fitoterapia, 79(4), 279-282. doi:10.1016/j. fitote.2008.01.007

Zandonadi, R. P., Botelho, R. B. A., Gandolfi, L., Ginani, J. S., Montenegro, F. M., & Pratesi, R. (2012). Green banana pasta: An alternative for gluten-free diets. Journal of the Academy of Nutrition & Dietetics, 112(7), 1068-1072. doi:10.1016/j.jand.2012.04.002

REVIEWER(S)

Darlene Strayer, RN, MBA, Cinahl Information Systems, Glendale, CA

Nursing Executive Practice Council, Glendale Adventist Medical Center, Glendale, CA

Bitter Melon

WHAT WE KNOW

Bitter melon (Momordica charantia; also known as bitter gourd, karela, ampalaya, pare, and balsam pear) is member of the Cucurbitaceae family, along with honeydew, cantaloupe, musk melon, and watermelon. The climbing perennial plant of the bitter melon produces an elongated, warty, green fruit that has a characteristically bitter flavor. Although not the most attractive or palatable of the melons, the seeds, fruit, leaves, and root of bitter melon have a long history of medicinal and culinary use. Bitter melon is commonly used in Indian cuisine and is often combined with garlic, chili peppers, and coconut milk. Bitter melon can be stuffed with various foods and spices, curried, or pickled. Bitter melon is a good source of fiber; vitamins K, A, C, B6, pantothenic acid, choline, and folate; the minerals iron, magnesium, phosphorus, calcium, and potassium; and many phytonutrients (i.e., beneficial, plant-derived chemicals). With anti-inflammatory and antioxidant properties, bitter melon provides many health benefits and has been used to treat gastrointestinal (GI) distress, ulcers, colitis, intestinal worms, diabetes, dyslipidemia (i.e., abnormal amount of fat in the blood), cancer, kidney stones, fever, liver disease, microbial infections, hypertension (i.e., high blood pressure), wounds, and psoriasis (i.e., skin disease). More research is needed regarding the effectiveness of bitter melon for these conditions because study results have been conflicting and inconclusive.

The most researched mechanism of bitter melon is its effect on blood glucose (i.e., blood sugar) levels.

Although this effect is not completely understood, bitter melon is thought to lower blood sugar in the following ways:

- Increases glucose utilization by the liver
- Inhibits two of the enzymes involved in the production of glucose from non-carbohydrate sources
- Improves glucose oxidation
- Enhances cellular uptake and release of glucose
- Increases insulin production in the pancreas

NUTRIENTS IN BITTER MELON

- Bitter melon is an excellent source of vitamin K, which acts as a coenzyme in maintaining normal levels of blood-clotting proteins and contributes to bone growth.
- The fat-soluble vitamin A (also called retinol) in bitter melon is required for vision, maintenance of the surface linings of the eyes and other epithelial tissue, proper bone growth, immune response, energy regulation, reproduction, embryonic development, and activation of gene expression.
- The water-soluble vitamin C in bitter melon neutralizes free radicals, protecting against inflammation and cellular damage. Adequate vitamin C intake is vital for proper immune system function and is associated with prevention of heart disease, stroke, and cancer.
- Vitamin B6 (also called pyridoxine) in bitter melon is required to facilitate the reactions of amino acid breakdown such as, the conversion of tryptophan to niacin, and is involved in the conversion of homocysteine to cysteine. Vitamin B6 is necessary for the synthesis of serotonin and dopamine, which are neurotransmitters required for nerve cell communication. By maintaining the lymphoid organs, vitamin B6 contributes to proper function of the immune system. Vitamin B6 is essential for the metabolism of amino acids, carbohydrates, and lipids and is important for the formation of red blood cells and hemoglobin, which carry oxygen to the tissues.
- Bitter melon contains pantothenic acid (also called vitamin B5), a water-soluble member of the B-complex vitamin family that contributes to the metabolism or breakdown of carbohydrates, proteins, and lipids. It plays a role in the synthesis

of acetylcholine, which is a neurotransmitter in the central and peripheral nervous systems.

- The B-complex vitamin choline in bitter melon metabolizes into betaine, which assists in the regulation of inflammation in the cardiovascular system by preventing elevated levels of homocysteine. Betaine is associated with reduced levels of the inflammatory markers C-reactive protein (CRP), interleukin-6, and tumor necrosis factor alpha.
- Bitter melon contains the water-soluble vitamin folate, which is essential for the production and maintenance of red blood cells. Folate is vital for the synthesis of deoxyribonucleic acid (DNA) and ribonucleic acid (RNA), the genetic code for the cells, and is important in the metabolism of homocysteine.
- The iron in bitter melon is vital for the synthesis of red blood cells and hemoglobin, which are necessary for cellular respiration and the transport of oxygen to the tissues. Iron supports immune function, is vital for cognitive development, contributes to energy metabolism, and regulates temperature.
- The magnesium in bitter melon balances the action of calcium in cells to regulate bone health and nerve and muscle tone. Magnesium maintains relaxation of the nerves and muscles, which contributes to the prevention of high blood pressure, muscle spasms, asthma, migraine headaches, general soreness, and fatigue.
- Phosphorous combined with calcium is important for the formation of bones and teeth, muscle contraction, and nerve conduction, and is essential for maintaining the structural integrity of cell membranes.
- Bitter melon contains calcium, which builds and maintains bones and teeth, regulates muscle contraction, conducts nerve impulses, activates enzymes for energy production and muscle contraction, assists with blood clotting, assists with vitamin B12 absorption, and maintains the structural integrity of intracellular membranes.
- The potassium in bitter melon supports normal cellular, nerve, and muscle function and helps to eliminate excess sodium from the body.

DIETARY INTAKE GUIDELINES

The safety of using bitter melon supplementation for more than 3 months has not been established. Common dosages of bitter melon that have been used in studies include the following:

- 50–100 mL of fresh juice consumed daily
- Encapsulated dry powder 3–15 g taken daily
- Standardized, encapsulated extract 100–200 mg taken 3 times daily

Bitter melon has been shown to induce abortion in animal studies. Because safety has not been established during pregnancy, bitter melon should not be taken by women who are pregnant. Due to its blood-sugar-lowering effects, bitter melon can potentiate the effectiveness of diabetes medications and insulin.

RESEARCH FINDINGS

Although many studies have been conducted to assess the safety and effectiveness of bitter melon for the treatment of diabetes and metabolic syndrome, results are conflicting and inconclusive. Many of the studies were flawed and weak according to expert reviewers, who recommend more clinical trials with better control and adequate sample sizes.

SUMMARY

Consumers should become knowledgeable about the physiologic benefits of consuming bitter melon. Bitter melon is a good source of fiber, many vitamins and minerals, and phytonutrients. Bitter melon provides many health benefits and has been used to treat gastrointestinal (GI) distress and disorders, diabetes, cancer, kidney stones, fever, liver disease, microbial infections, and hypertension. More research is needed regarding the effectiveness of bitter melon for these conditions because study results have been conflicting and inconclusive.

—*Cherie Marcel, BS*

REFERENCES

Bartkowski, A. M. (2010). What is bitter melon good for? Livestrong.com. Retrieved April 21, 2015, from http://www.livestrong.com/article/118191-bitter-melon-good/

Bitter melon. (n.d.). WebMD. Retrieved April 21, 2015, from http://www.webmd.com/vitamins-supplements/ingredientmono-795-BITTER%20MELON.aspx?activeIngredientId=795&activeIngredientName=BITTER%20MELON

Ilkay, J. (2011). Bitter melon. Fruit's role in diabetes management is promising but uncertain. Today's Dietitian, 13(7), 10-11.

Leung, L., Birtwhistle, R., Kotech, J., Hannah, S., & Cuthbertson, S. (2009). Anti-diabetic and hypoglycaemic effects of Momordica charantia (bitter melon): A mini review. British Journal of Nutrition, 102(12), 1703-1708. doi:10.1017/S0007114509992054

Momordica charantia (bitter melon). (2007). Alternative Medicine Review, 12(4), 360-363.

Nerurkar, P. V., Johns, L. M., Buesa, L. M., Kipyakwai, G., Volper, E., Sato, R., & Nerurkar, V. R. (2011). Momordica charantia (bitter melon) attenuates high-fat diet-associated oxidative stress and neuroinflammation. Journal of Neuroinflammation, 8, 64. doi:10.1186/1742-2094-8-64

Ooi, C. P., Yassin, Z., & Hamid, T. A. (2012). Momordica charantia for type 2 diabetes mellitus. Cochrane Database of Systematic Reviews, 8. Art. No.: CD007845. doi:10.1002/14651858.CD007845.pub3

Summers, A. R. B. (2010, March 23). Bitter melon nutrition. Livestrong.com. Retrieved April 21, 2015, from http://www.livestrong.com/article/89801-bitter-melon-nutrition/

Tsai, C. H., Chen, E. C., Tsay, H. S., & Huang, C. J. (2012). Wild bitter gourd improves metabolic syndrome: A preliminary dietary supplementation trial. Nutrition Journal, 11, 4. doi:10.1186/1475-2891-11-4

Wolf, N. (2011, May 18). What are the benefits of eating bitter gourd? Livestrong.com. Retrieved April 21, 2015, from http://www.livestrong.com/article/445901-what-are-the-benefits-of-eating-bitter-gourd/

REVIEWER(S)

Darlene Strayer, RN, MBA, Cinahl Information Systems, Glendale, CA

Nursing Executive Practice Council, Glendale Adventist Medical Center, Glendale, CA

Blackberry

WHAT WE KNOW

Blackberry (Rubus fruticosus) is a member of the Rosaceae (i.e., rose) family, along with nectarines, peaches, apricots, cherries, raspberries, and plums. Because of its growth in a characteristically thorny hedge, blackberry is also called brambleberry (i.e., meaning prickly berry). Technically, blackberry is not a berry but an aggregate fruit in which each blackberry is actually a grouping of tiny individual fruit orbs called drupelets;

each drupelet contains its own seed. A delicious culinary treat, the blackberry can be eaten raw, canned, dried, baked in pies and cobblers, made into jams and sauces, and blended in drinks. Beyond its value in cuisine, blackberry ranks first among fruits for its exceptional antioxidant properties. Blackberry possesses a wealth of nutrients, including vitamins C, E, and K; manganese; magnesium; folate; copper; potassium; fiber; and a diverse collection of phytonutrients (i.e., protective, plant-derived chemicals). These nutrients provide blackberry with powerful anti-inflammatory, antioxidant, anti-microbial, cancer-preventive, and cardio-protective activity. The leaves and other parts of the blackberry plant have been used to treat diarrhea, colitis, whooping cough, labor pain, psoriasis, burns, bleeding gums, and sore throat.

NUTRIENTS IN THE BLACKBERRY

- Blackberry contains many valuable phytonutrients that have antioxidant and anti-inflammatory activities, giving it great potential to prevent cancer and heart disease. Some of these phytonutrients include the following:
  o Anthocyanins: reddish-color pigments that have high antioxidant and anti-carcinogenic activity, promote urinary tract health, and support memory function. They also fight bacteria (e.g., Streptococcus) by disrupting bacterial cell membranes.
  o Flavonols: Quercetin provides strong antioxidant and anti-inflammatory protection and has antihistamine, antimicrobial, antidiabetic, and anti-carcinogenic properties.
  o Flavonoid glycosides: Inhibit cancer cell proliferation and exhibit antibiotic activity.
  o Tannins: Proanthocyanidins have antioxidant, antihistamine, anti-cancer, and cardioprotective properties.
  o Hydroxybenzoic acids: Ellagic acid exhibits anti-inflammatory properties and has been shown to reduce symptoms associated with Crohn's disease. Ellagic acid fends off carcinogens and slows cancer cell proliferation. Sylicyclic acid inhibits atherosclerosis (i.e. clogged arteries).
- The water-soluble vitamin C in blackberry neutralizes free radicals, protecting against inflammation and cellular damage. Adequate vitamin C intake is vital for proper function of the immune

system and has been associated with prevention of heart disease, stroke, and cancer.

- Blackberry contains vitamin E, which functions primarily as an antioxidant but also maintains cell membranes, assists in vitamin K absorption, and contributes to immune system function.
- The vitamin K in blackberry acts as a coenzyme in maintaining normal levels of blood clotting proteins and contributes to bone growth.
- Manganese, a trace mineral found in blackberry, is responsible for energy production, fatty acid synthesis, necessary cholesterol production, and protection against the damage caused by free-radicals.
- Blackberry contains magnesium, which balances the action of calcium in cells to regulate bone health and nerve and muscle tone. It maintains nerve and muscle relaxation which contributes to the prevention of high blood pressure, muscle spasms, asthma, migraine headaches, general soreness, and fatigue.
- Blackberry contains the water-soluble B vitamin folate, which is essential for the production and maintenance of red blood cells (RBCs). Folate is vital for the synthesis of deoxyribonucleic acid (DNA) and ribonucleic acid (RNA), the genetic code for the cells, and is important in the breakdown of the amino acid, homocysteine.
- Blackberry provides copper, which is a vital component of superoxide dismutase, an enzyme involved in energy production and antioxidant activity. It contributes to the action of lysyloxidase, an enzyme necessary for the cross-linking of collagen and elastin that allows flexibility in the blood vessels, bones, and joints. It also enhances the body's ability to use iron, preventing iron-deficiency anemia, ruptured blood vessels, irregular heartbeat, and infection.
- Blackberry contains potassium, which is an essential element for regulating acid-base balance, maintaining fluid balance, supporting muscle contraction and cardiac function, protein building and carbohydrate metabolism (i.e. breakdown), promoting cellular growth, and transmission of nerve impulses.
- Blackberry is a good source of dietary fiber, which binds and removes toxins from the colon, assists in glycemic (i.e. blood sugar) control, and reduces high cholesterol levels.

DIETARY INTAKE GUIDELINES

Blackberry may increase risk for kidney stones in individuals with a history of kidney stones because it contains a high amount of the chemical oxalate, which is a primary component of kidney stones. Oxalates can build up and crystallize in body fluids and cause health problems in individuals with pre-existing kidney or gallbladder dysfunction.

RESEARCH FINDINGS

- The polyphenols anthocyanidins and ellagitannins in blackberry slow the digestion of starch, protein, and oil, which helps to stabilize blood sugar. The proanthocyanidins in blackberry inhibit lipase, the intestinal enzyme necessary for fat digestion. Blackberry nectar has been shown to lower serum triglycerides and total cholesterol in hamsters with high cholesterol levels. These factors make blackberry a potential tool for the treatment and prevention of metabolic syndrome and related conditions, including insulin resistance, diabetes mellitus, hypertension, heart disease, and obesity.
- Researchers report that blackberry extract has powerful antiviral activity. In a recent study, topically applied blackberry extract effectively inhibited early stages of herpes simplex virus type 1 (HSV-1). These results highlight the possibility of using blackberry extract as a topical prophylactic and therapeutic agent for patients with HSV-1. Blackberry extract (BBE) has also exhibited antimicrobial action against periodontal pathogens and Streptococcus mutans (S. mutans). Researchers suggest that BBE has the potential to be a useful agent for the prevention and control of periodontitis and dental caries.

SUMMARY

Consumers should become knowledgeable about the physiologic effects of blackberry consumption. The blackberry contains many nutrients, such as, vitamins C, E, and K; manganese; magnesium; folate; copper; potassium; fiber; and numerous phytonutrients. The blackberry may help prevent heart disease, stroke, cancer, iron-deficiency anemia and support overall immune system function.

—*Cherie Marcel, BS*

REFERENCES

Danaher, R. J., Wang, C., Dai, J., Mumper, R. J., & Miller, C. S. (2011). Antiviral effects of blackberry extract against herpes simplex virus type 1. Oral Surgery, Oral Medicine, Oral Pathology, Oral Radiology & Endodontology, 112(3), e31-35. doi:10.1016/j.tripleo.2011.04.007

de Araujo, P. R., da Silva Santos, V., Rodrigues Machado, A., Gevehr Fernandes, C., Silva, J. A., & da Silva Rodrigues, R. (2011). Benefits of blackberry nectar (Rubus spp.) relative to hypercholesterolemia and lipid peroxidation. Nutricion Hospitalaria, 26(5), 984-990. doi:10.1590/S0212-16112011000500010

Dyer, M. H. (2014). What are the health benefits of blackberries?. Livestrong.com. Retrieved September 10, 2014, from http://www.livestrong.com/article/231114-what-are-the-health-benefits-of-blackberries/

The George Mateljan Foundation editorial team. (n.d.). Can you tell me what oxalates are and in which foods they can be found? The World's Healthiest Foods. Retrieved September 10, 2014, from http://www.whfoods.com/genpage.php?tname=george&dbid=48

Gonzalez, O. A., Escamilla, C., Danaher, R. J., Dai, J., Ebersole, J. L., Mumper, R. J., ... Miller, C. S. (2013). Antibacterial effects of blackberry extract target periodontopathogens. Journal of Periodontal Research, 48(1), 80-86. doi:10.1111/j.1600-0765.2012.01506.x

Keville, K. (2012). Herb profile: Medicinal berries. American Herb Association Quarterly Newsletter, 27(1), 3.

Verma, R., Gangrade, T., Punasiya, R., & Ghulaxe, C. (2014). Rubus fruticosus (blackberry) use as an herbal medicine. Pharmacognosy Reviews, 8(16). doi:10.4103/0973-7847.1347.134239

Zanteson, L. (2012). Blackberries: Summer's antioxidant splash. Environmental Nutrition, 35(7), 8.

REVIEWER(S)

Darlene Strayer, RN, MBA, Cinahl Information Systems, Glendale, CA

Nursing Executive Practice Council, Glendale Adventist Medical Center, Glendale, CA

Blueberry

WHAT WE KNOW

Blueberry, or *Vaccinium corymbosum*, is a small shrub that belongs to the Ericaceae family and the Vaccinium genus along with more than 450 other plants, including cranberry and bilberry. The fruit of the blueberry plant is a small bluish-purple berry that is sweet and slightly tart. Although it is delicious raw, blueberries are also greatly appreciated as a culinary element and is commonly used for sauces, jams, beverages, and baked goods. The blueberry contains vitamins C and K, manganese, fiber, and a special mix of polyphenolic phytochemicals (i.e., protective plant-derived chemicals) that have powerful antioxidant activity. Blueberry consumption is associated with a reduced risk of developing heart disease, cancer, and dementia, and has been linked to good health of the urinary tract.

NUTRIENTS IN THE BLUEBERRY

- Blueberries contain important phytochemicals such as chlorogenic acid, resveratrol, and anthocyanins, all of which exhibit antioxidant and anti-inflammatory activity
  —Anthocyanins, the pigments that give blueberry its bluish-purple color, are the blueberry's most abundant phytochemicals; their potent anti-inflammatory and antioxidant properties have great potential in the prevention of cancer, heart disease, and dementia. Anthocyanins also appear to reduce urinary tract pathogens by limiting the ability of bacteria to adhere to the mucosal lining of the bladder and urethra.

DIETARY INTAKE GUIDELINES

- Although there is no standardized dosage recommendation for medicinal intake of blueberry, manufacturers of dietary supplements recommend 1 tablespoon of dried blueberry powder, 200–400 mg of blueberry concentrate, or 8–10 teaspoons of blueberry concentrated liquid per day.
- Blueberry intake is generally considered safe when consumed in amounts that are normally found in food.
- There is some evidence that blueberry intake can lower blood glucose levels, and individuals who receive antidiabetic medications should exercise caution with blueberry intake.

RESEARCH FINDINGS

- Numerous studies have investigated the neuroprotective properties of blueberry. There is a great deal of evidence from animal studies that the polyphenols in blueberries have highly antioxidant functions as well as other protective actions. These polyphenols have been shown to improve intercellular signaling and brain function. These actions are associated with improved motor and cognitive performance, which can improve memory and potentially reverse some of the neurodegeneration seen in patients with Alzheimer's

disease, Parkinson's disease, or damage caused by a stroke. Although results of human studies are beginning to substantiate the results of many animal studies in showing that blueberry causes significant improvement in learning and memory, further human trials are needed before the clinical effectiveness of blueberry compounds and appropriate therapeutic strategies can be established.

- There is evidence that the blueberry-derived phytochemical actions of counteracting oxidative stress, reducing inflammation, and modulating cellular interactions play a protective role against vascular disease and cancer. In part, the prevention of vascular disease is attributed to the ability of these phytochemicals to inhibit damage caused by oxidative low-density lipoproteins (LDLs), cell changes, and cell apoptosis (i.e., programmed cell death). The potential cancer treating properties of blueberry can help prevent the spread of tumors. Further study is needed to examine this process.
- Researchers have noted the potential for a therapeutic role of blueberry in the treatment of metabolic syndrome and the related conditions of insulin resistance and diabetes mellitus, hypertension and heart disease, and obesity. Evidence suggests that the constituents of blueberry act to boost insulin sensitivity, lower LDL cholesterol and triglycerides, and improve leptin (i.e., hunger controlling hormone) sensitivity, which reduces appetite.

SUMMARY

Consumers should become knowledgeable about the physiologic benefits of blueberry consumption. Blueberries are a rich source of vitamins C and K, manganese, fiber, and phytochemicals. The antioxidant power of blueberries may help fight cancer, Alzheimer's disease, Parkinson's disease, and risk for developing heart disease and diabetes

—Cherie Marcel, BS

REFERENCES

Brewer, G. J., Torricelli, J. R., Lindsey, A. L., Kunz, E. Z., Neuman, A., Fisher, D. R., ... Joseph, J. A. (2010). Age-related toxicity of amyloid-beta associated with increased pERK and pCREB in primary hippocampal neurons: Reversal by blueberry extract. *Journal of Nutritional Biochemistry*, 21(10), 991-998. doi:10.1016/j.jnutbio.2009.08.005

Faloon, W. (2005). Blueberries — the world's healthiest food. *Life Extension, Winter: Special Edition*, 3-6.

Faria, A., Pestana, D., Teixeira, D., de Freitas, V., Mateus, N., & Calhau, C. (2010). Blueberry anthocyanins and pyruvic acid adducts: Anticancer properties in breast cancer cell lines. *Phytotherapy Research, 24*(12), 1862-1869. doi:10.1002/ptr.3213

Fuentealba, J., Dbarrart, A. J., Fuentes-Fuentes, M. C., Saez-Orellana, F., Quinones, K., Guzman, L., ... Aguayo, L. G. (2011). Synaptic failure and adenosine triphosphate imbalance induced by amyloid-beta aggregates are prevented by blueberry-enriched polyphenols extract. *Journal of Neuroscience Research, 89*(9), 1499-1508. doi:10.1002/ jnr.22679

Giacalone, M., Di Sacco, F., Traupe, I., Topini, R., Forfori, F., & Giunta, F. (2011). Antioxidant and neuroprotective properties of blueberry polyphenols: A critical review. *Nutritional Neuroscience, 14*(3), 119-125. doi:10.1179/1476830511Y.0000000007

Ilkay, J. (2010). Blueberry buzz — research investigates supplements' effects in multiple health conditions. *Today's Dietitian, 12*(7), 18.

Martineau, L. C., Couture, A., Spoor, D., Benhaddou-Andaloussi, A., Harris, C., Meddah, B., ... Haddad, P. S. (2006). Anti-diabetic properties of the Canadian lowbush blueberry Vaccinium angustifolium Ait. *Phytomedicine, 13*(9-10), 612-623. doi:10.1016/j.phymed.2006.08.005

Medline Plus Editorial Team. (2014, July). Blueberry. *MedlinePlus*. Retrieved November 4, 2015, from http://www.nlm.nih.gov/medlineplus/druginfo/natural/1013.html

Montgomery, V. (2011). Pick blueberries for brain defense — Blueberry defense against Alzheimer's disease. *Environmental Nutrition, 34*(1), 1, 6.

Neto, C. C. (2007). Cranberry and blueberry: Evidence for protective effects against cancer and vascular diseases. *Molecular Nutrition & Food Research, 51*(6), 652-664.

Parente, M. (2011). Report — Can blueberry extracts halt metabolic syndrome? *Life Extension, 17*(3), 1-7.

Stull, A. J., Cash, K. C., Johnson, W. D., Champagne, C. M., & Cefalu, W. T. (2010). Bioactives in blueberries improve insulin sensitivity in obese, insulin-resistant men and women. *Journal of Nutrition, 140*(10), 1764-1768. doi:10.3945/jn.110.125336

Vuong, T., Matar, C., Ramassamy, C., & Haddad, P. S. (2010). Biotransformed blueberry juice protects neurons from hydrogen peroxide-induced oxidative stress and mitogen-activated protein kinase pathway alterations. *British Journal of Nutrition, 104*(5), 656-663. doi:10.1017/S0007114510001170

REVIEWER(S)

Darlene Strayer, RN, MBA, Cinahl Information Systems, Glendale, CA

Nursing Executive Practice Council, Glendale Adventist Medical Center, Glendale, CA

Cantaloupe

WHAT WE KNOW

The melon that is commonly called a cantaloupe in the United States is actually a muskmelon (*Cucumis melo* var *reticulatus*), which is a member of the *Cucurbitaceae* family along with honeydew, watermelon, and bitter melon. The true cantaloupe (*Cucumis melo* var *cantalupensis*) is primarily grown in areas of the world other than the U.S., particularly the Mediterranean region; unlike the muskmelon, the true cantaloupe does not have the characteristic netting pattern on its rind. Hereafter, use of the term cantaloupe refers to the more familiar fruit, muskmelon. The creeping vine of the cantaloupe plant produces round fruits with thick rinds that are beige, netted, and slightly ribbed. The dense and juicy flesh of the cantaloupe varies in color depending on the variety. Probably the most familiar color is deep orange. "Jenny Lind" cantaloupes have a green flesh, while varieties such as "Athena" or "Ambrosia" have a more salmon-colored flesh. Hidden in the center of the cantaloupe is a hollow cavity filled with slimy, but edible, seeds. Cantaloupe is frequently eaten raw, but can also be used in drinks or made into dressings and sauces. Beyond its culinary value, the nutritional diversity of cantaloupe is noteworthy. Cantaloupe is a good source of fiber, potassium, magnesium, many valuable phytonutrients (i.e., beneficial, plant-derived chemicals), and the vitamins A, C, K, folate, B6, B3, and B1. These nutrients provide cantaloupe with antioxidant, anti-inflammatory, cancer-preventative, and cardio-protective properties.

NUTRIENTS IN CANTALOUPE

* Cantaloupe is rich in phytonutrients, including flavonoids, carotenoids, and tripterpenoids, which have strong anti-inflammatory and antioxidant properties
   —The carotenoids alpha-carotene, beta-carotene, and their derivatives lutein, beta-cryptoxanthin, and zeaxanthin exhibit antioxidant

properties and scavenge free radicals. They also protect the eyes from light-induced oxidation, which prevents macular degeneration, and inhibit atherosclerosis.

—The flavonoid luteolin is a potent antioxidant and anticarcinogenic compound.

—The triterpenoids cucurbitacin E and cucurbitacin B exhibit strong anti-inflammatory activity.

—Caffeic and ferulic acids exhibit anticarcinogenic, antimicrobial, and antiviral properties. These acids are believed to inhibit the build-up of low-density lipoprotein (LDL) cholesterol.

- The fat-soluble vitamin A in cantaloupe is required for vision, maintenance of the surface linings of the eyes and other epithelial tissue, proper bone growth, immune response, energy regulation, reproduction, embryonic development, and activation of gene expression.

- Cantaloupe is an excellent source of vitamin C, which neutralizes free radicals, protecting against inflammation and cellular damage. Adequate vitamin C intake is vital for immune system function and has been associated with the prevention of heart disease, stroke, and cancer.

- Vitamin K acts as a coenzyme to maintain normal levels of blood clotting proteins, and contributes to bone remodeling.

- Cantaloupe is a good source of several B-complex vitamins.

—Folate is a water-soluble B vitamin that is essential for the production and maintenance of red blood cells (RBCs). It is vital for the synthesis of deoxyribonucleic acid (DNA) and ribonucleic acid (RNA), the genetic code for the cells, and is also important in the metabolism of homocysteine, an amino acid.

—Vitamin B6 is required for the conversion of tryptophan to niacin, and is involved in the conversion of homocysteine to cysteine. It is also necessary for the synthesis of serotonin and dopamine, neurotransmitters required for nerve cell communication. By maintaining the lymphoid organs, vitamin B6 contributes to immune system function. Additionally, it is essential for the metabolism of amino acids, carbohydrates, and lipids, and is important for the formation of RBCs and hemoglobin, which carries oxygen to the tissues.

—Vitamins B1 and B3 create energy by aiding the metabolism or break down of carbohydrates, provide cardiovascular protection, maintain the nervous system, and support the production of RBCs, hormones, and necessary cholesterol.

- Potassium supports normal cellular, nerve, and muscle function and helps to eliminate excess sodium from the body

- The magnesium provided by cantaloupe balances the action of calcium in cells to regulate bone health and nerve and muscle tone. It maintains relaxation of nerves and muscles, which contributes to the prevention of high blood pressure, muscle spasm, asthma, migraine headache, general soreness, and fatigue.

DIETARY INTAKE GUIDELINES

- Cantaloupe is generally considered safe for consumption

- Melons can serve as a vehicle for Salmonella and Listeria. To avoid contamination when purchasing commercially grown melons, the US Federal Food and Drug Administration (FDA) advises the following precautions:

—Don't eat bruised melons

—Always wash hands with soap and hot water prior to handling melons

—Thoroughly clean the whole melon with a clean produce brush and tap water prior to cutting open

—Refrigerate the melon upon cutting and eat within 2 days

RESEARCH FINDINGS

A clinical trial was conducted to determine the effect of melon juice supplementation on perceived stress and fatigue based on the hypothesis that perceived stress is associated with oxidative stress. Researchers reported that the group who received the oral melon juice supplementation showed improvement in several signs and symptoms of stress and fatigue. A similar study that analyzed the effects of a gliadin-combined plant superoxide dismutase extract (i.e., antioxidant enzyme) on perceived fatigue in women aged 50–65 years found no notable improvement in the participants receiving the extract.

SUMMARY

Consumers should become knowledgeable about the physiologic benefits of the consumption of cantaloupe. Cantaloupe is a good source of fiber, potassium, magnesium, phytonutrients, and the vitamins A, C, K, folate, B6, B3, and B1. These nutrients may help improve immune and nervous system function, muscle and bone health and vision, while preventing the risk for developing cardiovascular disease, stroke and cancer.

—*Cherie Marcel, BS*

REFERENCES

The George Mateljan Foundation editorial team. (2012). The world's healthiest foods: Cantaloupe. Retrieved April 1, 2015, from http://www.whfoods.com/genpage.php? tname=foodspice&dbid=17

Houghton, C. A., Steels, E. L., Fassett, R. G., & Coombes, J. S. (2011). Effects of a gliadin-combined plant superoxide dismutase extract on self-perceived fatigue in women aged 50--65 years. *Phytomedicine*, 18(6), 521-526. doi:10.1016/j.phymed.2010.09.006

Liddell, A. (2013). The health benefits of melons. *Livestrong.com*. Retrieved April 1, 2015, from http://www.livestrong.com/article/407556-the-health-benefits-of-melons/

McCollum, J. T., Cronquist, A. B., Silk, B. J., Jackson, K. A., O'Connor, K. A., Costrove, S., ... Mahon, B. E. (2013). Multistate outbreak of listeriosis associated with cantaloupe. *New England Journal of Medicine*, 369(10), 944-953. doi:10.1056/NEJMoa1215837;

Milesi, M. A., Lacan, D., Brosse, H., Desor, D., & Notin, C. (2009). Effect of an oral supplementation with a proprietary melon juice concentrate (Extramel) on stress and fatigue in healthy people: A pilot, double-blind, placebo-controlled clinical trial. *Nutrition Journal*, 8, 40. doi:10.1186/1475-2891-8-40

Wright, H. (2008). Cantaloupe: Enjoy succulence with tad of caution. *Environmental Nutrition*, 31(7), 8.

Zevnik, N. (2012). Healing foods. Melon marvel. *Better Nutrition*, 74(7), 40-42.

REVIEWER(S)

Darlene Strayer, RN, MBA, Cinahl Information Systems, Glendale, CA

Nursing Executive Practice Council, Glendale Adventist Medical Center, Glendale, CA

Cherries

WHAT WE KNOW

The sweet, or wild, cherry (i.e., *Prunus avium*) and the sour, or tart, cherry (i.e., *Prunuscerasus*) are both derived from the wild cherries, which originated around 70 BC. Cherries are from the Rosaceae (i.e., rose) family, along with nectarines, peaches, apricots, and plums. Like their relatives, cherries are stone fruits, meaning they contain a stone, or pit, at their center. Cherries were highly valued by ancient Romans, Greeks, and Chinese royalty and are still considered a symbol for immortality in China. A delicious culinary treat, cherries can be eaten raw, canned, dried, baked in pies and cobblers, made into jams and sauces, or blended in drinks. Beyond their value in cuisine, cherries have been used medicinally since the 15th century. The inner bark of the wild cherry is frequently used in infusions, decoctions, cough syrup, and tinctures as a treatment for chest congestion. Cherry juice and sour cherries are appreciated for their pain-relieving benefits. Cherries possess many nutrients, including vitamin C, potassium, important polyphenolic phytonutrients (i.e., protective, plant-derived chemicals), and fiber. These nutrients provide cherries with powerful anti-inflammatory and pain relieving properties and cancer-preventive and cardioprotectiveactivity.

NUTRIENTS IN CHERRIES

- Cherries contain important phytonutrients such as quercetin, genistein, naringenin, chlorogenic acid, and the highly acclaimed anthocyanins, which have antioxidant, anti-inflammatory, antibiotic, and antimutagenic properties that protect deoxyribonucleic acid (DNA) against damage, enhance DNA repair, protect blood vessels from rupture, promote urinary tract health, and support memory function.

- The water-soluble vitamin C in cherries neutralizes free radicals, protecting against inflammation and cellular damage. Adequate vitamin C intake is vital for the proper function of the immune system and has been associated with the prevention of heart disease, stroke, and cancer.

- Cherries contain potassium, which is an essential element responsible for regulating acid-base balance, maintaining fluid balance, supporting

muscle contraction and cardiac function, contributing to protein synthesis (i.e., building) and carbohydrate metabolism (i.e., breakdown), promoting cellular growth, and promoting transmission of nerve impulses.
- Cherries are an excellent source of dietary fiber, which binds and removes toxins from the colon, assists in glycemic (i.e., blood sugar) control, and reduces high cholesterol levels.

DIETARY INTAKE GUIDELINES
- There is no standard dosage of cherries for treatment, but studies have used the equivalent of 8 oz/day of pure cherry juice or 45 cherries.
- The common dosage for Wild cherry bark is a standard infusion of 3–9g or 10–15 drops of tincture.
- Cherries contain sorbitol, a sugar alcohol that can trigger painful symptoms in individuals with irritable bowel syndrome (IBS).
- Consuming therapeutic doses of cherries could enhance the antithrombotic (i.e., reduced blood clotting) activity of the drug warfarin.
- Wild cherry could increase the effects of medications broken down by the liver, including the following:
  —Lovastatin (Mevacor)
  —Ketoconazole (Nizoral)
  —Itraconazole (Sporanox)
  —Fexofenadine (Allegra)
  —Triazolam (Halcion)

RESEARCH FINDINGS
- Cherries contain melatonin, tryptophan, and serotonin, which protect against free radicals and help to regulate sleep/wake cycles. Researchers report that cherries promote sleep and could be used to improve sleep patterns in older adults with sleep disturbances and insomnia.
- Researchers have determined that consuming the sweet Bing cherry can effectively lower certain inflammatory markers (e.g., C-reactive protein [CRP], nitric oxide) in healthy men and women. This anti-inflammatory activity is potentially useful for the management and prevention of inflammatory diseases (e.g., arthritis, cardiovascular disease).

- The results of numerous studies show that tart cherry consumption can prevent exercise-induced muscle damage and soreness and aid muscle recovery following strenuous exercise.
- Results of a study conducted on obese rats indicated that consumption of tart cherries reduced multiple characteristics of metabolic syndrome and significantly reduced inflammation, lowering the risk for developing diabetes mellitus, type 2 (DM2) and heart disease.

SUMMARY
Consumers should become knowledgeable about the physiologic risks and benefits of cherry consumption. Cherries contain many nutrients, including vitamin C, potassium, phytonutrients, and fiber, which provide cherries with powerful anti-inflammatory and pain relieving properties, as well as cancer-preventive and cardio-protective activity. People with IBS should be aware that cherries contain sorbitol, a sugar alcohol that can trigger painful symptoms in individuals with IBS. Consumers should be aware of the possible drug-nutrient interactions associated with cherries.

—*Cherie Marcel, BS*

REFERENCES
Bell, P.G., McHugh, M.P., Stevenson, E., & Howatson, G. (2014). The role of cherries in exercise and health. *Scandinavian Journal of Medicine & Science in Sports*, 24(3), 477-490. doi:10.1111/sms.12085

Blando, F., Gerardi, C., & Nicoletti, I. (2004). Sour cherry (Prunus cerasus L) anthocyanins as ingredients for functional foods. *Journal of Biomedicine & Biotechnology*, 2004(5), 253-258. doi:10.1155/S1110724304404136

Bowers, K. (2006). Breathe easy. *New Life Journal*, 39.

Bowtell, J. L., Sumners, D. P., Dyer, A., Fox, P., & Mileva, K. N. (2011). Montmorency cherry juice reduces muscle damage caused by intensive strength exercise. *Medicine & Science in Sports & Exercise*, 43(8), 1544-1551. doi:10.1249/MSS.0b013e31820e5adc

Connolly, D. A. J., McHugh, M. P., Padilla-Zakour, O. I., Carlson, L., & Sayers, S. P. (2006). Efficacy of tart cherry juice blend in preventing the symptoms of muscle damage. *British Journal of Sports Medicine*, 40(8), 679-683. doi:10.1136/bjsm.2005.025429

Gable, C. (2008). Why tart cherry is tops: Find out how the juice of these sweet summer jewels can help quell pain and inflammation. *Better Nutrition*, 70(7), 50.

Garrido, M., Paredes, S. D., Cubero, J., Lozano, M., Toribio-Delgado, A. F., Muñoz, J. L., ... Rodríguez, A. B. (2010). Jerte Valley cherry-enriched diets improve nocturnal rest and increase 6-Sulfatoxymelatonin and total antioxidant capacity in the urine of middle-aged and elderly humans. *Journals of Gerontology Series A: Biological Sciences & Medical Sciences, 65*(9), 909-914. doi:10.1093/gerona/glq099

Goodman, S. (2007). Cherries: Powerful pain relief, cancer defense, and neuroprotection. *Life Extension, 13*(12), 81-83.

Howatson, G., McHugh, M. P., Hill, J. A., Brouner, J., Jewell, A. P., van Someren, K. A., ... Howatson, S. A. (2010). Influence of tart cherry juice on indices of recovery following marathon running. *Scandinavian Journal of Medicine & Science in Sports, 20*(6), 843-852. doi:10.1111/j.1600-0838.2009.01005.x

Kelley, D. S., Adkins, Y., Reddy, A., Woodhouse, L. R., Mackey, B. E., & Erickson, K. L. (2013). Sweet bing cherries lower circulating concentrations of markers for chronic inflammatory diseases in healthy humans. *Journal of Nutrition, 143*(3), 340-344. doi:10.3945/jn.112.171371

Kelley, D. S., Rasooly, R., Jacob, R. A., Kader, A. A., & Mackey, B. E. (2006). Consumption of Bing sweet cherries lowers circulating concentrations of inflammation markers in healthy men and women. *The Journal of Nutrition, 136*(4), 981-986.

Neithercott, T. (2012). Foods that fight pain. *Prevention, 64*(9), 74-81.

Pigeon, W. R., Carr, M., Gorman, C., & Perlis, M. L. (2010). Effects of a tart cherry juice beverage on the sleep of older adults with insomnia: A pilot study. *Journal of Medicinal Food, 13*(3), 579-583. doi:10.1089/jmf.2009.0096

Sego, S. (2012). Alternative meds update: Tart cherry. *Clinical Advisor for Nurse Practitioners, 15*(5), 63-64.

Seymour, E. M., Lewis, S. K., Urcuyo-Llanes, D. E., Tanone, I. I., Kirakosyan, A., Kaufman, P. B., & Bolling, S. F. (2009). Regular tart cherry intake alters abdominal adiposity, adipose gene transcription, and inflammation in obesity-prone rats fed a high fat diet. *Journal of Medicinal Food, 12*(5), 935-942. doi:10.1089/jmf.2008.0270

WebMD editorial team. (2009). Wild Cherry: Uses, side effects, interactions, and warnings. WebMD. Retrieved February 27, 2015, from http://www.webmd.com/vitamins-supplements/ingredientmono-888-wild%20cherry.aspx?activeingredientid=888&activeingredientname=wild%20cherry

Zanteson, L. (2012). Pick cherries for peak nutrition. *Environmental Nutrition,* 8.

REVIEWER(S)

Darlene Strayer, RN, MBA, Cinahl Information Systems, Glendale, CA

Nursing Executive Practice Council, Glendale Adventist Medical Center, Glendale, CA

Coconut

WHAT WE KNOW

The coconut, or *Cocos nucifera* (which means nut-bearing monkey face), is a member of the palm, or *Arecaceae*, family. Coconut palms are native to Southeast Asia and have been utilized nutritionally and medicinally for centuries. Protected by a hard fuzzy shell, the interior of the coconut is a firm white flesh, or meat, that has a sweet flavor and an appealing aroma. Young green coconuts contain a sweet, watery liquid that is subsequently absorbed in the interior coconut flesh. Coconut water differs from coconut milk, which is made by squeezing and grating the mature flesh to form a creamy liquid. The creamy texture of coconut milk is due to its oil content. The oil is the fat in the coconut, which can be extracted from the flesh and used for frying, baking, and as a healing agent when applied topically.

- Although scientists have cautioned for years against use of coconut because of its high saturated fat content, experts now believe that the unique medium chain fatty acids lauric and caprylic acid that are found in coconut provide many health benefits, including boosting the immune system through antimicrobial and antiviral activity and improving blood cholesterol ratios. Coconut provides fiber, protein, potassium, magnesium, calcium, and vitamins B6, folate, thiamin, C, and E.

NUTRIENTS IN COCONUT

- Coconut is considered a functional food (i.e., a food that provides health benefits that exceed basic nutrition). Some of the nutrients found in the coconut include the following:
  —Coconut flesh contains about 9g of fiber/cup. Dietary fiber increases the volume of the intestinal contents, which decreases absorption of cholesterol. The added bulk promotes more regular bowel movements, promoting intestinal health.

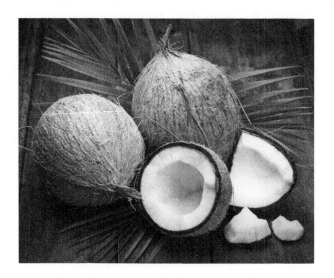

—The minerals potassium, magnesium, and calcium maintain homeostasis (i.e., regulated and stable conditions) in the cells, control blood pressure, promote bone and teeth formation, assist with production of blood cells, and support normal nerve and muscle function.

—Vitamin B6, or pyridoxine, is required for amino acid conversions of tryptophan to niacin, and is involved in the conversion of homocysteine to cysteine. Vitamin B6 is necessary for the synthesis of serotonin and dopamine, which are neurotransmitters that are essential for nerve cell communication. By maintaining the lymphoid organs, vitamin B6 contributes to healthy immune system function. It is essential for the metabolism of amino acids, carbohydrates, and lipids and is important for the formation of red blood cells and hemoglobin, which carries oxygen to the tissues

—Folate is essential for the production and maintenance of red blood cells, the metabolism of homocysteine (i.e., an amino acid), and the synthesis of deoxyribonucleic acid (DNA) and ribonucleic acid (RNA), the genetic code for the cells.

—Thiamine conducts the flow of electrolytes in and out of nerve and muscle cells, and contributes to the healthy function of the nervous system, the metabolism of carbohydrates, and the production of hydrochloric acid, a strong stomach acid, vital for digestion.

—The water-soluble vitamin C neutralizes free radicals, protecting against inflammation and cellular damage. Adequate vitamin C intake is vital to proper function of the immune system and is associated with the prevention of heart disease, stroke, and cancer.

—Vitamin E, a fat-soluble vitamin, functions primarily as an antioxidant but also maintains cell membranes, assists in vitamin K absorption, and contributes to healthy immune system function.

—The oil in coconut contains the fatty acids caprylic and lauric acid. These medium-chain triglycerides (MCTs) have antifungal, antibacterial, and antiviral properties, making them valuable contributors to a healthy immune system. MCTs are digested differently than other fats, serving as energy sources instead of fat storage, which helps stimulate metabolism, increase satiety (i.e., feeling full), and regulate blood glucose levels.

DIETARY INTAKE GUIDELINES

- Although the fat found in coconut has many health benefits, it is high in calories, which should be considered when including coconut in the diet. Overweight and obese individuals should use coconut sparingly. Coconut water is an exception because it contains no fat.

- Coconut is a significant source of dietary fat and cholesterol. Guidelines for dietary fat intake include the following: Reduce risk for CVD, cancer, DM2, and stroke by choosing unsaturated fats (including omega-3 fatty acid) and by limiting total fat intake to 30% or less of daily calories, limiting saturated fat (found in meat, whole milk, cream, butter, and cheese) to less than 10% of daily calories, and consuming less than 200 mg of cholesterol per day.

- There is no information in the medical literature regarding interactions of coconut and medications.

RESEARCH FINDINGS

- Coconut is used in folk medicine in rural Malaysia as treatment for malaria and fever. Scientists analyzed the phytochemical constituents (i.e., plant derived chemicals), parasite fighting activity, and risk for acute oral toxicity of the methanol white flesh extract of the coconut in order to determine if there is therapeutic validity for its use as an antimalarial remedy.

Although it could not be considered a cure for malaria, results of this study indicate that methanol white flesh extract of coconut does have an antimalarial effect.

• Researchers found in a pilot study that the coconut fragrance has a potentially beneficial effect on cardiovascular response to laboratory stress. Although further study is necessary, scientists consider that coconut aroma-therapy will become a useful tool in medicine, including that it could help to reduce cardiovascular stress during surgery.

SUMMARY

Consumers should become knowledgeable about the physiologic effects of coconut consumption. While coconut is a high-fat food, the unique medium chain fatty acids lauric and caprylic acid that are found in coconut provide many health benefits, including boosting the immune system through antimicrobial and antiviral activity and improving blood cholesterol ratios. Coconut provides fiber, protein, potassium, magnesium, calcium, and vitamins B6, folate, thiamin, C, and E. These nutrients may help prevent the risk of developing heart disease, stroke and cancer. Coconut is high in calories, which should be considered when including coconut in the diet.

—*Cherie Marcel, BS*

REFERENCES

Al-Adhroey, A. H., Nor, Z. M., Al-Mekhlafi, H. M., Amran, A. A., & Mahmud, R. (2011). Evaluation of the use of Cocos nucifera as antimalarial remedy in Malaysian folk medicine. *Journal of Ethnopharmacology, 134*(3), 988-991.

Amarasiri, W. A., & Dissanayake, A. S. (2006). Coconut fats. *Ceylon Medical Journal, 51*(2), 47-51.

Bowden, J. (2010). Break out of your shell. *Better Nutrition, 72*(3), 24-25.

Challem, J. (2009). Crazy for coconut water. *Better Nutrition, 71*(5), 46, 48.

Cullum-Dugan, D. (2014). Get the facts on coconut oil. *Environmental Nutrition, 37*(1), 6.

Gabbay, S. (2010). Coconut water: Elixir from the tropics. *Alive: Canada's Natural Health and Wellness Magazine, Nov*(337), 135.

Gursche, S. (2010). Ask the experts. *Alive: Canada's Natural Health and Wellness Magazine, Sep*(335), 29.

Helmer, J. (2007). Inside & out: Personal care. Cook and beautify with coconut oil. *Better Nutrition, 69*(3), 40, 42.

Kadey, M. (2010). Coconut water: The inside story. *Vegetarian Times, Feb*(374), 15.

Lomangino, K. (2012). Coconut oil and health: Assessing the evidence. *Clinical Nutrition Insight, 38*(12), 1-4.

Mezzacappa, E. S., Arumugam, U., Chen, S. Y., Stein, T. R., Oz, M., & Buckle, J. (2010). Coconut fragrance and cardiovascular response to laboratory stress: Results of pilot testing. *Holistic Nursing Practice, 24*(6), 322-332.

Turner, L. (2011). Off the shelf. Coo-coo for coconut. *Better Nutrition, 73*(4), 56-60.

Willett, W. C. (2011). Ask the doctor. I have started noticing more coconut oil at the grocery store and have heard it is better for you than a lot of other oils. Is that true?. *Harvard Health Letter, 36*(7), 7.

REVIEWER(S)

Darlene Strayer, RN, MBA, Cinahl Information Systems, Glendale, CA

Nursing Executive Practice Council, Glendale Adventist Medical Center, Glendale, CA

Cranberry

WHAT WE KNOW

Cranberry (also known as *Vaccinium macrocarpon, V. oxycoccus*, and *V. erythrocarpum*) is a small shrub that belongs to the Ericaceae family and the Vaccinium genus, along with blueberry, bilberry, and more than 450 other plants. When ripened, the fruit of the cranberry plant is a small, tart, red berry. Although it is perceived as unpleasant when eaten raw, the cranberry is commonly used to add flavor to sauces, jams, beverages, and baked goods. Beyond its value in food, cranberry is a good source of dietary fiber and valuable nutrients, including vitamin C, manganese, and a mix of polyphenolic phytochemicals (i.e., protective, plant-derived chemicals) that are associated with reduced risk of developing heart disease, cancer, urinary tract infections (UTIs), and periodontal disease.

NUTRIENTS IN THE CRANBERRY

• Cranberry contains the phytochemicals flavonols, flavan-3-ols, proanthocyanidin oligomers, anthocyanins, phenolic acids, triterpenoids, and carotenoids. These phytochemicals have antioxidant and anti-inflammatory activities, which give them great potential to fight cancer and heart disease and to prevent UTIs.

—The phenolic acids found in cranberry are thought to reduce risk for cardiovascular disease by inhibiting the oxidation of low density lipoproteins (LDL), interfering with blood clotting and lowering blood pressure. Other antithrombotic and anti-inflammatory activities are believed to be involved.

—Whole phenolic extracts of the cranberry have been shown to halt the cell cycle and induce apoptosis (i.e., natural cell death) inhibiting cell growth in certain tumors (e.g., tumors in the colon and prostate).

—Certain proanthocyanidins (e.g., A-type cranberry proanthocyanidins [AC-PACs]; commonly called A-type and PACs) in cranberries play a role in preventing bacterial infections of the urinary tract. PACs are able to inhibit the adhesion of bacteria (e.g., *Helicobacter pylori*, *Escherichia coli*) to the uroepithelial cells lining the bladder wall. Similar anti-adhesion mechanisms protect against periodontal disease.

DIETARY INTAKE GUIDELINES

- There is no standardized dosage recommended for medicinal intake of cranberry, although the following dosages have been used in studies:
  —Cranberry juice 1–10 oz/day in studies on preventing UTIs
  —Capsules in dosages of 300–400 mg/twice daily in studies on the treatment of diabetes mellitus, type 2 (DM2)
- Cranberry intake is generally considered safe when consumed by healthy individuals in amounts that are normally found in food.
- There is some concern that cranberry increases risk for kidney stones in individuals with a history of kidney stones because cranberry extract contains high amounts of oxalate, which is a primary component of kidney stones.
- Caution should be used by individuals taking warfarin (Coumadin), a medication used to slow blood clotting. Cranberry can increase the amount of time that warfarin is in the body, increasing risk for bruising and bleeding.

RESEARCH FINDINGS

- Study results have repeatedly documented the benefits of cranberry for the prevention of UTIs in women, men, and children. Although initially it was believed that cranberries exerted an antibiotic/antimicrobial effect on pathogens (i.e., disease-causing agents), subsequent research results revealed that the effectiveness of cranberry lies in the ability of its phytochemicals to prevent the adhesion of various pathogens to the uroepithelial cells of the bladder wall. This explains why cranberry consumption is a potentially effective prevention strategy but is not as successful in treatment of an existing UTI. Researchers report that in long-term studies, participants tend to stop drinking the cranberry juice, suggesting that it may not be palatable for long-term consumption, making it an undesirable strategy for long-term prevention. Efforts to replace cranberry juice with cranberry-containing tablets or capsules proved ineffective, possibly because these did not provide active ingredients with high enough potency.
- Similar mechanisms are noted in the role of cranberry in preventing periodontal disease. The constituents of cranberry decrease levels of *Streptococcus mutans* in saliva and inhibit adhesion of oral *Streptococci*. Cranberry polyphenols are highly effective in preventing harmful biofilm formation and inhibiting cysteine proteases of *Porphyromonas gingivalis*, a bacterium associated with chronic periodontitis.
- There is evidence that the cranberry- and blueberry-derived phytochemical action of counteracting oxidative stress, reducing inflammation, and modulating cellular interactions plays a protective role in preventing vascular disease and cancer. The prevention of vascular disease is attributed in part to the ability of these phytochemicals to inhibit damage caused by the oxidation of LDLs and cellular breakdown, inhibiting blood clotting, reducing blood pressure, and playing a role in anti-inflammatory activity. The potential chemopreventive properties of cranberry and blueberry include reducing the spread of tumor cells, although the ability to fight tumors depends on the bioavailability (i.e., amount the body is able to use) of the necessary phytochemicals

to the corresponding tissue. Further study is needed to examine this process.

- Researchers report that there is potential for a therapeutic role of cranberries in the treatment of metabolic syndrome and its related conditions of insulin resistance, DM2, hypertension, heart disease, and obesity. Evidence suggests that the constituents of cranberry reduce lipid oxidation, lower LDL cholesterol and triglycerides, and increase plasma antioxidant activity in women with metabolic syndrome.

SUMMARY

Consumers should become knowledgeable about the physiologic risks and benefits of cranberry consumption. Cranberries are a good source of dietary fiber and valuable nutrients, including vitamin C, manganese, and a mix of phytochemicals that are associated with reduced risk of developing heart disease, cancer, UTIs, and periodontal disease. Individuals that take warfarin (Coumadin), should be aware that cranberry can increase the amount of time that warfarin is in the body, increasing risk for bruising and bleeding. Individuals with a history of kidney stones should be aware that cranberry increases risk for kidney stones because cranberry extract contains high amounts of oxalate, a primary component of kidney stones.

—*Cherie Marcel, BS*

REFERENCES

Babich, H., Ickow, I. M., Weisburg, J. H., Zuckerbraun, H. L., & Schuck, A. G. (2012). Cranberry juice extract, a mild prooxidant with cytotoxic properties independent of reactive oxygen species. *Phytotherapy Research, 26*(9), 1358-1365. doi:10.1002/ptr.3735

Basu, A., Betts, N. M., Ortiz, J., Simmons, B., Wu, M., & Lyons, T. (2011). Low-energy cranberry juice decreases lipid oxidation and increases plasma antioxidant capacity in women with metabolic syndrome. *Nutrition Research, 31*(3), 190-196. doi:10.1016/j.nutres.2011.02.003

Beerepoot, M. A., Ter Riet, G., Nys, S., van der Wal, W. M., de Borgie, C. A., de Reijke, T. M., ... Geerlings, S. E. (2011). Cranberries vs antibiotics to prevent urinary tract infections: A randomized double-blind noninferiority trial in premenopausal women. *Archives of Internal Medicine, 171*(14), 1270-1278. doi:10.1001/archinternmed.2011.306

Efros, M., Bromberg, W., Cossu, L., Nakeleski, E., & Katz, A. E. (2010). Novel concentrated cranberry liquid blend, UTI-STAT with Proantinox, might help prevent recurrent urinary tract infections in women. *Urology, 76*(4), 841-845. doi:10.1016/j.urology.2010.01.068

Environmental Nutrition Editorial Team. (2012). The case of cranberry juice vs. UTI's. *Environmental Nutrition, 35*(11), 3.

Feldman, M., Weiss, E., Shemesh, M., Ofek, I., Bachrach, G., Rozen, R., ... Steinberg, D. (2009). Cranberry constituents affect fructosyltransferase expression in Streptococcus mutans. *Alternative Therapies in Health & Medicine, 15*(2), 32-38.

Gardner, E. (2014). The health properties of cranberry juice. *Nutrition Bulletin, 39*(2), 223-230. doi:10.1111/nbu.12093

Guay, D. R. P. (2009). Cranberry and urinary tract infections. *Drugs, 69*(7), 775-807. doi:10.2165/00003495-200969070-00002

Hamann, G. L., Campbell, J. D., & George, C. M. (2011). Warfarin-cranberry juice interaction. *Annals of Pharmacotherapy, 45*(3), e17. doi:10.1345/aph.1P451

Jepson, R. G., Williams, G., & Craig, J. C. (2012). The Cochrane Collaboration. Cranberries for preventing urinary tract infections (review). *John Wiley & Sons, Ltd., 10*, 80 pp.

Koo, H., Duarte, S., Murata, R. M., Scott-Anne, K., Gregoire, S., Watson, G. E., ... Vorsa, N. (2010). Influence of cranberry proanthocyanidins on formation of biofilms by Streptococcus mutans on saliva-coated apatitic surface and on dental caries development in vivo. *Caries Research, 44*(2), 116-126. doi:10.1159/000296306

La, V. D., Labrecque, J., & Grenier, D. (2009). Cytoprotective effect of proanthocyanidin-rich cranberry fraction against bacterial cell wall-mediated toxicity in macrophages and epithelial cells. *Phytotherapy Research, 23*(10), 1449-1452. doi:10.1002/ptr.2799

Lee, I. T., Chan, Y. C., Lin, C. W., Lee, W. J., & Sheu, W. H. (2008). Effect of cranberry extracts on lipid profiles in subjects with Type 2 diabetes. *Diabetic Medicine, 25*(12), 1473-1477. doi:10.1111/j.1464-5491.2008.02588.x

MacLean, M. A., Scott, B. E., Deziel, B. A., Nunnelley, M. C., Liberty, A. M., Gottschall-Pass, K. T., ... Hurta, R. A. R. (2011). North American cranberry (Vaccinium macrocarpon) stimulates apoptotic pathways in du145 human prostate cancer cells in vitro. *Nutrition & Cancer, 63*(1), 109-120. doi:10.1080/01635581.2010.516876

Mazokopakis, E. E., Karefilakis, C. M., & Starakis, I. K. (2009). Efficacy of cranberry capsules in prevention of urinary tract infections in postmenopausal women. *Journal of Alternative & Complementary Medicine*, *15*(11), 1155. doi:10.1089/acm.2009.0240

McMurdo, M. E., Argo, I., Phillips, G., Daly, F., & Davey, P. (2009). Cranberry or trimethoprim for the prevention of recurrent urinary tract infections? A randomized controlled trial in older women. *Journal of Antimicrobial Chemotherapy*, *63*(2), 389-395. doi:10.1093/jac/dkn489

Medline Plus Editorial Team. (2012, January 17). Cranberry. *MedlinePlus*. Retrieved October 9, 2014, from http://www.nlm.nih.gov/medlineplus/druginfo/natural/958.html

Micali, S., Isgro, G., Bianchi, G., Miceli, N., Calapai, G., & Navarra, M. (2014). Cranberry and recurrent cystitis: More than marketing? *Critical Reviews in Food Science & Nutrition*, *54*(8), 1063-1075. doi:10.1080/10408398.2011.625574

Nishizaki, N., Someya, T., Hirano, D., Fujinaga, S., Ohtomo, Y., Shimizu, T., ... Kaneko, K. (2009). Can cranberry juice be a substitute for cefaclor prophylaxis in children with visicoureteral reflux? *Pediatrics International*, *51*(3), 433-434. doi:10.1111/j.1442-200X.2009.02867.x

Pinzon-Arango, P. A., Liu, Y., & Camesano, T. A. (2009). Role of cranberry on bacterial adhesion forces and implications for Escherichia coli-uroepithelial cell attachment. *Journal of Medicinal Food*, *12*(2), 259-270. doi:10.1089/jmf.2008.0196

Ruel, G., Pomerleau, S., Couture, P., Lemieux, S., Lamarche, B., & Couillard, C. (2009). Plasma Matrix Metalloproteinase (MMP)-9 levels are reduced following low-calorie cranberry juice supplementation in men. *Journal of the American College of Nutrition*, *28*(6), 694-701.

Vidlar, A., Vostalova, J., Ulrichova, J., Student, V., Stejskal, D., Reichenbach, R., ... Simanesk, V. (2010). The effectiveness of dried cranberries (Vaccinium macrocarpon) in men with lower urinary tract symptoms. *British Journal of Nutrition*, *104*(8), 1181-1189. doi:10.1017/S0007114510002059

Wang, C., Yolitz, J., Alberico, T., Laslo, M., Sun, Y., Wheeler, C. T., ... Zou, S. (2014). Cranberry interacts with dietary macronutrients to promote healthy aging in Drosophila. *Journals of Gerontology Series A: Biological Sciences & Medical Sciences*, *69*(8), 945-954. doi:10.1093/Gerona/glt161

Yamanaka, A., Kouchi, T., Kasai, K., Kato, T., Ishihara, K., & Okuda, K. (2007). Inhibitory effect of cranberry polyphenol on biofilm formation and cysteine proteases of Porphyromonas gingivalis. *Journal of Periodontal Research*, *42*(6), 589-592. doi:10.1111/j.1600-0765.2007.00982.x

Yamanaka-Okada, A., Sato, E., Kouchi, T., Kimizuka, R., Kato, T., & Okuda, K. (2008). Inhibitory effect of cranberry polyphenol on cariogenic bacteria. *Bulletin of Tokyo Dental College*, *49*(3), 107-112. doi:10.2209/tdcpublication.49.107

REVIEWER(S)

Darlene Strayer, RN, MBA, Cinahl Information Systems, Glendale, CA

Nursing Executive Practice Council, Glendale Adventist Medical Center, Glendale, CA

Dragon Fruit

WHAT WE KNOW

- Dragon fruit (also called pitaya, pitahaya, nanettikafruit, and strawberry pear) refers to the fruit from a variety of cactus plants. The mildly sweet, seed-filled flesh of dragon fruit is similar in texture to the flesh of a kiwi, and is protected by a think, leathery skin that is similar to that of a pineapple. Dragon fruit can be eaten raw, dried, or mixed into sorbets and smoothies. Nutritionally, dragon fruit is a good source of fiber, several B vitamins, vitamins A and C, calcium, and phosphorus. There are 3 main types of dragon fruit:
  - Hylocereus undatus, or white pitaya, has pink, leathery skin and white flesh filled with tiny black seeds
  - Hylocereus polyrhizus, or red pitaya, has pink, leathery skin and red flesh filled with tiny black seeds
  - Selenicereus megalanthus, or yellow pitaya, has yellow, leathery skin and white flesh filled with tiny black seeds

NUTRIENTS IN DRAGON FRUIT

- Dragon fruit is a good source of fiber and provides several important vitamins and minerals, including the following:
  - —The B vitamins thiamin, riboflavin, and niacin work together to create energy by aiding

the metabolism (i.e., breakdown) of carbohydrates. They provide cardiovascular protection, maintain the nervous system, and support the production of red blood cells, hormones, and necessary cholesterol.

—Vitamin A, or retinol, is a fat-soluble vitamin that is required for vision, maintenance of the surface linings of the eyes and other epithelial tissue, proper bone growth, immune response, energy regulation, reproduction, embryonic development, and activation of gene expression.

—Vitamin C is a water-soluble vitamin that neutralizes free radicals, protecting against inflammation and cellular damage. Adequate vitamin C intake is necessary for the proper function of the immune system and has been associated with the prevention of heart disease, stroke, and cancer.

—Calcium builds and maintains bones and teeth, regulates muscle contraction, conducts nerve impulses, activates enzymes for energy production and muscle contraction, participates in blood clotting, assists with vitamin B12 absorption, and maintains the structural integrity of intracellular membranes.

—Phosphorous combines with calcium for the formation of bones and teeth, muscle contraction, and nerve conduction, and is essential for the structural integrity of cell membranes.

DIETARY INTAKE GUIDELINES

- There is no official recommendation specific to dragon fruit intake.
- A recent review of available literature found no information on dragon fruit toxicity.
- A recent review of the literature found no information regarding the interaction of dragon fruit with medications or other substances.

RESEARCH FINDINGS

- Researchers report that an aqueous extract of the fruit pulp of the dragon fruit was effective for controlling oxidative damage and reducing the aortic stiffness in diabetic rats.

SUMMARY

Consumers should become knowledgeable about the physiologic benefits of dragon fruit consumption. Drag-

on fruit is a good source of dietary fiber, several B vitamins, vitamins A and C, calcium, and phosphorus. These nutrients may help improve vision, metabolic processes, immune system function and the potential to decrease the risk of developing heart disease, stroke, and cancer.

—*Cherie Marcel, BS*

REFERENCES

Anand, S. K. R., Sattar, M. A., Abdullah, N. A., Abdulla, M. H., Salman, I. M., Rathore, H. A., & Johns, E. J. (2010). Effect of dragon fruit extract on oxidative stress and aortic stiffness in streptozotocin-induced diabetes in rats. *Pharmacognosy Research, 2*(1), 31-35.

Biala, D. (2011). Dragon fruit health benefits. *Livestrong.com.* Retrieved March 10, 2015, from http://www.livestrong.com/article/372456-dragon-fruit-health-benefits/

Coila, B. (2013). Dragon fruit nutrition. *Livestrong.com.* Retrieved March 10, 2015, from http://www.livestrong.com/article/81272-dragon-fruit-nutrition/

Shadix, K. (2010). Dragon fruit. *Today's Dietitian, 12*(6), 2p.

REVIEWER(S)

Darlene Strayer, RN, MBA, Cinahl Information Systems, Glendale, CA

Nursing Executive Practice Council, Glendale Adventist Medical Center, Glendale, CA

Elderberry

WHAT WE KNOW

European elderberry (*Sumbucus nigra*; also called black elder) has been used medicinally for centuries. Not to be confused with dwarf elder (*S. ebulus*), elderberry has been used as a treatment for the common cold, flu, arthritis, asthma, and constipation and as a topical ointment to aid in wound healing. The dark purple elderberry is rich in anthocyanins, carotenoids, and other phytonutrients (i.e., protective, plant-derived chemicals), which exhibit powerful anti-inflammatory, antioxidant, cancer-preventive, and cardioprotective activity. Other nutrients supplied by elderberry include vitamins C and B6, iron, potassium, calcium, phosphorous, and copper. Elderberry can be dried and prepared as a tea, or cooked as jams and syrups, but should not be eaten raw because raw or unripe elderberry contains a chemical similar to cyanide.

NUTRIENTS IN ELDERBERRY

- Elderberry contains flavonoids, which are phytonutrients that contain the color pigments red, yellow, and orange. Flavonoids protect blood vessels from rupture and exhibit antioxidant, antibiotic, and anti-inflammatory activity. Elderberry is specifically praised for the flavonoid anthocyanins.
  - —Anthocyanins contain reddish, blue, and purple color pigments and have high antioxidant and anti-carcinogenic activity. They promote urinary tract health, support memory function, and fight bacteria such as *Streptococcus* by disrupting bacterial cell membranes.
- The water-soluble vitamin C neutralizes free radicals, protecting against inflammation and cellular damage. Adequate vitamin C intake is vital for proper function of the immune system and has been associated with the prevention of heart disease, stroke, and cancer.
- The provitamin A carotenoid phytonutrients, which are required for vision, maintenance of the surface linings of the eyes and other epithelial tissue, proper bone growth, immune response, energy regulation, reproduction, embryonic development, and gene expression.
- Vitamin B6, or pyridoxine, is required for the conversion of tryptophan into niacin and is involved in the conversion of homocysteine to cysteine. It is also necessary for the synthesis of serotonin and dopamine, which are required for nerve cell communication. By maintaining the lymphoid organs, vitamin B6 contributes to the proper function of the immune system. Additionally, it is essential for the metabolism (i.e., breakdown) of amino acids, carbohydrates, and lipids and is important for the formation of red blood cells and Hgb.
- The iron provided by elderberry is vital for the synthesis of red blood cells and hemoglobin, which are necessary for cellular respiration and the transport of oxygen to the tissues. Iron also supports immune function, is vital for cognitive development, contributes to energy metabolism, and regulates temperature.
- Elderberry contains potassium, which is an essential element responsible for regulating acid-base balance, maintaining fluid balance, supporting muscle contraction and cardiac function, contributing to protein synthesis (i.e., building) and carbohydrate metabolism, promoting cellular growth, and promoting transmission of nerve impulses.
- Calcium builds and maintains bones and teeth, regulates muscle contraction, conducts nerve impulses, activates enzymes for energy production and muscle contraction, participates in blood clotting, assists with vitamin B12 absorption, and maintains the structural integrity of intracellular membranes.
- In combination with calcium, phosphorous assists in the formation of bones and teeth, muscle contraction, and nerve conduction and is essential for the structural integrity of cell membranes.
- Copper is a vital component of superoxide dismutase, an enzyme involved in energy production and antioxidant activity. Copper contributes to the action of lysyl oxidase, an enzyme necessary for the cross-linking of collagen and elastin, which allows flexibility in the blood vessels, bones, and joints. It also enhances the body's ability to use iron, preventing iron deficiency anemia, ruptured blood vessels, irregular heartbeat, and infection.

DIETARY INTAKE GUIDELINES

- Although there is no standard recommendation for elderberry dosage, a high anthocyanin elderberry extract of 6–13% at a dose of 250–500mg/day is commonly used.
- Elderberry-flower tea is made by steeping 3 to 5 g of dried flowers in 1 cup of boiling water and consumed three times a day.
- It is important that elderberry solutions are properly cooked and prepared. Raw and unripe elderberry fruits and the leaves and bark contain a chemical similar to cyanide and should not be eaten.
- Pregnant or breastfeeding women should not use medicinal elderberry solutions.
- There is some concern that elderberry can increase the risk for kidney stones in individuals with a history of kidney stones because they contain a high amount of the chemical oxalate, a primary component of kidney stones. Oxalates can build up and crystallize in body fluids and cause health problems in individuals with pre-existing kidney or gallbladder dysfunction.
- Elderberry can act as a diuretic (i.e., promotes the production of urine). Care should be taken when combining elderberry solutions with diuretic medications, including hydrochlorothiazide,

bumetanide (Burinex), furosemide (Lasix), amiloride (Midamor), and metolazone (Zaroxolyn).

- Elderberry can act as a laxative and should not be taken with other laxative medications.
- Elderberry can reduce blood levels of theophylline (TheoDur), a medication used to treat asthma.

RESEARCH FINDINGS

- There are many health claims and medicinal uses attributed to the consumption of elderberry, such as treatment for viral influenza infections, prevention of atherosclerotic and cardiovascular disease, and stress management.
- Results of some preliminary studies suggest that elderberry preparations can provide antioxidant, antiviral, antibiotic, anti-inflammatory, and anti-proliferative effects in vitro, but evidence is lacking. Researchers recommend more rigorous studies on these claims.

SUMMARY

Consumers should become knowledgeable about the physiologic effects of elderberry consumption. Elderberry is a good source of phytonutrients, vitamins C and B6, iron, potassium, calcium, phosphorous, and copper. These nutrients may help prevent cancer, stroke and heart disease. Elderberry helps support the immune system and some research suggests it may prevent bacterial and viral infections. Caution should be taken to properly cook elderberry due to the toxicity of raw fruits, leaves, and bark. Pregnant and breastfeeding women should not use medicinal elderberry solutions. Individuals with a high risk for kidney stones should avoid the use of medicinal elderberry due to its high content oxalate. Elderberry should not be taken with diuretics, laxatives, or the asthma medication theophylline (TheoDur).

—*Cherie Marcel, BS*

REFERENCES

Curtis, P. J., Kroon, P. A., Hollands, W. J., Walls, R., Jenkins, G., Kay, C. D., & Cassidy, A. (2009). Cardiovascular disease risk biomarkers and liver and kidney function are not altered in postmenopausal women after ingesting an elderberry extract rich in anthocyanins for 12 weeks. *Journal of Nutrition, 139*(12), 2266-2271. doi:10.3945/jn.109.113126

Ehrlich, S. D. (2013). Elderberry. *University of Maryland Medical Center.* Retrieved March 10, 2015, from http://www.umm.edu/altmed/articles/elderberry-002880.htm

The George Mateljan Foundation editorial team. (n.d.). Can you tell me what oxalates are and in which foods they can be found?. *The World's Healthiest Foods.* Retrieved March 10, 2015, from http://www.whfoods.com/genpage.php?tname=george&dbid=48

Johnson, K. (2012). Vitamins and supplements lifestyle guide: Elderberry. *WebMD.* Retrieved March 10, 2015, from http://www.webmd.com/vitamins-and-supplements/lifestyle-guide-11/supplement-guide-elderberry

Kilham, C. (2000). The healing powers of elderberry. *Total Health, 22*(5), 40-41.

Murkovic, M., Abuja, P. M., Bergmann, A. R., Zirngast, A., Adam, U., Winklhofer-Roob, B. M., & Toplak, H. (2004). Effects of elderberry juice on fasting and postprandial serum lipids and low-density lipoprotein oxidation in healthy volunteers: A randomized, double-blind, placebo-controlled study. *European Journal of Clinical Nutrition, 58*(2), 244-249. doi:10.1038/sj.ejcn.1601773

Natural and Alternative Treatments, DynaMed. (2013, August). Elderberry. Ipswich MA: EBSCO Information Services. Retrieved March 10, 2015, from http://therapy.epnet.com/ nat/nat.asp

Vanta, B. (2013, August 16). What are the health benefits of elderberry?. *Livestrong.com.* Retrieved March 10, 2015, from http://www.livestrong.com/article/376402-elderberry-extract-benefits/

Vlachojannis, J. E., Cameron, M., & Chrubasik, S. (2010). A systematic review on the sambuci fructus effect and efficacy profiles. *Phytotherapy Research, 24*(1), 1-8. doi:10.1002/ptr.2729

REVIEWER(S)

Darlene Strayer, RN, MBA, Cinahl Information Systems, Glendale, CA

Nursing Executive Practice Council, Glendale Adventist Medical Center, Glendale, CA

Fig

WHAT WE KNOW

Figs grow on the ficus tree, or Ficus carica, which is a member of the mulberry, or Moraceae, family. Mentioned in numerous ancient writings, the origin of the fig is thought to have been Egypt, followed by its appearance in ancient Greece and the Mediterranean. Currently, figs are predominately grown in California, Turkey, Greece, Portugal, and Spain, and are available in over 150 varieties (e.g., Black Mission, Kadota, Calimyrna, Brown Turkey, Adriatic). Commonly considered a fruit, the outer structure of the fig is technically a flower that is involuted (i.e., turned in on itself), forming a receptacle that is almost totally closed and has small flowers on the inner surface; the many seeds within the fig are technically the fruit. Depending on its variety, the smooth skin of the fig can be black, red, yellow, purple, pink, brown, green, and many variations of these colors. The deeper the color, the higher the concentration of antioxidants. The inner flesh of the fig is thick, sweet, and textured with many tiny seeds. The fig can be eaten raw, dried, baked in cookies, or used to make puddings and sauces. The fig is a good source of soluble and insoluble fiber, potassium, manganese, calcium, iron, vitamin B6, and important phytonutrients (i.e., protective, plant-derived chemicals) such as flavonoids. Together, these nutrients promote immune function and wound healing and provide preventative health benefits against heart disease, cancer, osteoporosis, and diabetes mellitus, type 2 (DM2).

NUTRIENTS IN FIG

- Fig contains many important phytonutrients, including the following:
  - —Flavonoids are the color pigments red, yellow, and orange, which protect blood vessels from rupturing and exhibit antioxidant, antibiotic, and anti-inflammatory activity.
    - –The flavonol quercetin provides strong antioxidant and anti-inflammatory protection. It also has antihistamine, antimicrobial, antidiabetic, and anti-carcinogenic properties.
    - –Anthocyanins, which are reddish color pigments, have high antioxidant and anticarcinogenic activity, promote urinary tract health, and support memory function.
- Fig is a good source of dietary fiber, including soluble fiber, which binds with water and slows the digestive process, allowing the body to better manage post-prandial (i.e., after eating) glucose and insulin responses. Fiber also increases the volume of the intestinal contents, which hinders the absorption of cholesterol. The added bulk leads to more regular bowel movements, promoting intestinal health.

- Fig provides valuable minerals, including the following:
  - —Potassium supports normal cellular, nerve, and muscle function and helps to eliminate excess sodium from the body.
  - —Calcium builds and maintains bones and teeth, regulates muscle contraction, conducts nerve impulses, activates enzymes for energy production and muscle contraction, assists in blood clotting function, assists with vitamin B12 absorption, and maintains the structural integrity of intracellular membranes.
  - —Manganese, a trace mineral, is responsible for energy production, fatty acid synthesis (i.e., building), essential cholesterol production, and protection against damage caused by free-radicals.
  - —Iron is vital for the synthesis of red blood cells and hemoglobin, which are necessary for cellular respiration and the transport of oxygen to the tissues. Iron also supports immune function, is vital for brain development, contributes to energy metabolism, and regulates temperature.
- Fig is a good source of vitamin B6, or pyridoxine, which is required for the conversion of tryptophan into niacin, and is involved in the conversion of homocysteine to cysteine. B6 is also necessary for the synthesis of serotonin and dopamine, which are neurotransmitters required for nerve cell communication. By maintaining the lymphoid organs, vitamin B6 contributes to healthy immune system function. Additionally, B6 is essential for the metabolism of amino acids, carbohydrates, and lipids, and is important in the formation of red blood cells and hemoglobin, which carries oxygen to the tissues.

DIETARY INTAKE GUIDELINES

There is no information in medical literature regarding recommended dosages of fig.

- Fig is not recommended for persons with a propensity for the formation of phytobezoar (i.e., abnormal compaction of ingested items in the gastrointestinal system, including leaves, skins, seeds, roots, stems, or other plant fibers). Individuals who have had surgery for peptic ulcer disease or stomach cancer or have lost normal pyloric function (i.e., control of contents leaving stomach and entering the intestines) are at elevated risk of developing phytobezoars.

- There is no information in medical literature regarding interactions of fig with medications.

RESEARCH FINDINGS

- There is evidence that the nutrients and phytochemicals found in fig counteract oxidative stress, reduce inflammation, and modulate cellular interactions, which play a protective role against cancer and heart disease. This is especially true of dried figs. Results of studies demonstrate that dried fig has over 6 times the antioxidant power of vitamin C, E, and beta-carotene. Test results also indicate that dried fig can boost the antioxidant activity in the blood by up to 18%.
- Researchers believe that the drying process used for the fig results in water and sugar loss, increasing phenol content of the fig.
- Researchers have found that fig leaf extracts exhibit strong anti-inflammatory activity and a neuroprotective effect. In the future, fig extracts may be used therapeutically to prevent and/or delay progression of neurodegenerative diseases such as Parkinson's disease.

SUMMARY

Consumers should become knowledgeable about the physiologic benefits of the consumption of figs. The fig is a good source of fiber, potassium, manganese, calcium, iron, vitamin B6, and important phytonutrients. These nutrients provide fig with strong antioxidant power, promote immune function, wound healing and may help prevent heart disease, cancer, osteoporosis, and type 2 diabetes.

—*Cherie Marcel, BS*

REFERENCES

Ahmed, F., Siddesha, J. M., Urooj, A., & Vishwanath, B. S. (2010). Radical scavenging and angiotensin converting enzyme inhibitory activities of standardized extracts of Ficus racemosa stem bark. *Phytotherapy Research, 24*(12), 1839-1843. doi:10.1002/ptr.3205

The George Mateljan Foundation. (n.d.). The world's healthiest foods: Figs. Retrieved March 10, 2015, from http://www.whfoods.com/genpage.php?tname=foodspice&dbid=24

Gilani, A. H., Mehmood, M. H., Janbaz, K. H., Khan, A. U., & Saeed, S. A. (2008). Ethnopharmacological studies on antispasmodic and antiplatelet activities of

Ficus carica. *Journal of Ethnopharmacology, 119*(1), 1-5. doi:10.1016/j.jep.2008.05.040

Houghton, V. (2006). Health & wellness. Dietary alternatives: Dried figs. *ACA News (American Chiropractic Association), 2*(4), 17.

Jung, H. W., Son, H. Y., Minh, C. V., Kim, Y. H., & Park, Y. K. (2008). Methanol extract of Ficus leaf inhibits the production of nitric oxide and proinflammatory cytokines in LPS-simulated microglia via the MAPK pathway. *Phytotherapy Research, 22*(8), 1064-1069. doi:10.1002/ptr.2442

Kruse, S. (2011). Fabulous figs. *IDEA Fitness Journal, 8*(7), 115.

Lansky, E. P., Paavilainen, H. M., Pawlus, A. D., & Newman, R. A. (2008). Ficus spp. (fig): Ethnobotany and potential as anticancer and anti-inflammatory agents. *Journal of Ethnopharmacology, 119*(2), 195-213. doi:10.1016/j.jep.2008.06.025

Puoci, F., Iemma, F., Spizzirri, U. G., Restuccia, D., Pezzi, V., Sirianni, R., & Picci, N. (2011). Antioxidant activity of a Mediterranean food product: "Fig syrup". *Nutrients, 3*(3), 317-329. doi:10.3390/nu3030317

Schepers, A. (2005). Go Figure. Ancient fruit of Biblical lore measures up in nutrition. *Environmental Nutrition, 28*(5), 8.

Slavin, J. L. (2006). Figs. *Nutrition Today, 41*(4), 180-184.

Yang, X. M., Yu, W., Ou, Z. P., Ma, H. L., Liu, W. M., & Ji, X. L. (2009). Antioxidant and immunity activity of water extract and crude polysaccharide from Ficus carica L. fruit. *Plant Foods for Human Nutrition, 64*(2), 167-173. doi:10.1007/s11130-009-0120-5

Zanteson, L. (2011). Figure figs into a healthy diet. *Environmental Nutrition, 34*(7), 8.

REVIEWER(S)

Darlene Strayer, RN, MBA, Cinahl Information Systems, Glendale, CA

Nursing Executive Practice Council, Glendale Adventist Medical Center, Glendale, CA

Grapefruit

WHAT WE KNOW

The grapefruit, or *Citrus paradisi*, is a 4–6 inch round, pinkish/yellow-skinned, citrus fruit with a combination of sweet and intensely tart flavor. Depending on the color of the flesh of the fruit, grapefruit are classified as white (also called blond), pink, or ruby. Grapefruit can be eaten raw, sectioned for inclusion in salads, drunk as juice, or added to drinks and foods as a tart flavoring agent. Botanists believe that the grapefruit resulted from a natural cross breeding between oranges and pomelos that occurred after the pomelos were brought to Barbados from Indonesia in the 17th century. Floridians began planting grapefruit groves in the 19th century and Florida remains a major producer of grapefruit along with California, Arizona, and Texas. Similar to other citrus fruits (e.g., oranges, lemons), grapefruit contains high levels of the antioxidant vitamin C and is rich in vitamin A, thiamin (B_1), pantothenic acid (B_5), potassium, fiber, and the phytonutrients (i.e., beneficial, plant-derived nutrients) limonoids and lycopene. These nutrients cause grapefruit to have antioxidant, antibiotic, and anticancer properties.

- Grapefruit contains the chemical compound furanocoumarin, which is known to interfere with the catabolism (i.e., break down of large molecules) of many medications (e.g., immune-suppressants, calcium channel blockers, statins), increasing their potency and potentially resulting in life-threatening complications.

NUTRIENTS IN GRAPEFRUIT

- The water-soluble vitamin C in grapefruit neutralizes free radicals, protecting against inflammation and cellular damage. Adequate vitamin C intake is vital for the proper function of the immune system and is associated with the prevention of heart disease, stroke, and cancer.
- Grapefruit is rich in vitamin A (i.e., retinol), a fat-soluble vitamin that is required for vision, maintenance of the surface lining of the eyes and other epithelial tissue, proper bone growth, normal immune response, energy regulation, reproduction, embryonic development, and activation of gene expression.
- The B-complex vitamins B1 and B5 create energy by aiding the metabolism (i.e., break down) of carbohydrates, provide cardiovascular protection, maintain the nervous system, and support the production of red blood cells, hormones, and necessary cholesterol.
- The potassium in grapefruit supports normal cellular, nerve, and muscle function and helps to eliminate excess sodium from the body.

- The soluble fiber in grapefruit binds with water and slows the digestive process, allowing better management of postprandial (i.e., after eating) glucose and insulin responses. Fiber increases the volume of the intestinal contents, which hinders the absorption of cholesterol. The added bulk promotes more regular bowel movements, promoting intestinal health.
- Grapefruit contain important phytonutrients, including limonoids, the flavonoid naringenin, and the carotenoid lycopene (lycopene is found only in pink or ruby grapefruit), which inhibit cancer cell proliferation, repair damaged deoxyribonucleic acid (DNA), and exhibit powerful antibiotic activity.

DIETARY INTAKE GUIDELINES

- Grapefruit can dangerously increase the potency of certain commonly prescribed pharmaceutical drugs, including the following:
  —Cyclosporine and other immunosuppressants (e.g., tacrolimus, siroliums, everolimus)
  —Calcium channel blockers (e.g., felodipine, verapamil, nifedipine)
  —Statin drugs (e.g., simvastatin, lovastatin, pravastatin, atorvastatin)
  —Antihistamines (e.g., terfenadine, fexofenadine)
  —The hormone estradiol
  —Antiretrovirals (e.g., saquinavir, indinavir)
  —The antidepressant sertraline
  —Central nervous system (CNS) agents (e.g., buspirone, alfentanil [oral preparation], dextromethorphan, fentanyl [oral preparation], ketamine [oral preparation], lurasidone, oxycodone, pimozide, quetiapine, ziprasidone)
  —Anticoagulants (e.g., apixaban, rivaroxaban)
  —Cytotoxics (e.g., nilotinib, lapatinib, crizontinib, dasatinib, erlotinib, everolimus, pazopanib, sunitinib, vandetanib, venurafenib)
  —Anti-infective agents (e.g., erythromycin, halofantrine, maraviroc, primaquine, quinine, rilpivirine)
  —The gastrointestinal agent domperidone
  —Agents used in treatment of abnormalities of the urinary tract (e.g., darifenacin, fesoterodine, solifenacin, silodosin, tamsulosin)
  —Cardiovascular agents (e.g., amiodarone, apixaban, clopidogrel, dronedarone, eplerenone, ticagrelor)

RESEARCH FINDINGS

- With the regular introduction of new medications, reports of adverse interactions of grapefruit with medication have increased. There are currently more than 85 medications that are known or suspected to interact with grapefruit, 43 of which can cause serious complications. Other citrus fruits such as sour oranges (also called bitter orange e.g., the Seville orange) have exhibited similar adverse interactions. It is important that clinicians remain informed of current information regarding potential interactions and educate their patients of risks.

- Grapefruit juice or grapefruit extract is commonly used in many U.S. manufactured soft drink beverages. A recent study identified at least 23 commonly consumed beverages that contained verifiable amounts of grapefruit, and more that possibly contained grapefruit.

- Although the 12-day Grapefruit Diet has been heralded since the 1930s as a miracle diet thought to burn fat and cause rapid weight loss, these claims are not supported by research. Individuals following the diet may lose weight temporarily due to its restrictive nature, but the weight loss is typically from loss of fluids and weight tends to be regained shortly after the diet ends.

- Grapefruit has been investigated for its potential role as an antidiabetic agent. In lab studies, grapefruit juice consumption has been associated with improved glucose and insulin levels. Authors of one study found that both whole grapefruit and grapefruit juice consumption were associated with improved insulin resistance.

- Results of some studies indicate an association between grapefruit intake and improved blood pressure and lipid profiles. Authors of one study noted that despite the lack of weight loss, there was a decrease in waist circumference in test subjects who consumed 1.5 grapefruits daily. Overall, the consensus among dietary professionals is that any short-term, highly restrictive, weight loss diet based on eating only one food item is probably unbalanced and has a high likelihood of long-term failure. Grapefruit is a very healthy food to include as part of one's diet along with many other fruits and vegetables.

SUMMARY

Consumers should become knowledgeable about the physiologic risks and nutritional benefits of grapefruit consumption. Certain medications may have potential harmful interactions with grapefruit. Elderly individuals on multiple medications, and liver cirrhosis patients are at especially increased risk of grapefruit and medication interaction. Grapefruit is a good source of vitamins, minerals, phytonutrients and fiber. These nutrients give grapefruit antioxidant, antibiotic, and anticancer properties. Research suggests that popular grapefruit diets do not produce long term weight loss results.

—Cherie Marcel, BS

REFERENCES

Auten, A. A., Beauchamp, L. N., Joshua Taylor, & Hardinger, K. L. (2013). Hidden sources of grapefruit in beverages: Potential interactions with immunosuppressant medications. *Hospital Pharmacy*, 48(6), 489-493. doi:10.1310/hpj4806-489

Bailey, D. G., Dresser, G., & Arnold, J. M. O. (2012). Grapefruit-medication interactions: Forbidden fruit or avoidable consequences? *CMAJ: Canadian Medical Association Journal*, 185(4), 309-316. doi:10.1503/cmaj.120951

Canadian Nursing Home editorial team. (2012). Grapefruit-drug interactions on the rise with providers unaware of the possible effect. *Canadian Nursing Home*, 23(4), 20.

Dow, C. A., Going, S. B., Chow, H. H., Patil, B. S., & Thomson, C. A. (2012). The effects of daily consumption of grapefruit on body weight, lipids, and blood pressure in healthy, overweight adults. *Metabolism: Clinical and Experimental*, 61(7), 1026-1035.

Fujioka, K., Greenway, F., Sheard, J., & Ying, Y. (2006). The effects of grapefruit juice on weight and insulin resistance: Relationship to the metabolic syndrome. *J Med Food*, 9(1), 49-54.

The George Mateljan Foundation Editorial Team. (n.d.). The world's healthiest foods: Grapefruit. Retrieved February 19, 2015, fromhttp://www.whfoods.com/genpage.php? tname=foodspice&dbid=25

Lutz, C. A., & Przytulski, K. R. (2011). medications and supplements. In *Nutrition & diet therapy* (5th ed., pp. 307). Philadelphia, PA: F. A. Davis Company.

Ojewole, P. M., & Ojewole, J. A. (2010). The grapefruit: An old wine in a new glass? Metabolic and cardiovascular perspectives. *Cardiovascular Journal of Africa*, 21(5), 280-285. doi:10.5830/CVJA-2010-012

Owira, P. M. O., & Ojewole, J. A. O. (2009). Grapefruit juice improves glycemic control but exacerbates metformin-induced lactic acidosis in non-diabetic rats. *Methods and Findings in Experimental and Clinical Pharmacology*, 31(9), 563-570.

Pirmohamed, M. (2013). Drug-grapefruit juice interactions. *BMJ: British Medical Journal*, 346(7890), 9.

Roth, S. L. (2011). Drug-nutrient interactions. In E. D. Schlenker, & S. L. Roth (Eds.), *Williams' essentials of nutrition and diet therapy* (10th ed., pp. 403). St. Louis, MO: Mosby, Inc, an affiliate of Elsevier Inc.

Schardt, D. (2012). Fruit with benefits: A tart cherry a day. *Nutrition Action Health Letter*, 39(2), 9-11.

Silver, H. J., Dietrich, M. S., & Niswender, K. D. (2011). Effects of grapefruit, grapefruit juice and water preloads on energy balance, weight loss, body composition, and cardiometabolic risk in free-living obese adults. *Nutrition & Metabolism*, 8(1), 8. doi:10.1186/1743-7075-8-8

Zelman, K. M. (2013). Weight loss & diet plans: The grapefruit diet. WebMD. Retrieved February 19, 2015, from http://www.webmd.com/diet/features/the-grapefruit-diet

REVIEWER(S)

Darlene Strayer, RN, MBA, Cinahl Information Systems, Glendale, CA

Nursing Executive Practice Council, Glendale Adventist Medical Center, Glendale, CA

Guava

WHAT WE KNOW

Guava, or *Psidium guajava*, is a tropical plant of Myrtaceae family that is native to Central and South America but now commonly grows in most of the world's tropical regions. Guava produces aromatic, round or pear-shaped yellow fruit with a flavor that ranges from acidic to very sweet. When guava is eaten raw, most persons remove the seeds and pulp. Guava is commonly cooked, which eliminates the aroma, which can be overpowering. Guava contains many nutrients, including vitamin C, calcium, potassium, carotenoids (i.e., plant pigments responsible for bright red, yellow and orange hues in many fruits and vegetables), folate, and fiber. The roots, bark, leaves, and fruit of the guava plant are commonly used by some populations for medicinal purposes. Crushed leaves are applied as treatment to wounds and sore joints, chewed as a pain reliever for toothache, and gargled in solution to treat sore gums. Guava root and bark are used to treat gastroenteritis and diarrhea. Other therapeutic uses of the guava plant are the treatment of cough, sore throat, vomiting, skin disease, nephritis, and cachexia.

NUTRIENTS IN GUAVA

- Guava contains important phytonutrients (i.e., beneficial plant-derived nutrients) such as ellagic acid, cyanidin, apigenin, lycopene, and quercetin, which have antioxidant, anti-inflammatory, antispasmodic (i.e., helps with muscle spasms), anti-proliferative (i.e., helps kill cancer cells), and antimicrobial properties.
- Vitamin C in guava neutralizes free radicals, protecting against inflammation and cellular damage. Adequate vitamin C intake is vital for proper function of the immune system and is associated with prevention of heart disease, stroke, and cancer.
- Guava is an excellent source of dietary fiber, which binds and removes toxins from the colon, assists in glycemic control, and reduces elevated cholesterol levels.
- The combination of vitamin C, potassium, and polyphenols in guava reduce triglyceride levels and prevent excessive platelet aggregation (i.e., blood clotting).

DIETARY INTAKE GUIDELINES

- A typical dosage of a guava leaf and/or twig decoction is 0.5–1 cup 3–5 times daily.
- Although no contraindications are specified for guava, because it is used by some populations to assist in evacuating the placenta following birth, avoiding medicinal doses of guava constituents during pregnancy is recommended.
- Although no interactions with medications have been documented, the high level of tannins found in guava leaf could theoretically decrease the therapeutic activity of alkaloid-based medications and herbs.

RESEARCH FINDINGS

- There is evidence that guava-derived nutrients and phytochemicals play a protective role against cancer. The potential chemopreventive and chemotherapeutic properties of guava are attributed in part to the ability of certain guava constituents (e.g., vitamin C, lycopene, apigenin) to:
  - —protect against DNA and cellular damage caused by oxidative stress
  - —reduce inflammation
  - —modulate cellular interactions
  - —prevent the proliferation of cancer cell lines
- Researchers report that guava leaf extract exhibits anti-diabetic properties by suppressing elevated glucose levels, and suggest that habitual ingestion such as drinking guava leaf tea with every meal can serve as alimentotherapy (i.e., dietary treatment) for the prevention of diabetes mellitus, type 2 (DM2).
  - —Guava leaf extract has also exhibited significant anti-inflammatory activity in both in vitro and in vivo studies, supporting theories that guava contains medicinal properties with the potential to treat inflammatory diseases.

SUMMARY

Consumers should become knowledgeable about the physiologic benefits of guava consumption. Guava can contribute to health because it contains many nutrients, including vitamin C, calcium, potassium, carotenoids, folate, and fiber. These nutrients may help relieve pain, sore throat, muscle spasms and vomiting, and prevent excessive blood clotting, while reducing risk of developing type 2 diabetes, heart disease, cancer and stroke. Avoiding medicinal doses of guava during pregnancy is recommended.

—*Cherie Marcel, BS*

REFERENCES

Birdi, T., Daswani, P., Brijesh, S., Tetali, P., Natu, A., & Antia, N. (2010). Newer insights into the mechanism of action of Psidium guajava L. leaves in infectious diarrhoea. *BMC Complementary & Alternative Medicine, 10*, 11.

Chen, K. C., Hsieh, C. L., Peng, C. C., Hsieh-Li, H. M., Chiang, H. S., Huang, K. D., & Peng, R. Y. (2007). Brain derived metastatic prostate cancer DU-145 cells are effectively inhibited in vitro by guava (Psidium guajava L.) leaf extracts. *Nutrition & Cancer, 58*(1), 93-106.

Chen, K., Peng, C., Chiu, W., Cheng, Y., Huang, G., Hsieh, C., & Peng, R. Y. (2010). Action mechanism and signal pathways of Psidium guajava L. aqueous extract in killing prostate cancer LNCaP cells. *Nutrition & Cancer, 62*(2), 260-270.

Deguchi, Y., & Miyazaki, K. (2010). Anti-hyperglycemic and anti-hyperlipidemic effects of guava leaf extract. *Nutrition & Metabolism, 7*, 10.

Hawrelak, J. (2003). Medicinal herb monograph: Guava (Psidium guajava). *Journal of the Australian Traditional-Medicine Society, 9*(1), 25-29.

Ipatenco, S. (2014, February 19). Is guava healthy? *Livestrong.com.* Retrieved June 18, 2015, from http://www.livestrong.com/article/409166-is-guava-healthy/

Jang, M., Jeong, S. W., Cho, S. K., Ahn, K. S., Lee, J. H., Yang, D. C., & Kim, J. C. (2014). Anti-inflammatory effects of an ethanolic extract of guava (Psidium guajava L.) leaves in vitro and in vivo. *Journal of Medicinal Food, 17*(6), 678-685. doi:10.1089/jmf.2013.2936

Owen, P. L., Martineau, L. C., Caves, D., Haddad, P. S., Matainaho, T., & Johns, T. (2008). Consumption of guava (Psidium guajava L.) and noni (Morinda citrifolia L.) may protect betel quid-chewing Papua New Guineans against diabetes. *Asia Pacific Journal of Clinical Nutrition, 17*(4), 635-643.

Roy, C. K., & Das, A. K. (2010). Hepatoprotective activity of some quercetin derivatives. *Internet Journal of Alternative Medicine, 8*(2), 8.

Ryu, N. H., Park, K., Kim, S., Yun, H., Nam, D., Lee, S., ... Ahn, K. S. (2012). A hexane fraction of guava leaves (Psidium guajava L.) induces anticancer activity by suppressing AKT/mammalian target of rapamycin/ribosomal p70 S6 kinase in human prostate cancer cells. *Journal of Medicinal Food, 15*(3), 231-241.

Sato, R., Dang, K. M., McPherson, B. G., & Brown, A. C. (2010). Anticancer activity of guava (Psidium guajava) extracts. *Journal of Complementary & Integrative Medicine, 7*(1), 12.

Shu, J., Chou, G., & Wang, Z. (2010). Two new benzophenone glycosides from the fruit Psidium guajava L. *Fitoterapia, 81*(6), 532-535.

REVIEWER(S)

Darlene Strayer, RN, MBA, Cinahl Information Systems, Glendale, CA

Nursing Executive Practice Council, Glendale Adventist Medical Center, Glendale, CA

Honeydew

WHAT WE KNOW

Honeydew melon (*Cucumis melo*; commonly called honeydew) is a variety of muskmelon and a member of the Cucurbitaceae family, along with watermelon, bitter melon, pumpkin, and cucumber. Originally known as the melon d'Antibesblancd'hiver (i.e., the white Antibes wintermelon), honeydew originated in southern France and Algeria centuries ago. The creeping vine of the honeydew plant produces round fruit with thick, white or green-tinged, waxy rinds. Considered the sweetest of the melons, the pale green or orange flesh of honeydew is creamy in texture, similar to its close relative, the cantaloupe. A delicious culinary treat, honeydew fruit is frequently eaten raw but can also be used in drinks, dressings, and sauces. Beyond its culinary value, honeydew is a good source of fiber; vitamins B1, B3, B5, B6, C, and K; folate; potassium; magnesium; copper; and valuable phytonutrients (i.e., beneficial, pant-derived chemicals), including zeaxanthin.

NUTRIENTS IN HONEYDEW

- Honeydew contains the phytonutrient zeaxanthin, a carotenoid that exhibits antioxidant properties and safeguards the eyes from light-induced oxidation, preventing age-related macular degeneration.
- Honeydew is a good source of vitamin C, which neutralizes free radicals, protecting against inflammation and cellular damage. Adequate vitamin C intake is vital for immune system function and is associated with the prevention of heart disease, stroke, and cancer.
- Vitamin K in honeydew acts as a coenzyme to maintain normal levels of blood clotting proteins and contributes to bone metabolism (i.e. break down).
- Honeydew is a good source of several B-complex vitamins:
  - —vitamins B1 and B3 create energy by aiding the metabolism of carbohydrates, provide cardiovascular protection, maintain the nervous system, and support the production of red blood cells, hormones, and necessary cholesterol.
  - —Folate is a B vitamin that is essential for the production and maintenance of red blood cells (RBCs). Folate is vital for the synthesis of deoxyribonucleic acid (DNA), the genetic code for the cells, and ribonucleic acid (RNA), and is important in the metabolism of homocysteine (i.e., an amino acid).
  - —Pantothenic acid, or vitamin B5, contributes to the metabolism of carbohydrates, proteins, and lipids. It also plays a role in the synthesis of acetylcholine, a neurotransmitter in the central and peripheral nervous systems.
  - —Vitamin B6, or pyridoxine, is required for the conversion of tryptophan to niacin and is involved in the conversion of homocysteine to cysteine. Vitamin B6 is necessary for the synthesis of serotonin and dopamine, which are neurotransmitters required for nerve cell communication. By maintaining the lymphoid organs, vitamin B6 contributes to immune system function. Vitamin B6 is essential for the metabolism of amino acids, carbohydrates, and lipids and is important for the formation of RBCs and hemoglobin, which carries oxygen to the tissues.
- Potassium in honeydew supports normal cellular, nerve, and muscle function and helps to eliminate excess sodium from the body.
- The magnesium provided by honeydew balances the action of calcium in cells to regulate bone health and nerve and muscle tone. It maintains relaxation of nerves and muscles, which contributes to the prevention of high blood pressure, muscle spasms, asthma, migraine headaches, general soreness, and fatigue.
- Copper is a vital component of superoxide dismutase (SOD), an enzyme involved in energy production and antioxidant activity. It contributes to the action of lysyl oxidase, an enzyme necessary for the cross-linking of collagen and elastin, which allows flexibility in the blood vessels, bones, and joints. It also enhances the body's ability to use iron, preventing iron-deficiency anemia, ruptured blood vessels, irregular heartbeat, and infection.

DIETARY INTAKE GUIDELINES

- There is no information in the literature regarding dosage and administration recommendations for honeydew.
- Melon rinds can serve as a vehicle for the bacteria *Salmonella* and *Listeria*. To avoid contamination when purchasing commercially grown melons,

the U.S. Federal Food and Drug Administration (FDA) advises the following precautions:
—Don't eat bruised melons
—Always wash hands with soap and hot water prior to handling melons
—Thoroughly clean the whole melon with a clean produce brush and tap water prior to cutting open

- Refrigerate the melon upon cutting and eat within 2 days.
- There is no information in the literature regarding interactions of honeydew with medications.

RESEARCH FINDINGS

- There is little published research in the literature regarding honeydew.
- A clinical trial was conducted to determine the effect of melon juice supplementation on perceived stress and fatigue based on the hypothesis that perceived stress is associated with oxidative stress. Researchers reported that the group that received the oral melon juice supplementation showed improvement in several signs and symptoms of stress and fatigue. A similar study, which analyzed the effects of a gliadin (wheat proteins)-combined plant SOD extract on perceived fatigue in women aged 50–65 years found no notable improvements in the participants receiving the extract.

SUMMARY

Consumers should become knowledgeable about the physiologic benefits of the consumption of honeydew. Honeydew is rich in vitamins, minerals, phytonutrients, and fiber. These nutrients assist with digestion, bone, muscle and eye health, as well as decrease risk of developing iron-deficiency anemia, heart disease, stroke, and cancer. Individuals should follow FDA precautions for avoiding contamination with *Salmonella* and *Listeria* when purchasing commercially grown melons.

—*Cherie Marcel, BS*

REFERENCES

Centers for Disease Control and Prevention. (2013). ListeriaListeria (Listeriosis). Retrieved May 7, 2015, from http://www.cdc.gov/listeria/

The editorial team of WebMD. (2014, June 3). Honeydew: 7 healthy facts. *WebMD*. Retrieved October 30, 2014, from http://www.webmd.com/food-recipes/features/honeydew-7-healthy-facts

Foodsafety.gov. (n.d.). Salmonella. Retrieved June 18, 2015, from http://www.foodsafety.gov/poisoning/causes/bacteriaviruses/salmonella/

The George Mateljan Foundation editorial team. (n.d.). The world's healthiest foods: How does honeydew compare to cantaloupe?. Retrieved October 30, 2014, from http:// whfoods.org/genpage.php?tname=dailytip&dbid=13&utm_source=rss_reader&utm_medium=rss&utm_campaign=rss_feed

Houghton, C. A., Steels, E. L., Fassett, R. G., & Coombes, J. S. (2011). Effects of a gliadin-combined plant superoxide dismutase extract on self-perceived fatigue in women aged 50--65 years. *Phytomedicine*, *18*(6), 521-526. doi:10.1016/j.phymed.2010.09.006

Ipatenco, S. (2013, December 18). Health benefits of eating honeydew melon. *Livestrong.com*. Retrieved October 30, 2014, from http://www.livestrong.com/article/340453-health-benefits-of-eating-honeydew-melon/

Liddell, A. (2013, December 18). The health benefits of melons. *Livestrong.com*. Retrieved from http://www.livestrong.com/article/407556-the-health-benefits-of-melons/

Milesi, M. A., Lacan, D., Brosse, H., Desor, D., & Notin, C. (2009). Effect of an oral supplementation with a proprietary melon juice concentrate (Extramel) on stress and fatigue in healthy people: A pilot, double-blind, placebo-controlled clinical trial. *Nutrition Journal*, 8, 40. doi:10.1186/1475-2891-8-40

REVIEWER(S)

Darlene Strayer, RN, MBA, Cinahl Information Systems, Glendale, CA
Nursing Executive Practice Council, Glendale Adventist Medical Center, Glendale, CA

Kiwi

WHAT WE KNOW

The most common variety of kiwi (also called kiwifruit; from the family Actinidiaceae) is the Hayward kiwi (from the plant *Actinidia deliciosa*), which is a small oval fruit with a fuzzy brown exterior and bright green flesh. Kiwi originated in China and was known as yang tao (i.e., strawberry peach) and Chinese gooseberry. Growers in New Zealand began calling it kiwifruit in 1962 as an attempt to improve its market appeal. The flavor of kiwi is an intense combination of sweetness

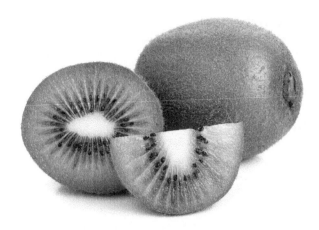

and tartness. Although the furry skin is edible, it is often removed to avoid the hairy texture. Smooth-skinned varieties of kiwi (e.g., the bite-sizedhardy kiwi; the silver vine kiwi) are currently available and have grown in popularity. Kiwi is eaten raw and should be eaten soon after cutting because it contains actinic and bromic acids, which are enzymes that act as food tenderizers and can cause the kiwi and any other food on the plate to become mushy. Kiwi contains many nutrients, including more vitamin C per ounce than an orange, more potassium than a banana, magnesium, folate, zinc, copper, vitamins E and K, lutein, fiber, and important polyphenolic phytonutrients (i.e., protective, plant-derived chemicals). Kiwi consumption is associated with a reduced risk of developing heart disease, stroke, asthma, macular degeneration, and cancer. In traditional Chinese medicine kiwi is used to treat cancers of the lung, liver, and stomach.

NUTRIENTS IN KIWI

- Kiwi contains important phytonutrients that have antioxidant, anti-inflammatory, and anti-mutagenic properties that protect cellular deoxyribonucleic acid (DNA) from damage and enhance DNA repair.

- The water-soluble vitamin C in kiwi neutralizes free radicals, protecting against inflammation and cellular damage. Adequate vitamin C intake is vital for proper function of the immune system and is associated with prevention of heart disease, stroke, and cancer.

- Kiwi is an excellent source of dietary fiber, which binds and removes toxins from the colon, assists in glycemic control, and reduces elevated cholesterol levels.

- The combination of vitamin C, potassium, and polyphenols found in kiwis reduce triglyceride levels and prevent excessive blood clotting.

RESEARCH FINDINGS

- There is evidence that the kiwi-derived nutrient and phytochemical actions of counteracting oxidative stress, reducing inflammation, and modulating cellular interactions play a protective role against vascular disease and cancer. The prevention of vascular disease is attributed, in part, to the ability of certain phytochemicals (e.g., flavonoids and carotenoids) and nutrients (e.g., vitamin C and potassium) to inhibit platelet aggregation (i.e., blood clotting) and lower serum lipid profiles. The potential chemo-preventive properties of kiwi involve the ability to protect against DNA and cellular damage caused by oxidative stress.

- Results of a 6-week study showed that daily consumption of 2 Hayward kiwis over a 4-week period shortens colon transit time, increases frequency of defecation, and improves bowel function in adults diagnosed with irritable bowel syndrome (IBS) with constipation. Researchers suggest that kiwi should be considered a safe and effective natural laxative for these individuals.

Results of a recent study indicate that sleep quality in adult subjects with self-reported sleep disturbances improved significantly following a 4-week trial of kiwi consumption. The regimen involved nightly intake of 2 kiwis 1 hour before bedtime. Improvement was seen in total sleep time as well as sleep efficiency. Researchers speculate that improvement could be due to the presence of folate and serotonin in kiwi. Serotonin is the end product of L-tryptophan metabolism, which is involved in rapid eye movement (REM) sleep.

SUMMARY

Consumers should become knowledgeable about the physiologic benefits of kiwi consumption. Kiwi is an excellent source of vitamin C and potassium and a good source of magnesium, folate, zinc, copper, vitamins E and K, fiber, and important phytonutrients. Kiwi consumption is associated with reduced risk of developing heart disease, stroke, asthma, macular degeneration, and cancer. Recent research suggests that kiwi may also work as a natural laxative and sleep aid.

—*Cherie Marcel, BS*

REFERENCES

Altshul, S. (2005). The kiwi kick. *Health*, 19(2), 54.

Chang, C. C., Lin, Y. T., Lu, Y. T., Liu, Y. S., & Liu, J. F. (2010). Kiwifruit improves bowel function in patients with irritable bowel syndrome with constipation. *Asia Pacific Journal of Clinical Nutrition*, 19(4), 451-457.

Chang, W. H., & Liu, J. F. (2009). Effects of kiwifruit consumption on serum lipid profiles and antioxidative status in hyperlipidemic subjects. *International Journal of Food Sciences & Nutrition*, 60(8), 709-716. doi:10.3109/09637480802063517

Collins, B. H., Horska, A., Hotten, P. M., Riddoch, C., & Collins, A. R. (2001). Kiwifruit protects against oxidative DNA damage in human cells and in vitro. *Nutrition & Cancer*, 39(1), 148-153. doi:10.1207/S15327914nc391_20

The George Mateljan Foundation editorial team. (n.d.). The world's healthiest foods: Kiwifruit. Retrieved June 23, 2015, fromhttp://www.whfoods.com/genpage.php? tname=foodspice&dbid=41

Latocha, P., Krupa, T., Wolosiak, R., Worobiej, E., & Wilczak, J. (2010). Antioxidant activity and chemical difference in fruit of different Actinidia sp. *International Journal of Food Sciences & Nutrition*, 61(4), 381-394. doi:10.3109/09637480903517788

Lee, D. E., Shin, B. J., Hur, H. J., Kim, J. H., Kim, J., Kang, N. J., & Lee, H. J. (2010). Quercetin, the active phenolic component in kiwifruit, prevents hydrogen peroxide-induced inhibition of gap-junction intercellular communication. *British Journal of Nutrition*, 104(2), 164-170. doi:10.1017/S0007114510000346

Lin, H., Tsai, P., Fang, S., & Liu, J. (2011). Effect of kiwifruit consumption on sleep quality in adults with sleep problems. *Asia Pacific Journal of Clinical Nutrition*, 20(2), 169-174.

Skinner, M. A., Loh, J. M., Hunter, D. C., & Zhang, J. (2011). Gold kiwifruit (Actinidia chinensis 'Hort16A') for immune support*Proceedings. of the Nutrition Society*, 70(2), 276-280. doi:10.1017/S0029665111110000048

Upton, J. (2009). Green or gold, kiwifruit deliver taste, nutrition. *Environmental Nutrition*, 32(1), 8.

Xu, H., Xu, H. E., & Ryan, D. (2009). A study of the comparative effects of Hawthorn fruit compound and simvastatin on lowering blood lipid levels. *American Journal of Chinese Medicine*, 37(5), 903-908. doi:10.1142/S0192415X09007302

REVIEWER(S)

Darlene Strayer, RN, MBA, Cinahl Information Systems, Glendale, CA

Nursing Executive Practice Council, Glendale Adventist Medical Center, Glendale, CA

Kumquat

WHAT WE KNOW

The kumquat, from the tree *Fortunella margarita Swingle*, is a small, orange, oval citrus fruit that looks like a tiny orange. Kumquat belongs to the Rutaceae family and is the smallest of the citrus fruits. Although kumquat can be eaten raw, including the skin, the intensely tart flavor results in the frequent use of kumquat in preserves. Kumquat is also frequently pickled and canned. Nutritionally, kumquat is high in fiber and provides calcium, riboflavin, the antioxidant vitamin C, and provitamin A carotenoids (i.e., beneficial plant-derived nutrients [i.e., phytonutrients] that serve as the precursors of vitamin A.

NUTRIENTS IN KUMQUAT

- Kumquat is a good source of the water-soluble vitamin C, which neutralizes free radicals, protecting against inflammation and cellular damage. Adequate vitamin C intake is vital for proper function of the immune system and is associated with prevention of heart disease, stroke, and cancer.

- The provitamin A carotenoids (e.g., beta-carotene) are precursors of vitamin A, or retinol, a fat-soluble vitamin that is required for vision, maintenance of the surface lining of the eyes and other epithelial tissue, bone growth, immune response, energy regulation, reproduction, embryonic development, and activation of gene expression.

- Kumquat provides calcium, which builds and maintains bones and teeth, regulates muscle contraction, conducts nerve impulses, activates enzymes for energy production and muscle contraction, participates in blood clotting, assists with vitamin B12 absorption, and maintains the structural integrity of intracellular membranes.

- Kumquat contains riboflavin, or vitamin B2, which is an essential micronutrient that catalyzes proteins for respiratory reactions in order to produce energy.

- Kumquat is a good source of dietary fiber, which promotes healthy digestion, allows for efficient postprandial management of glucose and insulin responses, and hinders the absorption of cholesterol.

RESEARCH FINDINGS

- Analysis of kumquat peel shows high antioxidant, antibacterial, and antifungal activity in the form of bioactive polyphenols (i.e., beneficial plant-derived chemicals). Researchers suggest further study into the possibility of its use in pharmaceutical and food applications.
- Researchers report the identification of kumquat active components may help prevent the spread of prostate cancer cells.

SUMMARY

Consumers should become knowledgeable about the nutritional composition and physiologic benefits of kumquat. Kumquats are a good source of fiber, calcium, riboflavin, vitamin C, and provitamin A carotenoids. These nutrients help with bone and muscle health, immune response and digestion, and may help reduce the risk of developing heart disease, stroke, and cancer.

—*Cherie Marcel, BS*

REFERENCES

Jayaprakasha, G. K., Murthy, K. N., Demarais, R., & Patil, B. S. (2012). Inhibition of prostate cancer (LNCaP) cell proliferation by volatile components from Nagami kumquats. *Planta Medica*, 78(10), 974-980. doi:10.1055/s-0031-1298619

McEvoy, K. (2015, January 28). The values of kumquats. Retrieved June 8, 2015, from http://www.livestrong.com/article/310690-nutritional-values-of-kumquats/

Sadek, E. S., Makris, D. P., & Kefalas, P. (2009). Polyphenolic composition and antioxidant characteristics of kumquat (Fortunella margarita) peel fractions. *Plant Foods for Human Nutrition*, 64(4), 297. doi:10.1007/s11130-009-0140-1

Wang, Y. W., Zeng, W. C., Xu, P. Y., Lan, Y. J., Zhu, R. X., Zhong, K., ... Gao, H. (2012). Chemical composition and antimicrobial activity of the essential oil of kumquat (Fortunella crassifolia Swingle) peel. *International journal of Molecular Sciences*, 13(3), 3382. doi:10.3390/ijms13033382

REVIEWER(S)

Darlene Strayer, RN, MBA, Cinahl Information Systems, Glendale, CA

Nursing Executive Practice Council, Glendale Adventist Medical Center, Glendale, CA

Lemon

WHAT WE KNOW

The lemon, the fruit from the *Citrus limon* tree, is a small, oval, yellow-skinned citrus fruit with an intensely tart flavor. Rarely eaten alone, lemons are frequently added to drinks or foods as a refreshing and tart flavoring agent. The Eureka and the Lisbon are the two primary types of sour lemons. The Eureka tends to have more texturized skin, a short neck at one end, and few seeds. The Lisbon has a smoother skin, no neck and usually no seeds. Sweeter varieties of lemons, such as the Meyer lemon, are also available and gaining in popularity. Lemons most likely originated in China or India, where they developed as a cross between the lime and the citron. Christopher Columbus brought lemons to the Americas, and currently many lemon groves are cultivated in Florida. One of the notable nutrients provided by lemons is the powerful antioxidant vitamin C. In the 1600s and 1700s the British Navy discovered that lemons and limes could prevent scurvy, a disease caused by the deficiency of vitamin C. Lemons also contain potassium, fiber, and valuable phytonutrients (i.e., beneficial, plant-derived nutrients). These nutrients cause lemons to have antioxidant, antibiotic, and anti-carcinogenic properties.

NUTRIENTS IN LEMON

- Lemons contain important phytonutrients, including limonin glucoside, which may decrease risk for cancers of the mouth, skin, lung, breast, stomach, and colon.
- The water-soluble vitamin C in lemons neutralizes free radicals, protecting against inflammation and cellular damage. Adequate vitamin C intake is vital for the proper function of the immune system and has been associated with the prevention of heart disease, stroke, and cancer.
- The potassium in lemons supports normal cellular, nerve, and muscle function; regulates blood pressure and heart rate; and helps to eliminate excess sodium from the body

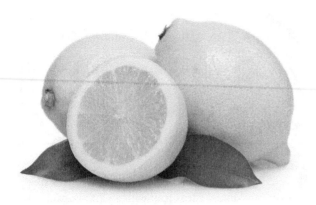

DIETARY INTAKE GUIDELINES

Lemons contain oxalates, which can crystallize in body fluids and cause health problems in individuals with pre-existing kidney or gallbladder dysfunction.

RESEARCH FINDINGS

Women have historically used lemon and lime juice as a form of vaginal douche, a practice that continues today, particularly by African women. Researchers have attempted to determine if this is an effective microbicidal treatment and, if so, what the safety parameters are. Studies indicate that a lemon concentration of up to 20% is likely safe for vaginal use, although concentrations less than 50% are ineffective for the prevention of human immunodeficiency virus (HIV) infection. Furthermore, concentrations over 50% have been shown to be toxic, exhibiting cytotoxicity to human cells, vaginal tissue, and beneficial vaginal bacteria (i.e., *Lactobacillus*). Scientists have also discovered that women who douche with citrus juices have a higher incidence of cervical cancer.

SUMMARY

Consumers should become knowledgeable about the physiologic risks and benefits of lemon consumption.

Lemons are a good source of vitamin C, potassium, fiber, and valuable phytonutrients, providing lemons with antioxidant, antibiotic, and anti-carcinogenic properties. Lemons may also help prevent heart disease, stroke, and cancer. Although lemons have been used around the world as a vaginal douche, research suggests that using the safe concentration is ineffective and higher levels may be toxic.

—*Cherie Marcel, BS*

REFERENCES

The George Mateljan Foundation. (n.d.). The world's healthiest foods: Lemon/limes. Retrieved June 23, 2015, fromhttp://www.whfoods.com/genpage.php?tname=foodspice&dbid=27

Hemmerling, A., Potts, M., Walsh, J., Young-Holt, B., Whaley, K., & Stefanski, D. A. (2007). Lime juice as a candidate microbicide? An open-label safety trial of 10% and 20% lime juice used vaginally. *Journal of Women's Health, 16*(7), 1041-1051. doi:10.1089/jwh.2006.0224

Lackman-Smith, C. S., Snyder, B. A., Marotte, K. M., Osterling, M. C., Mankowski, M. K., Jones, M., & Sanders-Beer, B. E. (2010). Safety and anti-HIV assessments of natural vaginal cleansing products in an established topical microbicides in vitro testing algorithm. *AIDS Research & Therapy, 7*, 22. doi:10.1186/1742-6405-7-22

Sagay, A. S., Imade, G. E., Onwuliri, V., Egah, D. Z., Grigg, M. J., Musa, J., ... Short, R. V. (2009). Genital tract abnormalities among female sex workers who douche with lemon/lime juice in Nigeria. *African Journal of Reproductive Health, 13*(1), 37-45.

Schepers, A. (2009). Pucker up for lemons and limes: Tart, refreshing and healthful. *Environmental Nutrition, 32*(6), 8.

REVIEWER(S)

Darlene Strayer, RN, MBA, Cinahl Information Systems, Glendale, CA

Nursing Executive Practice Council, Glendale Adventist Medical Center, Glendale, CA

Lime

WHAT WE KNOW

The lime, the fruit from the *Citrus aurantifolia* tree, is a small, oval or round, green-skinned citrus fruit with a slightly sweet and intensely tart flavor. Rarely eaten raw, limes are frequently added to drinks or foods as a flavoring agent. Although the lime is native to Asia, Christopher Columbus brought the lime to the Americas, and currently there are many lime groves in the United States. One of the notable nutrients in lime is the powerful antioxidant vitamin C. In the 1600s and 1700s, the British Navy discovered that lemon and lime prevented scurvy, a disease caused by deficiency of vitamin C. Lime also contains potassium, fiber, and valuable phytonutrients (i.e., beneficial, plant-derived nutrients). These nutrients cause the lime to have antioxidant, antibiotic, and anti-carcinogenic properties.

NUTRIENTS IN LIME

- Lime contains important phytonutrients, including flavonol glycosides, which inhibit cancer cell proliferation and exhibit antibiotic activity.
- The water-soluble vitamin C in lime neutralizes free radicals, protecting against inflammation and cellular damage. Adequate vitamin C intake is vital for proper immune system function and is associated with prevention of heart disease, stroke, and cancer.
- The potassium in lime supports normal cellular, nerve, and muscle function and helps to eliminate excess sodium from the body.

RESEARCH FINDINGS

- A clinical trial recently demonstrated that the regular intake of lime juice can reduce the severity of sickle cell anemia in children as evidenced by a lower rate of bone pain crises, fever, and hospitalization.
- Historically, women have used lime as a form of vaginal douche, a practice that continues today, particularly by African women. Researchers have attempted to determine if this is an effective microbicidal treatment and, if so, what the safety parameters are. Results of studies indicate that a lime concentration of up to 20% is likely safe for vaginal use, but concentrations over 50% have been shown to be toxic, exhibiting cytotoxicity to human cells, vaginal tissue, and *Lactobacillus* (i.e., beneficial vaginal bacteria). Scientists have discovered that women who douche with citrus juice have a higher incidence of cervical cancer.

SUMMARY

Consumers should become knowledgeable about the physiologic benefits of lime consumption.

Limes are a good source of vitamin C, potassium, fiber, and valuable phytonutrients, providing limes with antioxidant, antibiotic, and anti-carcinogenic properties. Limes may also help prevent heart disease, stroke, and cancer. Although limes have been used around the world as a vaginal douche, research suggests that using the safe concentration is ineffective and higher levels may be toxic.

—*Cherie Marcel, BS*

REFERENCES

Adegoke, S. A., Shehu, U. A., Mohammed, L. O., Sanusi, Y., & Oyelami, O. A. (2013). Influence of lime juice on the severity of sickle cell anemia. *Journal of Alternative & Complementary Medicine*, *19*(6), 588-592. doi:10.1089/acm.2012.0567

The George Mateljan Foundation. (n.d.). Lemon/limes. *The World's Healthiest Foods*. Retrieved June 23, 2015, from http://www.whfoods.com/genpage.php?tname=foodspice&dbid=27

Hemmerling, A., Potts, M., Walsh, J., Young-Holt, B., Whaley, K., & Stefanski, D. A. (2002). Lime juice as a candidate microbicide? An open-label safety trial of 10% and 20% lime juice used vaginally. *Journal of Women's Health*, *16*(7), 1041-1051. doi:10.1089/jwh.2006.0224

Lackman-Smith, C. S., Snyder, B. A., Marotte, K. M., Osterling, M. C., Mankowski, M. K., Jones, M., & Sanders-Beer, B. E. (2010). Safety and anti-HIV assessments of natural vaginal cleansing products in an established topical microbicides in vitro testing algorithm. *AIDS Research and Therapy*, *7*, 13. doi:10.1186/1742-6405-7-22

Sagay, A. S., Imade, G. E., Onwuliri, V., Egah, D. Z., Grigg, M. J., Musa, J., ... Short, R. V. (2009). Genital tract abnormalities among female sex workers who douche with lemon/lime juice in Nigeria. *African Journal of Reproductive Health*, *13*(1), 37-45.

Schepers, A. (2009). Pucker up for lemons and limes: Tart, refreshing and healthful. *Environmental Nutrition*, *32*(6), 8.

REVIEWER(S)

Darlene Strayer, RN, MBA, Cinahl Information Systems, Glendale, CA

Nursing Executive Practice Council, Glendale Adventist Medical Center, Glendale, CA

Loquat

WHAT WE KNOW

The loquat plant, or *Eriobotrya japonica*, a member of the Rosaceae family, is a shrub-like tree with large, glossy leaves and clusters of small, round fruit. Indigenous to China, the loquat fruit and leaves have been consumed in Asia for over 1,000 years. The loquat fruit is sweet and fleshy, similar in texture to an apricot but with smooth skin. The skin of the loquat can be ivory, yellow, orange, or red. Encased in the center of the fruit are large, smooth, round seeds. The loquat leaves are edible raw, but are typically used to make infusions or teas.

Practitioners of Chinese medicine use loquat leaf tea for the treatment of GI discomfort (e.g., diarrhea, upset stomach), cough, congestion, and diabetes, although there is no research to substantiate the efficacy of such treatment. Nutritionally, loquat fruit is rich in carotenoids, which are powerful antioxidants, and the leaves contain calcium, phosphorus, iron, potassium, and vitamins.

NUTRIENTS IN LOQUAT

- Loquat fruit contains the phytonutrients (i.e., beneficial, plant-derived chemicals) carotenoids, particularly in the skin of the orange- to red-colored fruits. Carotenoids provide the color pigment to yellow to red fruits. They assist in immune response and exhibit high antioxidant activity, preventing damage from harmful free radicals.
- The leaves of loquat contain valuable vitamins and minerals, including the following:
  —Vitamin C is a water-soluble vitamin that neutralizes free radicals, protecting against inflammation and cellular damage. Adequate vitamin C intake is vital for the proper function of the immune system and has been associated with the prevention of heart disease, stroke, and cancer.
  —Calcium builds and maintains bones and teeth, regulates muscle contraction, conducts nerve impulses, activates enzymes for energy production and muscle contraction, participates in blood clotting, assists with vitamin B12 absorption, and maintains the structural integrity of intracellular membranes.
  —Phosphorous combines with calcium for the formation of bones and teeth, muscle contraction, and nerve conduction, and is essential for the structural integrity of cell membranes.
  —Iron is necessary for the synthesis of red blood cells and Hgb, which are necessary for cellular respiration and the transport of oxygen to the tissues. Iron supports immune function, is important for cognitive development, contributes to energy metabolism, and regulates temperature.
  —Potassium supports normal cellular, nerve, and muscle function, and helps to eliminate excess sodium from the body.
  —Provitamin-A carotenoids (e.g., beta-carotene) are precursors of vitamin A, or retinol, a fat-soluble vitamin that is required for vision, maintenance of the surface lining of the eyes and other epithelial tissue, bone growth, immune response, energy regulation, reproduction, embryonic development, and activation of gene expression.

RESEARCH FINDINGS

- Researchers report that the methanol extract of loquat leaves and, to a lesser extent, the seeds, exhibited anti-metastatic effects against breast cancer cells. Study results indicated that the loquat extract impeded the adhesion, migration, and invasion of human breast cancer cells.

SUMMARY

Consumers should become knowledgeable about the physiologic effects of consuming loquat. Loquat fruit is a good source of carotenoids, and the leaves contain calcium, phosphorus, iron, potassium, and vitamin C. These nutrients help support the immune system, eye, bone and muscle health, and may decrease the risk of developing iron deficiency anemia, heart disease, stroke, and cancer. Historically, loquat infusions have been used to treat GI disorders and the common cold. Research suggests that loquat may help treat breast cancer.

—*Cherie Marcel, BS*

REFERENCES

Fu, X., Kong, W., Peng, G., Zhou, J., Azam, M., Xu, C., ... Chen, K. (2012). Plastid structure and carotenogenic gene expression in red- and white-fleshed loquat (Eriobotrya japonica) fruits. *Journal of Experimental Botany, 63*(1), 341-354. doi:10.1093/jxb/err284

Kim, M. S., You, M. K., Rhuy, D. Y., Kim, Y. J., Baek, H. Y., & Kim, H. A. (2009). Loquat (Eriobotrya japonica) extracts suppress the adhesion, migration and invasion of human breast cancer cell line. *Nutrition Research and Practice, 3*(4), 259. doi:10.4162/nrp.2009.3.4.259

Renee, J. (2015, January 29). The health benefits of making tea from loquat leaves. Livestrong.com. Retrieved June 8, 2015, from http://www.livestrong.com/article/557610-the-health-benefits-of-making-tea-from-loquat-leaves/

Zhou, C. H., Xu, C. J., Sun, C. D., Li, X., & Chen, K. S. (2007). Carotenoids in white- and red-fleshed loquat fruits. *Journal of Agricultural and Food Chemistry*, 55(19), 7822-7830. doi:10.1021/jf071273h

REVIEWER(S)
Darlene Strayer, RN, MBA, Cinahl Information Systems, Glendale, CA

Nursing Executive Practice Council, Glendale Adventist Medical Center, Glendale, CA

Lychee

WHAT WE KNOW

The lychee (from the tree *Litchi chinensis*; also called litchus) is a small, pinkish-red, oval fruit that grows on evergreen trees that are found primarily in China and Asia, but are also cultivated in Hawaii, California, and Florida. As it ripens, the skin of the lychee fruit dries into a rough, leathery rind, but the interior flesh remains sweet and juicy. Nutritionally, the lychee fruit is a good source of vitamin C and many minerals and phytonutrients (i.e., beneficial plant-derived nutrients). A large seed is found in the flesh of the lychee that is inedible whole but is frequently crushed into a powder and used in medicines or teas. There is no evidence of a health benefit for any of the current uses of lychee seeds.

NUTRIENTS IN LYCHEE

- Lychee fruit are rich in vitamin C, which is a water-soluble vitamin that neutralizes free radicals, protecting against inflammation and cellular damage. Adequate vitamin C intake is vital for the proper function of the immune system and has been associated with the prevention of heart disease, stroke, and cancer.
- Almost all essential minerals are found in lychee fruit in varying amounts:
    - Copper is a vital component of superoxide dismutase (SOD), an enzyme involved in energy production and antioxidant activity. It contributes to the action of lysyl oxidase, an enzyme necessary for the cross-linking of collagen and elastin. Elastin promotes flexibility in the blood vessels, bones, and joints. Copper enhances the body's ability to use iron, preventing iron-deficiency anemia, ruptured vessels, irregular heartbeat, and infection.
    - Potassium supports normal cellular, nerve, and muscle function and helps to eliminate excess sodium from the body.
    - Phosphorous combines with calcium to form bones and teeth, assists in muscle contraction and nerve conduction, and is essential for the structural integrity of cell membranes.
    - Magnesium balances the action of calcium in cells to regulate bone health and tone of nerves and muscles. It maintains relaxation of nerves and muscles, which contributes to the prevention of high blood pressure, muscle spasms, asthma, migraine headaches, general soreness, and fatigue.
    - Manganese is a trace mineral that has a role in energy production, fatty acid synthesis, cholesterol production, and protection against the damage caused by free radicals.
    - Iron is vital for the synthesis of red blood cells and hemoglobin, which are necessary for cellular respiration and the transport of oxygen to the tissues. Iron supports immune function, is vital for cognitive development, contributes to energy metabolism, and regulates temperature.
    - Selenium is an essential trace mineral that combines with proteins to create selenoproteins
- Selenoproteins are important antioxidant enzymes that protect cells from the damaging effects of free radicals, regulate thyroid function, and support the immune system.
- As a precursor to glutathione peroxidase, which is an antioxidant enzyme, selenium is believed to support lung health.
    - Calcium builds and maintains bones and teeth, regulates muscle contraction, conducts nerve impulses, activates enzymes for energy production and muscle contraction, participates in blood clotting, assists with vitamin B12 absorption, and maintains the structural integrity of intracellular membranes.
    - Zinc is an essential trace mineral that is involved in the activation of about 100 enzymes, supports the immune system and wound healing, and is essential for maintaining vision and the senses of smell and taste.

- Lychee fruit contains an important mixture of phytonutrients (referred to as oligonol, which acts as an antioxidant and anti-inflammatory agent) and has been shown to help fight obesity and liver damage.

RESEARCH FINDINGS

Results of many studies show that the phytonutrients, such as oligonol, found in lychee fruit and lychee fruit extracts are easy for the body to break down. Because of the proven antioxidant, anti-inflammatory, and liver and kidney protective activity of these phenolic compounds, researchers suggest that lychee extracts could be used for treating the complications of DM2 and other disease states related to inflammation and oxidation.

SUMMARY

Consumers should become knowledgeable about the physiologic effects of consuming lychee fruit. Lychee is a good source of vitamin C, many minerals, and phytonutrients. These nutrients help support healthy bone, muscle, thyroid, immune and lung health, and may decrease the risk of developing iron deficiency anemia, heart disease, stroke, and cancer. Research suggests lychee may be beneficial in treating type 2 diabetes and other inflammatory diseases.

—*Cherie Marcel, BS*

REFERENCES

Bhoopat, L., Srichairatanakool, S., Kanjanapothi, D., Taesotikul, T., Thanachai, H., & Bhoopat, T. (2011). Hepatoprotective effects of lychee (Litchi chinensis Sonn.): A combination of antioxidant and antio-apoptotic activities. *Journal of Ethnopharmacology, 136*(1), 55-66. doi:10.1016/j.jep.2011.03.061

Chen, Y. C., Lin, J. T., Lu, P. S., & Yang, D. J. (2011). Composition of flavonoids and phenolic acids in lychee (Litchi, Chinensis Sonn.) flower extracts and their antioxidant capacities estimated with human LDL, erythrocytes, and blood models. *Journal of Food Science, 76*(5), C724-C728. doi:1111/j.1750-3841.2011.02164.x

Joy, T. (2011). Nutritional value of lychee fruit. *Livestrong.com*. Retrieved June 8, 2015, from http://www.livestrong.com/article/496398-nutritional-value-of-lychee-fruit/

Kalgaonkar, S., Nishioka, H., Gross, H. B., Fujii, H., Keen, C. L., & Hackman, R. M. (2010). Bioactivity of a flavanol-rich lychee fruit extract in adipocytes and its effects on oxidant defense and indices of metabolic syndrome in animal models. *Phytotherapy Research, 24*(8), 1223-1228. doi:10.1002/ptr.3137

Kang, S. W., Hahn, J. K., Yang, S. M., Park, B. J., & Chul, L. S. (2012). Oligomerized lychee fruit extract (OLFE) and a mixture of vitamin C and E for endurance capacity in a double blind randomized controlled trial. *Journal of Clinical Biochemistry and Nutrition, 50*(2), 106-113. doi:10.3164/jcbn.11-46

Nishizawa, M., Hara, T., Miura, T., Fujita, S., Yoshigai, E., Ue, H., ... Isaka, T. (2011). Supplementation with a flavonol-rich lychee fruit extract influences the inflammatory status of young athletes. *Phytotherapy Research: PTR, 25*(10), 1486-1493. doi:10.1002/ptr.3430

Noh, J. S., Kim, H. Y., Park, C. H., Fujii, H., & Yokozawa, T. (2010). Hypolipidaemic and antioxidative effects of oligonol, a low-molecular-weight polyphenol derived from lychee fruit, on renal damage in type 2 diabetic mice. *British Journal of Nutrition, 104*(8), 1120-1128. doi:10.1017/S0007114510001819

Noh, J. S., Park, C. H., & Yokozawa, T. (2011). Treatment with oligonol, a low-molecular polyphenol derived from lychee fruit, attenuates diabetes-induced helpatic damage through regulation of oxidative stress and lipid metabolism. *The British Journal of Nutrition, 106*(7), 1013-1022. doi:10.1017/S0007114511001322

Sakurai, T., Nishioka, H., Fujii, H., Nakano, N., Kiaki, T., Radak, Z., ... Ohno, H. (2008). Antioxidative effects of a new lychee fruit-derived polyphenol mixture, oligonol, converted into a low-molecular form in adipocytes. *Bioscience, 72*(2), 463-476.

Thomas, J. (2013, August 16). Health benefits of lychee seeds. *Livestrong.com*. Retrieved June 8, 2015, from http://www.livestrong.com/article/433767-health-benefits-of-lychee-seeds/

REVIEWER(S)

Darlene Strayer, RN, MBA, Cinahl Information Systems, Glendale, CA

Nursing Executive Practice Council, Glendale Adventist Medical Center, Glendale, CA

Melon

WHAT WE KNOW

Melon is a group of fruits belonging to the gourd, or *Cucurbitaceae*, family. Melons include watermelon, cantaloupe, honeydew, and bitter melon. Melons are round or oblong fruits that grow on creeping vines. Melon tends to be low in calories, high in vitamins and minerals, and essentially free of fat.

NUTRIENTS IN MELON

- Watermelon, cantaloupe, honeydew, and bitter melon are all excellent sources of vitamin C, which neutralizes free radicals, protecting against inflammation and cellular damage. Adequate vitamin C intake is vital for immune system function and has been associated with the prevention of heart disease, stroke, and cancer.
- Melon also supplies several of the water-soluble B-complex vitamins
  —Folate is essential for the production and maintenance of red blood cells (RBCs). It is vital for building deoxyribonucleic acid (DNA) and ribonucleic acid (RNA), and is important in the breakdown of homocysteine (i.e., an amino acid).
  —Vitamin B5, or pantothenic acid, is essential for building and breaking down amino acids, carbohydrates, and lipids; is important for the formation of RBCs and hemoglobin, which carries oxygen to the tissues; and plays a role in building acetylcholine, a neurotransmitter in the central and peripheral nervous systems.
  —Vitamin B6, or pyridoxine, is required for the conversion of tryptophan to niacin and is involved in the conversion of homocysteine to cysteine. It is necessary for building the neurotransmitters serotonin and dopamine and maintains the lymphoid organs to promote immune system function.
  —Choline breaks down into betaine, which assists in the regulation of inflammation in the cardiovascular system by preventing elevated levels of homocysteine. Betaine is associated with reduced levels of inflammation markers.
  —Vitamins B1, or thiamin, and B3, or niacin, create energy by aiding the breakdown of carbohydrates, provide cardiovascular protection, maintain nervous system function, and support the production of RBCs, certain hormones, and cholesterol.
- The potassium provided by melon supports normal cellular, nerve, and muscle function and helps to eliminate excess sodium from the body.

- Melon supplies magnesium, which balances the action of calcium in cells to regulate bone health and nerve and muscle tone. It maintains relaxation of nerves and muscles, which contributes to the prevention of high blood pressure, muscle spasms, asthma, migraine headaches, general soreness, and fatigue.
- The provitamin A carotenoids in watermelon, cantaloupe, and bitter melon break down into the fat-soluble vitamin A, or retinol, which is required for vision, maintenance of the surface linings of the eyes and other epithelial tissue, proper bone growth, immune response, energy regulation, reproduction, embryonic development, and activation of gene expression.
- Cantaloupe, honeydew, and bitter melon contain the fat-soluble vitamin K, which acts as a coenzyme involved in maintaining normal levels of blood clotting proteins and contributes to bone building.

WATERMELON

As the name suggests, watermelon (*Citrullus lanatus*)is about 92% water. The crisp and juicy flesh of the watermelon ranges in color from pink to deep red and has a flavor that is sweet and refreshing. Traditionally, watermelon contained black seeds that were randomly occurring throughout the fruit, although seedless varieties have become increasingly available and account for 85% of all watermelon grown in the United States.

- Watermelon is a good source of amino acids, vitamins C, A, and B6, potassium, magnesium and many valuable phytonutrients (i.e., beneficial, plant-derived chemicals). These nutrients provide antioxidant, anti-inflammatory, cancer-preventive, and cardio-protective properties.
  —Watermelon is particularly noted for containing the carotenoid lycopene, a phytonutrient responsible for the pinkish-red color of the fruit. Lycopene inhibits the inflammatory process, neutralizes free radicals, impedes cancer cell proliferation (i.e., kills cancer cells), and repairs damaged DNA.
  —Cucurbitacin E, a phytonutrient called a triterpenoid, exhibits strong anti-inflammatory activity.
  —Watermelon is a good source of the amino acid citrulline, which metabolizes into the amino

acid arginine, which slows the formation of blood clots and reduces arterial congestion. Another byproduct of citrulline is nitric oxide (NO), a muscle relaxant.

CANTALOUPE

The melon referred to in the U.S. as the cantaloupe is actually a muskmelon (*Cucumis melo* var.*reticulatus*). The true cantaloupe (*Cucumis melo* var.*cantalupensis*) is primarily grown in other parts of the world, particularly the Mediterranean region, and does not have the netting pattern on the rind that is characteristic of muskmelon. Hereafter, the term cantaloupe refers to the more familiar muskmelon. The dense and juicy flesh of the cantaloupe varies in color depending on the variety. The most familiar color is deep orange. Jenny Lind cantaloupes have green flesh, and varieties such as Athena and Ambrosia have salmon-colored flesh. Hidden in the center of the cantaloupe is a hollow cavity filled with viscous seeds that are edible.

- Cantaloupe is a good source of fiber, vitamins A, C, K, B6, B3, and B1, folate, potassium, magnesium, and many valuable phytonutrients (e.g., flavonoids, carotenoids, and triterpenoids) that have strong anti-inflammatory and antioxidant properties.
  —The carotenoids alpha-carotene, beta-carotene, lutein, beta-cryptoxanthin, and zeaxanthin exhibit antioxidant properties and scavenge free radicals. They protect the eyes from light-induced oxidation, preventing macular degeneration, and inhibit atherosclerosis.
  —The flavonoid luteolin is a potent antioxidant and anti-carcinogenic compound.
  —The triterpenoids cucurbitacin E and cucurbitacin B exhibit strong anti-inflammatory activity.
  —Caffeic acid and ferulic acid exhibit anti-carcinogenic, anti-microbial, and anti-viral properties. These acids are believed to inhibit the buildup of low density lipoprotein (LDL) cholesterol (i.e., the "bad" cholesterol).

HONEYDEW

A close relative to the cantaloupe, honeydew (*Cucumis melo*) is a variety of muskmelon. Originally known as the melon d'Antibes blanc d'hiver (i.e., white Antibes wintermelon), honeydew originated centuries ago in southern France and Algeria. Considered the sweetest of the melons, the pale green and sometimes orange flesh of honeydew is creamy in texture.

- Honeydew is a good source of fiber, vitamins C, K, B1, B3, B5, and B6, folate, potassium, magnesium, copper, and valuable phytonutrients.
  —The carotenoid zeaxanthin exhibits antioxidant properties and protects the eyes from light-induced damage, preventing age related macular degeneration (AMD).
  —The copper in honeydew is a vital component of superoxide dismutase (SOD), an enzyme involved in energy production and antioxidant activity. It contributes to the action of lysyl oxidase, an enzyme necessary for the cross-linking of collagen and elastin, which allows flexibility in the blood vessels, bones, and joints. Copper enhances the body's ability to use iron, preventing iron-deficiency anemia, ruptured blood vessels, irregular heartbeat, and infection.

BITTER MELON

Bitter melon (*Momordica charantia*; also known as bitter gourd, karela, ampalaya, pare, and balsam pear) is a climbing perennial plant that produces an elongated, warty, green fruit with a characteristic bitter flavor. Although not the most attractive or palatable of the melons, the seeds, fruit, leaves, and root of bitter melon have a long history of medicinal and culinary use.

- Bitter melon is a good source of fiber, vitamins A C, B5, and B6, choline, folate, the minerals iron, magnesium, phosphorus, calcium, and potassium, and many valuable phytonutrients.
  —Iron is vital for the production of red blood cells (RBCs) and hemoglobin, which are necessary for energy production and the transport of oxygen to the tissues. Iron supports immune system function, is vital for cognitive development, contributes to energy building and breakdown, and regulates temperature.
  —Phosphorous combines with calcium in the formation of bones and teeth, muscle contraction, and nerve conduction. Phosphorous is essential for the structural integrity of cell membranes.
  —Calcium builds and maintains bones and teeth, regulates muscle contraction, conducts nerve impulses, activates enzymes for energy production and muscle contraction, participates in blood clotting, assists with vitamin B12 absorption, and maintains the structural integrity of intracellular membranes.

- Because it has anti-inflammatory and antioxidant properties, bitter melon provides a multitude of health benefits and has been used to treat gastrointestinal (GI) distress, ulcers, colitis, intestinal worms, diabetes, dyslipidemia, cancer, kidney stones, fever, liver disease, infections, hypertension, wounds, and psoriasis. More research is needed regarding the effectiveness of bitter melon for these uses because research results have been conflicting and inconclusive.
  —The most researched mechanism of bitter melon is its effect on blood glucose. Although not entirely understood, bitter melon is thought to lower blood glucose levels in the following ways:
    –It increases glucose use by the liver.
    –It inhibits two of the enzymes involved in building glucose in the body.
    –It improves glucose breakdown.
    –It enhances cellular uptake of glucose and promotes glucose release.
    –It increases insulin production.

DIETARY INTAKE GUIDELINES

- There is no officially recommended dosage for the use of melon, including watermelon, cantaloupe, and honeydew.
- Common dosages used for bitter melon administration include the following:
  —50–100 mL of fresh juice daily.
  —3–15 g of encapsulated dry powder daily.
  —100–200 mg of standardized, encapsulated extract 3 times daily.
- The safety of long-term use (i.e., using for more than 3 months) of bitter melon has not been established.
- Bitter melon has been shown to induce abortion in animal studies. Because safety has not been established during pregnancy, bitter melon should not be consumed by women who are pregnant.
- Melon can serve as a vehicle for *Salmonella* and *Listeria*. To avoid contamination when purchasing commercially grown melons, the U.S. Food and Drug Administration (FDA) advises the following precautions:
  —Don't eat bruised melons
  —Always wash hands with soap and hot water prior to handling melons
  —Thoroughly clean the whole melon with a clean produce brush and tap water prior to cutting open
  —Refrigerate the melon upon cutting and eat within 2 days
- Due to its blood glucose–lowering effects, bitter melon can increase the effects of anti-diabetic medications, including insulin.

RESEARCH FINDINGS

- A clinical trial was conducted to determine the effect of melon juice supplementation on perceived stress and fatigue based on the hypothesis that perceived stress is associated with oxidative stress. Researchers reported that the group receiving oral melon juice supplementation showed improvement in several signs and symptoms of stress and fatigue. However, a similar study found no notable improvements in perceived stress in the participants receiving the extract.
- Numerous studies have been conducted to determine the safety and effectiveness of bitter melon for the treatment of diabetes and metabolic syndrome, but results are conflictive and inconclusive. Many of the studies reviewed were flawed and weak according to researchers, who recommend further clinical trials with better controls and adequate sample sizes.

SUMMARY

Consumers should become knowledgeable about the physiologic effects of melon consumption. Melon is low in calories, high in vitamins, minerals, important phytonutrients, and essentially free of fat. These nutrients produce energy, combat oxidative stress, improve blood pressure, and may help treat type II diabetes. Follow the FDA precautions for avoiding contamination with *Salmonella* and *Listeria* when purchasing commercially grown melons. Bitter melon has been shown to induce abortion in animal studies, so bitter melon should not be consumed by women who are pregnant. Bitter melon may increase the effects of insulin, so individuals on insulin should use caution when consuming it.

—*Cherie Marcel, BS*

REFERENCES

Bartkowski, A. M. (2010). What is bitter melon good for? *Livewell.com*. Retrieved June 23, 2015, from http://livewell.jillianmichaels.com/bitter-melon-good-for-4954.html

Centers for Disease Control and Prevention. (2013). Listeria (Listeriosis). Retrieved May 7, 2015, from http://www.foodsafety.gov/poisoning/causes/bacteriaviruses/listeria/

The editorial team of Alternative Medicine Review. (2007). Momordica charantia (bitter melon). *Alternative Medicine Review*, *12*(4), 360-363.

Edward, J. (2013, October 12). Benefits of Watermelon for Men. *Livestrong.com*. Retrieved June 23, 2015, from http://www.livestrong.com/article/359133-watermelons-health-benefits-for-men/

Foodsafety.gov. (n.d.). Salmonella. Retrieved May 7, 2015, from http://www.foodsafety.gov/poisoning/causes/bacteriaviruses/salmonella/

The George Mateljan Foundation editorial team. (2012). The world's healthiest foods: Watermelon. Retrieved June 23, 2015, fromhttp://www.whfoods.com/genpage.php? tname=foodspice&dbid=31#healthbenefits

The George Mateljan Foundation editorial team. (2013). The world's healthiest foods: How does honeydew compare to cantaloupe?. Retrieved June 23, 2015, fromhttp:// whfoods.org/genpage.php?tname=dailytip&dbid=13&utm_source=rss_reader&utm_medium=rss&utm_campaign=rss_feed

The George Mateljan Foundation editorial team. (2014, February 25). The world's healthiest foods: Cantaloupe. Retrieved June 23, 2015, fromhttp://www.whfoods.com/ genpage.php?tname=foodspice&dbid=17#healthbenefits

Houghton, C. A., Steels, E. L., Fassett, R. G., & Coombes, J. S. (2011). Effects of a gliadin-combined plant superoxide dismutase extract on self-perceived fatigue in women aged 50--65 years. *Phytomedicine*, *18*(6), 521-526. doi:10.1016/j.phymed.2010.09.006

Ilkay, J. (2011). Bitter melon. Fruit's role in diabetes management is promising but uncertain. *Today's Dietitian*, *13*(7), 10-11.

Ipatenco, S. (2013, December 18). Health benefits of eating honeydew melon. *Livestrong.com*. Retrieved June 23, 2015, from http://www.livestrong.com/article/340453-health-benefits-of-eating-honeydew-melon/

Leung, L., Birtwhistle, R., Kotech, J., Hannah, S., & Cuthbertson, S. (2009). Anti-diabetic and hypoglycaemic effects of Momordica charantia (bitter melon): A mini review. *British Journal of Nutrition*, *102*(12), 1703-1708. doi:10.1017/S0007114509992054

Liddell, A. (2013, December 18). The health benefits of melons. *Livestrong.com*. Retrieved from http://www.livestrong.com/article/407556-the-health-benefits-of-melons/

Milesi, M. A., Lacan, D., Brosse, H., Desor, D., & Notin, C. (2009). Effect of an oral supplementation with a proprietary melon juice concentrate (Extramel) on stress and fatigue in healthy people: A pilot, double-blind, placebo-controlled clinical trial. *Nutrition Journal*, *8*, 40. doi:10.1186/1475-2891-8-40

Nerurkar, P. V., Johns, L. M., Buesa, L. M., Kipyakwai, G., Volper, E., Sato, R., ... Nerurkar, V. R. (2011). Momordica charantia (bitter melon) attenuates high-fat diet-associated oxidative stress and neuro-inflammation. *Journal of Neuroinflammation*, *8*, 64. doi:10.1186/1742-2094-8-64

Ooi, C. P., Yassin, Z., & Hamid, T. A. (2012). Momordica charantia for type 2 diabetes mellitus. *Cochrane Database of Systematic Reviews*, *8*. Art. No.: CD007845. doi:10.1002/14651858.CD007845.pub3

Ratini, M. (2015, January 23). Vitamins & supplements: Bitter melon. *WebMD*. Retrieved June 23, 2015, from http://www.webmd.com/vitamins-and-supplements/bitter-melon

Summers, A. R. B. (2010, March 23). Bitter melon nutrition. *Livestrong.com*. Retrieved June 23, 2015, from http://www.livestrong.com/article/89801-bitter-melon-nutrition/

Thompson, C. (2014, December 3). Honeydew: 7 healthy facts. *WebMD*. Retrieved June 23, 2015, from http://www.webmd.com/food-recipes/features/honeydew-7-healthy-facts

Tsai, C. H., Chen, E. C., Tsay, H. S., & Huang, C. J. (2012). Wild bitter gourd improves metabolic syndrome: A preliminary dietary supplementation trial. *Nutrition Journal*, *11*(1), 4. doi:10.1186/1475-2891-11-4

Wolf, N. (2011, May 19). What are the benefits of eating bitter gourd? *Livestrong.com*. Retrieved June 23, 2015, from http://www.livestrong.com/article/445901-what-are-the-benefits-of-eating-bitter-gourd/

Zevnik, N. (2012). Healing foods. Melon marvel. *Better Nutrition*, *74*(7), 40-42.

REVIEWER(S)

Darlene Strayer, RN, MBA, Cinahl Information Systems, Glendale, CA

Nursing Executive Practice Council, Glendale Adventist Medical Center, Glendale, CA

Papaya

WHAT WE KNOW

The papaya is the oval-shaped fruit of the *Carica papaya* plant, a member of the Caricaceae family. The skin of the papaya is greenish-yellow and the flesh is deep orange, pink, or yellow with a buttery texture and sweet, musky flavor. The gelatinous interior cavity of the papaya contains many round, black, peppery seeds. Although the seeds are edible, they are frequently overlooked because of their bitter taste. The flesh of papaya can be eaten raw, dried, diced into salsas, used in drinks, and made into jams and sauces. Papaya is a good source of fiber; vitamins C, E, and K; folate; potassium; and valuable phytonutrients (i.e., beneficial, plant-derived chemicals). The enzyme papain is often considered the most important nutritional element of papaya. Papaya has anti-inflammatory and antioxidant properties that provide health benefits, including improved gastrointestinal (GI) function, enhanced wound healing, relief of arthritic and myalgic pain, protection against macular degeneration, and reduced risk of heart disease and cancer.

NUTRIENTS IN PAPAYA

- Papaya contains the proteolytic (i.e., protein-digesting) enzyme papain, which exhibits anti-inflammatory properties that relieve the pain of inflamed joints, muscles, and soft tissue and promote healing following injury.
- Papaya is an excellent source of the provitamin A carotenoids, which are required for vision, maintenance of the surface linings of the eyes and other epithelial tissue, proper bone growth, immune response, energy regulation, reproduction, embryonic development, and gene expression.
- The water-soluble vitamin C in papaya neutralizes free radicals, protecting against inflammation and cellular damage. Adequate vitamin C intake is vital for immune system function and has been associated with the prevention of heart disease, stroke, and cancer.
- Papaya contains vitamin E, a fat-soluble vitamin that functions primarily as an antioxidant but also maintains cell membranes, assists in vitamin K absorption, and contributes to immune system function.
- The vitamin K in papaya acts as a coenzyme to maintain normal levels of blood-clotting proteins and contributes to bone growth.
- Papaya provides the water-soluble vitamin folate, which is essential for the production and maintenance of red blood cells (RBCs). It is vital for building deoxyribonucleic acid (DNA) and ribonucleic acid (RNA) and has an important role in the breakdown of homocysteine.
- Potassium, a mineral found in papaya, supports normal cellular, nerve, and muscle function and helps to eliminate excess sodium from the body.
- Papaya is a good source of dietary fiber, including soluble fiber, which binds with water and slows the digestive process; this allows better management of postprandial (i.e., after eating) glucose and insulin responses. Fiber increases the volume of intestinal contents, which hinders the absorption of cholesterol. The added bulk promotes more regular bowel movements, promoting intestinal health.

DIETARY INTAKE GUIDELINES

- There is no standard dosage for papaya.
- Persons with allergy to latex may also be allergic to papaya. Papayas contain chitinases, which are enzymes associated with latex-fruit allergy syndrome.
- Due to the blood-thinning potential of papain, eating large amounts of papaya should be avoided by persons with coagulation disorders.
- Due to the blood-thinning potential of papain, papaya should not be ingested by persons receiving blood thinners (e.g., heparin, salicylates, warfarin).

RESEARCH FINDINGS

- Evidence shows that the carotenoids provided by papaya are more bioavailable (i.e., more easily digested and absorbed) in humans than they are in tomato and carrot.
- Research results show that both unripe papaya extract and papaya latex (i.e., a protective milky exudate) can help protect against and heal gastric ulcers.

- Researchers demonstrated that a modified papaya extract promoted wound healing in patients with chronic skin ulceration. The extract caused vasodilation of the blood vessels (i.e., improved blood flow) around the wound, enabling it to heal. The anti-inflammatory activity of the papaya extract also promoted wound healing. Similar results have been reported regarding the use of papaya latex for the treatment of burns.

SUMMARY

Consumers should become knowledgeable about the physiologic benefits of papaya. Papaya is a good source of fiber, vitamins C, E, and K, folate, potassium, provitamin A carotenoids, and the enzyme papain. These nutrients may improve GI function, enhance wound healing, relieve pain, protect against macular degeneration, and reduce risk of heart disease and certain cancers. Individuals with coagulations disorders should avoid eating large amounts of papaya. Individuals on blood thinners should avoid papaya due to its blood-thinning potential. Individuals with a latex allergy may also be allergic to papaya.

—*Cherie Marcel, BS*

REFERENCES

Ezike, A. C., Akah, P. A., Okoli, C. O., Ezeuchenne, N. A., & Ezeugwu, S. (2009). Carica papaya (Paw-Paw) unripe fruit may be beneficial in ulcer. *Journal of Medicinal Food*, 12(6), 1268-1273. doi:10.1089/jmf.2008.0197

Gurung, S., & Skalko-Basnet, N. (2009). Wound healing properties of Carica papaya latex: In vitro evaluation in mice burn model. *Journal of Ethnopharmacology*, 121(2), 338-341.

Hall, S. (2010). Papaya power. *Health*, 24(4), 104.

Lissandrello, M. (2009). Papaya: Enhance digestion and soothe inflammation with this juicy gem. *Vegetarian Times*, (367), 32, 35.

Mello, V. J., Gomes, M. T. R., Lemos, F. O., Delfino, J. L., Andrade, S. P., Lopes, M. T., & Salas, C. E. (2008). The gastric ulcer protective and healing role of cysteine proteinases from Carica candamarcensis. *Phytomedicine*, 15(4), 237-244.

Mitchell, G. K. (2011). Clinical observations supporting a vasodilatory effect of the modified papaya extract OPAL001. *Wound Practice & Research*, 19(4), 190-195.

Russell, F. D., Windegger, T., Hamilton, K. D., & Cheetham, N. W. H. (2011). Effect of the novel wound healing agent, OPAL A on leukotriene B4 production in human neutrophils and 5-liboxygenase activity. *Wound Practice & Research*, 19(4), 200-203.

Schweiggert, R. M., Kopec, R. E., Villalobos-Guiterrez, M. G., Hogel, J., Quesada, S., Esquivel, P., ... Carle, R. (2014). Carotenoids are more bioavailable from papaya than from tomato and carrot in humans: A randomised cross-over study. *British Journal of Nutrition*, 111(3), 490-498.

The George Mateljan Foundation editorial team. (n.d.). The world's healthiest foods: Papaya. Retrieved June 23, 2015, fromhttp://www.whfoods.com/genpage.php? tname=foodspice&dbid=47

REVIEWER(S)

Darlene Strayer, RN, MBA, Cinahl Information Systems, Glendale, CA

Nursing Executive Practice Council, Glendale Adventist Medical Center, Glendale, CA

Peach

WHAT WE KNOW

The peach, from the trea *Prunus persica*, is a stone fruit from the Rosaceae (i.e., rose) family, along with nectarines, cherries, apricots, and plums. Its origins have been traced back to over 3,000 years ago, where it was believed to be a sacred plant that symbolized hope and longevity. Peaches are a delicious culinary treat that can be eaten raw, canned, or dried; baked in pies or cobblers; made into jams and sauces; or blended in drinks. There are over 4,000 varieties of peaches, which are categorized as clingstone (i.e., the flesh clings to the pit) and freestone (i.e., the flesh is free from the pit). Beyond its value in cuisine, the peach possesses a wealth of nutrients, including beta-carotene (i.e., a precursor of vitamin A), vitamin C, potassium, important polyphenolic phytonutrients (i.e., protective, plant-derived chemicals), and fiber. The soft, fuzzy skin of the peach is edible and contains more beta-carotene and vitamin C than the interior fleshy fruit.

NUTRIENTS IN PEACH

- Peaches contain important phytonutrients that have antioxidant, anti-inflammatory, and anti-mutagenic properties and act to protect deoxyribonucleic acid (DNA) against damage and enhance DNA repair.

- The water-soluble vitamin C in peaches neutralizes free radicals, protecting against inflammation and cellular damage. Adequate vitamin C intake is vital for proper immune system function and is associated with the prevention of heart disease, stroke, and cancer.
- The beta-carotene in peaches is a precursor of vitamin A, which provides antioxidant protection to the heart and promotes visual health. Studies have shown both beta-carotene and vitamin A play a preventive role against age-related macular degeneration (AMD).
- Peaches contain potassium, which is an essential element responsible for regulating acid-base balance, maintaining fluid balance, supporting muscle contraction and cardiac function, contributing to protein building and carbohydrate break down, promoting cellular growth, and promoting transmission of nerve impulses.
- Peaches are an excellent source of dietary fiber, which binds and removes toxins from the colon, assists in glucose control, and reduces high cholesterol levels.
- The beta-carotene, vitamin C, potassium, and polyphenols found in peaches work together to reduce triglycerides and prevent excessive platelet aggregation (i.e., blood clotting).

RESEARCH FINDINGS

Cisplatin, a highly effective chemotherapeutic agent carries a high risk of toxicity. Researchers report that peach flesh extract positively affected markers of toxicity (improved antioxidant levels and reduced cell damage) in mice. This suggests that peach can potentially be protective against cisplatin-induced toxicity in humans.

SUMMARY

Consumers should become knowledgeable about the physiologic benefits of peach consumption. Peach is a good source of beta-carotene, vitamin C, potassium, phytonutrients, and fiber. These nutrients improve vision, support the immune system, and reduce cholesterol and triglycerides, which may decrease the risk

for cardiovascular disease. Recent research indicates that peach has the potential to reduce chemotherapy toxicity.

—*Cherie Marcel, BS*

REFERENCES

Daniels-Zellar, D. (2006). Peach passion. *Vegetarian Journal, 25*(2), 6-9.

Lee, C. K., Park, K. K., Hwang, J. K., Lee, S. K., & Chung, W. Y. (2008). The extract of Prunus persica flesh (PPFE) attenuates chemotherapy-induced hepatotoxicity in mice. *Phytotherapy Research, 22*(2), 223-227.

Rossato, S. B., Haas, C., Raseira, M. C. B., Moreira, J. C. F., & Zuanazzi, J. A. S. (2009). Antioxidant potential of peels and fleshes of peaches from different cultivars. *Journal of Medicinal Food, 12*(5), 1119-1126. doi:10.1089/jmf.2008.0267

Schepers, A. (2004). Peaches, nectarines offer phytonutrient punch. *Environmental Nutrition, 27*(8), 8.

Zevnik, N. (2007). Summer's bounty.*Better Nutrition, 69*(6), 52-55.

REVIEWER(S)

Darlene Strayer, RN, MBA, Cinahl Information Systems, Glendale, CA
Nursing Executive Practice Council, Glendale Adventist Medical Center, Glendale, CA

Pears

WHAT WE KNOW

The most common type of pear, or *Pyrus communis*, is a fruit from the Rosaceae (i.e., rose) family, along with apples, cherries, peaches, apricots, and plums. Other common types of pears are the Asian pear (*Pyrus pyrifolia*) and the Siberian/Manchurian pear (*Pyrus ussuriensis*); worldwide, there are over 3,000 pear varieties, including Bartlett/Williams, Bosc, Comice, Concorde, Forelle, Green and Red Anjou, Seckel, and Starkrimson. The origin of pears has been traced to 1000 BC in Europe, Asia, and. Currently, pear trees are grown worldwide and contributes more than half of the world's supply of pears. Some types of pears are narrow at the stem and plump at the base, and others are round like an apple; depending on the type, pears are covered in green, gold, red, or brown skin. Pears can be eaten raw, canned, dried, baked in pastry, or made into jams and sauces. Although pears are a good source of fiber, vitamin C, and vitamin K, the many phytonutrients (i.e., protective, plant-derived chemicals) found in pears are considered their most important nutritional content. Pears have antihistamine, anti-inflammatory, and antioxidant properties and provide many health benefits, including prevention of allergic reactions, improved gastrointestinal function, and reduced risk for diabetes mellitus, type 2 (DM2), heart disease, and cancer (e.g., esophageal, gastric, and colon cancer).

NUTRIENTS IN PEARS

- The nutrient concentration is especially high in the skin of pears.
- Pears contain many important phytonutrients, including the following:
  - The flavonols quercetin, kaempferia, and isorhamnetin provide strong antioxidant and anti-inflammatory protection. They also have antihistamine, antimicrobial, anti-diabetic, and anti-carcinogenic properties.
  - The flavonols catechin and epicatechin are thought to decrease risk for cardiovascular disease (CVD) and hypertension by preventing the damage of low-density lipoproteins (LDLs), enhancing endothelium-dependent relaxation (i.e., relaxation of arteries), reducing inflammation, and preventing the formation of blood clots.
  - The hydroxybenzoic phenolic acids chlorogenic, gentisic, syringe, and vanillic acids exhibit anti-carcinogenic, antimicrobial, and antiviral properties. Hydroxybenzoic phenolic acids are also believed to inhibit the build-up of LDL cholesterol.
  - The carotenoids beta-carotene (i.e., a precursor to vitamin A), lutein, and zeaxanthin provide powerful antioxidant and anti-inflammatory activity.
  - The skin of red pear contains anthocyanins, which are reddish-color pigment that has high antioxidant and anticarcinogenic activity, promotes urinary tract health, and supports memory function.
- The water-soluble vitamin C in pear neutralizes free radicals, protecting against inflammation and cellular damage. Adequate vitamin C intake is vital for immune system function and has been associated with the prevention of heart disease, stroke, and cancer.
- Pears are a source of vitamin K, which acts as a coenzyme to maintain normal levels of blood clotting proteins and contributes to bone growth.
- Pears are a good source of dietary fiber, including soluble fiber, which binds with water and slows the digestive process; this allows the body to better manage postprandial (i.e., after eating) glucose and insulin responses. Fiber increases the volume of the intestinal contents, which hinders the absorption of cholesterol. The added bulk promotes more regular bowel movements, promoting intestinal health.

RESEARCH FINDINGS

There is evidence that the nutrients and phytochemicals in pears counteract oxidative stress, reduce inflammation, and control cellular interactions, all of which play a protective role against vascular disease and cancer. The prevention of vascular disease is attributed in part to the ability of the nutrients in pears (e.g., chlorogenic acid and vitamin C) to inhibit blood clotting and lower serum lipid profiles. Pears may help prevent cancer by its nutrients' ability to protect against DNA and cellular damage caused by oxidative stress, control carcinogen buildup, prevent inflammation, induce cancer cell death, and function as anti-mutagenic and anti-proliferative agents.

SUMMARY

Consumers should become knowledgeable about the physiologic benefits of the consumption of pears. Pears are a good source of fiber, vitamins C and K, and many phytonutrients. These nutrients may help prevent allergic reactions, improve digestion, and reduce the risk of developing type 2 diabetes, heart disease, and cancer.

—*Cherie Marcel, BS*

REFERENCES

Alvarez-Parrilla, E., De La Rosa, L. A., Legarreta, P., Saenz, L., Rodrigo-Garcia, J., & Gonzalez-Aguilar, G. A. (2010). Daily consumption of apple, pear and orange juice differently affects plasma lipids and antioxidant capacity of smoking and non-smoking adults. *International Journal of Food Sciences & Nutrition, 61*(4), 369-380. doi:10.3109/09637480903514041

Jio, S. (2006). Flavor. Shed pounds with pears: Take a bite of this sweet autumn fruit that can help you stay trim. *Health (Time Inc.), 20*(8), 147-148.

Palmer, S. (2009). Asian pears, a pear by any other name. *Environmental Nutrition, 32*(9), 8.

The George Mateljan Foundation editorial team. (n.d.). Pears. *The world's healthiest foods.* Retrieved December 2, 2015, from http://www.whfoods.com/genpage.php?tname=foodspice&dbid=28

Webster, S. T. (2010). Pears. *IDEA Fitness Journal, 7*(9), 61.

Zevnik, N. (2008). Pear affair. *Better Nutrition, 70*(12), 40, 42.

REVIEWER(S)

Darlene Strayer, RN, MBA, Cinahl Information Systems, Glendale, CA

Nursing Executive Practice Council, Glendale Adventist Medical Center, Glendale, CA

Pineapple

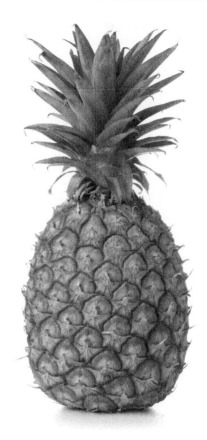

WHAT WE KNOW

The pineapple is a large fibrous fruit produced by the *Ananas comosus* plant, which is a member of the Bromeliaceae family. Although considered a single fruit, pineapple is actually formed from a grouping of many individual flower fruitlets that fuse together at a central, fibrous core. The scaly and spiny exterior of pineapple covers bright yellow, juicy flesh that has an intense flavor that is considered equally sweet and tart. The flesh of pineapple can be eaten raw, canned, dried, baked in pastry, used in drinks, or made into jams and sauces. Although pineapple is an excellent source of fiber, folate, manganese, copper, and vitamins C, B1, and B6, the most significant property of pineapple is that it contains the sulfhydryl-containing enzyme called bromelain. Pineapple has anti-inflammatory, antifungal, antitumor, fibrinolytic, coagulant, and antioxidant properties that provide many health benefits, including improved gastrointestinal (GI) function, enhanced wound healing, arthritic and myalgic pain relief, protection against macular degeneration, and reduced risk for obesity, diabetes mellitus, type 2 (DM2), heart disease, and cancer.

NUTRIENTS IN PINEAPPLE

- Bromelain is a powerful enzyme with proteolytic (i.e., protein-digesting) and nonproteolytic components that perform the following beneficial activities:
  - —Bromelain improves gastric motility and counter the harmful effects of intestinal pathogens (e.g., *Vibrio cholera, Escherichia coli*), promoting digestive health.
  - —Bromelain exhibits anti-inflammatory properties that relieve the pain of inflamed joints, muscles, and soft tissue and may prevent inflammation-induced chronic diseases such as atherosclerosis, inflammatory bowel disease (IBD), periodontal disease, arthritis, and cancer.
  - —Bromelain speeds the healing process following injury. Bromelain preparations are used to remove dead skin in the treatment of burns.
- The water-soluble vitamin C in pineapple neutralizes free radicals, protecting against inflammation and cellular damage. Adequate vitamin C

intake is vital for immune system function and has been associated with the prevention of heart disease, stroke, and cancer.

- Pineapple provides B-complex vitamins, which perform the following functions:
  —Vitamin B1, or thiamin, aids the breakdown of carbohydrates, provides cardiovascular protection, maintains the nervous system, and supports the production of red blood cells (RBCs), hormones, and cholesterol.
  —Vitamin B6, or pyridoxine, is essential for building and breaking down proteins, carbohydrates, and lipids and is important for the formation of RBCs and hemoglobin, which carries oxygen to the tissues. It is required for conversion of the amino acid tryptophan to niacin and homocysteine to cysteine and is necessary for building serotonin and dopamine, which are neurotransmitters required for nerve cell communication. By maintaining the lymphoid organs, vitamin B6 contributes to immune system function.
  —Folate is a water-soluble B vitamin that is essential for the production and maintenance of RBCs. It is vital for building deoxyribonucleic acid (DNA) and ribonucleic acid (RNA), and is also important in the breakdown of homocysteine.
- Manganese, a trace mineral found in pineapple, is involved in energy production, building fatty acids, cholesterol production, and protection against damage caused by free radicals.
- The copper in pineapple is a vital component of superoxide dismutase (SOD), which is an enzyme involved in energy production and antioxidant activity. It contributes to the action of lysyl oxidase, an enzyme necessary for the cross-linking of collagen and elastin, which allows flexibility in the blood vessels, bones, and joints. It also enhances the body's ability to use iron, preventing iron-deficiency anemia, ruptured blood vessels, irregular heart rate, and infection.
- Pineapple is a good source of dietary fiber, including soluble fiber, which binds with water and slows the digestive process, allowing the body to better manage postprandial (i.e., after eating) glucose and insulin responses. Fiber increases the volume of intestinal contents, which hinders the absorption of cholesterol. The added bulk promotes more regular bowel movements, promoting intestinal health.

DIETARY INTAKE GUIDELINES
- There is no standardized dosage recommendation for pineapple.
- As a precaution, pineapple and bromelain should not be used therapeutically by pregnant or breastfeeding women.
- Due to the blood-thinning potential of bromelain, pineapple is not recommended for persons with coagulation disorders.
- Pineapple can oppose the function of angiotensin-converting enzyme (ACE) inhibitors (e.g., lisinopril, ramipril).
- Due to the blood-thinning potential of bromelain, pineapple should not be used with anticoagulants (e.g., heparin, salicylates, warfarin).

RESEARCH FINDINGS
There is evidence that the bromelain in pineapple may fight cancer. Researchers report that bromelain induces apoptosis (i.e., natural cell death) in breast cancer cells, inhibits the growth of melanoma, and reduces tumor growth.

SUMMARY
Consumers should become knowledgeable about pineapple consumption and use. Pineapple is a good source of the enzyme bromelain, fiber, folate, manganese, copper, and vitamins C, B1, and B6. These nutrients may help improve GI function, enhance wound healing and eye health, relieve pain, as well as reduce risk for developing obesity, type II diabetes, and heart disease. Individuals with coagulation disorders should be aware that pineapple is not recommended due to its blood thinning potential. Consumers should be aware of the possible drug-nutrient interactions associated with pineapple.

—*Cherie Marcel, BS*

REFERENCES
Aiyegbusi, A. I., Duru, F. I., Anunobi, C. C., Noronha, C. C., & Okanlawon, A. O. (2011). Bromelain in the early phase of healing in acute crush Achilles tendon injury. *Phytotherapy Research*, 25(1), 49-52. doi:10.1002/ptr.3199

Báez, R., Lopes, M. T., Salas, C. E., & Hernández, M. (2007). In vivo antitumoral activity of stem pineapple (Ananas comosus) bromelain. *Planta Medica*, 73(13), 1377-1383.

Dhandayuthapani, S., Perez, H. D., Paroulek, A., Chinnakkannu, P., Kandalam, U., Jaffe, M., & Rathinavelu, A. (2012). Bromelain-induced apoptosis in GI-101 A breast cancer cells. *Journal of Medicinal Food, 15*(4), 344-349. doi:10.1089/jmf.2011.0145

Goodman, S. (2008). Powerful relief from inflammatory pain and other age-related disorders. *Life Extension, 14*(5), 24-30.

Michael, A., Hedayati, B., & Dalgleish, A. G. (2007). Disease regression in malignant melanoma: Spontaneous resolution or a result of treatment with antioxidants, green tea, and pineapple cores? A case report. *Integrative Cancer Therapies, 6*(1), 77-79.

Ospina, B. (2009). Patient primer. A focus on healthy eating to control inflammatory disease. *Case in Point, 7*(7), 52.

The Alternative Medicine Review editorial team. (2010). Bromelain monograph. *Alternative medicine Review, 15*(4), 361-368.

The George Mateljan Foundation editorial team. (n.d.). Pineapple. *The world's healthiest foods.* Retrieved June 18, 2015, from http://www.whfoods.com/genpage.php? tname=foodspice&dbid=34

Vukovic, L. (2007). Pineapple power. *Better Nutrition, 69*(7), 20-21.

REVIEWER(S)

Darlene Strayer, RN, MBA, Cinahl Information Systems, Glendale, CA

Nursing Executive Practice Council, Glendale Adventist Medical Center, Glendale, CA

Plum

WHAT WE KNOW

The plum, from the tree *Prunus domestica*, is a stone fruit of the Rosaceae (i.e., rose) family, along with peaches, nectarines, apricots, and cherries. There are over 2,000 varieties of the plum that are cultivated throughout the world; the United States, Russia, China, and Romania produce the majority of commercially grown plums. The plum is typically spherical or heart-shaped and has smooth, tight skin in a range of colors, including red, purple, green, and yellow. The juicy flesh of the plum also varies in color and is a sweet, tart, refreshing flavor. The plum can be eaten raw, canned, dried (i.e.,as prunes), baked in pies and tarts, and made into jams and sauces. The plum is rich in nutrients, including vitamins C, K, and A and potassium, tryptophan, and fiber. Plum is especially noted for its high content of the phytonutrients (i.e., beneficial, plant-derived chemicals) neochlorogenic acid and chlorogenic acid, which have potent antioxidant activity.

NUTRIENTS IN PLUM

- The plum is a good source of the antioxidants chlorogenic acid, which consists of caffeic acid and neochlorogenic acid.
  - —These phytonutrients have cancer-preventive antioxidant activity as demonstrated by their
    - –effective neutralization of damaging free radicals.
    - –protection of fats from damage. By inhibiting the damage to fats, chlorogenic and neochlorogenic acid prevent damage to neurons and cell membranes, which are largely composed of fats.
  - —Chlorogenic acid has been shown to increase insulin sensitivity and reduce blood glucose levels.
- The water-soluble vitamin C found in plum neutralizes free radicals, protecting against inflammation and cellular damage. Adequate vitamin C intake is vital for proper function of the immune system and has been associated with the prevention of heart disease, stroke, and cancer.
- The vitamin K in plum acts as a coenzyme in maintaining normal levels of blood-clotting proteins and contributes to bone growth.
- Vitamin A, or retinol, is a fat-soluble vitamin that is required for vision, maintenance of the surface linings of the eyes and other epithelial tissue, proper bone growth, immune response, energy regulation, reproduction, embryonic development, and activation of gene expression.
- Plum contains potassium, which is an essential element responsible for regulating acid-base balance, maintaining fluid balance, supporting muscle contraction and cardiac function, contributing to protein building and carbohydrate breakdown, promoting cellular growth, and promoting transmission of nerve impulses.
- Plum is a source of the amino acid tryptophan, which contributes to the synthesis of niacin and serotonin. Serotonin is thought to promote healthy sleep patterns and stabilize mood.

- Plum is a good source of dietary fiber, which binds and removes toxins from the colon, assists in glucose control, and reduces high cholesterol levels.

DIETARY INTAKE GUIDELINES

- There is no standard dosage recommended in the literature for plum.
- The consumption of plum may increase risk for kidney stones in individuals with a history of kidney stones because plum contains a high amount of the chemical oxalate, which is a primary component of kidney stones. Oxalates can build up and crystallize in body fluids and cause health compromise in individuals with pre-existing kidney or gallbladder dysfunction.

RESEARCH FINDINGS

- Dried plum (i.e., prune) juice is frequently used to relieve constipation and regulate bowel function. Researchers compared the effectiveness of consuming prune juice to consuming apple juice containing psyllium and found that prune juice was an acceptable alternative to psyllium as an effective treatment for stool softening and relief of constipation.
- Researchers have reported that plum extracts containing phytonutrients can promote bone formation in postmenopausal women and should be considered as an alternative treatment for the prevention and treatment of osteoporosis.

SUMMARY

Consumers should become knowledgeable about the physiologic risks and benefits of plum consumption. Plum is a good source of antioxidants, vitamins, minerals, and fiber. These nutrients improve bowel function, prevent cell damage, and improve blood glucose levels, which may help prevent cancer, heart disease, and type II diabetes. Individuals with a history of kidney stones should be aware that plum increases risk for kidney stones because plum contains high amounts of oxalate, a primary component of kidney stones.

—*Cherie Marcel, BS*

REFERENCES

Can you tell me what oxalates are and in which foods they can be found? (n.d.). *The George Mateljan Foundation editorial team.* Retrieved December

4, 2015, from http:// www.whfoods.com/genpage. php?tname=george&dbid=48

The George Mateljan Foundation editorial team. (n.d.). Plums & Prunes. *The World's Healthiest Foods.* Retrieved December 4, 2015, from http://www.whfoods.com/ genpage.php?tname=foodspice&dbid=35#descr

Cheskin, L. J., Mitola, A. H., Ridore, M., Kolge, S., Hwang, K., & Clark, B. (2009). A naturalistic, controlled, crossover trial of plum juice versus psyllium versus control for improving bowel function. *Internet Journal of Nutrition & Wellness, 7*(2). doi:10.5580/974

Are dried plums "super food" for increasing bone mineral density in postmenopausal women? (2011) *Lippincott's. Bone & Joint Newsletter, 17*(11), 127-128.

Arjmandi, B. H., Johnson, C. D., Campbell, S. C., Hooshmand, S., Chai, S. C., & Akhter, M. P. (2010). Combining fructooligosaccharide and dried plum has the greatest effect on restoring bone mineral density among select functional foods and bioactive compounds. *Journal of Medicinal Food, 13*(2), 312-319. doi:10.1089/jmf.2009.0068

Hooshmand, S., Chai, S. C., Saadat, R. L., Payton, M. E., Brummel-Smith, K., & Arjmandi, B. H. (2011). Comparative effects of dried plum and dried apple on bone in postmenopausal women. *British Journal of Nutrition, 106*(6), 923-930. doi:10.1017/S000711451100119X

Scott, S. M., & Knowles, C. H. (2011). Constipation: Dried plums (prunes) for the treatment of constipation. *Nature Reviews of Gastroenterology & Hepatology, 8*(6), 306-307. doi:10.1038/nrgastro.2011.82

Zanteson, L. (2012). Plum good for you. *Environmental Nutrition, 35*(9), 8.

Barclay, L. (2009). New strategies for optimizing bone strength. *Life Extension, 15*(4), 58-64.

Hooshmand, S., Brisco, J. R. Y., & Arjmandi, B. H. (2014). The effect of dried plum on serum levels of receptor activator of NF-kappaB ligand, osteoprotegerin and sclerostin in osteopenic postmenopausal women: A randomised controlled trial. *British Journal of Nutrition, 112*(1), 55-60. doi:10.1017/S0007114514000671

REVIEWER(S)

Darlene Strayer, RN, MBA, Cinahl Information Systems, Glendale, CA

Nursing Executive Practice Council, Glendale Adventist Medical Center, Glendale, CA

Pomegranate

WHAT WE KNOW

The pomegranate is the fruit of an ancient shrub, *Punica granatum*, of the Punicaceae family, that has a history of medicinal use. Ayurvedic medicine considers the pomegranate root, bark, flower buds, and leaves to be therapeutic. The round pomegranate fruit is encased in a thick, leathery, yellow and red skin that has a calyx at its base. The membranous interior is a labyrinth of white tissue that creates pockets filled with tart and juicy seeds. The seeds are the most commonly consumed portion of the pomegranate and comprise about half of the total weight of the fruit. Although the collection of the edible pomegranate seeds can be time consuming, in certain cultures it is viewed as a group activity that is part of the social dining experience. Pomegranate can be made into juice, jams, sauces, and wine. Pomegranate is a good source of fiber and contains many nutrients, including vitamin C, B-complex vitamins, calcium, phosphorous, iron, copper, potassium, and a diverse collection of phytonutrients (i.e., protective, plant-derived chemicals). These nutrients have powerful anti-inflammatory, antioxidant, antimicrobial, antifungal, antiviral, antispasmodic, anthelmintic, hypotensive, cancer-preventive, and cardio-protective activity. Historically, the pomegranate plant has been used to treat worm infestations, sore throat, hemorrhoids, diarrhea, bronchitis, periodontal disease, sore eyes, and hypertension.

NUTRIENTS IN POMEGRANATE

- Pomegranate contains many valuable phytonutrients that have antioxidant and anti-inflammatory activities that reduce risk for cancer and heart disease. Phytonutrients in pomegranate include the following:
  - Hydroxybenzoic acids: Punicalagin is an ellagitannin that breaks down into ellagic acid, which exhibits anti-inflammatory properties and has been shown to reduce symptoms of Crohn's disease. Ellagic acid also fights carcinogens and slows cancer cell proliferation (i.e., cancer cell growth).
  - Anthocyanins: reddish-color pigments that have high levels of antioxidant and anticarcinogenic activity. Anthocyanins promote urinary tract health, support memory function, and fight bacteria (e.g., *Streptococcus*) by disrupting bacterial cell membranes.
  - Flavonols: Quercetin and kaempferol provide strong antioxidant and anti-inflammatory protection and have antihistamine, antimicrobial, anti-diabetic, and anti-carcinogenic properties.
  - Flavonoid glycosides inhibit cancer cell proliferation and exhibit antibiotic activity.
  - Tannins have antioxidant, antihistamine, anticancer, and cardio-protective properties.
- The water-soluble vitamin C in pomegranate neutralizes free radicals, protecting against inflammation and cellular damage. Adequate vitamin C intake is vital for immune system function and is associated with prevention of heart disease, stroke, and cancer.
- Pomegranate is a source of the B-complex vitamins B1 (thiamin), B2 (riboflavin), and B3 (niacin), which help produce energy by building and breaking down carbohydrates, provide cardiovascular protection, maintain the nervous system, and support the production of red blood cells, hormones, and cholesterol.
- The calcium in pomegranate builds and maintains bones and teeth, regulates muscle contraction, promotes conduction of nerve impulses, activates enzymes for energy production and muscle contraction, participates in blood clotting, assists with vitamin B12 absorption, and maintains the structural integrity of intracellular membranes.
- Phosphorous combines with calcium for the formation of bones and teeth, muscle contraction, and nerve conduction and is essential for the structural integrity of cell membranes.
- The iron provided by pomegranate is vital for building red blood cells and hemoglobin, which are necessary for energy production and the transport of oxygen to the tissues. Iron also supports immune function, is vital for cognitive development, contributes to energy metabolism, and regulates temperature.
- Pomegranate provides copper, which is a vital component of superoxide dismutase (SOD), an enzyme involved in energy production and antioxidant activity. It contributes to the action of lysyl oxidase, an enzyme necessary for the cross-linking of collagen and elastin to allow flexibility in the blood vessels, bones, and joints. It also

enhances the body's ability to use iron, preventing iron-deficiency anemia, ruptured blood vessels, irregular heartbeat, and infection.

- Pomegranate contains potassium, which is an essential element for regulating acid-base balance, maintaining fluid balance, supporting muscle contraction and cardiac function, contributing to protein building and carbohydrate breakdown, promoting cellular growth, and promoting transmission of nerve impulses.
- Pomegranate is a good source of dietary fiber, which binds and removes toxins from the colon, assists in glucose control, and reduces high cholesterol levels.

RESEARCH FINDINGS

- There is evidence that regular consumption of pomegranate juice can result in improved lipid profiles and reduce systolic blood pressure in hypertensive individuals. Additionally, pomegranate seed oil has been shown to have favorable effects on glucose breakdown and serum lipid profiles. These factors make pomegranate a potential ingredient in the strategy for the treatment and prevention of metabolic syndrome and its related conditions: insulin resistance, diabetes mellitus, hypertension, heart disease, and obesity.
- The polyphenols in pomegranate inhibit blood clotting and improve function of arteries, preventing atherosclerosis and promoting cardiovascular health.
- The ellagitannins in pomegranate slow the digestion of starch, protein, and oil, which helps to stabilize blood glucose levels.
- Two major constituents of pomegranate juice, punicalagin and ellagic acid, inhibit the formation of harmful compounds that reduce blood flow. This may help prevent retinopathy, nephropathy, neuropathy, and atherosclerosis.
- Researchers report that pomegranate extract has powerful pro-apoptotic and anti-proliferative activity effects on breast and prostate cancer cells, and supplementation of pomegranate polyphenols can enhance these anti-cancer effects.

SUMMARY

Consumers should become knowledgeable about the physiologic benefits of pomegranate consumption. Pomegranate contains vitamin C, B-complex vitamins, calcium, phosphorous, iron, copper, potassium, fiber, and many antioxidant phytonutrients. These nutrients support the immune system, improve bone health, help with digestion, and may prevent cardiovascular disease and cancer.

—*Cherie Marcel, BS*

REFERENCES

Asgary, S., Sahebkar, A., Afshani, M. R., Keshvari, M., Haghjooyjavanmard, S., & Rafieian-Kopaei, M. (2014). Clinical evaluation of blood pressure lowering, endothelial function improving, hypolipidemic and anti-inflammatory effects of pomegranate juice in hypertensive subjects. *Phytotherapy Research*, 28(2), 193-199. doi:10.1002/ptr.4977

Bagri, P., Ali, M., Sultana, S., & Aeri, V. (2009). New sterols esters from the flowers of Punica granatum Linn. *Journal of Asian Natural Products Research*, 11(8), 710-715. doi:10.1080/10286020903004291

Dikmen, M., Ozturk, N., & Ozturk, Y. (2011). The antioxidant potency of Punica granatum L. fruit peel reduces cell proliferation and induces apoptosis on breast cancer. *Journal of Medicinal Food*, 14(12), 1638-1646. doi:10.1089/jmf.2011.0062

Dorsey, P. G., & Greenspan, P. (2014). Inhibition of non-enzymatic protein clycation by pomegranate and other fruit juices. *Journal of Medicinal food*, 17(4), 447-454. doi:10.1089/jmf.2013.0075

Hashemi, M., Kelishadi, R., Hashemipour, M., Zakerameli, A., Khavarian, N., Ghatrehsamani, S., & Poursafa, P. (2010). Acute and long-term effects of grape and pomegranate juice consumption on vascular reactivity in paediatric metabolic syndrome. *Cardiology in the Young*, 20(1), 73-77. doi:10.1017/S1047951109990850

Hong, M. Y., Seeram, N. P., & Heber, D. (2008). Pomegranate polyphenols down-regulate expression of androgen synthesizing genes in human prostate cancer cells overexpressing the androgen receptor. *Journal of Nutritional Biochemistry*, 19(12), 848-855. doi:10.1016/j.jnutbio.2007.11.006

Kahn, G. N., Gorin, M. A., Rosenthal, D., Pan, Q., Bao, L. W., Wu, Z. F., ... Merajver, S. D. (2009). Pomegranate fruit extract impairs invasion and motility in human breast cancer. *Integrative Cancer Therapies*, 8(3), 242-253. doi:10.1177/1534735409341405

Kelishadi, R., Gidding, S. S., Hashemi, M., Hashemipour, M., Zakerameli, A., & Poursafa, P. (2011). Acute and long term effects of grape and pomegranate juice consumption on endothelial dysfunction in pediatric metabolic syndrome. *Journal of Research in Medical Sciences, 16*(3), 245-253.

Kim, H. K., Baek, S. S., & Cho, H. Y. (2011). Inhibitory effect of pomegranate on intestinal sodium dependent glucose uptake. *American Journal of Chinese Medicine, 39*(5), 1015-1027. doi:10.1142/S0192415X11009378

Mattiello, T., Trifirò, E., Jotti, G. S., & Pulcinelli, F. M. (2009). Effects of pomegranate juice and extract polyphenols on platelet function. *Journal of Medicinal Food, 12*(2), 334-339. doi:10.1089/jmf.2007.0640

Mirmiran, P., Fazeli, M. R., Asghari, G., Shafiee, A., & Azizi, F. (2010). Effect of pomegranate seed oil on hyperlipidaemic subjects: A double-blind placebo-controlled clinical trial. *British Journal of Nutrition, 104*(3), 402-406. doi:10.1017/S0007114510000504

Rosenblat, M., & Aviram, M. (2011). Pomegranate juice protects macrophages from triglyceride accumulation: Inhibitory effect on DGAT1 activity and on triglyceride biosynthesis. *Annals of Nutrition & Metabolism, 58*(1), 1-9. doi:10.1159/000323096

Shema-Didi, L., Kristal, B., Sela, S., Geron, R., & Ore, L. (2014). Does pomegranate intake attenuate cardiovascular risk factors in hemodialysis patients? *Nutrition Journal, 13*(1), 18 pp. doi:10.1186/1475-2891-13-18

Turcotte, M. (2015, January 28). The health benefits of pomegranate seeds. *Livestrong.com*. Retrieved June 25, 2015, from http://www.livestrong.com/article/396484-pomegranate-health-skincare-benefits/

Shirode, A. B., Bharali, D. J., Nallanthighal, S., Coon, J. K., Mousa, S. A., & Reliene, R. (2015). Nanoencapsulation of pomegranate bioactive compounds for breast cancer chemoprevention. *International Journal of Nanomedicine, 10*, 475-484. doi:10.2147/IJN.S65145

REVIEWER(S)

Darlene Strayer, RN, MBA, Cinahl Information Systems, Glendale, CA

Nursing Executive Practice Council, Glendale Adventist Medical Center, Glendale, CA

Pumpkin

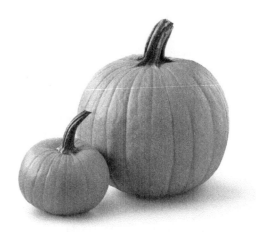

WHAT WE KNOW

The pumpkin is a nutrient-rich gourd of the Cucurbitaceae family, which includes cucumber and a variety of types of squash and melon. Pumpkins grow in a variety of shapes, sizes, and colors, but tend to be round and ribbed and to grow on creeping vines. They are encased in a thick outer skin that protects the fibrous and fleshy interior, which contains a cavity filled with seeds that are slimy. The flavor of pumpkin is moderately sweet, and pumpkin can be used in both sweet and savory recipes. There are many culinary uses of pumpkin, including in soups, breads, pastas, and pies. The seeds of the pumpkin can be roasted and provide many nutrients. Pumpkin seeds have been shown to exhibit disease-fighting activity against cardiovascular disease (CVD), osteoporosis, bladder dysfunction, anxiety, and arthritis. Although the seeds contain essential fatty acids, the flesh of the pumpkin is low in fat and calories and rich in vitamins, minerals, phytonutrients (i.e., beneficial plant-derived chemicals), and fiber.

NUTRIENTS IN PUMPKIN

* Nutrients in pumpkin and its seeds include the following:
  —Pumpkin is rich in carotenoids (e.g., beta-carotene, lutein), which are powerful antioxidants with anti-cancer activity. Carotenoids protect the eyes from age-related macular degeneration.
    –Provitamin A carotenoids, such as beta-carotene, are precursors of vitamin A, or retinol, a fat-soluble vitamin that is required for vision, maintenance of the surface lining of the eyes, bone growth, immune response, energy regulation, reproduction, embryonic development, and activation of gene expression.
  —Pumpkin is an excellent source of vitamin C, which neutralizes free radicals, protecting

against inflammation and cellular damage. Adequate intake of vitamin C is vital for immune system function and has been associated with prevention of heart disease, stroke, and cancer.

—The potassium in pumpkin supports normal cellular, nerve, and muscle function and helps to eliminate excess sodium from the body.

—Pumpkin, including the seeds, is a good source of dietary fiber, which binds and removes toxins from the colon, assists in glucose control, and reduces high cholesterol levels.

—Pumpkin seeds supply several B-complex vitamins, including the following:

–Folate is a B vitamin that is essential for the production and maintenance of red blood cells (RBCs). Folate is vital for building deoxyribonucleic acid (DNA; the genetic code for the cells) and ribonucleic acid (RNA), and is important in the metabolism of homocysteine, an amino acid.

–Vitamin B6 (pyridoxine) is required for the conversion of tryptophan to niacin and is involved in the conversion of homocysteine to cysteine. Vitamin B6 is also necessary for the synthesis of serotonin and dopamine, which are neurotransmitters required for nerve cell communication. By maintaining the lymphoid organs, vitamin B6 contributes to the proper function of the immune system. Vitamin B6 is essential for building and breaking down proteins, carbohydrates, and lipids and is important for the formation of RBCs and hemoglobin, which carries oxygen to the tissues.

–Vitamin B1 (thiamin), B2 (riboflavin), and B3 (niacin) create energy by aiding the breakdown of carbohydrates, provide cardiovascular protection, help maintain the nervous system, and support the production of RBCs, hormones, and cholesterol.

—Pumpkin seeds are rich in magnesium, which balances the action of calcium in cells to regulate bone health and nerve and muscle tone. Magnesium maintains relaxation of the nerves and muscles, which contributes to the prevention of high blood pressure, muscle

spasms, asthma, migraine headaches, general soreness, and fatigue.

—Pumpkin seeds are a good source of manganese, which is a trace mineral involved in energy production, fatty acid building, cholesterol production, and protection against the damage caused by free radicals.

—In combination with calcium, the phosphorous in pumpkin seeds assists in the formation of bones and teeth, muscle contraction, and nerve conduction and is essential for the structural integrity of cell membranes.

—Pumpkin seeds contain copper, which is a vital component of superoxide dismutase (SOD), an enzyme involved in energy production and antioxidant activity. Copper contributes to the action of lysyl oxidase, an enzyme necessary for the cross-linking of collagen and elastin, which allows flexibility in blood vessels, bones, and joints. Copper enhances the body's ability to use iron, preventing iron-deficiency anemia, ruptured blood vessels, irregular heartbeat, and infection.

—The essential trace element zinc in pumpkin seeds supports immune system function and wound healing, and is essential for maintaining vision and the senses of smell and taste.

—The iron in pumpkin seeds is vital for the synthesis of RBCs and hemoglobin, which are necessary for energy production and the transport of oxygen to the tissues. Iron supports immune function, is vital for cognitive development, contributes to energy building and breakdown, and regulates temperature.

—Pumpkin seeds contain protein. Protein is present in every cell in the human body and is vital to the development and maintenance of skin, muscles, organs, and glands.

—Pumpkin seeds contain essential fatty acids, which contribute to blood clotting and are necessary for brain development, providing energy to the body, assisting the absorption of fat-soluble vitamins, and controlling inflammation.

RESEARCH FINDINGS

Researchers report that pumpkin seed oil exhibits antihypertensive and cardio-protective activity. The consumption of pumpkin seed oil was shown to lower blood pressure and improve blood lipid profiles in post-menopausal women; it was also effective in reducing menopausal symptoms such as hot flashes, headaches, joint pain, and depression.

SUMMARY

Consumers should become knowledgeable about the physiologic benefits of the consumption of pumpkin. Pumpkin is rich a good source of vitamins, minerals, phytonutrients, and fiber. These nutrients have been shown to exhibit disease-fighting activity against cardiovascular disease, osteoporosis, bladder dysfunction, anxiety, and arthritis.

—*Cherie Marcel, BS*

REFERENCES

El-Mosallamy, A. E., Sleem, A. A., Abdel-Salam, O. M., Shaffie, N., & Kenawy, S. A. (2012). Antihypertensive and cardioprotective effects of pumpkin seed oil. *Journal of Medicinal Food, 15*(2), 180-189. Advance online publication. doi:10.1089/jmf.2010.0299

Gamonski, W. (2012). Super foods: The true potency of the pumpkin seed. *Life Extension, 18*(10), 95-98.

The George Mateljan Foundation editorial team. (2012). Pumpkin seeds. *The World's Healthiest Foods.* Retrieved June 15, 2015, from http://www.whfoods.com/genpage.php? tname=foodspice&dbid=82

Golub, C. (2007). Carve out nutrients from colorful pumpkin. *Environmental Nutrition, 30*(10), 8.

Gossell-Williams, M., Hyde, C., Hunter, T., Simms-Stewart, D., Fletcher, H., McGrowder, D., & Walters, C. A. (2011). Improvement in HDL cholesterol in postmenopausal women supplemented with pumpkin seed oil: Pilot study. *Climacteric, 14*(5), 558-564.

Gossell-Williams, M., Lyttle, K., Clarke, T., Gardner, M., & Simon, O. (2008). Supplementation with pumpkin seed oil improves plasma lipid profile and cardiovascular outcomes of female non-ovariectomized and ovariectomized Sprague-Dawley rats. *Phytotherapy Research, 22*(7), 873-877. doi:10.1002/ptr.2381

Kwon, Y. I., Apostolidis, E., Kim, Y. C., & Shetty, K. (2007). Health benefits of traditional corn, beans, and pumpkin: In vitro studies for hyperglycemia and hypertension management. *Journal of Medicinal Food, 10*(2), 266-275.

Magee, E. (2006). Vine ripe. Pumpkin seed power. *Better Nutrition, 68*(10), 58-59.

Marano, H. E. (2009). Smashing pumpkins: With its antioxidants and rich flavor, pumpkin deserves more than dessert. *Psychology Today, 42*(6), 55.

Neithercott, T. (2009). Food for thought. The best of the harvest. Squash is a sweet seasonal treat. *Diabetes Forecast, 62*(10), 35-38.

Raymond, S. (2009). Sensational squash: Autumn's nutritional superstar. *Alive: Canada's Natural Health & Wellness Magazine,* (324), 130-133.

Stein, N. (2014, March 1). What are the health benefits of pumpkins? *Livestrong.com.* Retrieved June 15, 2015, from http://www.livestrong.com/article/412480-what-are-the-health-benefits-of-pumpkins/

REVIEWER(S)

Darlene Strayer, RN, MBA, Cinahl Information Systems, Glendale, CA

Nursing Executive Practice Council, Glendale Adventist Medical Center, Glendale, CA

Raspberry

WHAT WE KNOW

The raspberry is a member of the Rosaceae (i.e., rose) family, along with nectarines, peaches, apricots, cherries, blackberries, and plums. Although there are over 200 species of raspberry in the genus *Rubus*, most of the commercially grown varieties can be categorized as red, black, or purple raspberry. Known as aggregate fruits, each raspberry is actually a grouping of tiny individual fruit orbs called drupelets, and each drupelet has its own seed. Raspberry is considered by most to be the third most popular berry after strawberry and blueberry. A delicious culinary treat, the raspberry can be eaten raw, canned, dried, baked in pies and cobblers, made into jams and sauces, and blended in drinks. Beyond its value in cuisine, raspberry has many nutrients, including vitamins

C, E, and K and manganese, magnesium, folate, copper, potassium, fiber, and a diverse collection of phytonutrients (i.e., protective, plant-derived chemicals). These nutrients provide the raspberry with powerful anti-inflammatory, antioxidant, antimicrobial, cancer-preventive, and cardio-protective activity. Black raspberry has about 3 times more antioxidants than blueberry. The leaves and other parts of the raspberry plant have been used to treat sore throat, diarrhea, intestinal parasites, hemorrhoids, diabetes, rheumatism, and the discomforts of menstruation and pregnancy.

NUTRIENTS IN RASPBERRY

- Raspberry contains many valuable phytonutrients, which have antioxidant and anti-inflammatory activities that have great potential in preventing cancer and heart disease. These phytonutrients include the following:
  - —Anthocyanins: Reddish color pigments that have high antioxidant and anti-carcinogenic activity, promote urinary tract health, and support memory function. They also fight bacteria such as *Streptococcus* species by disrupting bacterial cell membranes.
  - —Flavonols: Quercetin and kaempferol provide strong antioxidant and anti-inflammatory protection. They also have antihistamine, antimicrobial, anti-diabetic, and anti-carcinogenic properties.
  - —Flavonols: Epicatechin and catechin are thought to decrease risk factors for cardiovascular disease (CVD) and hypertension by preventing the damage to low-density lipoproteins (LDLs), enhancing endothelium-dependent relaxation (i.e., relaxes arteries), reducing inflammation, and inhibiting excess blood clotting.
  - —Flavonoid glycosides: Inhibit cancer cell proliferation (i.e., cancer cell growth) and exhibit antibiotic activity.
  - —Tannins: Proanthocyanidins have antioxidant, antihistamine, anti-cancer, and cardio-protective properties.
  - —Hydroxybenzoic acids: Gallic acid is an antioxidant that has demonstrated the ability to prevent proliferation of prostate cancer cells. Chlorogenic acid acts as an antimicrobial and antiviral agent. Ellagic acid exhibits anti-inflammatory properties and has been shown to reduce symptoms associated with Crohn's disease. Ellagic acid also repels carcinogens and slows cancer cell proliferation.
  - —Hydroxycinnamic acids: Caffeic acid exhibits anti-carcinogenic, antimicrobial, and antiviral properties. It is also believed to inhibit the buildup of LDL cholesterol.
  - —Stilbenoids: Resveratrol prevents damage to blood vessels, lowers LDL cholesterol, and inhibits blood clots.

- The water-soluble vitamin C in raspberry neutralizes free radicals, protecting against inflammation and cellular damage. Adequate vitamin C intake is vital for the proper function of the immune system and has been associated with the prevention of heart disease, stroke, and cancer.
- Raspberry contains vitamin E, which functions primarily as an antioxidant but also maintains cell membranes, assists in vitamin K absorption, and contributes to normal immune system function.
- The vitamin K in raspberry acts as a coenzyme involved in maintaining normal levels of blood clotting proteins and contributes to bone building.
- Manganese, a trace mineral found in raspberries, is responsible for energy production, fatty acid production, cholesterol production, and protection against damage caused by free radicals.
- Raspberry contains magnesium, which balances the action of calcium in cells to regulate bone health and nerve and muscle tone. Magnesium maintains relaxation of the nerves and muscles, which contributes to the prevention of high blood pressure, muscle spasms, asthma, migraine headaches, general soreness, and fatigue.
- The water-soluble B vitamin folate is provided by raspberry and is essential for the production and maintenance of red blood cells (RBCs). Folate is vital for the production of deoxyribonucleic acid (DNA) and ribonucleic acid (RNA), and is also important in the production of homocysteine (i.e., an amino acid).
- Raspberry provides copper, a vital component of superoxide dismutase (SOD), which is an enzyme involved in energy production and antioxidant activity. Copper contributes to the action of lysyl oxidase, an enzyme necessary for the cross-linking of collagen and elastin to allow flexibility in the blood vessels, bones, and joints. Copper also enhances the body's ability to use iron, preventing iron-deficiency anemia, ruptured blood vessels, irregular heartbeat, and infection.
- Raspberry contains potassium, which is an essential element responsible for regulating acid-base balance, maintaining fluid balance, supporting muscle contraction and cardiac function,

contributing to protein production and carbohydrate breakdown, promoting cellular growth, and transmitting nerve impulses.

- Raspberry is a good source of dietary fiber, which binds and removes toxins from the colon, assists in glucose control, and reduces high cholesterol levels.

DIETARY INTAKE GUIDELINES

- There is some concern that the raspberry may increase the risk of kidney stones in individuals with a history of kidney stones because it contains a high amount of the chemical oxalate, a primary component of kidney stones. Oxalates can build up and crystallize in body fluids and cause health problems in individuals with preexisting kidney or gallbladder dysfunction.

RESEARCH FINDINGS

- Researchers suggest that raspberries in the form of food are a more reliable source of raspberry-derived phenolics than dietary supplements because U.S. dietary supplements are not regulated with the same degree of oversight as foods.
- The anthocyanidins and ellagitannins in raspberry are able to slow the digestion of starch, protein, and oil, which helps stabilize blood sugar. The proanthocyanidins in raspberry inhibit lipase, the intestinal enzyme necessary for fat digestion. These factors make raspberry a potential tool for the treatment and prevention of metabolic syndrome and the related conditions of insulin resistance, diabetes mellitus, hypertension, heart disease, and obesity.
- Many studies over the past 15 years have provided evidence that raspberry may prevent and treat numerous cancers, including cancers of the mouth, breast, liver, and colon.

SUMMARY

Consumers should become knowledgeable about the physiologic risks and benefits of raspberry. Raspberry is a good source of vitamins C, E, and K, manganese, magnesium, folate, copper, potassium, fiber, and many antioxidant-rich phytonutrients. These nutrients can help fight cancer cells and lower cholesterol, blood pressure, and blood sugar, which may decrease risk for developing cardiovascular disease, diabetes, and cancer. Individuals with a history of kidney stones may want to avoid raspberries due to their high concentration of oxalates.

—*Cherie Marcel, BS*

REFERENCES

Broihier, K. (2007). Red or black, raspberries ripe with phytonutrients. *Environmental Nutrition, 30*(6), 8.

The George Mateljan Foundation Editorial Team. (2012). The world's healthiest foods: Raspberries. The World's Healthiest Foods. Retrieved June 29, 2015, fromhttp:// www.whfoods.com/genpage. php?tname=foodspice&dbid=39

God, J., Tate, P. L., & Larcom, L. L. (2010). Red raspberries have antioxidant effects that play a minor role in the killing of stomach and colon cancer cells. *Nutrition Research, 30*(11), 777-782. doi:10.1016/j.nutres.2010.10.004

Keville, K. (2012). Herb profile: Medicinal berries. *American Herb Association Quarterly Newsletter, 27*(1), 3.

Keville, K. (2011). Herb profile: Raspberry (Rubus species). *American Herb Association Quarterly Newsletter, 26*(3), 3.

Lee, J. (2014). Marketplace analysis demonstrates quality control standards needed for black raspberry dietary supplements. *Plant Foods for Human Nutrition, 69*(2), 161-167. doi:10.1007/s11130-014-0416-y

Zanteson, L. (2011). Raspberries, rich in nutrients and flavor. *Environmental Nutrition, 34*(8), 8.

Zikri, N. N., Riedl, K. M., Wang, L. S., Lechner, J., Schwartz, S. J., & Stoner, G. D. (2009). Black raspberry components inhibit proliferation, induce apoptosis, and modulate gene expression in rat esophageal epithelial cells. *Nutrition & Cancer, 61*(6), 816-826. doi:10.1080/01635580903285148

REVIEWER(S)

Darlene Strayer, RN, MBA, Cinahl Information Systems, Glendale, CA

Nursing Executive Practice Council, Glendale Adventist Medical Center, Glendale, CA

Rhubarb

WHAT WE KNOW

Rhubarb, or *Rheum rhabarbarum*, is a vegetable from the *Picornaviridae*, or buckwheat, family that has celery-like stalks that are streaked in red, pink, and green. Rhubarb has a tart flavor and requires the addition of sugar to be considered edible in a pie. Rhubarb is a good source of fiber, vitamins K and C, potassium, manganese, calcium, and many phytonutrients (i.e., beneficial, plant-derived chemicals). The nutrients in rhubarb have antioxidant, anti-inflammatory, and anti carcinogenic properties. For more than 5,000 years, the root and stalks of rhubarb have been used for medicinal purposes, including for the treatment of menopausal signs and symptoms, hypertension, indigestion, and hemorrhoids. The leaves of the rhubarb plant are toxic due to high levels of oxalic acid.

NUTRIENTS IN RHUBARB

- Rhubarb contains many valuable phytonutrients that have antioxidant and anti-inflammatory activities, which reduce risk for cancer and heart disease. Phytonutrients in rhubarb include the following:
    - Anthocyanins, which are reddish-color pigments that have high antioxidant and anti-carcinogenic activity, promote urinary tract health, support memory function, and fight bacteria (e.g., *Streptococcus*) by disrupting bacterial cell membranes.
    - The anthraquinone emodin exhibits anti-inflammatory activity, induces apoptosis (i.e., natural cell death), and inhibits cancer cell proliferation (i.e., slows cancer cell growth).
    - The xanthophylls lutein and zeaxanthin exhibit antioxidant properties, scavenging free radicals. They also protect the eyes from light-induced damage, promote eye health, and inhibit atherosclerosis.
- The vitamin K in rhubarb acts as a coenzyme to maintain normal levels of blood-clotting proteins and contributes to bone growth.
- The water-soluble vitamin C in rhubarb neutralizes free radicals, which protects against inflammation and cellular damage. Adequate vitamin C intake is important for normal immune system function and is associated with reduced risk of heart disease, stroke, and cancer.
- Rhubarb contains potassium, which is an essential element for regulating acid-base balance, maintaining fluid balance, supporting muscle contraction and cardiac function, contributing to protein production and carbohydrate breakdown, promoting cellular growth, and promoting transmission of nerve impulses.

- Manganese, a trace mineral in rhubarb, is responsible for energy production, fatty acid production, necessary cholesterol production, and protection from damage caused by free radicals.
- The calcium in rhubarb builds and maintains bones and teeth, regulates muscle contraction, promotes conduction of nerve impulses, activates enzymes for energy production and muscle contraction, participates in blood clotting, assists with vitamin B12 absorption, and maintains the structural integrity of intracellular membranes.
- Rhubarb is a good source of dietary fiber, which binds and removes toxins from the colon, assists in glucose control, and reduces high cholesterol levels.

DIETARY INTAKE GUIDELINES

- The leaves of rhubarb contain high levels of oxalates and should not be eaten. Consuming a large amount of rhubarb leaves can cause burning in the mouth and difficulty breathing.
- Rhubarb can interact with digoxin (Lanoxin) to increase adverse effects of digoxin.
- Rhubarb can interact with corticosteroids such that potassium stores become depleted.
- Rhubarb can enhance the function of stimulant laxatives.
- Rhubarb can increase the effects of warfarin (Coumadin).

RESEARCH FINDINGS

- Researchers report that the rhubarb constituent aloe-emodin is able to decrease pro-inflammatory cytokine production cells by inhibiting signaling pathways that create cytokines, which makes it a potentially valuable anti-inflammatory pharmaceutical agent for the treatment of inflammatory diseases.
- Results of a randomized controlled trial indicate that rhubarb is an effective treatment for alleviating the symptoms of primary dysmenorrhea without notable side effects.
- Evidence supports the use of rhubarb extract for the treatment of menopausal signs and symptoms. Researchers report that rhubarb extract is effective in alleviating the vasomotor signs and symptoms (commonly called hot flashes) of menopause, suggesting that it is a safe alternative to hormone therapy.

SUMMARY

Consumers should become knowledgeable about the physiologic effects of rhubarb. Rhubarb is a good source of vitamins K and C, potassium, manganese, calcium, fiber, and many antioxidant-rich phytonutrients. These nutrients support healthy digestion, fight inflammation, and support muscle function, and may help prevent cardiovascular disease, cancer, and symptoms associated with menopause. The leaves of the rhubarb plant contain high levels of oxalates and should not be eaten. Consumers should be aware of the drug-nutrient interactions associated with rhubarb.

—Cherie Marcel, BS

REFERENCES

Durkin, P. (2012). Rhubarb: Not just for pies anymore. *Alive: Canada's Natural Health & Wellness Magazine*, (356), 102-107.

The editorial team of WebMD. (n.d.). Rhubarb. *WebMD*. Retrieved June 22, 2015, from http://www.webmd.com/vitamins-supplements/ingredientmono-214-rhubarb.aspx?activeIngredientId=214&activeIngredientName=rhubarb&source=1

Heller, J. L., & Zieve, D. (2013). Rhubarb leaves poisoning. *MedlinePlus*. Retrieved June 22, 2015, from http://www.nlm.nih.gov/medlineplus/ency/article/002876.htm

Hu, B., Zhang, H., Meng, X., Wang, F., & Wang, P. (2014). Aloe-emodin from rhubarb (Rheum rhabarbarum) inhibits lipopolysaccharide-induced inflammatory responses in RAW264.7 macrophages. *Journal of Ethnopharmacology*, 153(3), 846-853. doi:10.1016/j.jep.2014.03.059

Ipatenco, S. (2013). The health benefits of rhubarb. Livestrong.com. Retrieved June 22, 2014, from http://www.livestrong.com/article/403208-the-health-benefits-of-rhubarb/

Kaszkin-Bettag, M., Beck, S., Richardson, A., Heger, P. W., & Beer, A. M. (2008). Efficacy of the special extract ERr 731 from rhapontic rhubarb for menopausal complaints: A 6-month open observational study. *Alternative Therapies in Health & Medicine*, 14(6), 32-38.

Kaszkin-Bettag, M., Ventskovskiy, B. M., Solskyy, S., Beck, S., Hasper, I., Kravchenko, A., & Heger, P. W. (2009). Confirmation of the efficacy of Err 731 in perimenopausal women with menopausal symptoms. *Alternative Therapies in Health & Medicine*, 15(1), 24-34.

Rehman, H., Begum, W., Anjum, F., Tabasum, H., & Zahid, S. (2015). Effect of rhubarb (Rheum emodi) in primary dysmenorrhea: A single-blind randomized controlled trial. *Journal of Complementary & Integrative Medicine*, 12(1), 61-69. doi:10.1515/jcim-2014-0004

Zanteson, L. (2011). Nutrition is "in the pink" with rhubarb. *Environmental Nutrition*, 34(4), 8.

REVIEWER(S)

Darlene Strayer, RN, MBA, Cinahl Information Systems, Glendale, CA

Nursing Executive Practice Council, Glendale Adventist Medical Center, Glendale, CA

Sour Cherry

WHAT WE KNOW

The sour, or tart, cherry (*Prunus cerasus*) is a descendant of the wild cherries that originated around 70 BC. Sour cherries are from the Rosaceae (i.e., rose) family, along with nectarines, peaches, apricots, and plums. Like their relatives, cherries are stone fruits, meaning they contain a stone, or pit, at their center. Cherries were highly valued by ancient Romans, Greeks, and Chinese royalty, and are considered a symbol for immortality in China today. A delicious culinary treat, sour cherries are frequently dried, baked in pies and cobblers, and made into jams and sauces. Beyond their value in cuisine, cherries have been used medicinally since the 15th century. They possess a wealth of nutrients, including vitamin C, potassium, important polyphenolic phytonutrients (i.e., protective, plant-derived nutrients), and fiber. Sour cherries are particularly praised for their high content of anthocyanins, which exhibit potent antioxidant activity. All of these nutrients provide sour cherries with powerful anti-inflammatory, antiviral, antioxidant, antibiotic, and pain relieving properties; sour cherries also have cancer-preventive and cardio-protective activity.

NUTRIENTS IN SOUR CHERRY

* Sour cherry contains important phytonutrients such as quercetin, genistein, naringenin, chlorogenic acid, and the highly acclaimed anthocyanins, which have antioxidant, anti-inflammatory, antibiotic, and anti-mutagenic properties, acting to protect deoxyribonucleic acid (DNA) against damage, enhance DNA repair, protect

blood vessels from rupture, promote urinary tract health, and support memory function.

- Sour cherry contains melatonin, which protects against free radicals and helps to regulate sleep/wake cycles.
- The water-soluble vitamin C in sour cherry neutralizes free radicals, protecting against inflammation and cellular damage. Adequate vitamin C intake is vital for the proper function of the immune system and has been associated with the prevention of heart disease, stroke, and cancer.
- Sour cherry contains potassium, which is an essential element responsible for regulating acid-base balance, maintaining fluid balance, supporting muscle contraction and cardiac function, contributing to protein building and carbohydrate breakdown, promoting cellular growth, and promoting transmission of nerve impulses.
- Sour cherry is an excellent source of dietary fiber, which binds and removes toxins from the colon, assists in glucose control, and reduces high cholesterol levels.

DIETARY INTAKE GUIDELINES

- There is no standard dosage of sour cherry for treatment, but studies have used the equivalent of 8 oz/day of pure cherry juice or 45 cherries.
- Sour cherry contains sorbitol, a sugar alcohol that can trigger painful symptoms in individuals with irritable bowel syndrome (IBS).
- Consuming therapeutic doses of cherry could enhance the blood-thinning activity of the drug warfarin.

RESEARCH FINDINGS

- The melatonin, serotonin, and tryptophan found in cherry can promote healthy nocturnal sleep cycles. Researchers suggest that cherry may be useful therapeutic tools for improving sleep patterns in older adults with sleep disturbances and insomnia.
- Results of a study conducted on obese rats indicated that consumption of sour cherries reduced multiple risks associated with developing metabolic syndrome and significantly reduced inflammation, lowering the risk for developing type II diabetes and heart disease. Specifically, sour cherry consumption was associated with reductions in body weight, abdominal fat, blood lipids, fasting glucose levels, and inflammation.

- The results of numerous studies show that tart cherry consumption can prevent exercise-induced muscle damage and soreness and aid muscle recovery following strenuous exercise.

SUMMARY

Consumers should become knowledgeable about the physiologic risks and benefits of sour cherry consumption. Sour cherry is a good source of dietary fiber, vitamin C, potassium, and many phytonutrients, including anthocyanins. These nutrients are anti-inflammatory, fight viruses and bacteria, and relieve pain, and may help decrease the risk of developing cancer and cardiovascular disease. Individuals with IBS should avoid sour cherry because it contains sorbitol, which can trigger painful symptoms in individuals with IBS. Consumers should be aware of drug-nutrient interactions associated with sour cherry.

—*Cherie Marcel, BS*

REFERENCES

Blando, F., Gerardi, C., & Nicoletti, I. (2004). Sour cherry (Prunus cerasus L) anthocyanins as ingredients for functional foods. *Journal of Biomedicine & Biotechnology*, *2004*(5), 253-258. doi:10.1155/S1110724304404136

Bowtell, J. L., Sumners, D. P., Dyer, A., Fox, P., & Mileva, K. N. (2011). Montmorency cherry juice reduces muscle damage caused by intensive strength exercise. *Medicine & Science in Sports & Exercise*, *43*(8), 1544-1551. doi:10.1249/MSS.0b013e31820e5adc

Connolly, D. A. J., McHugh, M. P., & Padilla-Zakour, O. I. (2006). Efficacy of tart cherry juice blend in preventing the symptoms of muscle damage. *British Journal of Sports Medicine*, *40*(8), 679-683.

Gable, C. (2008). Why tart cherry is tops: Find out how the juice of these sweet summer jewels can help quell pain and inflammation. *Better Nutrition*, *70*(7), 50.

Goodman, S. (2007). Cherries: Powerful pain relief, cancer defense, and neuroprotection. *Life Extension*, *13*(12), 81-83.

Howatson, G., McHugh, M. P., Hill, J. A., Brouner, J., Jewell, A. P., van Someren, K. A., ... Howatson, S. A. (2010). Influence of tart cherry juice on indices of recovery following marathon running. *Scandinavian Journal of Medicine & Science in Sports*, *20*(6), 843-852. doi:10.1111/j.1600-0838.2009.01005.x

Neithercott, T. (2012). Foods that fight pain. *Prevention*, *64*(9), 74-81.

Pigeon, W. R., Carr, M., Gorman, C., & Perlis, M. L. (2010). Effects of a tart cherry juice beverage on the sleep of older adults with insomnia: A pilot study. *Journal of Medicinal Food*, *13*(3), 579-583. doi:10.1089/jmf.2009.0096

Sego, S. (2012). Alternative meds update: Tart cherry. *Clinical Advisor for Nurse Practitioners*, *15*(5), 63-64.

Seymour, E. M., Lewis, S. K., Urcuyo-Llanes, D. E., Tanone, I. I., Kirakosyan, A., Kaufman, P. B., & Bolling, S. F. (2009). Regular tart cherry intake alters abdominal adiposity, adipose gene transcription, and inflammation in obesity-prone rats fed a high fat diet. *Journal of Medicinal Food*, *12*(5), 935-942. doi:10.1089/jmf.2008.0270

Zanteson, L. (2012). Pick cherries for peak nutrition. *Environmental Nutrition*, May, 8.

REVIEWER(S)

Darlene Strayer, RN, MBA, Cinahl Information Systems, Glendale, CA

Nursing Executive Practice Council, Glendale Adventist Medical Center, Glendale, CA

Strawberry

WHAT WE KNOW

There are over 600 varieties of strawberry, which are from the genus *Fragaria*. The strawberry is a member of the Rosaceae (i.e., rose) family along with nectarines, peaches, apricots, cherries, raspberries, and plums. Although the wild strawberry (*Fragaria vesca*) has existed for at least 2,000 years, commercially grown strawberries (*Fragaria ananassa* and *Fragaria virginiana*) have only been cultivated for about 300 years. With its sweet flavor and fragrance, this red, heart-shaped fruit is the most popular berry fruit in the world. Strawberries can be eaten raw, canned, dried, baked into pies or cobblers, made into jams and sauces, or blended into drinks. Beyond its value in cuisine, strawberry ranks fourth (following blackberries, cranberries, and raspberries) among fruits as a source of antioxidants. Strawberry possesses a wealth of nutrients, including vitamins C and K, manganese, folate, iodine, potassium, magnesium, omega-3 fatty acids, fiber, and a diverse collection of phytonutrients (i.e., protective, plant-derived chemicals). These nutrients provide strawberry with powerful anti-inflammatory, antioxidant, cancer-preventive, and cardio-protective activity. Strawberry has exhibited powerful cardiovascular support; improved

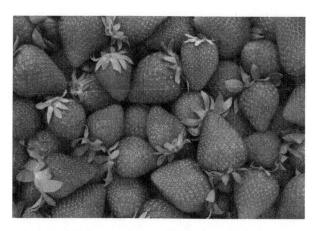

blood sugar regulation, reducing risk for diabetes mellitus, type 2 (DM2); and contributed to the prevention of cancers of the breast, colon, cervix, and esophagus.

NUTRIENTS IN STRAWBERRY

- Strawberry contains many valuable phytonutrients with antioxidant and anti-inflammatory activities, giving the strawberry great potential in reducing risk for cancer and heart disease. Some of these phytonutrients include the following:
  —Anthocyanins: Reddish-color pigments that have high antioxidant and anti-carcinogenic activity, promote urinary tract health, and support memory function. They also fight bacteria, such as *Streptococcus*, by disrupting bacterial cell membranes.
  —Flavonols: Quercetin, kaempferol, epicatechins, gallocatechins, catechins, and procyanidins provide strong antioxidant and anti-inflammatory protection. They also have antihistamine, antimicrobial, anti-diabetic, and anti-carcinogenic properties.
  —Hydroxybenzoic acids: Gallic acid is an antioxidant that has demonstrated the ability to prevent the cell proliferation of prostate cancer cells (i.e., prevents cancer cell growth). Ellagic acid exhibits anti-inflammatory properties and has been shown to reduce symptoms associated with Crohn's disease. Ellagic acid also fights carcinogens and slows cancer cell proliferation. Salicylic acid inhibits atherosclerosis.
  —Hydroxycinnamic acids: Exhibits anti-carcinogenic, antimicrobial, and antiviral properties. It is also believed to inhibit the buildup of LDL cholesterol.

—Stilbenes: Resveratrol prevents damage to blood vessels, lowers LDL cholesterol, and inhibits blood clots.

—Tannins: Have antioxidant, antihistamine, anti-cancer, and cardio-protective properties.

- The water-soluble vitamin C in strawberry neutralizes free radicals, protecting against inflammation and cellular damage. Adequate vitamin C intake is vital for the proper function of the immune system and has been associated with the prevention of heart disease, stroke, and cancer.

- The vitamin K in strawberry acts as a coenzyme involved in maintaining normal levels of blood clotting proteins and contributes to bone growth.

- Manganese, a trace mineral found in strawberry, is responsible for energy production, fatty acid production, necessary cholesterol production, and protection against the damage caused by free radicals.

- The trace mineral iodine in strawberry supports thyroid gland function and has antifungal, antimicrobial, and antibacterial activity.

- Strawberry contains magnesium, which balances the action of calcium in cells to regulate bone health, nerves, and muscle tone. It keeps the nerves and muscles relaxed, which contributes to the prevention of high blood pressure, muscle spasms, asthma, migraine headaches, general soreness, and fatigue.

- The water-soluble B vitamin folate in strawberry is essential for the production and maintenance of red blood cells. It is vital for the production of deoxyribonucleic acid (DNA) and ribonucleic acid (RNA), the genetic code for the cells, and is also important in the production of homocysteine (i.e., an amino acid).

- Strawberry contains potassium, which is an essential element responsible for regulating acid-base balance, maintaining fluid balance, supporting muscle contraction and cardiac function, contributing to protein building and carbohydrate breakdown, promoting cellular growth, and promoting transmission of nerve impulses.

- Strawberry is a good source of dietary fiber, which binds and removes toxins from the colon, assists in glucose control, and reduces high cholesterol levels.

- The essential omega-3, or alpha-linolenic, fatty acids in strawberry support cardiovascular function and reduce the risk for Alzheimer's disease.

DIETARY INTAKE GUIDELINES

- There is some concern that strawberry can increase the risk of kidney stones in individuals with a history of kidney stones because strawberry contains a high amount of the chemical oxalate, which is a primary component of kidney stones. Oxalates can build up and crystallize in body fluids and cause health problems in individuals with preexisting kidney or gallbladder dysfunction.

RESEARCH FINDINGS

- Anthocyanins and ellagitannins, types of polyphenols found in strawberry, are able to slow the digestion of starch, protein, and oil, which helps to stabilize blood sugar. Strawberry has also been shown to improve antioxidant status and reduce cell damage and inflammatory response in patients with type II diabetes, and lower cholesterol and reduce risk factors (e.g., dyslipidemia) for cardiovascular disease, stroke, and DM2 in obese persons. These factors make strawberry a potential tool for the treatment and prevention of metabolic syndrome and its related conditions insulin resistance, type II diabetes, hypertension, heart disease, and obesity.

SUMMARY

Consumers should become knowledgeable about the physiologic effects of strawberry consumption. Strawberry is a good source of vitamins C and K, manganese, folate, iodine, potassium, magnesium, omega-3 fatty acids, fiber, and many phytonutrients. These nutrients provide powerful cardiovascular support, improve blood sugar regulation, reduce risk for DM2, and contribute to the prevention of cancers of the breast, colon, cervix, and esophagus. Individuals with a history of kidney stones should be aware that strawberry increases risk for kidney stones because it contains high amounts of oxalate, a primary component of kidney stones.

—*Cherie Marcel, BS*

REFERENCES

Basu, A., Fu, D. X., Wilkinson, M., Simmons, B., Wu, M., Betts, N. M., & Lyons, T. J. (2010). Strawberries decrease atherosclerotic markers in subjects with metabolic syndrome. *Nutrition Research*, 30(7), 462-469. doi:10.1016/j.nutres.2010.06.016

Edirisinghe, I., Banaszewski, K., Cappozzo, J., Sandhya, K., Ellis, C. L., Tadapaneni, R., & Burton-Freeman, B. M. (2011). Strawberry anthocyanin and its association with postprandial inflammation and insulin. *British Journal of Nutrition*, 106(6), 913-922. doi:10.1017/S0007114511001176

The George Mateljan Foundation editorial team. (n.d.). Can you tell me what oxalates are and in which foods they can be found?. *The World's Healthiest Foods*. Retrieved March 5, 2015, from http://www.whfoods.com/genpage.php?tname=george&dbid=48

The George Mateljan Foundation editorial team. (n.d.). Strawberries. *The World's Healthiest Foods*. Retrieved March 5, 2015, from http://www.whfoods.com/genpage.php? tname=foodspice&dbid=32

Giampieri, F., Tulipani, S., Alvarez-Suarez, J. M., Quiles, J. L., Mezzetti, B., & Battino, M. (2012). The strawberry: Composition, nutritional quality, and impact on human health. *Nutrition*, 28(1), 9-19. doi:10.1016/j.nut.2011.08.009

Henning, S. M., Seeram, N. P., Zhang, Y., Gao, K., Lee, R. P., Wang, D. C., & Heber, D. (2010). Strawberry consumption is associated with increased antioxidant capacity in serum. *Journal of Medicinal Food*, 13(1), 116-122. doi:10.1089/jmf.2009.0048

Keville, K. (2012). Herb profile: Medicinal berries. *American Herb Association Quarterly Newsletter*, 27(1), 3.

Moazen, S., Amani, R., Homayouni, R. A., Shahbazian, H., Ahmadi, K., & Taha Jalali, M. (2013). Effects of freeze-dried strawberry supplementation on metabolic biomarkers of atherosclerosis in subjects with type 2 diabetes: A randomized double-blind controlled trial. *Annals of Nutrition & Metabolism*, 63(3), 256-264. doi:10.1159/000356053

Sesso, H. D., Gaziano, J. M., Jenkins, D. J., & Buring, J. E. (2007). Strawberry intake, lipids, C-reactive protein, and the risk of cardiovascular disease in women. *Journal of the American College of Nutrition*, 26(4), 303-310. doi:10.1080/07315724.2007.10719615

Tulipani, S., Mezzetti, B., & Battino, M. (2009). Impact of strawberries on human health: Insight into marginally discussed bioactive compounds for the Mediterranean diet. *Public Health Nutrition*, 12(9A), 1656-1662. doi:10.1017/S1368980009990516

Zunino, S. J., Parelman, M. A., Freytag, T. L., Stephensen, C. B., Kelley, D. S., Mackey, B. E., & Bonnel, E. L.

(2012). Effects of dietary strawberry powder on blood lipids and inflammatory markers in obese human subjects. *British Journal of Nutrition*, 108(5), 900-909. doi:10.1017/S000711451100602

REVIEWER(S)

Darlene Strayer, RN, MBA, Cinahl Information Systems, Glendale, CA

Nursing Executive Practice Council, Glendale Adventist Medical Center, Glendale, CA

Tomatoes

WHAT WE KNOW

Tomatoes are technically the berries of the *Lycopersicon esculentum* (i.e., *Solanum lycopersicum*) plant, which is a member of the *Solanaceae* (i.e., solanoid, or "nightshade") family. There are over 1,000 different varieties of tomatoes that vary in size from small cherry tomatoes to large beefsteak tomatoes. They can be yellow, green, orange, purple, brown, and red, and are typically round or oval but some varieties are more flattened in shape, grooved, and/or knotty. Tomatoes have a sweet, acidic, and somewhat tart flavor and are typically categorized as a vegetable for culinary use. They can be eaten raw, separately or in salads, stewed, sautéed, dried, sauced, or juiced. Nutritionally, tomatoes have been referred to as a "super food" due to their high content of nutrients. They are a rich source of the antioxidant vitamins, C and E, and provide many phytonutrients (i.e., beneficial, plant-derived chemicals). Consuming tomatoes has been associated with improved bone density and reduced risk for cardiovascular disease (CVD), cancer, and neurologic diseases (e.g., Alzheimer's disease).

NUTRIENTS IN TOMATOES

- Tomatoes are a good source of health-promoting vitamins and minerals, including the following:
  —Vitamin C is a water-soluble vitamin that neutralizes free radicals, protecting against inflammation and cellular damage. Adequate vitamin C intake is important for the proper function of the immune system and has been associated with the prevention of heart disease, stroke, and cancer.
  —Vitamin E is a fat-soluble vitamin that functions primarily as an antioxidant, but also maintains cell membranes, assists in vitamin

K absorption, and contributes to immune system function.

—Vitamin K acts as a coenzyme in helping maintain normal levels of blood clotting proteins, and contributes to bone growth.

—The B vitamin pyridoxine is required for the conversion of tryptophan into niacin, and is involved in the conversion of homocysteine to cysteine. It supports the production of serotonin and dopamine, which are neurotransmitters required for nerve cell communication. By maintaining lymphoid organs, pyridoxine contributes to immune system function.

—The B vitamins thiamin, folate, and niacin create energy by aiding the breakdown of carbohydrates. They provide cardiovascular protection, maintain the nervous system, and support the production of red blood cells, hormones, and necessary cholesterol.

—The B vitamin choline produces the metabolite betaine, which assists in the regulation of inflammation in the cardiovascular system by preventing elevated levels of homocysteine. Betaine is associated with reduced levels of the inflammatory markers C reactive protein (CRP), interleukin-6, and tumor necrosis factor-alpha (TNF-α).

—Potassium supports normal cellular, nerve, and muscle function, and helps to eliminate excess sodium from the body.

—Manganese is a trace mineral that is responsible for energy production, fatty acid production, necessary cholesterol production, and protection against the damage caused by free radicals.

—Copper is an important component of superoxide dismutase, which is an enzyme involved in energy production and antioxidant activity. Copper contributes to the action of lysyl oxidase, an enzyme necessary for the cross-linking of collagen and elastin that allows flexibility in the blood vessels, bones, and joints. Copper enhances the body's ability to use iron, preventing iron-deficient anemia, ruptured vessels, irregular heartbeat, and infection.

—Magnesium balances the action of calcium in cells for the regulation of bone health and tone of nerves and muscles. Copper maintains relaxation of nerves and muscles, which

contributes to the prevention of high blood pressure, muscle spasms, asthma, migraine headaches, general soreness, and fatigue.

—Phosphorous combines with calcium for the formation of bones and teeth, muscle contraction, and nerve conduction, and is essential for the structural integrity of cell membranes.

—Iron is essential for the production of red blood cells and hemoglobin, which are necessary for energy production and transport of oxygen to the tissues. Iron supports immune function, is essential for cognitive development, contributes to energy production, and regulates temperature.

• Tomatoes are a powerful source of valuable phytonutrients such as flavanone, flavonols, hydroxycinnamic acids, carotenoids, glycosides, and fatty acid derivatives. These phytonutrients are potent antioxidants that are known to support cardiovascular health, protect against cancer, and support the health of the bones, liver, kidneys and bloodstream. Some notable phytonutrients in tomatoes include the following:

—The carotenoids lycopene, lutein, and zeaxanthin are antioxidants that inhibit the inflammatory process, neutralize free radicals, impede cancer cell proliferation (i.e., prevents cancer cell growth), and repair damaged deoxyribonucleic acid (DNA). They prevent atherosclerosis and protect the eyes from light-induced damage, promoting eye health.

–Pro-vitamin A carotenoids (e.g., beta-carotene) are the precursors for vitamin A, or retinol, a fat-soluble vitamin that is required for vision, maintenance of the surface lining of the eyes and other epithelial tissue, bone growth, immune response, energy regulation, reproduction, embryonic development, and activation of gene expression.

—The flavonols rutin, quercetin, and kaempferol provide strong antioxidant and anti-inflammatory protection. They have antihistamine, antimicrobial, anti-diabetic, and cancer-fighting properties.

—The hydroxycinnamic acid caffeic acid exhibits cancer-fighting, antimicrobial, and antiviral properties. Caffeic acid is believed to inhibit the build-up of low-density lipoprotein (LDL) cholesterol (i.e., the "bad" cholesterol).

- Tomatoes are a source of the amino acid tryptophan, which contributes to the synthesis of niacin and serotonin. Serotonin is thought to promote healthy sleep patterns and stabilize mood.

RESEARCH FINDINGS
- Results of many studies show that consumption of tomatoes/other foods containing lycopene is associated with decreased risk for several types of cancer, including ovarian, gastric, pancreatic, and prostate cancer. Researchers report that consuming tomatoes could significantly decrease the risk for prostate cancer in particular because lycopene tends to concentrate in prostate tissues. This cancer-protective effect appears to be stronger if tomatoes are processed into sauces, juices, or pastes because these processes allow the phytonutrients to be released and easily absorbed.
- Authors of a 2-year comparative study of juices made from organic and nonorganic tomatoes in Poland reported that the organically cultivated tomato juice contained more phytonutrients than the non-organically cultivated juice. However, researchers also noted that the juice produced in 2008 contained more carotenoids and flavonoids than the juice produced in 2009, indicating that the phytonutrient composition was more dramatically affected by the year of cultivation than by the method of cultivation.

RELATED GUIDELINES
A review of available literature revealed no dietary guidelines regarding dietary consumption of tomatoes

SUMMARY
Consumers should become knowledgeable about the physiologic effects of consuming tomatoes. Tomatoes are a good source of powerful antioxidants, vitamins, minerals, and phytonutrients. These nutrients improve bone density, promote eye health, and reduce risk for CVD, cancer, and neurologic diseases.

—*Cherie Marcel, BS*

REFERENCES

AICR editorial staff. (2014, November 18). Foods that fight cancer? Tomatoes. *American Institute for Cancer Research*. Retrieved March 6, 2015, from http://www. aicr.org/foods-that-fight-cancer/foodsthatfightcancer_ tomatoes.html

Basu, A., & Imrhan, V. (2007). Tomatoes versus lycopene in oxidative stress and carcinogenesis: Conclusions from clinical trials. *European Journal of Clinical Nutrition, 61*(3), 295-303. doi:10. 1038/ sj.ejcn.1602510

Durkin, P. (2008). Health from the vine: Tomatoes are nutritional all-stars. *Alive: Canada's Natural Health & Wellness Magazine*. Retrieved March 6, 2015, from http:// www.alive.com/articles/view/21981/ health_from_the_vine

Eat right to fight cancer: Tomatoes. (2011). *Oncology Nutrition Connection, 19*(2), 16-18.

Hallmann, E., Lipowski, J., Marszalek, K., & Rembialkowska, E. (2013). The seasonal variation in bioactive compounds content in juice from organic and non-organic tomatoes. *Plant Foods for Human Nutrition* , *68*(2), 171-176. doi:10.1007/ s11130-013-0352-2

Kavanaugh, C. J., Trumbo, P. R., & Ellwood, K. C. (2007). The U. S. Food and Drug Adminstration's evidence-based review for qualified health claims: Tomatoes, lycopene, and cancer. *JNCI: Hournal of the National Cancer Institute, 99*(14), 1074-1085.

Palmer, S. (2012). Can tomatoes slice prostate cancer risk?. *Today's Dietitian, 14*(6), 20-25.

The George Mateljan Foundation editorial staff. (n.d.). The world's healthiest foods: Tomatoes. *World's Healthiest Foods*. Retrieved March 6, 2015, from http:// www.whfoods.com/genpage. php?tname=foodspice&dbid=44

Tomatoes lower men's stroke risk. (2013). *Tufts University Health & Nutrition Letter, 30*(11), 1-3.

REVIEWER(S)

Darlene Strayer, RN, MBA, Cinahl Information Systems, Glendale, CA
Nursing Executive Practice Council, Glendale Adventist Medical Center, Glendale, CA

Watermelon

WHAT WE KNOW
Watermelon (*Citrullis lanatus*) is member of the *Cucurbitaceae* family along with honeydew, cantaloupe, musk melon, and bitter melon. Worldwide, there are hundreds of varieties of watermelon. The creeping vine of the watermelon plant produces large, round, oblong, or spherical fruit with a thick, green rind. Watermelon is about

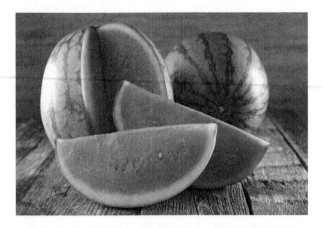

92% water, which gives the flesh a juicy and refreshing quality. The crisp flesh of the watermelon ranges in color from pink to a deep red and has a sweet flavor. Although watermelon traditionally contained black seeds that were spaced randomly throughout the flesh, seedless varieties have become increasingly available and account for 85% of all watermelon that is currently grown in the United States. Watermelon is frequently eaten raw, but can also be canned, used in drinks, pickled, and made into dressings and sauces. Watermelon is a good source of amino acids; potassium; magnesium; many valuable phytonutrients (i.e., beneficial, pant-derived chemicals), including lycopene and pro-vitamin A carotenoids; and vitamins C and B6. These nutrients provide watermelon with antioxidant, anti-inflammatory, cancer-preventive, and cardio-protective properties.

NUTRIENTS IN WATERMELON

- Watermelon is rich in phytonutrients, including flavonoids, carotenoids, and tripterpenoids, which have strong anti-inflammatory and antioxidant properties.
  - Watermelon is particularly noted for containing the carotenoid lycopene, which is responsible for the pinkish-red color of the fruit. Lycopene inhibits the inflammatory process, neutralizes free radicals, impedes cancer cell proliferation (e.g., in prostate cancer), repairs damaged deoxyribonucleic acid (DNA), and is a powerful antioxidant.
  - The pro-vitamin A carotenoids (e.g., beta-carotene) are the precursors for vitamin A, or retinol, a fat-soluble vitamin that is required for vision, maintenance of the surface lining of the eyes and other epithelial tissue, bone growth, immune response, energy regulation, reproduction, embryonic development, and activation of gene expression.
  - The tripterpenoid cucurbitacin E in watermelon exhibits strong anti-inflammatory activity.
- Watermelon is a good source of the amino acid citrulline, which metabolizes to the amino acid arginine, which slows the formation of blood clots and relaxes the arteries. Another byproduct of citrulline is nitric oxide (NO), a muscle relaxant.
- Watermelon is an excellent source of vitamin C, which neutralizes free radicals, protecting against inflammation and cellular damage. Adequate vitamin C intake is important for immune system function and has been associated with the prevention of heart disease, stroke, and cancer.
- Vitamin B6 is required for the conversion of tryptophan to niacin, and is involved in the conversion of homocysteine to cysteine. It is necessary for the synthesis of serotonin and dopamine, which are neurotransmitters required for nerve cell communication. By maintaining the lymphoid organs, vitamin B6 contributes to the proper function of the immune system. It is essential for building and breaking down amino acids, carbohydrates, and lipids, and is important for formation of red blood cells and hemoglobin, which carries oxygen to the tissues.
- Potassium supports normal cellular, nerve, and muscle function and helps eliminate excess sodium from the body.
- The magnesium provided by watermelon balances the action of calcium in cells to regulate bone health and tone of nerves and muscles. It maintains relaxation of nerves and muscles, which contributes to the prevention of high blood pressure, muscle spasm, asthma, migraine headache, general soreness, and fatigue.

RESEARCH FINDINGS

- A clinical trial was conducted to determine the effect of melon juice supplementation on perceived stress and fatigue based on the hypothesis that perceived stress is associated with oxidative stress. Researchers reported that the group receiving oral melon juice supplementation showed improvement in several signs and symptoms of stress and fatigue. However, a similar study found no notable improvements in perceived stress in the participants receiving the extract.

- Researchers conducted a study measuring the effect of watermelon supplementation on arterial stiffness in obese postmenopausal women with hypertension. Results of the study showed that watermelon supplementation can reduce aortic systolic blood pressure and arterial stiffness by lowering the pressure wave reflection amplitude.

SUMMARY

Consumers should become knowledgeable about the physiologic benefits of consuming watermelon. Watermelon is a good source of powerful antioxidants, vitamins, minerals, and phytonutrients. These nutrients support eye health, lower blood pressure, and may help prevent cancer and heart disease.

—*Cherie Marcel, BS*

REFERENCES

Figueroa, A., Wong, A., Hooshmand, S., & Sanchez-Gonzalez, M. A. (2013). Effects of watermelon supplementation on arterial stiffness and wave reflection amplitude in postmenopausal women. *Menopause* (10723714), 20(5), 573-577. doi:10.1097/GME.0b013e3182733794

Edward, J. (2013, October 12). Benefits of watermelon for men. *Livestrong.com*. Retrieved March 17, 2015, from http://www.livestrong.com/article/359133-watermelons-health-benefits-for-men/

Houghton, C. A., Steels, E. L., Fassett, R. G., & Coombes, J. S. (2011). Effects of a gliadin-combined plant superoxide dismutase extract on self-perceived fatigue in women aged 50--65 years. *Phytomedicine*, 18(6), 521-526. doi:10.1016/j.phymed.2010.09.006

Liddell, A. (2013, December 18). The health benefits of melons. Livestrong.com. Retrieved March 17, 2015, from http://www.livestrong.com/article/407556-the-health-benefits-of-melons/

Milesi, M. A., Lacan, D., Brosse, H., Desor, D., & Notin, C. (2009). Effect of an oral supplementation with a proprietary melon juice concentrate (Extramel) on stress and fatigue in healthy people: A pilot, double-blind, placebo-controlled clinical trial. *Nutrition Journal*, 8, 40. doi:10.1186/1475-2891-8-40

The George Mateljan Foundation editorial team. (2011). The world's healthiest foods: Watermelon. Retrieved May 17, 2015, fromhttp://www.whfoods.com/genpage.php? tname=foodspice&dbid=31

REVIEWER(S)

Darlene Strayer, RN, MBA, Cinahl Information Systems, Glendale, CA

Nursing Executive Practice Council, Glendale Adventist Medical Center, Glendale, CA

Wild Cherry

WHAT WE KNOW

The wild, or sweet, cherry (*Prunus avium*) is a descendant of the wild cherries that originated around 70 BC. Wild cherry is from the Rosaceae (i.e., rose) family, along with nectarines, peaches, apricots, and plums. Like their relatives, cherries are stone fruits, meaning they contain a stone, or pit, at their center. Cherries were highly valued by ancient Romans, Greeks, and Chinese royalty, and are considered a symbol for immortality in China today. One example of a wild cherry is the popular Bing cherry, known for its candy-sweet flavor and robust size. Wild cherries are delicious when eaten raw, but can also be canned, dried, baked in pies and cobblers, made into jams and sauces, and blended in drinks. Beyond their value in cuisine, cherries have been used medicinally since the 15th century. They possess a wealth of nutrients, including vitamin C, potassium, fiber, and important polyphenolic phytonutrients (i.e., protective, plant-derived nutrients) such as the highly praised anthyocyanins, which exhibit potent antioxidant activity. All of these nutrients provide wild cherries with powerful anti-inflammatory, antiviral, antioxidant, antibiotic, and pain-relieving properties; cherries also have cancer-preventive and cardio-protective activity. Wild cherry bark is appreciated for its medicinal properties. The inner bark of the wild cherry can be used in infusions, decoctions, cough syrup, and tinctures as a treatment for chest congestion.

NUTRIENTS IN WILD CHERRY

- Wild cherry contains important phytonutrients such as quercetin, genistein, naringenin, chlorogenic acid, and the highly acclaimed anthocyanins, which have antioxidant, anti-inflammatory, antibiotic, and anti-mutagenic properties, acting to protect deoxyribonucleic acid (DNA) against damage, enhance DNA repair, protect blood vessels from rupture, promote urinary tract health, and support memory function.

- Wild cherry contains melatonin, tryptophan, and serotonin, which protect against free radicals and help regulate sleep/wake cycles.
- The water-soluble vitamin C in wild cherry neutralizes free radicals, protecting against inflammation and cellular damage. Adequate vitamin C intake is vital for the proper function of the immune system and has been associated with the prevention of heart disease, stroke, and cancer.
- Wild cherry contains potassium, which is an essential element responsible for regulating acid-base balance, maintaining fluid balance, supporting muscle contraction and cardiac function, contributing to protein building and carbohydrate breakdown, promoting cellular growth, and promoting transmission of nerve impulses.
- Wild cherry is an excellent source of dietary fiber, which binds and removes toxins from the colon, assists in glucose control, and reduces high cholesterol levels.
- Wild cherry bark is thought to provide medicinal benefits as an expectorant (i.e., cough medicine), antispasmodic, antiseptic, antitussive, and soother of respiratory nerves, but more research is needed to confirm these benefits.

DIETARY INTAKE GUIDELINES

- There is no standard dosage of cherry for treatment, but studies have used the equivalent of 8 oz/day of pure cherry juice or 45 cherries.
- The common dosage for wild cherry bark is a standard infusion of 3–9g or 10–15 drops of tincture.
- Consuming therapeutic doses of cherries could enhance the blood thinning activity of the drug warfarin.
- Wild cherry could increase the effects of medications that are broken down by the liver, including the following:
  —Lovastatin (Mevacor)
  —Ketoconazole (Nizoral)
  —Itraconazole (Sporanox)
  —Fexofenadine (Allegra)
  —Triazolam (Halcion)

RESEARCH FINDINGS

- Researchers have determined that consuming Bing cherry can effectively lower certain inflammatory markers (e.g., C-reactive protein, nitric oxide) in healthy men and women. This anti-inflammatory activity is potentially useful for the management and prevention of inflammatory diseases (e.g., arthritis, cardiovascular disease).
- The results of numerous studies show that cherry consumption can prevent exercise-induced muscle damage and soreness and aid muscle recovery following strenuous exercise.
- Researchers report that consumption of the wild cherry grown in Jerte Valley, Spain can improve sleep and prevent oxidation. They suggest that the melatonin, tryptophan, and serotonin found in cherries promotes healthy nocturnal sleep cycles and that cherries could be useful therapeutic tools for improving sleep patterns in older adults with sleep disturbances and insomnia.

SUMMARY

Consumers should become knowledgeable about the physiologic risks and benefits of wild cherry consumption. Wild cherry is a good source of vitamin C, potassium, fiber, and important phytonutrients, including anthyocyanins. These nutrients are anti-inflammatory, antiviral, antioxidant, and antibiotic, relieve pain, and may help prevent cancer and cardiovascular disease. Consuming therapeutic doses of wild cherry can enhance the blood thinning activity of the drug warfarin. Wild cherry consumption could increase the effects of medications that are broken down by the liver.

—*Cherie Marcel, BS*

REFERENCES

Bowers, K. (2006). Breathe easy. *New Life Journal*, 39.

Garrido, M., Paredes, S. D., Cubero, J., Lozano, M., Toribio-Delgado, A. F., Munoz, J. L., & Rodriguez, A. B. (2010). Jerte Valley cherry-enriched diets improve nocturnal rest and increase 6-sulfatoxymelatonin and total antioxidant capacity in the urine of middle-aged and elderly humans. *Journals of Gerontology Series A: Biological Sciences & Medical Sciences*, 65A(9), 909-914. doi:10.1093/gerona/glq099

Goodman, S. (2007). Cherries: Powerful pain relief, cancer defense, and neuroprotection. *Life Extension*, 13(12), 81-83.

Kelley, D. S., Rasooly, R., Jacob, R. A., Kader, A. A., & Mackey, B. E. (2006). Consumption of Bing sweet cherries lowers circulating concentrations of inflammation markers in healthy men and women. *The Journal of Nutrition*, 136(4), 981-986.

Neithercott, T. (2012). Foods that fight pain. *Prevention*, *64*(9), 74-81.

Pigeon, W. R., Carr, M., Gorman, C., & Perlis, M. L. (2010). Effects of a tart cherry juice beverage on the sleep of older adults with insomnia: A pilot study. *Journal of Medicinal Food*, *13*(3), 579-583. doi:10.1089/jmf.2009.0096

Spitalnick, A. (2011). This just in: Bing cherries. *Vegetarian Times*, *37*(6), 16.

WebMD Editorial Team. (2014, November 19). Wild cherry: Uses, side effects, interactions, and warnings. *WebMD*. Retrieved March 24, 2015, from http://www.webmd.com/vitamins-supplements/ingredient-mono-888-wild+cherry.aspx?activeIngredientId=888&activeIngredientName=wild+cherry&source=1

Zanteson, L. (2012). Pick cherries for peak nutrition. *Environmental Nutrition*, 8.

REVIEWER(S)

Darlene Strayer, RN, MBA, Cinahl Information Systems, Glendale, CA

Nursing Executive Practice Council, Glendale Adventist Medical Center, Glendale, CA

VEGETABLES

Artichoke

WHAT WE KNOW

The artichoke, or *Cynara*, is an ancient perennial thistle plant from the sunflower, or *Asteraceae* family. Although native to the Mediterranean, the globe variety *Cynara scolymus* is grown primarily along the California coast and is currently the most commonly eaten artichoke. The silvery-green artichoke plant produces large green and, in some varieties, purple-tinged flower buds that are commonly recognized as the artichoke. Appreciated as a culinary delicacy, artichoke is not easy to prepare or eat, but its flavor is undeniable and it contains valuable nutrition. Artichoke is rich in fiber and provides nutrients such as iron, magnesium, phosphorous, potassium, calcium, and vitamins C, K, and folate. Artichoke is a notable source of phytonutrients (i.e., beneficial, plant-derived nutrients), especially cynarin and silymarin. Together, these nutrients provide the artichoke with antioxidant and anti-inflammatory properties that prevent heart disease, and multiple types of cancer (e.g., prostate, breast, and leukemia) and promote optimal liver, gallbladder, and overall digestive health.

NUTRIENTS IN ARTICHOKE

- Artichoke is rich in many phytochemicals, including the following:
  - —Cynarin and silymarin have strong antioxidant properties and are believed to aid in the regeneration of liver tissue.
  - —Luteolin is a potent antioxidant and anti-carcinogenic compound.
  - —Anthocyanins, which reddish color pigments that have high antioxidant and anticarcinogenic activity, promote urinary tract health and support memory function.
  - —The flavonoids quercetin and rutin function as anti-inflammatory agents, promote vascular health, and exhibit anti-carcinogenic activity.

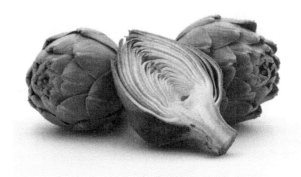

  - —Caffeic and chlorogenic acids exhibit anti-carcinogenic, anti-microbial and anti-viral properties. These acids are also believed to inhibit the build-up of LDL cholesterol (i.e., the "bad" cholesterol).
  - —Gallic acid is an antioxidant that has demonstrated the ability to prevent proliferation of prostate cancer cells.
- Artichoke contains vitamin K, which acts as a coenzyme in maintaining normal levels of blood clotting proteins and contributes to bone metabolism.
- Artichoke contains the immunity-enhancing antioxidant vitamin C, which aids in the absorption of iron.
- Some of the minerals found in artichoke include magnesium, phosphorous, potassium, calcium, manganese, copper, and iron. These provide many health benefits, including maintaining cell regulation, controlling blood pressure, promoting bone formation, assisting with wound healing, and promoting blood cell production.
- Artichokes contain insulin, a polyfructan carbohydrate that serves as a prebiotic with the ability to promote the growth of intestinal flora (i.e., beneficial bacteria in the intestines).
- Artichokes are a good source of dietary fiber, including soluble fiber, which binds with water and slows the digestive process, allowing the body to better manage postprandial (i.e., after eating)

glucose and insulin responses. Fiber increases the volume of the intestinal contents, which hinders the absorption of cholesterol. The added bulk also leads to more regular bowel movements, promoting intestinal health.

RESEARCH FINDINGS

- Results of many studies confirm the powerful antioxidant and anti-inflammatory properties of artichoke. Research results show that artichoke protects the liver by protecting liver cells, and inducing death of liver cancer cells. Similarly, study results support the claim that artichoke contains compounds that induce break down of leukemia cells as well as breast and prostate cancer cells.

- Artichoke leaf extract (ALE) has demonstrated the ability to reduce plasma cholesterol in persons with high cholesterol. Researchers suggest that ALE presents a well tolerated, effective treatment option for high cholesterol and suggest further research in this area.

- Researchers observed that ALE contains compounds (i.e., cynarin and cyanidin) that down-regulate the expression of inducible nitric oxide synthase (iNOS) in the smooth muscle cells of the coronary vascular system. Nitric oxide (NO) is usually produced by endothelial-type nitric oxide synthase (eNOS), but conditions of inflammation, sepsis, or oxidative stress induce iNOS, which can result in the production of large amounts of NO, leading to vascular dysfunction. This study provides evidence that ALE compounds possess therapeutic potential in the treatment of vascular dysfunction.

- Although it has been theorized that ALE can be used to treat symptoms of alcohol-induced hangover results of a double-blind, crossover, placebo-controlled study showed that ALE provided no more benefit than a placebo.

SUMMARY

Consumers should become knowledgeable about the physiologic effects of artichoke consumption. Artichokes are a good source of fiber, iron, magnesium, phosphorous, potassium, calcium, and vitamins C, K, and folate. Artichoke is a notable source of phytonutrients, especially cynarin and silymarin. The nutritional benefits of consuming artichokes include, preventing heart disease, and multiple types of cancer (e.g., prostate, breast, and leukemia) and promoting optimal liver, gallbladder, and overall digestive health.

—*Cherie Marcel, BS*

REFERENCES

Artichoke extract to treat alcohol-induced hangover. (2004). *ACOG Clinical Review, 9*(4), 11-12.

Bowden, J., & Bessinger, J. (2011). World's healthiest foods. At the "heart" of spring. *Better Nutrition, 73*(5), 54.

Bundy, R., Walker, A. F., Middleton, R. W., Wallis, C., & Simpson, H. C. R. (2008). Artichoke leaf extract (Cynara scolymus) reduces plasma cholesterol in otherwise healthy hypercholesterolemic adults: A randomized, double blind placebo controlled trial. *Phytomedicine, 15*(9), 668-675. doi:10.1016/j.phymed.2008.03.001

Eder, C. (2011). The amazing artichoke. *Life Extension, 17*(11), 1-3.

Joy, J. F., & Haber, S. L. (2007). Alternative therapies. Clinical uses of artichoke leaf extract. *American Journal of Health-System Pharmacy, 64*(18), 1904, 1906-1909. doi:10.2146/ajhp070013

Keller, A. C. (2013). Artichoke leaf extract improves HDL cholesterol levels in patients with hypercholesterolemia. *HerbalGram*, (30).

Miadokova, E., Nadova, S., Vlckova, V., Duhova, V., Kopaskova, M., Cipak, L., & Grancai, D. (2008). Antigenotoxic effect of extract from Cynara cardunculus L. *Phytotherapy Research, 22*(1), 77-81. doi:10.1002/ptr.2268

Miccadei, S., Di Venere, D., Cardinali, A., Romano, F., Durazzo, A., Foddai, M. S., & Maiani, G. (2008). Antioxidative and apoptotic properties of polyphenolic extracts from edible part of artichoke (Cynara scolymus L.) on cultured rat hepatocytes and on human hepatoma cells. *Nutrition and Cancer, 60*(2), 276-283. doi:10.1080/01635580801891583

Nadova, S., Miadokova, E., Mucaji, P., Grancai, D., & Cipak, L. (2008). Growth inhibitory effect of ethyl acetate-soluble fraction of Cynara cardunculus L. in leukemia cells involves cell cycle arrest, cytochrome c release and activation of caspases. *Phytotherapy Research, 22*(2), 165-168. doi:10.1002/ptr.2263

Nilsen, E. S., Sæterdal, I., & Underland, V. (2011). Artichoke leaf extract for hypercholesterolemia. *Alternative Therapies in Health and Medicine, 17*(6), 18-20.

Palmer, S. (2010). Getting to the heart of artichokes. *Environmental Nutrition, 33*(7), 8.

Ramnani, P., Gaudier, E., Bingham, M., van Bruggen, P., Tuohy, K. M., & Gibson, G. R. (2010). Prebiotic effect of fruit and vegetable shots containing Jerusalem artichoke inulin: A human intervention study. *British Journal of Nutrition, 104*(2), 233-240. doi:10.1017/S000711451000036X

Rondanelli, M., Giacosa, A., Opizzi, A., Faliva, M. A., Perna, S., Riva, A., ... Bombardelli, E. (2013). Beneficial effects of artichoke leaf extract supplementation on increasing HDL-cholesterol in subjects with primary mild hypercholesterolaemia: A double-blind, randomized, placebo-controlled trial. *International Journal of Food Sciences & Nutrition, 64*(1), 7-15. doi:10.3109/09637486.2012.700920

Wider, B., & Bundy, R. (2008). Cynara scolymus (artichoke) yields modest reductions of plasma total cholesterol. *Focus on Alternative and Complementary Therapies, 13*(4), 259-260. doi:10.1211/fact.13.4.0009

Wider, B., Pittler, M. H., Thompson-Coon, J., & Ernst, E. (2013). Artichoke leaf extract for treating hypercholesterolaemia. *Cochrane Database of Systematic Reviews,* 3. Art. No.: CD003335. doi:10.1002/14651858.CD003335

Xia, N., Pautz, A., Wallscheid, U., Reifenberg, G., Forstermann, U., & Li, H. (2014). Artichoke, cynarin and cyanidin downregulate the expression of inducible nitric oxide synthase in human coronary smooth muscle cells. *Molecules (Basel, Switzerland), 19*(3), 3654-3668. doi:10.3390/molecules19033654

REVIEWER(S)

Darlene Strayer, RN, MBA, Cinahl Information Systems, Glendale, CA

Nursing Executive Practice Council, Glendale Adventist Medical Center, Glendale, CA

Asparagus

WHAT WE KNOW

Asparagus, or *Asparagus officinalis*, is an ancient perennial garden vegetable from the lily, or *Liliaceae* family, which is native to Europe, Asia, and North Africa. Although about 300 varieties of asparagus exist, only 20 varieties are edible. Asparagus has long fibrous spears that are topped with tightly budded heads and has a flavor that is rich and earthy. Appreciated as a culinary delicacy, asparagus can be eaten raw or cooked. Green is the most common color variety of asparagus, but asparagus is also available in the more delicate white and purple varieties. Asparagus also has a long history of medicinal uses, particularly in the treatment of digestive conditions. Asparagus is rich in fiber and provides a wealth of nutrients such as folate, iron, magnesium, phosphorous, potassium, calcium, sodium, zinc, and vitamins B, C, E, and K. Asparagus is also a good source of phytochemicals (i.e., beneficial, plant-derived chemicals), including beta carotene and chlorophyll. Together these nutrients cause asparagus to have antioxidant, anti-carcinogenic, antimicrobial, and anti-inflammatory properties, which promote optimal digestive health and reduce risk for diabetes mellitus, heart disease, and cancer.

NUTRIENTS IN ASPARAGUS

- Asparagus is rich in many phytochemicals, including the following:
  - —Beta-carotene, a precursor to vitamin A, which provides powerful antioxidant, anti-viral, and anti-inflammatory activity. There is evidence to suggest that high dietary intake of beta-carotene can play a preventative role against developing cervical cancer.
  - —Saponins (i.e., naturally occurring detergents) such as sarsasapogenin, asparanin A, protodioscin, and diosgenin, which have strong antimicrobial, anti-inflammatory, and antioxidant properties.
  - —The flavonoids quercetin, rutin, kaempferol, and isorhamnetin, which inhibit tumor growth, reduce inflammation, and stimulate the production of detoxifying enzymes.
  - —Chlorophyll (i.e., the green pigment in asparagus), which is a powerful anti-carcinogen that protects DNA from damaging aflatoxins, potentially preventing cancers of the liver, skin, and colon.
- Asparagus contains vitamin K, which acts as a coenzyme involved in maintaining normal levels of blood clotting proteins and assists in bone metabolism.
- Asparagus contains many immune-enhancing antioxidants such as vitamins C and E, zinc, manganese, selenium, and glutathione (GSH). Additional health benefits associated with these nutrients include the following:
  - —Vitamin C aids in the absorption of iron.

—Vitamin E maintains cell membranes and assists in vitamin K absorption.

—Zinc promotes wound healing and is essential for maintaining vision, smell, and taste.

—Manganese is responsible for energy production, fatty acid synthesis, and essential cholesterol production.

—Selenium combines with proteins to create selenoproteins, which regulate thyroid function.

—GSH supports the liver in detoxification.

- Other minerals found in asparagus include magnesium, phosphorous, potassium, calcium, sodium, and iron. These minerals provide many health benefits, including maintaining homeostasis within the cells, controlling blood pressure, assisting with bone formation, promoting wound healing, and assisting with blood cell production.

- Asparagus contains inulin, a polyfructan carbohydrate that serves as a prebiotic with the ability to promote the growth of intestinal flora (i.e., beneficial bacteria in the intestines).

- Asparagus is a good source of dietary fiber, including soluble fiber, which binds with water and slows the digestive process, allowing the body to better manage postprandial (i.e., after eating) glucose and insulin responses. Fiber increases the volume of the intestinal contents, which hinders the absorption of cholesterol. The added bulk leads to more regular bowel movements, promoting intestinal health.

DIETARY INTAKE GUIDELINES

- Asparagus contains purines, which form uric acid when broken down; uric acid build-up can result in gout and kidney stones in at-risk persons. For this reason, persons with kidney damage or gout should limit consumption of asparagus.

- Asparagus contains chlorophyll, which can increase the skin's sensitivity to sunlight.

- Asparagus consumption frequently results in the harmless reaction of strong smelling urine. There is no danger associated with this phenomenon.

RESEARCH FINDINGS

- Results of many studies confirm the powerful antioxidant and anti-inflammatory potential of asparagus. Asparagus has been found to play a role in preventing cellular damage induced by stress and free radicals, and has demonstrated protective action of the liver (e.g., prevents hepatocarcinogenesis) and kidney (e.g., inhibiting acetaminophen toxicity). Extracts of asparagus have been shown to induce natural death of colon cancer cells.

- Results of a study conducted at the University of California, Davis (UC Davis) showed that an enzyme found in the stalk of asparagus is able to degrade malathion, a common nontoxic pesticide. Researchers suggest that including asparagus with malathion-treated foods could reduce the total amount of pesticides consumed.

SUMMARY

Consumers should become knowledgeable about the physiologic effects of asparagus. Asparagus is a good source of fiber, folate, iron, magnesium, phosphorous, potassium, calcium, sodium, zinc, vitamins B, C, E, and K, and phytochemicals (e.g., beta carotene and chlorophyll). The nutritional benefits of consuming asparagus include, promoting optimal digestive health and reducing risk for diabetes mellitus, heart disease, and cancer. Persons with gout, kidney failure, or a propensity for kidney stones should be aware that asparagus contains purines, which form uric acid when broken down; uric acid build-up can result in gout and kidney stones.

—*Cherie Marcel, BS*

REFERENCES

Agrawal, A., Sharma, M., Rai, S. K., Singh, B., Tiwari, M., & Chandra, R. (2008). The effect of the aqueous extract of the roots of Asparagus racemosus on hepatocarcinogenesis initiated by diethylnitrosamine. *Phytotherapy Research*, 22(9), 1175-1182. doi:10.1002/ptr.2391

Bhutani, K. K., Paul, A. T., Fayad, W., & Linder, S. (2010). Apoptosis inducing activity of steroidal constituents from Solanum xanthocarpum and Asparagus racemosus. *Phytomedicine*, 17(10), 789-793. doi:10.1016/j.phymed.2010.01.017

Chrubasik, S., Droste, C., Dragano, N., Glimm, E., & Black, A. (2006). Effectiveness and tolerability of the herbal mixture Asparagus P on blood pressure in treatment-requiring antihypertensives. *Phytomedicine*, 13(9-10), 740-742. doi:10.1016/j.phymed.2006.01.009

Dartsch, P. C. (2008). Effect of Asparagus-P on cell metabolism of cultured kidney and inflammation-mediating cells. *Phytotherapy Research, 22*(11), 1477-1481. doi:10.1002/ ptr.2497

Dartsch, P. C. (2008). The potential of Asparagus-P to inactivate reactive oxygen radicals. *Phytotherapy Research, 22*(2), 217-222. doi:10.1002/ptr.2293

Editorial staff at WebMD. (n.d.). Chlorophyll. Retrieved February 24, 2015, from http://www.webmd.com/vitamins-supplements/ingredientmono-712-chlorophyll. aspx?activeingredientid=712&activeingredientname= chlorophyll

The George Mateljan Foundation. (n.d.). The world's healthiest foods: Asparagus. Retrieved February 24, 2015, fromhttp://whfoods.org/genpage.php? tname=foodspice&dbid=12

Hewawasam, R. P., Jayatilaka, K. A. P., & Pathirana, C. (2008). Effect of Asparagus falcatus on acetaminophen toxicity in mice: A comparison of antioxidative effect with N-acetyl cysteine. *Journal of Dietary Supplements, 5*(1), 1-19. doi:10.1080/19392010802328933

Jian, R., Zeng, K., Li, J., Li, N., Jiang, Y., & Tu, P. (2013). Anti-neuroinflammatory constituents from Asparagus cochinchinensis. *Fitoterapia, 84*(1), 80-84. doi:10.1016/ j.fitote.2012.10.011

Kanwar, A. S., & Bhutani, K. K. (2010). Effects of Chlorophytum arundinaceum, Asparagus adscendens and Asparagus racemosus on pro-inflammatory cytokine and corticosterone levels produced by stress. *Phytotherapy Research, 24*(10), 1562-1566. doi:10.1002/ptr.3218

Largeman, F. A. (2005). Food: Super stalks. Tender and delicious, asparagus reigns as the queen of spring veggies. *Health, 19*(2), 163-164.

Tonn, S. (2004). Aspiring to asparagus: Healthful reasons to savour the flavour of this luxurious vegetable. *Alive: Canada's Natural Health and Wellness Magazine,* (261), 72-73.

Tsu-Tsair, N. (2014). Asparagus extract for heart, kidney and immune functions. *Nutritional Perspectives: Journal of the Council on Nutrition, 37*(3), 27-36.

REVIEWER(S)

Darlene Strayer, RN, MBA, Cinahl Information Systems, Glendale, CA

Nursing Executive Practice Council, Glendale Adventist Medical Center, Glendale, CA

Broccoli

WHAT WE KNOW

Broccoli, which means "flowering top of cabbage," is a species of cabbage called *Brassica olacerea,* which is of the *Brassicaceae,* also called *Cruciferea,* family (i.e., the mustard family), which contains what are commonly referred to as cruciferous vegetables. Other cruciferous vegetables include cabbage, cauliflower, kale, mustard, Brussels sprouts, and cress, all of which offer many nutritional and medicinal benefits. Broccoli possesses many nutrients, including calcium, selenium, vitamins C and K, fiber, valuable secondary metabolites (referred to as glucosinolates), and other bioactive components (e.g., flavonoids). These nutrients regulate enzymes, control the cell cycle and apoptosis (i.e., genetically programmed cell death), and prevent oxidation. Broccoli consumption is associated with reduced risk of developing hypertension, atherosclerosis, and coronary heart disease, and with prevention of cancers of the lung, pancreas, bladder, prostate, thyroid, skin, colon, and stomach.

NUTRIENTS IN BROCCOLI

- Broccoli is a source of the sulfur-containing glucosinolates (i.e., healthy chemicals of pungent plants) and S-methyl cysteine sulfoxide (i.e., sulfur containing non-essential amino acid), which appear to have anti-carcinogenic and therapeutic actions:
  —Glucoraphanin is the principal glucosinolate in broccoli. It is hydrolyzed (i.e., broken down) by the enzyme myrosinase into the isothiocyanate sulforaphane, which has strong anti-carcinogenic action.
  —Glucosinolates and sulforaphane inhibit growth and kill multiple strains of *Helicobacter pylori,* a bacterium known to cause gastric ulcers and increase the risk for gastric cancer.
- Broccoli florets contain the polyphenolic flavonoids quercetin 3-O-sophoroside and kaempferol 3-O-sophoroside, which have high antioxidant activity.
- Broccoli is a good source of fat-soluble vitamin K, which acts as a coenzyme and is involved in maintaining normal levels of blood clotting proteins and contributing to bone metabolism. Broccoli is rich in carotenoids and the vitamins C, thiamine,

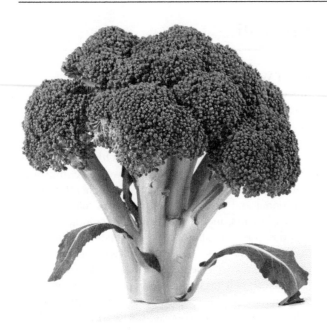

folate, and riboflavin, and provides powerful anti-oxidant activity.

- Minerals found in broccoli include sodium, potassium, calcium, magnesium, chloride, phosphorous, sulfur, and the trace minerals iron, zinc, copper, manganese, chromium, and selenium. These provide many health benefits, including maintaining cell homeostasis (i.e., regularity), controlling blood pressure, and assisting with bone formation, wound healing, and blood cell production. Even the micronutrients serve a valuable purpose; chromium and selenium improve blood sugar control in overweight persons with diabetes mellitus, type 2 (DM2).

RECOMMENDED DIETARY INTAKE

- There is no standardized dosage recommended for broccoli, although research results show that consumption of 3–5 servings of broccoli per week reduces risk for cancer.
- Broccoli has not been associated with toxicity or adverse reactions.

RESEARCH FINDINGS

- Results of many studies confirm that broccoli, along with other cruciferous vegetables, has many anti-carcinogenic activities. It is clear that the isothiocyanate sulforaphane is a major contributor

to this effect, but the overall benefit of cancer-fighting nutrients found in broccoli is established. Scientists have attempted to understand each of these nutrients and phytochemicals in order to explain how they work together or possibly, against each other. Studying individual nutrients and phytochemicals is difficult because dietary and lifestyle variations are affected by outside influences such as environment, economy, and culture

- —A 12-week clinical trial that included 291 participants from a region of China characterized by high levels of airborne pollutants revealed that consuming a daily dose of a broccoli sprout-derived beverage containing 600 mol glucoraphanin and 40 mol solforaphane was associated with significant detoxication of the airborne pollutants, benzene and acrolein metabolites, potentially attenuating the long-term health risks of such pollutants.

- Study results show that isolated components of broccoli have specific medicinal benefits and can be used in conjunction with other treatment for a greater effect. For example, broccoli preparations of sulforaphane combined with 17-demethoxygeldanamycin (17-AAG) inhibit pancreatic tumor growth by more than 70% compared with 50% suppression using 17-AAGalone.

- Results of a study on the safety of broccoli sprout extract found no evidence of toxicity or adverse effects in healthy volunteers after receiving repeated doses of calibrated extract. Results of a similar study comparing different dosages of glucoraphanin extracted from broccoli showed that glucoraphanin can be safely used in concentrations as high as 60 mg/kg, which is a sufficient dose to enhance the liver and lung activity associated with the antioxidant and anti-carcinogenic effect of glucoraphanin.

SUMMARY

Consumers should become knowledgeable about the physiologic benefits of broccoli consumption. Broccoli is a good source of many nutrients, including calcium, selenium, vitamins C and K, fiber, secondary metabolites, such as glucosinolates, and other bioactive components, such as flavonoids. Broccoli consumption is associated with reduced risk of developing heart disease and many cancers.

—*Cherie Marcel, BS*

REFERENCES

Dye, D. (2011). Broccoli compound goes after cancer cells. *Life Extension*, 17(10), 24.

Dye, D. (2010). In the news. New research contributes to the understanding of how I3C blocks cancer cells. *Life Extension*, 16(10), 22.

Egner, P. A., Chen, J. G., Zarth, A. T., Ng, D. K., Wang, J. B., Kensler, K. H., ... Kensler, T. W. (2014). Rapid and sustainable detoxication of airborne pollutants by broccoli sprout beverage: Results of a randomized clinical trial in China. *Cancer Prevention Research*, 7(8), 813-823. doi:10.1158/1940-6207.CAPR-14-0103

Finkle, J. (2011). In the news. Basis for broccoli'scancer-fighting ability revealed. *Life Extension*, 16(6), 23.

Herr, I., & Buchler, M. W. (2010). Dietary constituents of broccoli and other cruciferous vegetables: Implications for prevention and therapy of cancer. *Cancer Treatment Reviews*, 36(5), 377-383. doi:10.1016/j.ctrv.2010.01.002

James, D., Devaraj, S., Bellur, P., Lakkanna, S., Vicini, J., & Boddupalli, S. (2012). Novel concepts of broccoli sulforaphanes and disease: Induction of phase II antioxidant and detoxification enzymes by enhanced-glucoraphanin broccoli. *Nutrition Reviews*, 70(11), 654-665. doi:10.1111/j.1753-4887.2012.00532.x

Li, Y., & Zhang, T. (2013). Targeting cancer stem cells with sulforaphane, a dietary component from broccoli and broccoli sprouts. *Future Oncology*, 9(8), 1097-1103. doi:10.2217/fon.13.108

Li, Y., Zhang, T., Schwartz, S. J., & Sun, D. (2011). Sulforaphane potentiates the efficacy of 17-allylamino 17-demethoxygeldanamycin against pancreatic cancer through enhanced abrogation of Hsp90 chaperone function. *Nutrition & Cancer*, 63(7), 1151-1159. doi:10.1080/01635581.2011.596645

Murugan, S. S., Balakrishnamurthy, P., & Mathew, Y. J. (2007). Antimutagenic effect of broccoli flower head by the Ames Salmonella reverse mutation assay. *Phytotherapy Research*, 21(6), 545-547. doi:10.1002/ptr.2104

Riso, P., Martini, D., Visioli, F., Martinetti, A., & Porrini, M. (2009). Effect of broccoli intake on markers related to oxidative stress and cancer risk in healthy smokers and nonsmokers. *Nutrition & Cancer*, 61(2), 232-237. doi:10.1080/01635580802425688

Shapiro, T. A., Fahey, J. W., Dinkova-Kostova, A. T., Holtzclaw, W. D., Stephenson, K. K., Wade, K. L., ... Talalay, P. (2006). Safety, tolerance, and metabolism of broccoli sprout glucosinolates and isothiocyanates: A clinical phase I study. *Nutrition & Cancer*, 55(1), 53-62. doi:10.1207/s15327914nc5501_7

USDA Natural Resources Conservation Service. (n.d.). Classification for Kingdom Plantae down to Genus Brassica L. Retrieved March 10, 2015, from http://plants.usda.gov/ java/ClassificationServlet?source=display&classid=BRASS2

Vasanthi, H. R., Mukherjee, S., & Das, D. K. (2009). Potential health benefits of broccoli – A chemico-biological overview. *Mini Reviews in Medicinal Chemistry*, 9(6), 749-759. doi:10.2174/138955709788452685

REVIEWER(S)

Darlene Strayer, RN, MBA, Cinahl Information Systems, Glendale, CA

Nursing Executive Practice Council, Glendale Adventist Medical Center, Glendale, CA

Cabbage

WHAT WE KNOW

Cabbage, or brassica, is a member of the *Brassica oleracea* genus, and the *Brassicaceae*, or *Cruciferae*, family (more commonly referred to as cruciferous vegetables). Other cruciferous vegetables include broccoli, cauliflower, kale (also called wild cabbage), mustard, Brussels sprouts, and cress, all of which offer many nutritional and medicinal benefits. Cabbage contains many nutrients, including minerals (e.g., calcium and selenium), vitamins C and K, and fiber as well as valuable secondary metabolites (called glucosinolates) and other bioactive components (e.g., flavonoids). These nutrients regulate enzymes, control the cell cycle, and prevent oxidation, making cruciferous vegetables, especially broccoli, important in the prevention of cancer and heart disease.

NUTRIENTS IN CABBAGE

- Cabbage is a source of the sulfur-containing phytochemicals glucosinolates and S-methyl cysteine sulphoxide, whose degradation products, isothiocyanates, appear to have chemo-preventive and therapeutic activity.
  —Glucoraphanin is the principal glucosinolate in cabbage. It is hydrolyzed (i.e., broken down) by the enzyme myrosinase into the isothiocyanate sulforaphane, which has strong anti-carcinogenic action.

—Glucosinolates and sulforaphane inhibit the growth of and kill multiple strains of *Helicobacter pylori*, a bacteria known to cause gastric ulcers and increase risk for gastric cancer.

- Cabbage contains the polyphenolic flavonoids anthocyanins, which have high antioxidant activity.
- Cabbage is a good source of the fat-soluble vitamin K, which acts as a coenzyme in maintaining normal levels of blood clotting proteins and contributes to bone metabolism. Cabbage has powerful antioxidant properties because it is rich in carotenoids and the vitamins C, thiamine, folate, and riboflavin.
- Minerals found in cabbage include potassium, calcium, and phosphorous along with the trace mineral manganese. These minerals provide many health benefits, including maintaining homeostasis (i.e., regularity) within the cells, controlling blood pressure, promoting bone formation, wound healing, and blood cell production.

RESEARCH FINDINGS

- Results of many studies confirm that cabbage, along with other cruciferous vegetables, has vast anti-carcinogenic activities. Although scientists attempt to understand each of the nutrients and phytochemicals in these vegetables to help explain how they work together or possibly against each other, this is difficult to study in humans because of dietary and lifestyle variations that are affected by outside influences such as environment, economy, and culture.

SUMMARY

Consumers should become knowledgeable about the physiologic benefits of cabbage consumption. Cabbage is a good source of calcium, selenium, vitamins C and K, fiber, glucosinolates, and flavonoids. These nutrients help with digestion and maintain healthy cells, which contributes to the prevention of cancer and heart disease.

—*Cherie Marcel, BS*

REFERENCES

Arnell, N. M. (2011). Is cabbage the ultimate anti-cancer food? *NaturalNews.com*. Retrieved May 6, 2015, from http://www.naturalnews.com/032377_cabbage_anti-cancer_food.html

Botts, B. (2012). Cabbage & company. *Organic Gardening*, 59(2), 52-57.

Consumption of raw or short-cooked cabbage may lower breast cancer risk. (2005). *Oncology News International*, 14(12), 43, 50.

Finkel, J. (2011). In the news - Basis for broccoli'scancer-fighting ability revealed. *Life Extension*, (May), 23.

The George Mateljan Foundation. (n.d.). The world's healthiest foods: Cabbage. Retrieved May 6, 2015, fromhttp://www.whfoods.com/genpage.php?tname=foodspice&dbid=19

Herr, I., & Buchler, M. W. (2010). Dietary constituents of broccoli and other cruciferous vegetables: Implications for prevention and therapy of cancer. *Cancer Treatment Reviews*, 36(5), 377-383. doi:10.1016/j.ctrv.2010.01.002

Noh, J. S., Choi, H., & Song, Y. O. (2013). Beneficial effects of the active principle component of Korean cabbage kimchi via increasing nitric oxide production and suppressing inflammation in the aorta of apoE knockout mice. *British Journal of Nutrition*, 109(1), 17-24. doi:10.1017/S0007114512000633

Szaefer, H., Licznerska, B., Krajka-Kuzniak, V., Bartoszek, A., & Baer-Dubowska, W. (2012). Modulation of CYP1A1, CYP1A2, and CYP1B1 expression by cabbage juices and indoles in human breast cell lines. *Nutrition & Cancer*, 64(6), 879-888. doi:10.1080/01635581.2012.690928

REVIEWER(S)

Darlene Strayer, RN, MBA, Cinahl Information Systems, Glendale, CA

Nursing Executive Practice Council, Glendale Adventist Medical Center, Glendale, CA

Carrot

WHAT WE KNOW

The carrot, or *Daucus carota*, is a member of the *Apiaceae*, or *Umbelliferae*, family, which includes parsley, anise, dill, caraway, celery, and fennel. Although the long, pointed, orange root of the carrot is most familiar, carrot roots were originally yellow, red, or purple. In the 17th century, Dutch growers are believed to have cultivated orange carrots in honor of William I, Prince of Orange (also called William the Silent and a German nobleman by birth), who fought for Dutch independence. Carrots are high in fiber and loaded with powerful nutrients such as vitamins K, C, E, B6, thiamin, niacin, and riboflavin as well as potassium, manganese, molybdenum, and phosphorous. The carrot contains many phytonutrients (i.e., beneficial, plant-derived chemicals), including carotenoids, hydroxycinnamic acids, and anthocyanins. These combined nutrients reduce inflammation, inhibit aggregation of red blood cells, and prevent oxidation, resulting in reduced risk of heart disease. Additionally, carrot is believed to support eye health and reduce risk of colon cancer. Carrot can be eaten raw, pickled, or cooked. While most persons enjoy the sweet and colorful root of the carrot, the greens are also edible and have a fresh and slightly bitter flavor. Whole cooked carrots retain 25% more nutrients than chopped cooked carrots.

NUTRIENTS IN CARROT

- Carrot is rich in the carotenoids, alpha- and beta-carotene (i.e., a pre-cursor to vitamin A), and lutein, as well as vitamins C and E, which provide powerful antioxidant and anti-inflammatory activity.
- Minerals found in carrot include potassium, magnesium, phosphorous and trace minerals molybdenum and manganese. These provide many health benefits, including maintaining cells, controlling blood pressure, promoting wound healing, and assisting blood cell production.
- Carrot is a good source of dietary fiber, which binds with water and slows the digestive process, allowing the body to better manage post-prandial (i.e., after eating) glucose and insulin responses. Fiber also increases the volume of the intestinal contents, which hinders the absorption of cholesterol. The added bulk leads to more regular bowel movements, promoting intestinal health. There is some evidence that carrot fiber contains pectin polysaccharides (i.e., a type of fiber), which provide extra health benefits such as protection against colon cancer and promotion of cardiovascular health.

DIETARY INTAKE GUIDELINES

—Excessive ingestion of carrots can result in hypercarotenemia, a harmless condition in which carotenoid pigments are collected in the fatty tissue, causing the skin to turn yellow or orange, particularly on the palms of the hands and soles of the feet.

—Stopping of excessive carrot consumption will resolve toxicity. As the carotenoids leave the system, the hyperpigmentation will fade.

RESEARCH FINDINGS

- Researchers have found that carrot is especially protective of cardiovascular health. Results of one study revealed that drinking 16 fluid ounces of fresh carrot juice per day increases the total antioxidant level of the blood and decreases lipid peroxidation (i.e., cell damage).
- Including carrot in meals increases satiety (i.e., feeling full) and reduces subsequent intake according to researchers. Eating whole or blended carrots as part of a mixed meal appears to enhance fullness and result in long-term lower food intake. Scientists believe this effect is due to both the physical structure and the fiber content of the carrots, and that including the carrot in meal planning is important in a diet designed to lower overall energy intake.
- Researchers report that the content of phenolic compounds of carrot varies according to root color and origin. In the study, carrots with purple roots contained close to 9 times the amount of phenolic compounds of other root colors, while red carrots exhibited more antioxidant activity than orange, yellow, or white carrots. Scientists noted that carrots of Asian origin were more likely to be red or purple, while those of Western origin were mainly orange. Researchers have also found that extracts from black carrot tissue have potent anticancer activity, and could potentially be used as an agent for the treatment of brain cancer without causing harm to healthy cells.

SUMMARY

Consumers should become knowledgeable about the physiologic benefits of the consumption of carrot. Carrot is a good source of fiber, vitamins K, C, E, B6, thiamin, niacin, and riboflavin, as well as potassium, manganese, molybdenum, phosphorous, and many phytonutrients (e.g., carotenoids, hydroxycinnamic acids, and anthocyanins). These nutrients are beneficial because they inhibit inflammation, support eye health, and reduce risk of heart disease and colon cancer.

—*Cherie Marcel, BS*

REFERENCES

Carrot cooking. (2010). *IDEA Fitness Journal*, 7(3), 52.

Dye, D. (2011). Broccoli compound goes after cancer cells. *Life Extension*, 17(10), 24.

Dye, D. (2010). New research contributes to the understanding of how I3C blocks cancer cells. *Life Extension, 16*(10), 22.

The George Mateljan Foundation. (n.d.). The world's healthiest foods: Carrots. Retrieved February 27, 2015, fromhttp://www.whfoods.com/genpage.php?tname=foodspice&dbid=21

Leja, M., Kaminska, I., Kramer, M., Maksylewicz-Kaul, A., Kammerer, D., Carle, R., & Baranski, R. (2013). The content of phenolic compounds and radical scavenging activity varies with carrot origin and root color. *Plant Foods for Human Nutrition, 68*(2), 163-170. doi:10.1007/s11130-013-0351-3

Matthews, G. (2011). Cranberries & carrots: Add colour to your celebration. *Alive: Canada's Natural Health and Wellness Magazine,* (348), 120-132.

McKevith, B. (2005). A carrot a day to keep cancer away? *Nutrition Bulletin, 30*(2), 117-119.

Moorhead, S. A., Welch, R. W., Barbara, M., Livingstone, E., McCourt, M., Burns, A. A., & Dunne, A. (2006). The effects of the fibre content and physical structure of carrots on satiety and subsequent intakes when eaten as part of a mixed meal. *British Journal of Nutrition, 96*(3), 587-595.

Potter, A. S., Foroudi, S., Stamatikos, A., Patil, B. S., & Deyhim, F. (2011). Drinking carrot juice increases total antioxidant status and decreases lipid peroxidation in adults. *Nutrition Journal, 10,* 96.

Sevimli-Gur, C., Cetin, B., Akay, S., Gulce-Iz, S., & Yesil-Celiktas, O. (2013). Extracts from black carrot tissue culture as potent anticancer agents. *Plant Foods for Human Nutrition, 68*(3), 293-298. doi:10.1007/s11130-013-0371-z

Wageesha, N. D., Ekanayake, S., Jansz, E. R., & Lamabadusuriya, S. (2011). Studies on hypercarotenemia due to excessive ingestion of carrot, pumpkin and papaw. *International Journal of Food Sciences and Nutrition,* 20-25. doi:10.3109/09637486.2010.511164

REVIEWER(S)

Darlene Strayer, RN, MBA, Cinahl Information Systems, Glendale, CA

Nursing Executive Practice Council, Glendale Adventist Medical Center, Glendale, CA

Celery

WHAT WE KNOW

Celery, or *Apium graveolens*, is a member of the Apiaceae, or Umbelliferae, family, which includes parsley, anise, dill, and fennel. Although it is a good source of vitamin K, celery is relatively low in most vitamins and minerals compared with other vegetables. It is, however, rich in phytonutrients, including phthalides, quercetin, apigenin, and luteolin, which have antioxidant, anti-inflammatory, antispasmodic, and anti-carcinogenic properties. Celery is believed to relieve indigestion, reduce inflammation, and serve as a diuretic. It has been used to treat gastrointestinal (GI) disorders, bronchitis, asthma, and liver and spleen diseases.

NUTRIENTS IN CELERY

- The active components of celery are found throughout the plant structure. These include phytonutrients such as phthalides, quercetin, apigenin, and luteolin.
  - Apigenin has been shown to reduce the size of prostate tumors.
  - Celery extract appears to increase liver production of enzymes that remove toxins from the body.
  - Luteolin is believed to be a potent anti-carcinogenic compound.
  - Phthalides have hypotensive properties (i.e., lowers blood pressure).

DIETARY INTAKE GUIDELINES

- There is no recommended dosage for medicinal administration of celery.
- Celery is reported to be a major food allergen in many European countries.
- Treatment of adverse reactions is achieved by discontinuing celery intake and by treating the signs and symptoms of the allergic reaction.

RESEARCH FINDINGS

- Researchers studying celery extract for its mosquito-repellent properties in comparison with commercial, synthetic repellents found that celery exhibited mild bug-repelling properties. During the 6 months of the study, no adverse effects were observed on the skin from the topical application of celery extract. Celery application was considered a potent mosquito repellent in this study and can be a good alternative to commercial repellents.

- Celery seed extracts have bactericidal action against *Campylobacter jejuni*, *Escherichia coli*, *Listeria monocytogenes*, *Salmonella enterica*, and *Helicobacter pylori*. In a recent study of the gastric antiulcer, anti-secretory, and cell-protective properties of celery in rats, celery extract significantly protected the lining of the stomach. Researchers attribute this activity to the anti-inflammatory and antioxidant properties of celery. With its gastric-protective potential and its low risk of adverse reactions, celery may prove to be a useful agent in the treatment and prevention of gastric ulcers and other GI disorders.

SUMMARY

Consumers should become knowledgeable about the physiologic effects of celery. Celery is a good source of many phytonutrients, which reduce muscle spasms, fight inflammation, and may prevent cancer.

—*Cherie Marcel, BS*

REFERENCES

Al-Howiriny, T., Alsheikh, A., Alqasoumi, S., Al-Yahya, M., ElTahir, K., & Rafatullah, S. (2010). Gastric antiulcer, antisecretory and cytoprotective properties of celery (Apium graveolens) in rats. *Pharmaceutical Biology*, 48(7), 786-793. doi:10.3109/13880200903280026

Fæste, C. K., Jonscher, K. R., Sit, L., Klawitter, J., Løvberg, K. E., & Moen, L. H. (2010). Differentiating cross-reacting allergens in the immunological analysis of celery (Apium graveolens) by mass spectrometry. *Journal of AOAC International*, 93(2), 451-461.

Gamonski, W. (2012, November). Super foods. Time to celebrate celery. *Life Extension Magazine*, 5 pp.

Hermann, M. (2006). Celery deceptively rich in phytonutrients. *Environmental Nutrition*, 29(12), 8.

Powanda, M. C., & Rainsford, K. D. (2011). A toxicological investigation of a celery seed extract having anti-inflammatory activity. *Inflammopharmacology*, 19(4), 227-233. doi:10.1007/s10787-010-0049-1

Sowbhagya, H. B. (2014). Chemistry, technology, and nutraceutical functions of celery (Apium graveolens L.): An overview. *Critical Reviews in Food Science & Nutrition*, 54(3), 389-398. doi:10.1080/10408398.2011.586740

Tuetun, B., Choochote, W., Kanjanapothi, D., Rattanachanpichai, E., Chaithong, U., Chaiwong, P., & Pitasawat, B. (2005). Repellent properties of celery, Apium graveolens L., compared with commercial repellents, against mosquitoes under laboratory and field conditions. *Tropical Medicine & International Health*, 10(11), 1190-1198. doi:10.1111/j.1365-3156.2005.01500.x

REVIEWER(S)

Darlene Strayer, RN, MBA, Cinahl Information Systems, Glendale, CA

Nursing Executive Practice Council, Glendale Adventist Medical Center, Glendale, CA

Eggplant

WHAT WE KNOW

Eggplant (*Solanum melongena*) is widely considered a vegetable but is technically a fruit from the nightshade, or *Solanaceae* family. Other members of the nightshade family include tomato, bell pepper, and potato. Although eggplant is most frequently depicted having a deep purple color, the glossy skin of the eggplant can be lavender, jade green, orange, yellow, or white depending on the eggplant variety. The spongy, pale-colored flesh in all varieties of eggplant is relatively consistent in flavor, color, and texture. There is a mild bitter taste to eggplant, which is easily offset by the addition of salt; otherwise, the mellow flavor of eggplant tends to adopt the flavors of the ingredients that are added to it; this quality and its spongy texture allows for eggplant to be a good substitute for meat. Eggplant can be sautéed, grilled, roasted, steamed, or baked. Nutritionally, eggplant is very low in calories, a good source of fiber, and rich in phytonutrients (i.e., beneficial, plant-derived chemicals).

NUTRIENTS IN EGGPLANT

- Eggplant contains a variety of valuable phytonutrients, including the following:
  —Nasunin is a flavonoid with powerful antioxidant activity that protects cell membranes from free radical-induced damage. Nasunin has been shown to protect brain cell membranes and binds to iron, preventing the undesirable accumulation of iron.
  —Caffeic and chologenic acid are phenolic compounds that exhibit anti-mutagenic,

anti-microbial, and antiviral properties. They are believed to inhibit the build-up of low density lipoprotein (LDL) cholesterol (i.e., the "bad" cholesterol).

DIETARY INTAKE GUIDELINES

- Because eggplant contains oxalate, which is a primary component of kidney stones, individuals who are prone to developing kidney stones should be cautioned about consuming large quantities of eggplant.

RESEARCH FINDINGS

- A cross-sectional study was conducted to determine the prevalence of food allergy to eggplant in India. Although many subjects reported having an adverse reaction to eating eggplant, specific protein allergens were rarely detected. Immunoglobulin E (IgE)-mediated eggplant allergy was estimated to be present in about 0.8% of the population, with a higher predominance in women. Researchers speculate that allergic reactions that were unrelated to specific protein allergens were possibly the result of the pharmacologic action of histamine and other non-protein components.

SUMMARY

Consumers should become knowledgeable about the physiologic risks and benefits associated with eggplant. Eggplant is a good source of phytonutrients that prevent inflammation, lower LDL cholesterol, and prevent gene mutation. Individuals with an allergy or sensitivity to eggplant should avoid eating eggplant-containing dishes, and possibly other members of the nightshade family. Individuals with history of kidney stones should avoid eating large quantities of eggplant.

—*Cherie Marcel, BS*

REFERENCES

Eggplant: Superfood? (2010). *Running & FitNews, 28*(3), 17-20.

The George Mateljan Foundation editorial team. (n.d.). The world's healthiest foods: Eggplant. Retrieved March 12, 2015, from http://www.whfoods.com/genpage.php? tname=foodspice&dbid=22#healthbenefits

Harish Babu, B. N., Mahesh, P. A., & Venkatesh, Y. P. (2008). A cross-sectional study on the prevalence of food allergy to eggplant (Solanum melongena L.) reveals female predominance. *Clinical and Experimental Allergy: Journal of the British Society for Allergy and Clinical Immunology, 38*(11), 1795. doi:10.1111/j.1365-2222.2008.03076.x

Lofshult, D. (2009). The elegant eggplant. *IDEA Fitness Journal, 6*(10), 62.

Zevnik, N. (2009). Eat smart. Exceptional eggplant. *Better Nutrition, 71*(1), 52-53.

REVIEWER(S)

Darlene Strayer, RN, MBA, Cinahl Information Systems, Glendale, CA

Nursing Executive Practice Council, Glendale Adventist Medical Center, Glendale, CA

Fennel

WHAT WE KNOW

Fennel, or *Foeniculum vulgare*, is a member of the Umbelliferae family, along with parsley, carrots, dill, cumin, and coriander. Fennel has a pale green bulb, celery-like stalk, and a wispy, gnarled leaf. It is both appreciated and avoided because of its distinctive scent of licorice. Nutritionally, it is an excellent source of vitamin C, folic acid, potassium, and fiber. Fennel is also a source of many trace minerals including calcium, chromium, copper, iron, magnesium and zinc. In Greek mythology, fennel was called "marathon" and was considered to be the stalk that carried the gods' gift of knowledge to man. Modern civilizations use fennel for a variety of purposes, including as an effective insect repellent. Medicinally, fennel is included in a variety of cough syrups as an expectorant and decongestant and is believed to alleviate indigestion and bad breath. Topically, it can be used as an astringent or made into an eyewash or salve to treat conjunctivitis and sore eyes.

NUTRIENTS IN FENNEL

- The active components of fennel are found in the seeds, bulbs, stalks, and leaves; these include the flavonoids rutin, quercetin, and multiple kaempferol glycosides, which provide strong antioxidant activity. Anethole is the primary phytonutrient in fennel's volatile oil.
    - —Anethole appears to reduce inflammation and have anti-carcinogenic properties.

- Fennel is claimed to have anti-inflammatory, antioxidant, antiseptic, anti-carcinogenic, and diuretic properties. It is also thought to promote lactation, prevent blood clots, lower blood pressure, relieve hangover, and suppress appetite.

DIETARY INTAKE GUIDELINES

- A typical dosage is 1 cup of freshly brewed tea 2–3 times daily. The tea is prepared by steeping 10 mL of crushed fennel seeds in 250 mL of boiling water for 10–15 minutes, then straining.
- An eyewash can be made by infusing ½ cup of crushed seeds in 1–2 cups of cold water for about 1 hour, then straining. This infusion can also be used as a gargle for sore throat.
- As a precaution, women who are pregnant should not use fennel in medicinal doses because of its potential to induce abortion.

RESEARCH FINDINGS

- Results of a study in mice revealed the potential of fennel to inhibit the cognitive decline in dementia and Alzheimer's disease, possibly due to its anti-inflammatory properties.
- In a comparison of the effectiveness of fennel and mefenamic acid, a nonsteroidal anti-inflammatory drug (NSAID), on the management of dysmenorrhea, fennel was shown to be as effective as mefenamic acid in reducing pain and improving energy. A separate study of the effectiveness of fennel in the treatment of the symptoms of dysmenorrhea revealed that treatment with fennel capsules reduced nausea and weakness, and improved feelings of well-being.
- Researchers evaluated the effectiveness of a topical fennel gel as treatment for hirsutism (i.e., unwanted hair growth) on 44 women with mild to moderate idiopathic hirsutism and concluded that the fennel gel effectively decreased hair thickness.
- Researchers have reported evidence of antioxidant and anti-carcinogenic properties in the volatile oil of fennel. One report stated that the fennel oil exhibited antitumor effects and reduced oxidative stress in the cells of mice, and suggested that it may have anticancer potential against breast and liver cancer. In addition, researchers observed strong free radical scavenging activity and reported that fennel could be used as

a safe and effective food preservative in addition to its antimicrobial activities.

SUMMARY

Consumers should become knowledgeable about the physiologic effects of fennel. Fennel is a good source of powerful phytonutrients that help reduce blood pressure, inflammation, and risk of cancer. Pregnant women should not use medicinal doses of fennel.

—*Cherie Marcel, BS*

REFERENCES

Akha, O., Rabiei, K., Kashi, Z., Bahar, A., Zaeif-Khorasani, E., Kosaryan, M., ... Emadian, O. (2014). The effect of fennel (Foeniculum vulgare) gel 3% in decreasing hair thickness in idiopathic mile to moderate hirsutism, A randomized placebo controlled clinical trial. *Caspian Journal of Internal Medicine, 5*(1), 26-29.

Badgujar, S. B., Patel, V. V., & Bandivdekar, A. H. (2014). Foeniculum vulgare Mill: A review of its botany, phytochemistry, pharmacology, contemporary application, and toxicology. *BioMed Research International, 2014.* doi:10.1155/2014/842674

Burnett, B. (2008). Fennel: Good health, great taste. *Alive: Canada's Natural Health & Wellness Magazine,* (311), 154-156.

Cetin, B., Ozer, H., Cakir, A., Polat, T., Dursun, A., Mete, E., & Ekinci, M. (2010). Antimicrobial activities of essential oil and hexane extract of Florence fennel [Foeniculum vulgare var. azoricum (Mill.) Thell.] against foodborne microorganisms. *Journal of Medicinal Food, 13*(1), 196-204. doi:10.1089/jmf.2008.0327

Ghodsi, Z., & Asltoghiri, M. (2014). The effect of fennel on pain quality, symptoms, and menstrual duration in primary dysmenorrhea. *Journal of Pediatric and Adolescent Gynecology, 27*(5), 283-286. doi:10.1016/j.jpag.2013.12.003

Griffin, A. (2008). Flavor-filled fennel. *Better Nutrition, 70*(2), 74, 76-77.

Fennel. (2002). In F. Hoffmann, & M. Manning (Eds.), *Herbal medicine and botanical medical fads* (pp. 73-74). Binghamton, NY: The Haworth Press, Inc.

Joshi, H., & Parle, M. (2006). Cholinergic basis of memory-strengthening effect of Foeniculum vulgare Linn. *Journal of Medicinal Food, 9*(3), 413-417. doi:10.1089/jmf.2006.9.413

Maguire, C. (2007). Humble fennel. *Natural Health and Vegetarian Life,* 24.

Mohamad, R. H., El-Bastawesy, A. M., Abdel-Monem, M. G., Noor, A. M., Al-Mehdar, H. A. R., Sharawy, S. M., & El-Merzabani, M. M. (2011). Antioxidant and anticarcinogenic effects of methanolic extract and volatile oil of fennel seeds (Foeniculum vulgare). *Journal of Medicinal Food*, *14*(9), 986-1001. doi:10.1089/jmf.2008.0255

Nejad, V. M., & Asadipour, M. (2006). Comparison of the effectiveness of fennel and mefenamic acid on pain intensity in dysmenorrhoea. *Easter Mediterranean Health Journal*, *12*(3-4), 423-427.

Robbers, J., & Tyler, V. E. (1999). Fennel. In *Tyler's herbs of choice the therapeutic use of phytomedicinals* (pp. 72). Binghamton, NY: The Haworth Press, Inc.

Wilde, B. (2007). Fennel. *Organic Gardening*, *54*(3), 26-27.

Zanteson, L. (2011). The finer side of fennel. *Environmental Nutrition*, *34*(2), 8.

REVIEWER(S)

Darlene Strayer, RN, MBA, Cinahl Information Systems, Glendale, CA

Nursing Executive Practice Council, Glendale Adventist Medical Center, Glendale, CA

Garlic

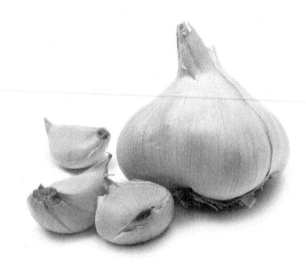

WHAT WE KNOW

Garlic, or *Allium sativum*, is a sulfur-containing bulb from the Amaryllidaceae or Liliaceae family. Other names for garlic include ail, allium, camphor of the poor, da-sua, knoblauch, la-suan, nectar of the gods, poor man's treacle, rustic treacle, and stinking rose. Alliin, one of the many compounds of garlic, converts to allicin, which is responsible for the characteristic odor of garlic. Although garlic is generally appreciated as a culinary seasoning, it has historically been used medicinally, both orally and topically. Some of its uses are as treatment for arthrosclerosis, hyperlipidemia, and hypertension. Garlic is also noted for its antithrombotic effects, chemopreventive potential, and antimicrobial action. While regular garlic intake has obvious benefits, consuming too much raw garlic can result in abdominal discomfort, flushing, rapid pulse, and insomnia. Care must also be taken when topical garlic is used as a treatment, as it has been reported to result in skin irritation, blistering, and in some cases, third-degree burns. Discontinuing the use of garlic usually resolves the adverse effects, and if skin damage has occurred, such as with a burn, it must also be treated, as needed.

NUTRIENTS IN GARLIC

* The suspected active components of garlic are sulfur derivatives (e.g., alliin, allicin) that have a strong odor and are found in the bulb and cloves. Because of this, odorless preparations of garlic are thought to be ineffective.
* Garlic exhibits strong potential as an antithrombotic (i.e., prevents blood clots), hypotensive (i.e., lowers blood pressure), and lipid-lowering agent, and has anti-microbial, antifungal, antiviral, and insecticidal properties.
* Garlic exhibits antibacterial activity with demonstrated effectiveness in fighting *Helicobacter pylori*, a bacterium responsible for most cases of ulcers.
* Garlic has shown anti-tumorigenic and chemopreventive activity, especially against gastric and colorectal cancer. Researchers believe that garlic detoxifies carcinogens by reducing inflammation, sulfur compound binding, or antioxidant activity.

DIETARY INTAKE GUIDELINES

* Oral: While there is no set dosage recommendation, clinical trials have used garlic extract 600–1,200 mg divided into 3 daily doses. Fresh garlic, 1 clove/day, has also been used.
* Topical: For the treatment of tinea infections (i.e., fungal infections such as ringworm or athlete's foot), clinical trials have used the garlic

constituent ajoene as a 0.4% cream or a 0.6–1% gel applied twice a day for 1 week.

- Some common, relatively minor adverse reactions to garlic consumption include pungent breath and body odor, burning of the mouth, and gastrointestinal (GI) discomfort (e.g., heartburn, gas, nausea, vomiting, and diarrhea). These signs and symptoms develop more frequently in persons who are not accustomed to eating garlic and in persons who ingest raw garlic.
- As a precaution, women who are pregnant should not use garlic in medicinal doses. In theory, large amounts of garlic can cause uterine contractions, although there are no published reports of adverse effects in mothers or infants resulting from garlic ingestion.
- In some cases, applying garlic topically irritates the skin, causes blistering, and/or results in third-degree burns.
- Garlic is known to exhibit blood-thinning activity, which may increase the risk of bleeding; stopping garlic consumption at least 7 days prior to surgery is recommended.
- Garlic can enhance the effects of blood thinning agents (e.g., warfarin, aspirin, clopidogrel, enoxaparin).
- Garlic may enhance the effects (both positive and negative) of glucose-lowering drugs or insulin.
- There is concern that garlic may decrease the effectiveness of cyclosporine to subtherapeutic levels, potentially resulting in transplant rejection.
- Large amounts of garlic intake on can potentially reduce the effectiveness of some birth control pills that contain estrogen.
- Garlic can affect enzymes in the liver that are responsible for removing certain medications from the body; this can impact the effectiveness of chemotherapy and some medications used for HIV/ AIDS.

RESEARCH FINDINGS

- Results of several studies have shown that garlic has a potentially protective role against hepatitis. Aged black garlic, which has strong antioxidant properties, was studied for the prevention of alcohol-induced liver damage in rats with promising results. Another study revealed similar results with fresh garlic extract tested on mice that were given acetaminophen at toxic levels.

- Research regarding the effectiveness of garlic in lowering cholesterol has produced mixed results. Some study results show modest improvement in cholesterol reduction, while others show no significant effect. Similar results have been reported for the use of garlic in the treatment of hypertension. While some researchers suggest that garlic contributes to a reduction of blood pressure for individuals with hypertension, others believe that evidence to recommend garlic for antihypertensive use in daily practice is lacking. Overall, the benefits of garlic may be too small to be clinically significant.
- Garlic constituents have exhibited effectiveness in fighting cancer cells in laboratory experiments. However, definitive evidence that garlic reduces cancer risk is mixed. Although researchers state that the evidentiary support was very limited, a cancer risk analysis using the United States Food and Drug Administration (FDA) evidence-based review system reported that garlic consumption appears to be protective against cancers of the stomach, colon, prostate, esophagus, larynx, mouth, ovaries, and kidneys.

SUMMARY

Consumers should become knowledgeable about the physiologic effects of garlic. Garlic is a good source of alliin, which converts to allicin. These compounds exhibit strong potential as blood-thinning, blood pressure-lowering, and lipid-lowering agents, and have antimicrobial, antifungal, antiviral, and insecticidal properties. Individuals who are scheduled for surgery should avoid garlic consumption for at least 7 days prior to surgery. Individuals who take blood-thinning agents should be aware that garlic can enhance the effects of these medications, increasing risk for bruising and bleeding. Garlic can decrease the effectiveness of cyclosporine, potentially resulting in transplant rejection.

—*Cherie Marcel, BS*

REFERENCES

Alpers, D. H. (2009). Garlic and its potential for prevention of colorectal cancer and other conditions. *Current Opinion in Gastroenterology, 25*(2), 116-121. doi:10.1097/ MOG.0b013e32831ef221

Budoff, M. J., Ahmadi, N., Gul, K. M., Liu, S. T., Flores, F. R., Tiano, J., & Tsimikas, S. (2009). Aged garlic extract supplemented with B vitamins, folic acid and L-arginine retards the progression of sub-clinical atherosclerosis: A randomized clinical trial. *Preventive Medicine, 49*(2-3), 101-107. doi:10.1016/j.ypmed.2009.06.018

Editorial staff at American Cancer Society. (2008). Garlic. *The American Cancer Society.* Retrieved March 3, 2015, from http://www.cancer.org/treatment/ treatmentsand-sideeffects/complementaryandalternativemedicine/dietandnutrition/garlic

El-Sabban, F., & Abouazra, H. (2008). Effect of garlic on atherosclerosis and its factors. *Eastern Mediterranean Health Journal, 14*(1), 195-205.

Ernst, E., & Posadzki, P. (2012). Can garlic-intake reduce the risk of cancer? A systematic review of randomised controlled trials. *Focus on Alternative & Complementary Therapies, 17*(4), 192-196. doi:10.1111/fct.12000

Ezeala, C. C., Nweke, I. N., Unekwe, P. C., El-Safty, I. A., & Nwaegerue, E. J. (2009). Fresh garlic extract protects the liver against acetaminophen-induced toxicity. *Internet Journal of Nutrition & Wellness, 7*(1), 9p.

Gilbert, J. A. (2011). Metabolic stress. In E. D. Schlenker & S. L. Roth (Eds.), *Williams' essentials of nutrition and diet therapy* (10th ed., pp. 373, 387). St. Louis, MO: Mosby Elsevier.

Khoo, Y. S. K., & Aziz, Z. (2009). Garlic supplementation and serum cholesterol: A meta-analysis. *Journal of Clinical Pharmacy & Therapeutics, 34*(2), 133-145. doi:10.1111/j.1365-2710.2008.00998.x

Kim, J. Y., & Kwon, O. (2009). Garlic intake and cancer risk: An analysis using the Food and Drug Administration'sevidence-based review system for the scientific evaluation of health claims. *American Journal of Clinical Nutrition, 89*(1), 257-264. doi:10.3945/ajcn.2008.26142

Kim, M. H., Kim, M. J., Lee, J. H., Han, J. I., Kim, J. H., Sok, D., & Kim, M. R. (2011). Hepatoprotective effect of aged black garlic on chronic alcohol-induced liver injury in rats. *Journal of Medicinal Food, 14*(7/8), 732-738. doi:10.1089/jmf.2010.1454

Nagini, S. (2008). Cancer chemoprevention by garlic and its organosulfur compounds-panacea or promise?. *Anti-Cancer Agents in Medicinal Chemistry, 8*(3), 313-321. doi:10.2174/187152008783961879

National Institutes of Health. (2014, August 21). Garlic. *MedlinePlus.* Retrieved February 4, 2015, from http://www.nlm.nih.gov/medlineplus/druginfo/natural/300.html

Reinhart, K. M., Coleman, C. I., Teevan, C., Vachhani, P., & White, C. M. (2008). Effects of garlic on blood pressure in patients with and without systolic hypertension: A meta-analysis. *Annals of Pharmacotherapy, 42*(12), 1766-1771. doi:10.1345/aph.1L319

Reinhart, K. M., Talati, R., White, C. M., & Coleman, C. I. (2009). The impact of garlic on lipid parameters: A systematic review and meta-analysis. *Nutrition Research Reviews, 22*(1), 39-48. doi:10.1017/S0954422409350003

Ried, K., Frank, O. R., & Stocks, N. P. (2013). Aged garlic extract reduces blood pressure in hypertensives: A dose-response trial. *European Journal of Clinical Nutrition, 67*(1), 64-70. doi:10.1038/ejcn.2012.178

Simons, S., Wollersheim, H., & Thien, T. (2009). A systematic review on the influence of trial quality on the effect of garlic on blood pressure. *The Netherlands Journal of Medicine, 67*(6), 212-219.

Stabler, S. N., Tejani, A. M., Huynh, F., & Fowkes, C. (2012). Garlic for the prevention of cardiovascular morbidity and mortality in hypertensive patients. *Cochrane Database of Systematic Reviews,* Issue 8. Art. No.: CD007653. doi:10.1002/14651858.CD007653.pub2

REVIEWER(S)

Darlene Strayer, RN, MBA, Cinahl Information Systems, Glendale, CA

Nursing Executive Practice Council, Glendale Adventist Medical Center, Glendale, CA

Kale

WHAT WE KNOW

Kale (i.e., *Brassica oleracea var. Acephala*; also called wild cabbage) is a member of the Brassicaceae, or Cruciferae, family; members of this family are commonly referred to as cruciferous vegetables. Other cruciferous vegetables include broccoli, cauliflower, mustard, cress, and Brussels sprouts, all of which have many nutritional and medicinal benefits. The thick, curly, ruffled leaves of kale can be green, purple, or white and branch out from a central fibrous stalk. The flavor of kale varies from peppery to almost sweet depending on the variety of kale and the weather during its cultivation. Kale can be sautéed, steamed, baked, eaten raw as a salad green, and blended as an ingredient of juice. However it is consumed, kale provides many nutrients and health benefits. Nutrients found in kale include vitamins A, B1, B2, B3, B6, C, E, and K; folate; and minerals such as manganese, copper, calcium, potassium, iron, magnesium, and phosphorous. Kale is rich in fiber and many phytonutrients (i.e., beneficial plant-derived chemicals). Kale has antioxidant, anti-inflammatory, anti-cancer, and cardio-protective properties.

NUTRIENTS IN KALE

- Kale contains many powerful antioxidants and anti-inflammatory properties in the form of vitamins, minerals, and phytonutrients, including the following:
  - —Kale is a great source of vitamin K and one serving contains over 1,300% of the recommended daily intake. Vitamin K produces blood-clotting proteins and contributes to bone building.
  - —Kale contains provitamin A carotenoids, which serve as precursors for vitamin A, or retinol, in the human body. Vitamin A is a fat-soluble vitamin that is required for vision, maintenance of the surface lining of the eyes and other epithelial tissue, proper bone growth, immune response, energy regulation, reproduction, embryonic development, and gene expression.
  - —Vitamin C is a water-soluble vitamin that neutralizes free radicals, protecting against inflammation and cellular damage. Adequate vitamin C intake is essential for proper function of the immune system and is associated with the prevention of heart disease, stroke, and cancer.
  - —Vitamin E is a fat-soluble vitamin that functions primarily as an antioxidant but also maintains cell membranes, assists in vitamin K absorption, and contributes to immune system function.
  - —Vitamin B6, or pyridoxine, is required for the conversion of tryptophan to niacin and is involved in the conversion of homocysteine to cysteine. It supports the synthesis of serotonin and dopamine, which are neurotransmitters required for nerve cell communication. By maintaining lymphoid organs, vitamin B6 contributes to proper function of the immune system.
  - —The B vitamins thiamin (B1), riboflavin (B2), and niacin (B3) create energy by aiding in the production and breakdown of carbohydrates, lipids, proteins, and alcohol. They provide cardiovascular protection, maintain the nervous system, and support the production of red blood cells (RBCs), hormones, and cholesterol.
  - —Folate is a B vitamin that is essential for the production and maintenance of RBCs. It is essential for the production of deoxyribonucleic acid (DNA), the genetic code for the cells, and ribonucleic acid (RNA), and is important in the production of the amino acid homocysteine.
  - —Manganese is a trace mineral that is responsible for energy production, fatty acid production, cholesterol production, and protection against the damage caused by free radicals.
  - —Copper is an important component of superoxide dismutase (SOD), which is an enzyme involved in energy production and antioxidant activity. Copper contributes to the action of lysyl oxidase, an enzyme necessary for the cross-linking of collagen and elastin, which allows flexibility in the blood vessels, bones, and joints. Copper enhances the body's ability to use iron, preventing iron-deficiency anemia, ruptured vessels, irregular heartbeat, and infection.
  - —The calcium in kale is important for building and maintaining bones and teeth. Calcium regulates muscle contraction, conducts nerve impulses, activates enzymes for energy production and muscle contraction, participates in blood clotting, assists with vitamin B12 absorption, and maintains the structural integrity of intracellular membranes.
  - —Potassium supports normal cellular, nerve, and muscle function, and helps to eliminate excess sodium from the body.
  - —Iron is vital for the production of RBCs and hemoglobin, which are necessary for energy production and the transport of oxygen to the tissues. Iron supports immune function, is essential for mental development, contributes to energy production, and regulates temperature.
  - —Magnesium balances the action of calcium in cells for the regulation of bone health, nerve tone, and muscle tone. It maintains relaxation of the nerves and muscles, which contributes to the prevention of high blood pressure, muscle spasms, asthma, migraine headaches, general soreness, and fatigue.

—Phosphorous combines with calcium for the formation of bones and teeth, muscle contraction, and nerve conduction and is essential for the structural integrity of cell membranes.

—Kale is a source of the amino acid tryptophan, which contributes to the synthesis of niacin and serotonin. Serotonin is thought to promote healthy sleep patterns and stabilize mood.

—Kale is a good source of dietary fiber, which binds and removes toxins from the colon, assists in glucose control, and reduces high cholesterol levels.

—Kale is an excellent source of valuable phytonutrients, including glucosinolates, carotenoids, and 45 different flavonoids. These nutrients are potent antioxidants that are known to support cardiovascular health, protect against cancer, regulate blood glucose levels, and promote the health of the bones, liver, kidneys, and blood.

–The flavonoids quercetin and kaempferol provide strong antioxidant and anti-inflammatory protection. They have antihistamine, antimicrobial, anti-diabetic, and anti-carcinogenic properties.

–The carotenoids lutein and beta-carotene are antioxidants that inhibit the inflammatory process, neutralize free radicals, impede cancer cell proliferation (i.e., kills cancer cells), and repair damaged DNA. They prevent atherosclerosis and safeguard the eyes from light-induced damage.

DIETARY INTAKE GUIDELINES

- There is no information in the literature regarding an official recommendation for the intake of kale.
- A recent review of available literature found no information on kale deficiency.
- A recent review of available literature found no information on kale toxicity.
- Because kale is a substantial source of vitamin K, which can interfere with the effectiveness of blood-thinning medications (e.g., warfarin), individuals receiving blood thinners should be educated regarding the implications of including kale in their diet.
  —Results of a randomized, controlled trial showed that dietary intake of vitamin K does not need to be limited in persons receiving

warfarin therapy if consistent, moderate intake of vitamin K is maintained. Consistent vitamin K consumption prevents large fluctuations in intake and supports optimal blood clotting management.

- Kale may increase risk for kidney stones in individuals with a history of kidney stones because it contains a high amount of oxalate, which is a primary component of kidney stones. Oxalate can build up, crystallize in body fluids, and cause stones in individuals with preexisting kidney or gallbladder dysfunction.

RESEARCH FINDINGS

- Researchers have investigated the impact of the intake of oxalate on the absorption of the nutrients magnesium and iron by comparing meals containing spinach (which is higher in oxalate) and meals containing kale (which is lower in oxalate).
  —Results of one study indicated that the magnesium absorbed from the meal with spinach was about 35% lower than that of the meal with kale.
  —The results of a study evaluating the influence of oxalate on the absorption of iron indicated that although iron absorption was lower in the meal with spinach than in the meal with kale, the difference was not statistically significant. Researchers suggested that the impact of oxalate on iron absorption was minor.

SUMMARY

Consumers should become knowledgeable about the physiologic risks and benefits of kale consumption. Kale is a good source of fiber, vitamins B1, B2, B3, B6, C, E, and K, folate, minerals, including manganese, copper, calcium, potassium, iron, magnesium, and phosphorous, and many phytonutrients, including provitamin A carotenoids. These nutrients support the immune system and eye health, contribute to blood clotting, and may help prevent cancer and heart disease. Individuals with a history of kidney stones should be aware that kale may increase risk for developing kidney stones. Individuals on blood thinners should be aware of kale's ability to counteract blood-thinning medications.

—Cherie Marcel, BS

REFERENCES

Bohn, T., Davidsson, L., Walczyk, T., & Hurrell, R. F. (2004). Fractional magnesium absorption is significantly lower in human subjects from a meal served with an oxalate-rich vegetable, spinach, as compared with a meal served with kale, a vegetable with low oxalate content. *British Journal of Nutrition, 91*(4), 601-606. doi:10.1079/BJN20031081

Gebuis, E. P., Rosendaal, F. R., van Meegen, E., & der Meer, F. J. (2011). Vitamin K1 supplementation to improve the stability of anticoagulation therapy with vitamin K antagonists: A dose-finding study. *Haematologica, 96*(4), 583-589.

Gennant Bonsmann, S. S., Walczyk, T., Renggli, S., & Hurrell, R. F. (2008). Oxalic acid does not influence nonhaem iron absorption in humans: A comparison of kale and spinach in meals. *European Journal of Clinical Nutrition, 62*(3), 336-341.

The George Mateljan Foundation editorial team. (n.d.). Can you tell me what oxalates are and in which foods they can be found? The World's Healthiest Foods. Retrieved August 20, 2013, from http://www.whfoods.com/genpage.php?tname=george&dbid=48

The George Mateljan Foundation editorial team. (n.d.). Kale. *The World's Healthiest Foods*. Retrieved August 20, 2013, from http://www.whfoods.com/genpage.php? tname=foodspice&dbid=38

Laifer, S. (2008). Kale: Powerful cancer protection and healthy eye and heart benefits. *Life Extension, 14*(7), 89-91.

Zelman, K. M. (2014, June 19). The truth about Kale. *WebMD*. Retrieved June 8, 2015, from http://www.webmd.com/food-recipes/features/the-truth-about-kale

REVIEWER(S)

Darlene Strayer, RN, MBA, Cinahl Information Systems, Glendale, CA

Nursing Executive Practice Council, Glendale Adventist Medical Center, Glendale, CA

Onion

WHAT WE KNOW

The onion, or *Allium cepa*, is a bulb from the Alliaceae family along with garlic, shallots, leeks, and chives. Onions are thought to be native to Asia and the Middle East, and have been a significant part of the human diet for over 5,000 years. There are many varieties of onion, which vary in color, size, and flavor. Spring and summer onions (e.g., Maui Sweet Onion, Vidalia, Walla Walla), which are grown in warmer weather, have a sweet flavor. The onions grown in colder weather are called storage onions, which have a more pungent flavor and include white, yellow, red, and Spanish onions. Unlike garlic, which produces many small bulbs, the onion plant produces a single bulb made of many layered rings and is cloaked in a thin skin that is peeled off before use. The crisp and juicy rings of the onion can be eaten raw as a topping or sautéed to add flavor to various foods. Nutritionally, onions are a good source of vitamin C and are rich in a variety of sulfur-containing compounds and phytonutrients (i.e., beneficial, plant-derived chemicals), which support bone health and provide cancer-preventive, anti-inflammatory, antibacterial, antioxidant, and cardiovascular benefits.

NUTRIENTS IN ONION

- Onion contains sulfur, which is required for the production of connective tissue and is necessary for bone health. The sulfur-containing compounds in onions exhibit anti-clotting and cholesterol-lowering activity in the blood.
  - —Onion is a sulfur-containing compound in onions that helps reduce inflammation by inhibiting the activity of macrophages (i.e., overactive inflammatory cells).
- Onions are rich in the flavonoid quercetin and in other bioavailable polyphenols that act as antioxidants and help reduce inflammation. These compounds exhibit antihistamine, antimicrobial, anti-diabetic, and cancer-protective properties.
- Among other vitamins and minerals (e.g., folate, manganese, potassium), onions are a good source of vitamin C, a water-soluble vitamin that neutralizes free radicals, protecting against inflammation and cellular damage. Adequate vitamin C intake is necessary for the proper function of the immune system and has been associated with prevention of heart disease, stroke, and cancer.

DIETARY INTAKE GUIDELINES

- Most of the results of studies conducted on the health benefits of onion consumption have shown that health benefits are only significant with daily consumption of at least ½ cup of onion.

- There are no reported risks of interactions between onions and medications or other substances.

RESEARCH FINDINGS

- Daily onion consumption appears to improve bone density in perimenopausal (i.e., women near the age of menopause) and postmenopausal non-Hispanic White women, reducing their risk for hip fracture by over 20% compared to women in the same demographic who never eat onions.
- Results of several studies indicate that frequent onion consumption reduces the risk of cardiovascular disease (CVD), heart attack, and damage caused by toxic substances reaching the brain when reduced blood flow to the brain is present. Researchers suggest that this effect is most likely due to the sulfur-containing compounds and phytonutrients found in onions.
- Researchers conducted a study of the effects of raw red onion consumption on metabolic features (e.g., blood sugar, triglycerides, cholesterol) of overweight and obese women with polycystic ovary syndrome (PCOS). Researchers reported that total cholesterol and low-density lipoprotein (LDL) cholesterol levels decreased significantly in the women who consumed a high amount of raw red onion every day for 8 weeks (compared with a 'low-onion' control group). Further research is recommended.

SUMMARY

Consumers should become knowledgeable about the physiologic benefits of onion consumption. Onion is a good source of minerals, vitamin C, and a variety of sulfur-containing compounds and phytonutrients. These nutrients support bone health and provide cancer-preventive, anti-inflammatory, antibacterial, antioxidant, and cardiovascular benefits.

—*Cherie Marcel, BS*

REFERENCES

Cook, T. M. (2006). The allium twins. *Homeopathic Heritage, 31*(10), 25-28.

Ebrahimi-Mamaghani, M., Saghafi-Asl, M., Pirouzpanah, S., & Asghari-Jafarabadi, M. (2014). Effects of raw red onion consumption on metabolic features in overweight or obese women with polycystic ovary syndrome: A randomized controlled clinical trial. *The Journal of Obstetrics and Gynaecology Research, 40*(4), 1067-1076. doi:10.1111/ jog.12311

Galeone, C., Tavani, A., Pelucchi, C., Negri, E., & La Vecchia, C. (2009). Allium vegetable intake and risk of acute myocardial infarction in Italy. *European Journal of Nutrition, 48*(2), 120-123. doi:10.1007/ s00394-008-0771-2

Hubbard, G. P., Wolffram, S., de Vos, R., Bovy, A., Gibbins, J. M., & Lovegrove, J. A. (2006). Ingestion of onion soup high in quercetin inhibits platelet aggregation and essential components of the collagen-stimulated platelet activation pathway in man: A pilot study. *British Journal of Nutrition, 96*(3), 482-488.

Hyun, S. W., Jang, M., Park, S. W., Kim, E. J., & Jung, Y. S. (2013). Onion (Allium cepa) extract attenuates brain edema. *Nutrition, 29*(1), 244-249. doi:10.1016/ j.nut.2012.02.017

Leser, M., & Reddin, K. (2011). Eat right to fight cancer. Onions in a cancer prevention diet. *Oncology Nutrition Connection, 19*(1), 15-18.

Matheson, E. M., Mainous, A. G., III, & Carnemolla, M. A. (2009). The association between onion consumption and bone density in perimenopausal and postmenopausal non-Hispanic white women 50 years and older. *Menopause, 16*(4), 756-759. doi:10.1097/ gme.0b013e31819581a5

Riley, T. (2007). Super foods. The healthy onion: Helping to fight cancer and cardiovascular disease. *Life Extention, 13*(10), 93-95.

The George Mateljan Foundation editorial team. (n.d.). The world's healthiest foods: Onions. Retrieved November 16, 2015, fromhttp://www.whfoods.com/ genpage.php? tname=foodspice&dbid=45

REVIEWER(S)

Darlene Strayer, RN, MBA, Cinahl Information Systems, Glendale, CA

Nursing Executive Practice Council, Glendale Adventist Medical Center, Glendale, CA

Potatoes

WHAT WE KNOW

Potatoes, or *Solanum tuberosum*, are members of the nightshade, or Solanaceae, family, along with tomatoes, eggplants, peppers, and tomatillos. There are about 100 varieties of potatoes, including small fingerling potatoes, medium-sized Yukon gold potatoes and red potatoes, and very large Russet potatoes. Potatoes vary in color from light beige to dark purple. Cook potatoes have a smooth and creamy texture and a mild, neutral flavor; potatoes have been considered a "comfort food" in the human diet for about 7,000 years. Although technically a tuber vegetable, potatoes are categorized as a starch due to their high carbohydrate content. Potatoes can be baked, mashed, fried, boiled, and used in soups, casseroles, and patties. Potatoes are a good source of vitamins C and B6 (pyridoxine), potassium, manganese, the amino acid tryptophan, and fiber. They provide a variety of phytonutrients (i.e., beneficial, plant-derived chemicals) such as carotenoids, flavonoids, caffeic acid, and patatin.

NUTRIENTS IN POTATOES

- Potatoes contain nutrients that have strong antioxidant, anti-inflammatory, anticancer, and cardio-protective properties.
  - —Vitamin C is a water-soluble vitamin that neutralizes free radicals, protecting against inflammation and cellular damage. Adequate vitamin C intake is vital for proper function of the immune system and has been associated with prevention of heart disease, stroke, and cancer.
  - —The B vitamin pyridoxine is required for the conversion of tryptophan to niacin and is involved in the conversion of homocysteine to cysteine. It also supports the synthesis of serotonin and dopamine, which are neurotransmitters required for nerve cell communication. By maintaining lymphoid organs, pyridoxine contributes to the proper function of the immune system.
  - —Potassium supports normal cellular, nerve, and muscle function and helps to eliminate excess sodium from the body.
  - —Manganese is a trace mineral that is responsible for energy production, fatty acid production, cholesterol production, and protection against the damage caused by free radicals.
  - —Copper is a vital component of superoxide dismutase, which is an enzyme involved in energy production and antioxidant activity. Copper contributes to the action of lysyl oxidase, an enzyme necessary for the cross-linking of collagen and elastin to allow flexibility in blood vessels, bones, and joints. Copper enhances the body's ability to use

iron, preventing iron-deficiency anemia, ruptured vessels, irregular heartbeat, and infection.
  - —Potatoes are a source of the amino acid tryptophan, which contributes to the synthesis of niacin and serotonin. Serotonin is thought to promote healthy sleep patterns and stabilize mood.
  - —The phytonutrients found in potatoes vary with the color. For example, purple potatoes contain more anthocyanins than white potatoes. However, all potatoes provide a collection of potent phytonutrients that protect against cardiovascular disease (CVD), respiratory conditions, cancer, and hypertension.

DIETARY INTAKE GUIDELINES

- There are no recommendations for daily intake of potatoes in the literature.
- There is no information in the literature regarding potato deficiency.
- Except when organically grown, potatoes frequently have pesticide residues. Pesticides have been documented to impede the ability of the liver to process toxins, the ability of nerves to conduct messages to the brain, and the ability of the cells to create energy.
- Potatoes contain the amino acid asparagine; when heated to a high temperature, asparagine can form the carcinogen acrylamide. Cooking methods such as frying, baking, or broiling have been reported to produce acrylamide. French fries and potato chips have been found to contain more acrylamide than other foods.
  - —Blanching potatoes before frying and drying potatoes in a hot air oven after frying can decrease the formation of acrylamide.
- No information was found in the literature regarding risk for interactions of potatoes and medications.

RESEARCH FINDINGS

- Researchers analyzed the bioavailability of vitamin C from processed potatoes and found that the vitamin C in mashed potatoes and potato chips was effectively absorbed in the intestine after human consumption. Researchers concluded that potatoes are a good nutritional source of vitamin C.

SUMMARY

Consumers should become knowledgeable about the physiologic effects of consuming potatoes. Potatoes are a good source of vitamins C and B6, potassium, manganese, tryptophan, fiber, and a variety of phytonutrients. These nutrients contribute to energy production, support the immune system, and may prevent cardiovascular disease and cancer. Cooking methods such as frying, baking, and broiling have been reported to produce the carcinogen acrylamide. French fries and potato chips have been found to contain more acrylamide than other foods.

—*Cherie Marcel, BS*

REFERENCES

Kondo, Y., Higashi, C., Iwama, M., Ishihara, K., Handa, S., Mugita, H., ... Ishigami, A. (2012). Bioavailability of vitamin C from mashed potatoes and potato chips after oral administration in healthy Japanese men. *British Journal of Nutrition*, 107(6), 885-892. doi:10.1017/S0007114511003643

National Cancer Institute editorial team. (2008). Acrylamide in food and cancer risk. *National Cancer Institute at the National Institutes of Health*. Retrieved June 3, 2015, from http://www.cancer.gov/cancertopics/factsheet/Risk/acrylamide-in-food

Palmer, S. (2010). Purple potatoes serve up royal nutrition. *Environmental Nutrition*, 33(9), 8.

Sandon, L. (2012). In praise of potatoes. *Bottom Line Health*, 26(3), 15.

Seal, C. J., de Mul, A., Eisenbrand, G., Haverkort, A. J., Franke, K., Lalljie, S. P. D., ... Wilms, L. (2008). Risk-benefit considerations of mitigation measures on acrylamide content of foods – a case study on potatoes, cereals and coffee. *British Journal of Nutrition*, (Suppl 2), S21-S46. doi:10.1017/S0007114508965314

The George Mateljan Foundation editorial staff. (n.d.). The world's healthiest foods: Potatoes. Retrieved June 3, 2015, from http://www.whfoods.com/genpage.php?tname=foodspice&dbid=48

The George Mateljan Foundation editorial staff. (n.d.). The world's healthiest foods: What is acrylamide and how is it involved with food and health? Retrieved June 3, 2015, from http://www.whfoods.com/genpage.php?tname=george&dbid=260

The goodness in potatoes. (2010). *Food Today*, 2-3.

Weichselbaum, E. (2010). An overview of the role of potatoes in the UK diet. *Nutrition Bulletin*, 35(3), 195-206. doi:10.1111/j.1467-3010.2010.01845.x

REVIEWER(S)

Darlene Strayer, RN, MBA, Cinahl Information Systems, Glendale, CA

Nursing Executive Practice Council, Glendale Adventist Medical Center, Glendale, CA

Seaweed

WHAT WE KNOW

Seaweed (also called sea vegetables) are not weeds or vegetables and are technically classified as algae. Categorized by color as brown, red, or green, there are thousands of varieties of seaweeds growing in both fresh-and saltwater lakes and seas. While relatively new to the cuisine of Western cultures, the Japanese have included seaweed in their diet for centuries. The rich content of minerals derived from seawater, vitamins, and phytonutrients (i.e., beneficial, plant-derived chemicals) in seaweed exhibit anti-inflammatory, anti-mutagenic, anticoagulant, antithrombotic, and antiviral activities. Some of the most widely used varieties of seaweed include the following:

- Nori is best known for its use in making sushi rolls. Nori is naturally dark purple to black in color but turns phosphorescent green when toasted.
- Kelp can range in color from light brown to dark green and is frequently used in flake form.
- Hijiki is black and wiry and has a strong flavor.
- Kombu is very dark in color and is frequently used in strips or sheets, or as a flavoring agent in soups.
- Wakame is similar to Kombu and is commonly used to make miso soup.
- Arame is a lacy, delicate seaweed that has a mild and somewhat sweet flavor.
- Dulse is a chewy, reddish-brown seaweed.

NUTRIENTS IN SEAWEED

- Seaweed derives many minerals from the water as it grows, making it an excellent source of most of the minerals required for human vitality. Seaweed provides sodium, calcium, magnesium, potassium, chlorine, sulfur, phosphorus, iron, zinc, copper, selenium, molybdenum, fluoride, manganese, boron, nickel, and cobalt. Seaweed is a source of iodine.
  —Iodine is a trace mineral that supports the function of the thyroid gland and has antifungal, antimicrobial, and antibacterial activities.

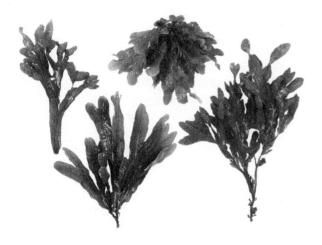

—Magnesium balances the action of calcium in cells for the regulation of bone health and tone in nerves and muscles. It maintains relaxation of nerves and muscles, which contributes to the prevention of high blood pressure, muscle spasms, asthma, migraine headaches, general soreness, and fatigue.

—Calcium builds and maintains bones and teeth, regulates muscle contraction, conducts nerve impulses, activates enzymes for energy production and muscle contraction, participates in blood clotting, assists with vitamin B12 absorption, and maintains the structural integrity of intracellular membranes.

—Iron is vital for the production of red blood cells and hemoglobin, which are necessary for energy production and the transport of oxygen to the tissues. Iron supports immune function, is necessary for cognitive development, contributes to energy production, and regulates temperature.

- Seaweed contains unique phytonutrients, including fucoidans (i.e., sulfated polysaccharides), which are starch-like compounds that contain sulfur atoms. Fucoidans have powerful anti-inflammatory, anticancer, anticoagulant, antithrombotic, and antiviral properties.
- Seaweed is a good source of vitamin K, which acts as a coenzyme involved in maintaining normal levels of blood clotting proteins and contributes to bone building. Measurable amounts of the antioxidant vitamins C and E are found in seaweed.
- The B vitamins folate, riboflavin, and pantothenic acid are present in seaweed. These vitamins

contribute to the production and breakdown of carbohydrates, proteins, and lipids; provide cardiovascular protection; maintain the nervous system; and contribute to the production of acetylcholine, deoxyribonucleic acid (DNA) and ribonucleic acid (RNA).

DIETARY INTAKE GUIDELINES

- Seaweed has a great capacity for absorbing and retaining minerals from the water in which it grows. This can pose a risk if the water is contaminated because seaweed absorbs unwanted elements such as arsenic, lead, and cadmium. It has been determined that all seaweed contains traces of arsenic, and hijiki has the highest capacity for arsenic absorption. Because of this, it is advised to avoid consumption of hijiki unless it is verified to contain very low levels of arsenic and is certified as organic.

RESEARCH FINDINGS

- Metabolic syndrome is increasing in most developed nations except for parts of Asia where seaweed is a dietary staple. Researchers conducting a study to determine if seaweed consumption prevents metabolic syndrome concluded that consuming 4–6 grams of seaweed per day, which is typical in Japan, appears to be associated with a lower incidence of metabolic syndrome.
- Epidemiologic study results show that Japanese women who consume high amounts of seaweed have significantly lower rates of breast cancer than women who consume a typically Western diet (e.g., containing "fast foods"). Results of several scientific studies show preventive and potentially therapeutic activity of several varieties of seaweed against mammary gland tumors and breast cancer. Similar findings have been reported regarding the therapeutic potential of the constituents of seaweed against hepatocarcinoma (i.e., liver cancer).

SUMMARY

Consumers should become knowledgeable about the risks and benefits of seaweed consumption. Seaweed is a good source of minerals, vitamins, and phytonutrients. These nutrients exhibit anti-inflammatory, antimutagenic, anticoagulant, antithrombotic, and antiviral activities. Seaweed can absorb and retain unwanted elements such as arsenic, lead, and cadmium, from the water in which it grows. Individuals should avoid consumption of hijiki unless it is verified to contain very low levels of arsenic and is certified as organic.

—*Cherie Marcel, BS*

REFERENCES

Abascal, K., & Yarnell, E. (2001). Herbs and breast cancer: Research review of seaweed, rosemary, and ginseng. *Alternative & Complementary Therapies*, 7(1), 32-36. doi:10.1089/107628001300000705

Bae, S. J., & Choi, Y. H. (2007). Methanol extract of the seaweed Gloiopeltis furcata induces G2/M arrest and inhibits cyclooxygenase-2 activity in human hepatocarcinoma HepG2 cells. *Phytotherapy Research*, 21(1), 52-57.

Corleone, J. (2010). The nutritional value of seaweed. Livestrong.com. *Livestrong.com*. Retrieved February 18, 2015, from http://www.livestrong.com/article/300690-the-nutritional-value-of-seaweed/

Edwards, G. F. (2007). Seaweed: Herb of the ocean. *Herb Quarterly*, 28-31.

The George Mateljan Foundation editorial team. (n.d.). Sea vegetables. *The World's Healthiest Foods*. Retrieved March 3, 2015, from http://www.whfoods.com/genpage.php? tname=foodspice&dbid=135

SHamsabadi, F. T., Khoddami, A., Fard, S. G., ABdullah, R., Othman, H. H., & Mohamed, S. (2013). Comparison of Tamoxifen with edible seaweed (Eucheuma cottonii L.) extract in suppressing breast tumor. *Nutrition & Cancer*, 65(2), 255-262. doi:10.10 80/01635581.2013.756528

Silberlicht, C. (2007). Healing foods. Under the sea: Savor seaweed in far more places than the sushi bar. *Alternative Magazine*, 43-46.

Teas, J., Baldeón, M. E., Chiriboga, D. E., Davis, J. R., Sarriés, A. J., & Braverman, L. E. (2009). Could dietary seaweed reverse the metabolic syndrome? *Asia Pacific Journal of Clinical Nutrition*, 18(2), 145-154.

Yang, Y. J., Nam, S. J., Kong, G., & Kim, M. K. (2010). A case-control study on seaweed consumption and the risk of breast cancer. *British Journal of Nutrition*, 103(9), 1345-1353. doi:10.1017/S0007114509993242

REVIEWER(S)

Darlene Strayer, RN, MBA, Cinahl Information Systems, Glendale, CA

Nursing Executive Practice Council, Glendale Adventist Medical Center, Glendale, CA

Spinach

WHAT WE KNOW

Spinach, or *Spinacia* oleracea, is a member of the *Amaranthaceae-Chenopodiaceae* family, which includes Swiss chard, quinoa and beets. The delicate, spade-shaped, bright green leaves of spinach have a savory flavor with a hint of bitterness that becomes more pronounced when cooked. Spinach leaves can be sautéed, steamed, baked, eaten raw as a salad green, and blended as an ingredient in a recipe for juice. However it is consumed, spinach provides many nutrients and health benefits. Nutrients found in spinach include vitamins K, C, E, B6, B2, B1, B3, and folate and minerals such as manganese, magnesium, iron, calcium, potassium, copper, phosphorous and selenium. Spinach is rich in fiber and many phytonutrients (i.e., beneficial plant-derived chemicals), including pro-vitamin A carotenoids. Spinach has antioxidant, anti-inflammatory, anti-cancer, and cardio-protective properties.

NUTRIENTS IN SPINACH

- Spinach contains many powerful antioxidants and has anti-inflammatory properties in the form of vitamins, minerals, and phytonutrients, including the following:
  - Spinach is a good source of vitamin K and contains over 1,000% of the recommended daily intake of vitamin K per cup of cooked spinach leaves. Vitamin K maintains normal levels of blood clotting proteins and contributes to bone building.
  - One cup of cooked spinach provides over 300% of the recommended daily intake of vitamin A, or retinol, in the form of pro-vitamin A carotenoids. Vitamin A is a fat-soluble vitamin that is required for vision, maintenance of the surface lining of the eyes and other epithelial tissue, proper bone growth, immune response, energy regulation, reproduction, embryonic development, and gene expression.
  - Vitamin C is a water-soluble vitamin that neutralizes free radicals, protecting against inflammation and cellular damage. Adequate vitamin C intake is essential for proper function of the immune system and is associated with the prevention of heart disease, stroke, and cancer.

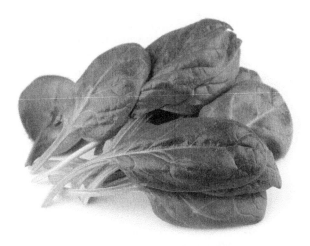

—Vitamin E is a fat-soluble vitamin that functions primarily as an antioxidant but also maintains cell membranes, assists in vitamin K absorption, and contributes to immune system function.

—Vitamin B6, or pyridoxine, is required for the conversion of tryptophan to niacin and is involved in the conversion of homocysteine to cysteine. It supports the synthesis of serotonin and dopamine, which are neurotransmitters required for nerve cell communication. By maintaining lymphoid organs, pyridoxine contributes to proper function of the immune system.

—The B vitamins thiamin (B1), riboflavin (B2), and niacin (B3) create energy by aiding the production and breakdown of carbohydrates, lipids, proteins, and alcohol. They provide cardiovascular protection, maintain nervous system function, and support the production of red blood cells (RBCs), hormones, and necessary cholesterol.

—Folate is a water-soluble B vitamin that is essential for the production and maintenance of RBCs. It is essential for the production of deoxyribonucleic acid (DNA) and ribonucleic acid (RNA), the genetic code for the cells, and is important in the metabolism of the amino acid homocysteine.

—Manganese is a trace mineral that is responsible for energy production, fatty acid production, necessary cholesterol production, and protection against the damage caused by free radicals.

—Magnesium balances the action of calcium in cells for the regulation of bone health and tone in nerves and muscles. It maintains relaxation of the nerves and muscles, which contributes to the prevention of high blood pressure, muscle spasms, asthma, migraine headaches, general soreness, and fatigue.

—Iron is important for the production of RBCs and hemoglobin, which are necessary for energy production and the transport of oxygen to the tissues. Iron supports immune function, is essential for mental development, contributes to energy production, and regulates temperature.

—The calcium in spinach is important for building and maintaining bones and teeth. Calcium regulates muscle contraction, conducts nerve impulses, activates enzymes for energy production and muscle contraction, participates in blood clotting, assists with vitamin B12 absorption, and maintains the structural integrity of intracellular membranes.

—Potassium supports normal cellular, nerve, and muscle function, and helps to eliminate excess sodium from the body.

—Copper is an important component of superoxide dismutase, which is an enzyme involved in energy production and antioxidant activity. Copper contributes to the action of lysyl oxidase, an enzyme necessary for the cross-linking of collagen and elastin, which allows flexibility in the blood vessels, bones, and joints. Copper enhances the body's ability to use iron, preventing iron-deficiency anemia, ruptured vessels, irregular heartbeat, and infection.

—Phosphorous combines with calcium for the formation of bones and teeth, muscle contraction, and nerve conduction, and is essential for the structural integrity of cell membranes.

—Selenium combines with proteins to create selenoproteins, which regulate thyroid function.

—Spinach is a source of the amino acid tryptophan, which contributes to the synthesis of niacin and serotonin. Serotonin is thought to promote healthy sleep patterns and stabilize mood.

—Spinach is a good source of dietary fiber, which binds and removes toxins from the colon, assists in glucose control, and reduces high cholesterol levels.

—Spinach is an excellent source of valuable phytonutrients, including carotenoids and flavonoids. These nutrients are potent antioxidants that are known to support cardiovascular health, protect against cancer, regulate blood glucose levels, and promote the health of the bones, liver, kidneys, and blood.

–The flavonoids quercetin and kaempferol provide strong antioxidant and anti-inflammatory protection. They have antihistamine, antimicrobial, anti-diabetic, and anti-carcinogenic properties

–The carotenoids lutein, zeaxanthin, and beta-carotene are antioxidants that inhibit the inflammatory process, neutralize free radicals, impede cancer cell proliferation, and repair damaged DNA. They prevent atherosclerosis and safeguard the eyes from light-induced damage.

DIETARY INTAKE GUIDELINES

- There is no information in the literature regarding an official recommendation for the intake of spinach
- A recent review of available literature found no information on spinach deficiency
- A recent review of available literature found no information on spinach toxicity
- Because spinach is a substantial source of vitamin K, which can interfere with the effectiveness of blood-thinning medications (e.g., warfarin), individuals receiving blood thinners should be educated regarding the implications of including spinach in their diet.

  —Results of a randomized, controlled trial showed that dietary intake of vitamin K does not need to be limited in persons receiving warfarin therapy if consistent, moderate intake of vitamin K is maintained. Consistent vitamin K consumption prevents large fluctuations in intake and supports optimal coagulation management.

- Spinach may increase risk for kidney stones in individuals with a history of kidney stones because it contains a high amount of oxalates, which are primary components of kidney stones. Oxalates can build up, crystallize in body fluids, and cause stones in individuals with preexisting kidney or gallbladder dysfunction.

RESEARCH FINDINGS

- Researchers have investigated the impact of the intake of oxalates on the absorption of the nutrients magnesium and iron by comparing meals containing spinach, which is higher in oxalates, and meals containing kale, which is lower in oxalates

  —Results of one study indicated that the magnesium absorbed from the meal with spinach was about 35% less than that absorbed from the meal with kale.

  —The results of a study evaluating the influence of oxalates on the absorption of iron indicated that although iron absorption was lower in the meal with spinach than in the meal with kale, the difference was not statistically significant. Researchers suggested that the impact of oxalates on iron absorption was minor.

SUMMARY

Consumers should become knowledgeable about the physiologic risks and benefits of spinach. Spinach is a good source of powerful antioxidants, vitamins, minerals, and phytonutrients. These nutrients support healthy blood clotting, prevent eye damage, and may help prevent heart disease and cancer. Individuals with a history of kidney stones should avoid spinach consumption due to the high oxalate content. Individuals taking blood thinning medications should be aware of the counteracting effect of spinach consumption.

—*Cherie Marcel, BS*

REFERENCES

Bohn, T., Davidsson, L., Walczyk, T., & Hurrell, R. F. (2004). Fractional magnesium absorption is significantly lower in human subjects from a meal served with an oxalate-rich vegetable, spinach, as compared with a meal served with kale, a vegetable with low oxalate content. *British Journal of Nutrition*, 91(4), 601-606. doi:10.1079/BJN20031081

Gebuis, E. P., Rosendaal, F. R., van Meegen, E., & der Meer, F. J. (2011). Vitamin K1 supplementation to improve the stability of anticoagulation therapy with vitamin K antagonists: A dose-finding study. *Haematologica*, 96(4), 583-589.

The George Mateljan Foundation editorial team. (n.d.). Can you tell me what oxalates are and in which foods they can be found? *World's Healthiest Foods*. Retrieved March 5, 2015, from http://www.whfoods.com/genpage.php?tname=george&dbid=48

The George Mateljan Foundation editorial team. (n.d.). Spinach. *The World's Healthiest Foods*. Retrieved March 5, 2015, from http://www.whfoods.com/gen-page.php? tname=foodspice&dbid=43

Gennant Bonsmann, S. S., Walczyk, T., Renggli, S., & Hurrell, R. F. (2008). Oxalic acid does not influence nonhaem iron absorption in humans: A comparison of kale and spinach in meals. *European Journal of Clinical Nutrition, 62*(3), 336-341.

Moser, B., Szekeres, T., Bieglmayer, C., Wagner, K., Misik, M., Kundi, M., ... Knasmueller, S. (2011). Impact of spinach consumption on DNA stability in peripheral lymphocytes and on biochemical blood parameters: Results of a human intervention trial. *European Journal of Nutrition, 50*(7), 587-594. doi:10.1007/s00394-011-0167-6

Palmer, S. (2009). Spinach flexes its might nutrition muscle. *Environmental Nutrition, 32*(3), 8.

REVIEWER(S)

Darlene Strayer, RN, MBA, Cinahl Information Systems, Glendale, CA

Nursing Executive Practice Council, Glendale Adventist Medical Center, Glendale, CA

Squash

WHAT WE KNOW

Squash are a group of nutrient-rich gourds from the *Cucurbitaceae* family, which includes melon and cucumber. As a group, squash tend to be round, oblong, or spherical and grow on creeping vines. They are encased in a thick outer skin that protects their fleshy interior and seeds. The types of squash include summer, winter, butternut, spaghetti, acorn, pumpkin, delicata, and kabocha squash. Culinary uses for squash include soups, breads, sautés, salads, and desserts. Squash types vary in level of sweetness, softness, and juiciness when ripe. Squash is essentially free of fat and low in calories, and is rich in vitamins, minerals, phytonutrients (i.e., beneficial plant-derived nutrients), and fiber.

NUTRIENTS IN SQUASH

Nutrients in squash include the following:

—Squash provide pro-vitamin A carotenoids (e.g., beta-carotene), which are powerful antioxidants with anti-cancer activity, and protect the eyes from damage. Carotenoids are converted to vitamin A in the body. Vitamin A is required for vision, maintenance of the surface lining of the eyes and other epithelial tissue, proper bone growth, immune response, energy regulation, reproduction, embryonic development, and activation of gene expression.

—Squash is an excellent source of vitamin C, which neutralizes free radicals, protecting against inflammation and cellular damage. Adequate intake of vitamin C is vital for immune system function and has been associated with prevention of heart disease, stroke, and cancer.

—The potassium provided by squash supports normal cellular, nerve, and muscle function and helps to eliminate excess sodium from the body.

—Squash is a good source of dietary fiber, which binds and removes toxins from the colon, assists in glucose control, and reduces high cholesterol levels.

DIETARY INTAKE GUIDELINES

• There is no officially recommended dosage for the therapeutic use of squash in the literature.

• Squash intake is generally considered safe when consumed by healthy individuals in amounts that are normally served as food.

• There is concern that squash may increase risk for kidney stones in individuals with a history of kidney stones because squash contains measurable amounts of the chemical oxalate, which is a primary component of kidney stones.

• There are no reported interactions between squash and medications.

• Researchers have reported that squash better retains antioxidant activity if steamed than if boiled or microwaved.

SUMMARY

Consumers should become knowledgeable about the physiologic benefits of the consumption of squash. Squash is a good source of vitamin C, potassium, carotenoids and fiber. These nutrients support the immune system, regulate blood pressure, improve GI health and may help reduce the risk of developing heart disease, stroke and cancer. Individuals with a history of kidney stones should know that squash intake can increase risk of kidney stones.

—Cherie Marcel, BS

REFERENCES

The George Mateljan Foundation editorial team. (2012). Squash, summer. *World's healthiest foods*. Retrieved March 5, 2015, from http://www.whfoods.com/genpage.php? tname=foodspice&dbid=62

Neithercott, T. (2009). Food for thought. The best of the harvest. Squash is a sweet seasonal treat. *Diabetes Forecast*, 62(10), 35-38.

Raymond, S. (2009). Sensational squash: Autumn's nutritional superstar. *Alive: Canada's Natural Health & Wellness Magazine*, (324), 130-133.

Riccardi, V. A. (2011). Butternut squash. *Vegetarian Times*, (388), 60-63.

Salat, H. (2005). Beyond the great pumpkin: Winter squash is as versatile as it is power-packed. *Health*, 19(9), 153-154, 156.

REVIEWER(S)

Darlene Strayer, RN, MBA, Cinahl Information Systems, Glendale, CA

Nursing Executive Practice Council, Glendale Adventist Medical Center, Glendale, CA

Sweet Potatoes

WHAT WE KNOW

The sweet potato, or *Ipomoea batatas*, is a nutrient-rich root vegetable from the *Convolvulaceae* family, and is one of the earliest vegetables known to be consumed by humans. Despite their name, sweet potatoes are not in the same family as traditional potatoes and are not related to yams; in North America, however, the common orange-colored variety of sweet potato is commonly referred to as a "yam," a name given to it in the mid-20th century in an attempt to distinguish it from the popular white-fleshed sweet potato. There are about 400 different varieties of sweet potatoes, and their skin and flesh colors are varying shades of white, yellow, pink, orange, red, and purple. Sweet potatoes are shaped similarly to common potatoes, but can be longer, knobby, and pointed at each end. Sweet potatoes can be baked, boiled, roasted, and steamed, all of which result in a sweet and creamy culinary dish. Nutritionally, sweet potatoes are rich in vitamins, minerals, and phytonutrients (i.e., beneficial, plant-derived chemicals), and are ranked among the most nutritious vegetables in the world. No other vegetable has a higher pro-vitamin A content than sweet potatoes, and they are an excellent source of many other antioxidants.

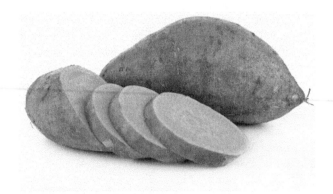

NUTRIENTS IN SWEET POTATOES

* Sweet potatoes contain many powerful antioxidants and anti-inflammatories in the form of vitamins, minerals, and phytonutrients, including the following:
  —Sweet potatoes provide over 400% of the daily value of vitamin A in the form of pro-vitamin A carotenoids (e.g., beta-carotene). Pro-vitamin A carotenoids are the precursors to vitamin A, or retinol, which is a fat-soluble vitamin that is required for vision, maintenance of the surface lining of the eyes and other epithelial tissue, bone growth, immune response, energy regulation, reproduction, embryonic development, and activation of gene expression.
  —Vitamin C is a water-soluble vitamin that neutralizes free radicals, protecting against inflammation and cellular damage. Adequate vitamin C intake is necessary for the proper function of the immune system and has been associated with the prevention of heart disease, stroke, and cancer.
  —The B vitamin pyridoxine is required for the conversion of tryptophan into niacin, and is involved in the conversion of homocysteine to cysteine. It also supports the synthesis of serotonin and dopamine, which are neurotransmitters required for nerve cell communication. By maintaining lymphoid organs, pyridoxine contributes to the proper function of the immune system.
  —The B vitamin niacin creates energy by aiding the production and breakdown of carbohydrates, lipids, proteins, and alcohol. It provides cardiovascular protection, maintains the

nervous system, and supports the production of red blood cells, hormones, and necessary cholesterol.

—Sweet potatoes are a source of the amino acid tryptophan, which contributes to the synthesis of niacin and serotonin. Serotonin is thought to promote healthy sleep patterns and stabilize mood.

—Manganese is a trace mineral that is responsible for energy production, fatty acid production, necessary cholesterol production, and protection against the damage caused by free radicals.

—Potassium supports normal cellular, nerve, and muscle function, and helps to eliminate excess sodium from the body.

—Copper is a vital component of superoxide dismutase, an enzyme involved in energy production and antioxidant activity. Copper contributes to the action of lysyl oxidase, which is an enzyme necessary for the cross-linking of collagen and elastin to allow flexibility in blood vessels, bones, and joints. Copper enhances the body's ability to use iron, preventing iron-deficiency anemia, ruptured vessels, irregular heartbeat, and infection.

—Along with carotenoids, sweet potatoes are an excellent source of phytonutrients such as glycosides, anthocyanin, and proanthocyanidins. These nutrients are potent antioxidants that are known to support cardiovascular health, protect against cancer, regulate blood glucose, and promote the health of the bones, liver, kidneys, and bloodstream.

DIETARY INTAKE GUIDELINES

- No information was found in the literature regarding recommended daily intake of sweet potatoes.
- There is no information in the literature regarding risk of interaction between sweet potatoes and medications.
- Sweet potatoes may increase risk for kidney stones in individuals with a history of kidney stones because they contain a moderate amount of oxalates, which are primary components of kidney stones. Oxalates can build up, crystallize in body fluids, and cause stones in individuals with preexisting kidney or gallbladder dysfunction.

RESEARCH FINDINGS

- Sweet potatoes grow worldwide and throughout the year, making them a valuable resource in the prevention of hunger and malnutrition in famine-plagued countries. Researchers have reported that providing at-risk populations with the ability to grow sweet potatoes is effective in preventing vitamin A deficiency and other complications of malnutrition.

SUMMARY

Consumers should become knowledgeable about the physiologic effects of consuming sweet potatoes. Sweet potatoes are a good source of fiber, amino acids, vitamins (e.g., C, B-complex), minerals (e.g., magnesium, copper, potassium), and phytonutrients (e.g., pro-vitamin A carotenoids). These nutrients support eye health, regulate blood glucose, and may protect against heart disease and cancer. Individuals with a history of kidney or gallbladder dysfunction should know that consumption of large amounts of sweet potatoes might increase the risk of developing kidney stones.

—*Cherie Marcel, BS*

REFERENCES

Bhide, M. (2006). Sweet potatoes. *Better Nutrition*, 68(2), 28-30.

Campbell, M. (2010). Sweet potato nutrition data. *Livestrong.com*. Retrieved January 20, 2014, from http://www.livestrong.com/article/297519-sweet-potato-nutrition-data/

The George Mateljan Foundation editorial staff. (n.d.). Can you tell me what oxalates are and in which foods they can be found?. *The World's Healthiest Foods*. Retrieved March 6, 2015, from http://www.whfoods.com/genpage.php?tname=george&dbid=48

The George Mateljan Foundation editorial staff. (n.d.). Sweet potatoes. *The World's Healthiest Foods*. Retrieved March 6, 2015, from http://www.whfoods.com/genpage.php? tname=foodspice&dbid=64#healthbenefits

Haskell, M. J., Hamil, K. M., Hassan, F., Peerson, J. M., Hossain, M. I., Fuchs, G. J., & Brown, K. H. (2004). Daily consumption of Indian spinach (Basella alba) or sweet potatoes has a positive effect on total-body vitamin A stores in Bangladeshi men. *The American Journal of Clinical Nutrition*, 80(3), 705.

Low, J. W., Arimond, M., Osman, N., Cunguara, B., Zano, F., & Tschirley, D. (2007). A food-based approach introducing orange-fleshed sweet potatoes increased vitamin A intake and serum retinol concentrations in young children in rural Mozambique. *The Journal of Nutrition, 137*(5), 1320-1327.

Palmer, S. (2009). Sweet potatoes glow with health and flavor. *Environmental Nutrition, 32*(12), 8.

REVIEWER(S)

Darlene Strayer, RN, MBA, Cinahl Information Systems, Glendale, CA

Nursing Executive Practice Council, Glendale Adventist Medical Center, Glendale, CA

Turnips

WHAT WE KNOW

Turnips, or *Brassica rapa*, are white or yellow bulbous root vegetables that belong to the *Brassica*, or *Cruciferae*, family. Other cruciferous vegetables include kale, collards, cabbage, and broccoli. Turnips are mildly bitter and savory in flavor and can be baked, sautéed, or boiled and are used in a similar manner as potatoes. Although the turnip bulb is most commonly used for cooking, the leaves of the turnip (also called turnip greens) are gaining popularity due to their high nutrient content. The turnip root is an excellent source of vitamin C and fiber. The leaves have many vitamins, minerals, and phytonutrients (i.e., beneficial, plant-derived chemicals), which have powerful antioxidant and anti-inflammatory properties. The consumption of turnip greens has been associated with the prevention of cancer of the bladder, breast, colon, lung, prostate, and ovaries.

NUTRIENTS IN TURNIPS

- Turnips provide vitamin C, which is a water-soluble vitamin that neutralizes free radicals, protecting against inflammation and cellular damage. Adequate vitamin C intake is vital for the proper function of the immune system and has been associated with the prevention of heart disease, stroke, and cancer.
- Turnip greens contain vitamin C and many other vitamins, minerals, and phytonutrients, including the following:
  - Vitamin K acts as a coenzyme involved in maintaining normal levels of blood clotting proteins, and contributes to bone building.

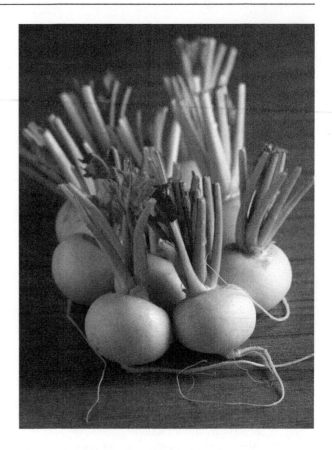

- Vitamin E is a fat-soluble vitamin that functions primarily as an antioxidant, but also maintains cell membranes, assists in vitamin K absorption, and contributes to the immune system.
- The B vitamins thiamin, riboflavin, folate, and niacin create energy by aiding the breakdown of carbohydrates. They provide cardiovascular protection, maintain the nervous system, and support the production of red blood cells, hormones, and necessary cholesterol.
- The B vitamin pantothenic acid is important in the production of acetylcholine, a neurotransmitter in the central and peripheral nervous systems.
- The B vitamin pyridoxine is required for the conversion of tryptophan into niacin, and is involved in the conversion of homocysteine to cysteine. It supports the production of serotonin and dopamine, which are neurotransmitters required for nerve cell communication. By maintaining lymphoid organs, pyridoxine contributes to the proper function of the immune system.

—Manganese is a trace mineral that is responsible for energy production, fatty acid production, necessary cholesterol production, and protection against the damage caused by free radicals.

—Calcium builds and maintains bones and teeth, regulates muscle contraction, conducts nerve impulses, activates enzymes for energy production and muscle contraction, participates in blood clotting, assists with vitamin B12 absorption, and maintains the structural integrity of intracellular membranes.

—Copper is a vital component of superoxide dismutase, an enzyme involved in energy production and antioxidant activity. It contributes to the action of lysyl oxidase, an enzyme necessary for the cross-linking of collagen and elastin, which allows flexibility in the blood vessels, bones, and joints. Copper enhances the body's ability to use iron, preventing iron-deficient anemia, ruptured vessels, irregular heartbeat, and infection.

—Potassium supports normal cellular, nerve, and muscle function, and helps to eliminate excess sodium from the body.

—Magnesium balances the action of calcium in cells for the regulation of bone health and tone of nerves and muscles. It maintains relaxation of nerves and muscles, which contributes to the prevention of high blood pressure, muscle spasms, asthma, migraine headaches, general soreness, and fatigue.

—Iron is necessary for the production of red blood cells and hemoglobin, which are necessary for energy production and the transport of oxygen to the tissues. Iron supports immune function, is necessary for cognitive development, contributes to energy production, and regulates temperature.

—Phosphorous combines with calcium for the formation of bones and teeth, muscle contraction, and nerve conduction, and is essential for the structural integrity of cell membranes.

—The amino acid tryptophan contributes to the synthesis of niacin and serotonin. Serotonin is thought to promote healthy sleep patterns and stabilize mood.

—The pro-vitamin A carotenoids (e.g., beta-carotene) are the precursors for vitamin A, or retinol, a fat-soluble vitamin that is required for vision, maintenance of the surface lining of the eyes and other epithelial tissue, bone growth, immune response, energy regulation, reproduction, embryonic development, and activation of gene expression.

—The phytonutrients hydroxycinnamic acid, quercetin, myricetin, isohamnetin, and kaempferol are potent antioxidants.

—The phytonutrient glucosinolate can be converted into isothiocyanates, which have cancer-preventing and anti-inflammatory activity.

RESEARCH FINDINGS

Recent review of the literature has found no new or updated research evidence regarding turnips.

SUMMARY

Consumers should become knowledgeable about the physiologic effects of consuming turnips. Turnips are a good source of vitamin C and fiber, and turnip greens contain many vitamins, minerals, and phytonutrients, which have powerful antioxidant and anti-inflammatory properties. These nutrients contribute to bone and muscle health, immune support and improved mood, and may help prevent many types of cancer, heart disease and stroke.

—*Cherie Marcel, BS*

REFERENCES

Bosley, E. (2013). Turnips. *Delicious Living, 29*(1), 58.

Golub, C. (2007). Be thankful for turnips: November nutrition. *Environmental Nutrition, 30*(11), 8.

The George Mateljan Foundation editorial staff. (n.d.). The world's healthiest foods: Turnip greens. *World's Healthiest Foods*. Retrieved March 16, 2015, from http:// www.whfoods.com/genpage. php?tname=foodspice&dbid=144

Zevnik, N. (2012). Healing Foods. Turnip temptation. *Better Nutrition, 74*(3), 54.

REVIEWER(S)

Darlene Strayer, RN, MBA, Cinahl Information Systems, Glendale, CA

Nursing Executive Practice Council, Glendale Adventist Medical Center, Glendale, CA

Watercress

WHAT WE KNOW

Watercress, or *Nasturtium officinale*, is a member of the cabbage, or Brassicaceae, family, also known as the cruciferous vegetable family, which includes bok choy, cauliflower, collards, broccoli, and mustard greens. It is a powerful antioxidant and a substantial source of many nutrients, including vitamins K and C, as well as beta-carotene, folic acid, calcium, phosphorus, iron, and fiber. Watercress is also a valuable source of phytonutrients, such as lutein, zeaxanthin, rutin, glucinolates, and nasturtiin, the precursor to phenethyl isothiocyanate (PEITC), a major cancer-fighting compound. As one of the first leafy greens to be consumed by humans, watercress has a long history, both in culinary use and medicinally. It has been used to treat gout, congestion, headaches, eczema and dermatitis, canker sores and mouth pain, anemia, rickets, cardiac disease, poor eyesight, and diminished lactation.

NUTRIENTS IN WATERCRESS

- The many active components of watercress are found primarily in its leaves.
- Watercress plays a major role in cancer prevention. Evidence indicates that it lowers the risk of prostate, colon, lung and breast cancers.
  - Watercress increases the antioxidants in the blood (e.g., lutein, beta-carotene, rutin) and prevents deoxyribonucleic acid (DNA) damage.
  - The phytonutrient nasturtiin is a precursor to PEITC, which inhibits enzymes that activate carcinogens and induces enzymes that rid the body of carcinogens.
- Lutein and zeaxanthin appear to reduce the risk of eye damage and help to protect skin, slowing the aging process and possibly reducing the risk of skin cancer.
- Watercress provides vitamin K, folic acid, iron, phosphorous, and calcium, promoting health and function of the bones and heart.

DIETARY INTAKE GUIDELINES

- Although there is no set recommendation for dosage, a tea or juice extract made from watercress leaves is commonly used for treating gout or mucous congestion. Watercress infusions can also be used as topical treatment of eczema or dermatitis, and are made by boiling the leaves in water, straining, and refrigerating before use.
- Individuals with hyperthyroidism should avoid watercress due to its high iodine content.
- There are no adverse reactions of watercress with medications reported in the literature.

RESEARCH FINDINGS

- Results of many studies regarding the effect of watercress consumption on the risk of developing cancer show that watercress is a powerful anti-carcinogenic agent; study results indicate that there is risk reduction for developing breast, lung, prostate, and colon cancer. Scientists continue to investigate what components of watercress are responsible for this risk reduction, how the components function, and what other types of cancer are affected. Recently, researchers reported that watercress is able to decrease damage to DNA and increase carotenoid concentrations in blood, both of which reduce cancer risk.
- Results of another study indicate that watercress and other cruciferous vegetables induce detoxification in the bloodstream.
- Researchers investigating the effect of crude watercress extract on human colon cancer cells concluded that watercress was protective against development and growth of cancer cells.

SUMMARY

Consumers should become knowledgeable about the physiologic effects of watercress. Watercress is a good source of vitamins K and C, beta-carotene, folic acid, calcium, phosphorus, iron, fiber, and many antioxidant-rich phytonutrients. These nutrients support the immune system, bone health, and may help prevent cancer. Individuals with hyperthyroidism should avoid watercress.

—*Cherie Marcel, BS*

REFERENCES

Boyd, L. A., McCann, M. J., Hashim, Y., Bennett, R. N., Gill, C. I. R., & Rowland, I. R. (2006). Assessment of the anti-genotoxic, anti-proliferative, and anti-metastatic potential of crude watercress extract in human colon cancer cells. *Nutrition & Cancer, 55*(2), 232-241.

Burns, S. (2011). Wonderful watercress: Pungent, peppery, and good for your skin. *Skin Deep, 9*(3), 11.

Dye, D. (2007). In the news. Watercress consumption prevents DNA damage. *Life Extension, 13*(6), 18.

Fogarty, M. C., Hughes, C. M., Burke, G., Brown, J. C., & Davison, G. W. (2013). Acute and chronic watercress supplementation attenuates exercise-induced peripheral mononuclear cell DNA damage and lipid peroxidation. *British Journal of Nutrition, 109*(2), 293-301. doi:10.1017/S0007114512000992

Gill, C. I. R., Haldar, S., Boyd, L. A., Bennett, R., Whiteford, J., Butler, M., & Rowland, I. R. (2007). Watercress supplementation in diet reduces lymphocyte DNA damage and alters blood antioxidant status in healthy adults. *American Journal of Clinical Nutrition, 85*(2), 504-510.

Watercress. (2002). In F. Hoffmann, & M. Manning (Eds.), *Herbal medicine and botanical medical fads* (pp. 212-213). Binghamton, NY: The Haworth Press, Inc.

Hoffmann, T., Kuhnert, A., Schubert, A., Gill, C., Rowland, I. R., Pool-Zobel, B. L., & Glei, M. (2009). Modulation of detoxification enzymes by watercress: In vitro and in vivo investigations in human peripheral blood cells. *European Journal of Nutrition, 48*(8), 483-491.

Raymond, S. (2011). Wonderful watercress: A cancer-fighting superstar. *Alive: Canada's Natural Health & Wellness Magazine,* (342), 142-145.

Rose, P., Huang, Q., Ong, C. N., & Whiteman, M. (2005). Broccoli and watercress suppress matrix metalloproteinase-9 activity and invasiveness of human MDA-MB-231 breast cancer cells,h. *Toxicology and Applied Pharmacology, 209*(2), 105-113.

Tsoukanelis, E. A. (2007). Watercress: Benefits for cancer protection, vision, and heart health. *Life Extension, 13*(11), 87-89.

REVIEWER(S)

Darlene Strayer, RN, MBA, Cinahl Information Systems, Glendale, CA

Nursing Executive Practice Council, Glendale Adventist Medical Center, Glendale, CA

Wheat Grass

WHAT WE KNOW

Wheatgrass, or *Triticum aestivum*, is a member of the Paceae (i.e., Gramineae) family. As its name indicates, wheat grass is the young grass shoot that is grown from wheat seeds. Many individuals consider wheat grass to be nutritionally potent and have therapeutic potential; wheat grass is most commonly used in juice as a supplement or as a naturopathic medicine. There is no scientific evidence to support the many claims of therapeutic properties attributed to wheat grass, but it is dense with nutrients (e.g., vitamins C and E; iron; calcium; magnesium; beta-carotene; and amino acids) that exhibit antioxidant, anti-inflammatory, antibacterial, and cancer-preventative properties.

NUTRIENTS IN WHEAT GRASS

- Adequate studies in humans are lacking and the medicinal use of wheat grass is not recommended; proponents of wheat grass claim that its use promotes oral health, prevents infections, detoxifies cancer-causing substances, and can be used to treat the following conditions:
  —Ulcerative colitis (UC)
  —Hypercholesterolemia
  —Anemia
  —Diabetes mellitus, type 2 (DM2)
  —Hypertension
  —Wounds
- Wheat grass is rich in the following nutrients:
  —The water-soluble vitamin C neutralizes free radicals, protecting against inflammation and cellular damage. Adequate vitamin C intake is vital for immune system function and has been associated with the prevention of heart disease, stroke, and cancer.
  —Vitamin E is a fat-soluble vitamin that functions as an antioxidant and contributes to the maintenance of cell membranes, vitamin K absorption, and proper immune function.
  —Iron is vital for the production of red blood cells and hemoglobin, which are necessary for energy production and the transport of oxygen to the tissues. Iron supports immune function, is vital for cognitive development, contributes to energy production, and regulates temperature.
  —Calcium builds and maintains bones and teeth, regulates muscle contraction, conducts nerve impulses, activates enzymes for energy production and muscle contraction, participates in blood clotting, assists with vitamin B12 absorption, and maintains the structural integrity of intracellular membranes.

—Magnesium balances the action of calcium in cells to regulate bone health and nerve and muscle tone. Magnesium maintains relaxation of the nerves and muscles, which contributes to the prevention of high blood pressure, muscle spasms, asthma, migraine headaches, general soreness, and fatigue.

—Pro-vitamin A carotenoids (e.g., beta-carotene) are the precursors for vitamin A, or retinol, a fat-soluble vitamin that is required for vision, maintenance of the surface lining of the eyes and other epithelial tissue, bone growth, immune response, energy regulation, reproduction, embryonic development, and activation of gene expression.

RESEARCH FINDINGS

- Researchers report that wheat grass exhibits therapeutic potential for treatment of patients with low hemoglobin levels in patients who may need blood transfusions. Although results of 2 studies showed that patients who were treated with wheat grass required less frequent blood transfusions, authors of a third study concluded that wheat grass therapy for the duration of 1 year was not effective in reducing the requirement for blood transfusion.

- A study was conducted to determine if wheat grass is an effective adjuvant treatment for patients with distal ulcerative colitis. Twenty-one patients participated in the study, which showed that wheat grass juice was associated with significant improvement in overall disease activity and severity. No serious side effects were noted.

SUMMARY

Consumers should become knowledgeable about the nutritional composition and physiologic effects of wheat grass. Wheat grass is a good source of vitamins, minerals, and phytonutrients. These nutrients support the immune system, promote bone and blood health, and exhibit antioxidant, anti-inflammatory, antibacterial, and cancer-preventative properties. Recent research findings suggest wheat grass may help reduce symptoms associated with ulcerative colitis.

—*Cherie Marcel, BS*

REFERENCES

American Cancer Society. (2008). Wheatgrass. Retrieved March 17, 2015, from http://www.cancer.org/treatment/treatmentsandsideeffects/complementaryandalternativemedicine/dietandnutrition/wheatgrass

Ben-Arye, E., Goldin, E., Wengrower, D., Stamper, A., Kohn, R., & Berry, E. (2002). Wheat grass juice in the treatment of active distal ulcerative colitis: A randomized double-blind placebo-controlled trial. *Scandinavian Journal of Gastroenterology*, 37(4), 444.

Choudhary, D. R., Naithani, R., Panigrahi, I., Kumar, R., Mahapatra, M., Pati, H. P., ... Choudhry, V. P. (2009). Effect of wheat grass therapy on transfusion requirement in beta-thalassemia major. *Indian Journal of Pediatrics*, 76(4), 375-376. doi:10.1007/s12098-009-0004-6

Crawford, L. H. (2000). Immune boosting wheat grass. *Nutritional Perspectives: Journal of the Council on Nutrition*, 23(4), 11-12.

Marawaha, R. K., Bansal, D., Kaur, S., & Trehan, A. (2004). Wheat grass juice reduces transfusion requirement in patients with thalassemia major: A pilot study. *Indian Pediatrics*, 41(7), 716.

Singh, K., Pannu, M. S., Singh, P., & Singh, J. (2010). Effect of wheat grass tablets on the frequency of blood transfusions in Thalassemia Major. *Indian Journal of Pediatrics*, 77(1), 90. doi:10.1007/s12098-010-0002-8

Wheatgrass. (n.d.). *WebMD*. Retrieved March 17, 1970, from http://www.webmd.com/vitamins-supplements/ingredientmono-1073-WHEATGRASS.aspx?activeIngredientId=1073&activeIngredientName=WHEATGRASS

REVIEWER(S)

Darlene Strayer, RN, MBA, Cinahl Information Systems, Glendale, CA

Nursing Executive Practice Council, Glendale Adventist Medical Center, Glendale, CA

Wild Yam

WHAT WE KNOW

Wild yam is a perennial turberous creeping vine. The leaves are broad and heart-shaped with a fuzzy underside, and the plant has bunches of small flowers that range from greenish-white to greenish-yellow in color.

The pale brown, knotty rhizome (i.e., root stalk) is the source of most medicinal preparations that contain wild yam. Although there are more than 600 species in the wild yam (*Discoreaceae*) family, most are too bitter for consumption and fewer than 20 varieties are known to be edible. Not to be confused with yellow yam or sweet potato, wild yam (*Dioscorea villosa*), a tuberous plant appreciated for its starchy rhizome, has a long history of medicinal use for the treatment of such ailments as joint pain, muscle spasms, diverticulosis, and menopause.

NUTRIENTS IN WILD YAM

* The primary bioactive chemical in wild yam is the phytoestrogen diosgenin. In laboratories, diosgenin is made into steroids such as estrogen and dehydro-epiandrosterone (DHEA) for use in preparations for hormone therapy. Unprocessed wild yam is not an effective substitute for estrogen or DHEA.

DIETARY INTAKE GUIDELINES

* There is no official recommended dosage for wild yam.
* Wild yam can cause vomiting if consumed in large quantities.
* There are no known interactions with medications, herbs, or other foods.

RESEARCH FINDINGS

* Researchers report that wild yam extract has potential anti-carcinogenic activity by causing cell death of breast cancer cells. It is unclear if this is due to estrogenic or to nonhormonal activity of the phytochemicals in the wild yam extract.

SUMMARY

Consumers should become knowledgeable about the consumption of wild yams. Wild yam is a good source of diosgenin, a phytonutrient used for hormone therapy. Wild yam is known to help treat joint pain, muscle spasms, diverticulosis, and menopause symptoms.

—*Cherie Marcel, BS*

REFERENCES

Brinker, F. (2008). Wild yam – Sorting out the species. *Journal of the American Herbalists Guild*, 8(2), 3-13.

Ehrlich, S. D. (2013, May 7). Wild yam. *University of Maryland Medical Center*. Retrieved from http://www.umm.edu/altmed/articles/wild-yam-000280.htm

DeVries, L. (2013, August 16). Wild yam properties. Retrieved March 17, 2015, from http://www.livestrong.com/article/458158-wild-yam-properties/

Park, M., Kwon, H., Ahn, W., Bae, S., Rhyu, M., & Lee, Y. (2009). Estrogen activities and the cellular effects of natural progesterone from wild yam extract in MCF-7 human breast cancer cells. *American Journal of Chinese Medicine*, 37(1), 159-167. doi:10.1142/S0192415X09006746

Sego, S. (2012). Alternative meds update. Wild yam. *Clinical Advisor for Nurse Practitioners*, 15(2), 100-102.

REVIEWER(S)

Darlene Strayer, RN, MBA, Cinahl Information Systems, Glendale, CA

Nursing Executive Practice Council, Glendale Adventist Medical Center, Glendale, CA

GRAINS

Bread

WHAT WE KNOW

As one of the most ancient prepared foods consumed by humans, bread has become a primary source of food for people worldwide. There are many methods for preparing bread, but the basic ingredients are flour or meal combined with milk or water to form dough, which is then baked. Bread can be made from rye, cornmeal, and other grains, but is most commonly made with wheat flour. The nutritional value of wheat varies greatly depending on the degree of its refinement. In its unprocessed state (i.e., whole wheat), which includes the bran and germ, wheat contains a multitude of valuable nutrients, including vitamins B1, B2, B3, and E, manganese, magnesium, calcium, phosphorus, zinc, copper, iron, and tryptophan. It is also a fantastic source of dietary fiber. However, in the United States, most of the wheat used in the production of breads has been processed into a 60% extraction (i.e., 40% of the original wheat, including the bran and germ, has been removed), bleached white flour. This degree of refinement strips the wheat of over half of its nutritional value, which is why, in 1941, the U.S. decided to "enrich" white flour with vitamins B1, B2, B3, and iron. Even with this refortification, white flour is dramatically inferior to 100% whole-wheat in its nutritional contribution. In fact, regular consumption of bread and other foods made from refined grain has been associated with weight gain, increased risk for insulin resistance and diabetes mellitus, type-2 (DM2), and cardiovascular disease, while consumption of whole grain bread has proven protective against these conditions. A few of the nutritional benefits gained from consuming 100% whole-wheat bread include lowering cholesterol and blood pressure, slowing the absorption of glucose and stabilizing blood sugar levels, and supporting bowel regularity.

NUTRIENTS IN BREAD

- Whole-wheat bread typically provides 2 g of dietary fiber/slice. Some benefits of dietary fiber include the following:
  - —It binds with water and slows the digestive process, thus allowing the body to better manage postprandial (i.e., after eating) glucose and insulin responses.
  - —It is able to increase the volume of the intestinal contents, which hinders the absorption of cholesterol. The added bulk also promotes more regular bowel movements, promoting intestinal health.
- Wheat contains vitamins B1, B2, and B3, which create energy by aiding the breakdown of carbohydrates, provide cardiovascular protection, maintain the nervous system, and support the production of red blood cells, hormones, and necessary cholesterol.
- Whole-wheat contains betaine, a metabolite of choline, which has been shown to reduce inflammation.
- Whole-wheat has numerous phytonutrients (i.e., beneficial plant-derived chemicals), which serve as antioxidants, have anti-cancer properties, and reduce inflammation. One important phytonutrient in whole-wheat is the lignan, enterolactone, which has estrogen-like effects. Increasing serum levels of enterolactones may help to protect against heart disease as well as hormone-dependent cancers such as breast and prostate cancers.
- Wheat germ is rich in vitamin E, a fat-soluble vitamin which functions primarily as an antioxidant, but also serves to maintain cell membranes, assist in vitamin K absorption, and contribute to the immune system.

DIETARY INTAKE GUIDELINES

- The United States Food and Drug Administration (FDA) recommends 25–30grams of dietary fiber intake per day, the amount provided in about 2 cups of 100% whole wheat flour.

RESEARCH FINDINGS

- Researchers have found that the dietary fiber in wheat has the ability to promote the growth of beneficial bacteria (i.e., flora) in the intestines.

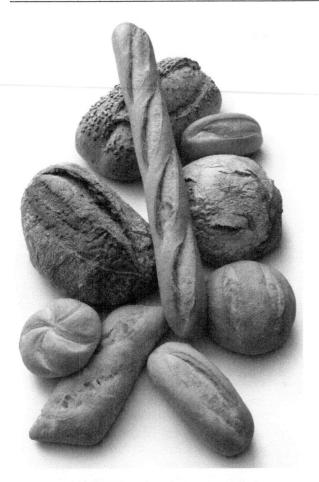

This prebiotic action increases the formation of fermentation products, such as the short-chain fatty acids (SCFAs), butyrate, propionate, and acetate, which inhibit the growth and induce death of cancerous cells in the colon. At the same time, these SCFAs serve as an energy source to normal cells, enhancing their survival.

- Diets high in simple carbohydrates, such as those made from refined wheat flour, are associated with dyslipidemia (i.e., high levels of cholesterol and triglycerides) and diabetes. Even whole grains have a relatively high glycemic index (i.e., elevated blood sugar after eating), which can cause elevated blood sugar resulting in the increased production of insulin. Researchers report that reformulating refined bread products with the use of composite flours (i.e., flours from other starches such as sweet potato) has the potential to reduce the postprandial glycemic response. However, it is still vital to emphasize that diet

modification, for the prevention of obesity, heart disease, and diabetes, should be well-rounded, including unsaturated fats, lean proteins, and fruits and vegetables, as well as whole grains.

SUMMARY

Consumers should become knowledgeable about the physiologic risks and benefits of bread. Whole wheat bread is a good source of fiber, B vitamins, and phytonutrients. These nutrients promote gastrointestinal health, reduce inflammation, lower blood pressure, and may help prevent cardiovascular disease and type 2 diabetes. Research suggests that diets high in refined wheat flour are associated with higher risk of high cholesterol and diabetes.

—*Cherie Marcel, BS*

REFERENCES

Bodinham, C. L., Hitchen, K. L., Youngma, P. J., Frost, G. S., & Robertson, M. D. (2011). Short-term effects of whole-grain wheat on appetite and food intake in healthy adults: A pilot study. *British Journal of Nutrition*, 106(3), 327-330. doi:10.1017/S0007114511000225

Borowicki, A., Michelmann, A., Stein, K., Scharlau, D., Scheu, K., Obst, U., & Glei, M. (2011). Fermented wheat aleurone enriched with probiotic strains IGG and Bb12 modulates markers of tumor progression in human colon cells. *Nutrition and Cancer*, 63(1), 151-160. doi:10.1080/01635581.2010.516874

Borowicki, A., Stein, K., Scharlau, D., Scheu, K., Brenner-Weiss, G., Obst, U., & Glei, M. (2010). Fermented wheat aleurone inhibits growth and induces apoptosis in human HT29 colon adenocarcinoma cells. *British Journal of Nutrition*, 103(3), 360-369. doi:10.1017/S0007114509991899

Burton, P. M., Monro, J. A., Alvarez, L., & Gallagher, E. (2011). Glycemic impact and health: New horizons in white bread formulations. *Critical Reviews in Food Science & Nutrition*, 51(10), 965-982. doi:10.1080/10408398.2010.491584

German, J. B., & Dillard, C. J. (2004). Saturated fats: What dietary intake? *American Journal of Clinical Nutrition*, 80(3), 550-559.

Gil, A., Ortega, R. M., & Maldonado, J. (2011). Wholegrain cereals and bread: A duet of the Mediterranean diet for the prevention of chronic diseases. *Public Health Nutrition*, 14(12), 2316-2322. doi:10.1017/S1368980011002576

Porter, L. (2011). Health benefits of 100% wheat bread. *Livestrong.com*. Retrieved March 10, 2015, from http://www.livestrong.com/article/486218-health-benefits-of-100-percent-wheat-bread/

Schlormann, W., Hiller, B., Jahns, F., Zoger, R., Hennemeier, I., Wilhelm, A., ... Glei, M. (2012). Chemopreventive effects of in vitro digested and fermented bread in colon cells. *European Journal of Nutrition*, 51(7), 827-839. doi:10.1007/s00394-011-0262-8

The world's healthiest foods: Wheat. (n.d.). *George Mateljan Foundation*. Retrieved March 10, 2015, from http://www.whfoods.com/genpage.php? tname=foods pice&dbid=66#safetyissues

Tighe, P., Duthie, G., Vaughan, N., Brittenden, J., Simpson, W. G., Duthie, S., ... Thies, F. (2010). Effect of increased consumption of whole-grain foods on blood pressure and other cardiovascular risk markers in healthy middle-aged persons: A randomized controlled trial. *American Journal of Clinical Nutrition*, 92(4), 733-740. doi:10.3945/ ajcn.2010.29417

Walton, G. E., Lu, C., Trogh, I., Arnaut, F., & Gibson, G. R. (2012). A randomised, double-blind, placebo controlled cross-over study to determine the gastrointestinal effects of consumption of arabinoxylan-oligosaccharides enriched bread in healthy volunteers. *Nutrition Journal*, 11, 36. doi:10.1186/1475-2891-11-36

Wilson, M. G. (2008). *Fiber*. Retrieved March 10, 2015, from http://www.merckmanuals.com/home/au/sec12/cH152/cH152d.html

REVIEWER(S)

Darlene Strayer, RN, MBA, Cinahl Information Systems, Glendale, CA

Nursing Executive Practice Council, Glendale Adventist Medical Center, Glendale, CA

Breakfast Cereals

WHAT WE KNOW

More than half of all adults in the United States are classified as overweight or obese, which puts them at risk for diabetes mellitus, type-2(DM2), cardiovascular disease (CVD), and cancer. One simple strategy for achieving and managing a healthy bodyweight is to eat breakfast, including cereal, as part of the daily meal plan. Breakfast is considered the meal that breaks the fast that occurs throughout the night. It has been called the most important meal of the day and has proven to play a significant role in overall nutrient consumption, energy balance, and weight management.

- Evidence indicates that fortified breakfast cereals make a significant contribution to the nutrient intake of persons in industrialized countries. Nutritional quality varies widely among breakfast cereals; some are heavily processed and high in sugar, and others contain whole grains, fruits, and nuts. Many of the cereals that are marketed to children (e.g., cereals with high sugar content) contain less nutrition than those. marketed to adults/
    —Reading labels can help to identify which breakfast cereals are healthier than others. Key elements to look for on cereal labels include the following:
      –To be sure that the cereal is a good source of whole grains, look for the word "whole" in the first two grains listed in the ingredients.
        –Exceptions to this include rolled oats, oat flakes, bran, and wheat germ, which are not technically considered whole grains but are high in fiber, protein, and other nutrients.
        –Choose cereals that list higher amounts (e.g., 3–5 grams/serving) of dietary fiber in the "Nutrition Facts" list.
      –Learn to identify added sugar in the ingredient list. Common terms for sugar include granulated sugar, brown sugar, corn syrup, honey, maple syrup, dextrose, fructose, sucrose (i.e., glucose and fructose combined, commonly called table sugar) maltose, molasses, lactose, evaporated cane juice, and fruit juice.

NUTRIENTS IN BREAKFAST CEREAL

- Breakfast cereal is often fortified with nutrients that are considered to be under-consumed by most persons. The most common fortified nutrients in breakfast cereals are the B-complex vitamins.
    —The B-complex vitamins create energy by aiding the breakdown of carbohydrates, lipids, proteins, and alcohol. They provide cardiovascular protection, maintain the nervous system, and support the production of red blood cells, hormones, and necessary cholesterol.
- Breakfast cereal can be a good source of dietary fiber, which binds and removes toxins from the colon, suppresses appetite, assists in glucose control, and reduces high cholesterol levels.

DIETARY INTAKE GUIDELINES

- Although there is no official recommendation for breakfast cereal consumption, breakfast cereal can be a significant source of dietary fiber.
  - —The United States Food and Drug Administration (USFDA) recommends a daily intake of 35 or more grams of fiber.
- A recent review of available literature found no information on breakfast cereal deficiency or toxicity.
- A recent review of the literature found no information on the interaction of breakfast cereal with medications or other substances.

RESEARCH FINDINGS

- Researchers consistently report that persons who consume breakfast, including breakfast cereal, are less likely to be overweight or obese, tend to have a lower body mass index (BMI; i.e., a measure of body weight in relation to height) and are more likely to consume a balanced diet with higher daily nutrient intake than those who do not eat breakfast. Researchers state that individuals who regularly eat whole grain breakfast cereal have a lower risk for developing hypertension or heart failure than those who do not consume whole grain cereal for breakfast.
- Researchers have conducted numerous studies examining the potential of oats in the prevention and treatment of metabolic syndrome and its related conditions of insulin resistance, DM2, hypertension, heart disease, and obesity. Authors of these studies have consistently documented results regarding the ability of oat-derived beta-glucan (i.e., a type of fiber found in oats) to reduce blood cholesterol and fasting blood glucose levels, enhance satiety, and improve fasting lipid levels. The antioxidants found in oats, including vitamin E and the phytonutrients (i.e., beneficial plant-derived chemicals) that are unique to oats, the avenanthramides (Avns), are believed to protect cells from free radical damage, act as anti-inflammatory agents, and contribute to the flow-mediated vessel dilation and hypotensive effects of oats, preventing the development of atherosclerosis and providing significant cardiovascular protection. Regular consumption of oat cereal has been shown to improve the success of weight loss, especially as

assessed by smaller waist circumference, when oat cereal is included in a dietary program for weight loss.
- Researchers studied the effects of the availability of high- and low-sugar cereals on children's breakfast-eating behavior. Results of the study indicated that children who were served high-sugar cereals consumed more total sugar with poorer overall nutritional quality at breakfast than those who received low-sugar cereals. Researchers reported that both groups of children were happy with their cereal options, suggesting that children do not need to be offered high-sugar cereal in order to happily consume breakfast cereal. Offering children low-sugar cereal options would provide them with a healthier breakfast.
- Evidence shows that individuals who regularly consume ready-to-eat breakfast cereal also have a higher intake of milk and calcium than those who do not.

SUMMARY

Consumers should become knowledgeable about the physiologic effects of consuming breakfast cereal. Fortified breakfast cereal is a good source of B-complex vitamins and dietary fiber. When milk is used with breakfast cereal, individuals receive a higher intake of calcium as well. Breakfast, including cereal, can be an important part of a heart-healthy diet for the goal of achieving and maintaining a healthy weight. Individuals should choose breakfast cereals that are low in sugar and high in fiber, and read labels to help make healthier breakfast cereal choices.

—*Cherie Marcel, BS*

REFERENCES

Ashwell, M., & Hunty, A. (2012). How does breakfast help manage bodyweight? *Nutrition Bulletin*, 37(4), 395-397. doi:10.1111/j.1467-3010.2012.01994.x

Costain, L. (2011). Breakfast: Getting to the 'weight' of the matter. *Primary Care Women's Health Journal*, 3(2), 85-87.

De la Hunty, A., & Ashwell, M. (2007). Are people who regularly eat breakfast cereals slimmer than those who don't? A systematic review of the evidence. *Nutrition Bulletin*, 32(2), 118-128. doi:10.1111/j.1467-3010.2007.00638.x

Djousse, L., & Gaziano, J. M. (2007). Breakfast cereals and risk of heart failure in the Physicians' Health

Study I. *Archives of Internal Medicine, 167*(19), 2080-2085. doi:10.1002/smi.1390

Harris, J. L., Schwartz, M. B., Ustjanauskas, A., Ohri-Vachaspati, P., & Brownell, K. D. (2011). Effects of serving high-sugar cereals on children's breakfast-eating behavior. *Pediatrics, 127*(1), 71-76. doi:10.1542/peds.2010-0864

Holzmeister, L. A. (2010). Supermarket smarts. Hot and cold breakfast cereals. *Diabetes Self-Management, 27*(1), 59, 61-65.

Kochar, J., Gaziano, J. M., & Djousse, L. (2012). Breakfast cereals and risk of hypertension in the Physicians' Health Study I. *Clinical Nutrition, 31*(1), 89-92. doi:10.1016/ j.clnu.2011.08.001

Lyly, M., Ohls, N., Lahteenmaki, L., Salmenkallio-Marttila, M., Liukkonen, K., Karhunen, L., & Poutanen, K. (2010). The effect of fibre amount, energy level and viscosity of beverages containing oat fibre supplement on perceived satiety. *Food & Nutrition Research, 54*, 1-8. doi:10.3402/fnr.v54i0.2149

Maki, K. C., Beiseigel, J. M., Jonnalagadda, S. S., Gugger, C. K., Reeves, M. S., Farmer, M. V., ... Rains, T. M. (2010). Whole-grain ready-to-eat oat cereal, as part of a dietary program for weight loss, reduces low-density lipoprotein cholesterol in adults with overweight and obesity more than a dietary program including low-fiber control foods. *Journal of the American Dietetic Association, 110*(2), 205-214. doi:10.1016/j.jada.2009.10.037

Meydani, M. (2009). Potential health benefits of avenanthramides of oats. *Nutrition Reviews, 67*(12), 731-735. doi:10.1111/j.1753-4887.2009.00256.x

Othman, R., Moghadasian, M. H., & Jones, P. J. H. (2011). Cholesterol-lowering effects of oat beta-glucan. *Nutrition Reviews, 69*(6), 299-309. doi:10.1111/j.1753-4887.2011.00401.x

Schwartz, M. B., Vartanian, L. R., Wharton, C. M., & Brownell, K. D. (2008). Examining the nutritional quality of breakfast cereals marketed to children. *Journal of the American Dietetic Association, 108*(4), 702-705.

Song, W. O., Chun, O. K., Kerver, J., Cho, S., Chung, C. E., & Chung, S. (2006). Ready-to-eat breakfast cereal consumption enhances milk and calcium intake in the US population. *Journal of the American Dietetic Association, 106*(11), 1783-1789. doi:10.1016/j.jada.2006.08.015

Sucrose. (2003). *Virtual Chembook. Elmhurst College.* Retrieved from http://www.elmhurst.edu/~chm/vchembook/546sucrose.html

Tighe, P., Duthie, G., Vaughan, N., Brittenden, J., Simpson, W. G., Duthie, S., ... Thies, F. (2010). Effect of increased consumption of whole-grain foods on blood pressure and other cardiovascular risk markers in healthy middle-aged persons: A randomized controlled trial. *American Journal of Clinical Nutrition, 92*(4), 733-740. doi:10.3945/ ajcn.2010.29417

REVIEWER(S)

Darlene Strayer, RN, MBA, Cinahl Information Systems, Glendale, CA

Nursing Executive Practice Council, Glendale Adventist Medical Center, Glendale, CA

Corn

WHAT WE KNOW

Corn (also called maize and Zea mays), from the grasses family Poaceae (also known as Gramineae), is technically a fruit although it is commonly classified as a grain. The domestication of corn occurred in 9000–8000 BC in Mexico and Central America, where it became the staple food for the Mayan and Olmec civilizations by 1500 BC. Although yellow corn is typically the most familiar in the United States, there are over 100 varieties of corn in colors of white, pink, red, blue, purple, and black. Some of the nutritional merits of corn include the B-complex vitamins B1, B5, niacin, and folic acid;

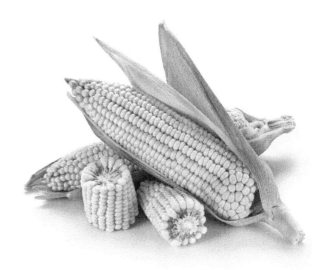

vitamin C; manganese; and many phytonutrients (i.e., beneficial plant-based chemicals). Each color variety of corn has a unique set of phytonutrients. For example, yellow corn contains a high amount of carotenoids, while blue corn is a great source of the flavonoid pigment anthocyanin. Corn also provides 5–6 g of protein per cup and is an excellent source of dietary fiber. The nutritional benefits of corn consumption include lowering cholesterol and blood pressure, slowing the absorption of glucose and stabilizing blood glucose levels, increasing satiety, and increasing bowel regularity. Corn silk, which is usually discarded prior to consumption, can be used in a tea to treat urinary tract discomfort and as a diuretic. Corn is commonly consumed as whole kernels on or cut off the cob, popped corn, and in ground meal, grits, and syrup.

NUTRIENTS IN CORN

- Corn provides 4.6 g of fiber per cup. Some benefits of dietary fiber include
  - binding with water and slowing the digestive process, which allows for better management of postprandial (i.e., after eating) glucose levels and insulin responses.
  - increasing the volume of intestinal contents, which hinders the absorption of cholesterol and promotes regular bowel movements, improving intestinal health.
- Corn is a good source of many antioxidant phytonutrients that are uniquely represented in each variety of corn
  - Yellow corn is high in the carotenoids lutein and zeaxanthin, which enhance the immune system, fight free radicals, protect against cancer, and reduce the risk of cataracts and eye damage.
  - Blue corn is high in anthocyanins, the flavonoids responsible for the blue color. Anthocyanins are powerful antioxidants with anti-inflammatory properties that protect connective tissue from damage.
  - Purple corn is high in protocatechuic acid, a hydroxybenzoic acid with strong antioxidant activity.
  - Other phytonutrients found in all varieties of corn include beta-carotene, caffeic acid, coumaric acid, ferulic acid, syringic acid, and vanillic acid.

- Corn contains the B-complex vitamins thiamine, folic acid, pantothenic acid, riboflavin, B6, and niacin, which create energy by aiding the breakdown of carbohydrates, providing cardiovascular protection, maintaining the nervous system, and supporting the production of red blood cells, hormones, and necessary cholesterol.

DIETARY INTAKE GUIDELINES

- The U.S. Food and Drug Administration (FDA) recommends 3 or more grams of soluble fiber intake per day, which is the amount provided in about 2 1/2 cups of cooked corn grits.

RESEARCH FINDINGS

- Corn is a major food staple in Africa, Central America, China, and Russia. Researchers are evaluating the use of fortified corn as a medium for supplementation in order to improve the status of undernourished populations in certain geographic locations, including rural areas of Africa, where households have poor access to nutritious foods. The corn is fortified with certain nutrients, including iron, zinc, ascorbic acid, copper, selenium, riboflavin, and vitamins A, B6, B12 and E. Infants, children, and adolescents provided with the fortified corn meal showed improvement in weight gain, motor development, and iron status. Researchers have noted similar results when studying the use of quality protein corn, which is corn fortified with the amino acids lysine and tryptophan.
- Results of several recent studies show that corn fibers, corn silk extract, and phytonutrients (particularly of purple corn) have therapeutic effects on persons with metabolic syndrome, diabetes mellitus, type 2 (DM2), and obesity. All types of corn-based dietary fibers are digested slowly and appear to improve postprandial glycemic control and insulin response. In addition, purple corn reduces high leptin levels in animals.
- Corn is used to make corn syrup (or glucose syrup) by a process of mixing corn starch with dilute hydrochloric acid and heating the mixture under pressure to form a glucose syrup. High-fructose corn syrup (HFCS) is distinct from corn syrup in that it requires the enzymatic conversion of some of the glucose into fructose, creating a highly sweetened syrup that is commonly used in soft drinks and processed food products. Unlike

glucose, fructose cannot be stored as glycogen to be used as energy; if consumed in large amounts, fructose is likely to be converted to fat by the liver. Fat that is synthesized by the liver is released into the bloodstream as very low density lipoproteins (VLDL), which is a form of cholesterol known to contribute to cardiovascular disease (CVD).

—HFCS and sucrose (i.e., table sugar) both contain a high amount of fructose. Scientists have studied HFCS in comparison to sucrose to determine the impact each has on metabolic health parameters (e.g., weight, lipid profiles, blood pressure) and have found them to impact metabolic health in similar ways. Both sucrose and HFCS have been shown to be significantly, positively associated with risk for CVD, hyperinsulinemia, and DM2. Researchers believe this to be due to the fructose content of each, as glucose has not been associated with changes in lipid profiles. Based on current evidence, researchers suggest that clinicians inform patients about the health impact of both sucrose and HFCS, emphasizing the significance of fructose-content in sweetened foods and drinks; and to comply with the current recommendation by the American Heart Association (AMA) to limit the consumption of added sugar to 100 calories/day for women and 150 calories/day for men.

SUMMARY

Consumers should become knowledgeable about the physiologic benefits of corn consumption. Corn is a good source of B-complex vitamins, vitamin C, manganese, phytonutrients (e.g., carotenoids, flavonoids), fiber, and protein. These nutrients can help lower cholesterol and blood pressure, control and stabilize glucose levels, increase satiety, and improve gastrointestinal health.

—*Cherie Marcel, BS*

REFERENCES

Akalu, G., Taffesse, S., Gunaratna, N. S., & De Groote, H. (2010). The effectiveness of quality protein maize in improving the nutritional status of young children in the Ethiopian highlands. *Food & Nutrition Bulletin, 31*(3), 418-430.

Bruton-Seal, J. (2011). Kitchen medicine. *Share Guide, 25.*

Ells, L. J., Seal, C. J., Kettlitz, B., Bal, W., & Mathers, J. C. (2005). Postprandial glycaemic, lipaemic and haemostatic responses to ingestion of rapidly and slowly digested starches in healthy young women. *British Journal of Nutrition, 94*(6), 948-955. doi:10.1079/BJN20051554

Faber, M., Kvalsvig, J. D., Lombard, C. J., & Benade, A. J. S. (2005). Effect of a fortified maize-meal porridge on anemia, micronutrient status, and motor development of infants. *American Journal of Clinical Nutrition, 82*(5), 1032-1039.

The George Mateljan Foundation editorial team. (n.d.). The world's healthiest foods: Corn. Retrieved March 6, 2015, fromhttp://www.whfoods.com/genpage.php?tname=foodspice&dbid=90

Gitau, R., Makasa, M., Kasonka, L., Sinkala, M., Chintu, C., Tomkins, A., ... Filteau, S. (2005). Maternal micronutrient status and decreased growth of Zambian infants born during and after the maize price increases resulting from the southern African drought of 2001-2002. *Public Health Nutrition, 8*(7), 837-843. doi:10.1079/PHN2005746

Guo, J., Liu, T., Han, L., & Liu, Y. (2009). The effects of corn silk on glycaemic metabolism. *Nutrition & Metabolism, 6,* 47. doi:10.1186/1743-7075-6-47

Johnson, R. J., Lanaspa, M. A., Roncal-Jimenez, C., & Sanchez-Lozada, L. G. (2012). Effects of excessive fructose intake on health. *Annals of Internal Medicine, 156*(12), 905-906. doi:10.7326/0003-4819-156-12-201206190-00024

Kendall, C. W., Esfahani, A., Hoffman, A. J., Evans, A., Sanders, L. M., Josse, A. R., ... Potter, S. M. (2008). Effect of novel maize-based dietary fibers on postprandial glycemia and insulinemia. *Journal of the American College of Nutrition, 27*(6), 711-718. doi:10.1080/07315724.2008.10719748

Li, S., Nugroho, A., Rocheford, T., & White, W. S. (2010). Vitamin A equivalence of the beta-carotene in beta-carotene-biofortified maize porridge consumed by women. *American Journal of Clinical Nutrition, 92*(5), 1105-1112. doi:10.3945/ajcn.2010.29802

Lieberman, S. (2007). The antioxidant power of purple corn: A research review. *Alternative & Complementary Therapies, 13*(2), 107-110.

Lopez-Martinez, L. X., Parkin, K. L., & Garcia, H. S. (2011). Phase II-inducing, polyphenols content and antioxidant capacity of corn (Zea mays L.) from phenotypes of white, blue, red, and purple corns processed into masa and tortillas. *Plant Foods for Human Nutrition, 66*(1), 41-47. doi:10.1007/s11130-011-0210-z

Lowndes, J., Sinnett, S., Pardo, S., Nguyen, V. T., Melanson, K. J., Zhiping, Y., ... Rippe, J. M. (2014). The effect of normally consumed amounts of sucrose or high fructose corn syrup on lipid profiles, body composition and related parameters in overweight/obese subjects. *Nutrients, 6*(3), 1128-1144. doi:10.3390/nu6031128

Nesamvuni, A. E., Vorster, H. H., Margetts, B. M., & Kruger, A. (2005). Fortification of maize meal improved the nutritional status of 1-3-year-old African children. *Public Health Nutrition, 8*(5), 461-467. doi:10.1079/PHN2005782

Ogunlade, A. O., Kruger, H. S., Jerling, J. C., Smuts, C. M., Covic, N., Hanekom, S. M., ... Kvalsvig, J. (2011). Point-of-use micronutrient fortification: Lessons learned in implementing a preschool-based pilot trial in South Africa. *International Journal of Food Science & Nutrition, 62*(1), 1-16. doi:10.3109/09637486.2010.495710

Othman, R., Moghadasian, M. H., & Jones, P. J. H. (2011). Cholesterol-lowering effects of oat beta-glucan. *Nutrition Reviews, 69*(6), 299-309. doi:10.1111/j.1753-4887.2011.00401.x

Seal, A., Kafwembe, E., Kassim, I. A. R., Hong, M., Wesley, A., Wood, J., ... van den Briel, T. (2008). Maize meal fortification is associated with improved vitamin A and iron status in adolescents and reduced childhood anemia in food aid-dependant refugee population. *Public Health Nutrition, 11*(7), 720-728. doi:10.1017/S1368980007001486

Sobel, L. L., & Dalby, E. (2014). Sugar or high fructose corn syrup – what should nurses teach patients and families? *Worldviews on Evidence-Based Nursing, 11*(2), 126-132. doi:10.1111/wvn.12027

REVIEWER(S)

Darlene Strayer, RN, MBA, Cinahl Information Systems, Glendale, CA

Nursing Executive Practice Council, Glendale Adventist Medical Center, Glendale, CA

Oats

WHAT WE KNOW

The oat, or *Avena sativa*, from the grasses family Poaceae, is a hardy cereal grain that is grown for its seeds, which are usually hulled and roasted, although dehulled oats (called groats) are used in some food products. Oats were

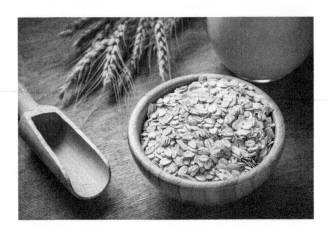

used in medicine to treat neuralgia, diabetes mellitus (DM), heart disease, and other conditions before they were considered a food source. In fact, oats were more commonly used to feed livestock than humans. Even now, oats are the preferred food for horses and other livestock, but oats are now commonly eaten by humans.

- Oats are noted to have more benefit than other common cereal grains (e.g., wheat, rice, rye) because of their rich nutritional profile. They have a third more protein and four times the fat (primarily unsaturated) of most grains. Although oats contain less starch than other cereals, they are an excellent source of dietary fiber, most notably the soluble fiber beta-glucan. Nutrients found in oats include vitamin E; the B vitamins riboflavin, thiamin, folate, and pantothenic acid; an array of minerals, including manganese, selenium, phosphorous, and zinc; and important phenolic phytonutrients (i.e., protective, plant-derived chemicals). Phytonutrients that are unique to oats are the avenanthramides (Avns), which have powerful antioxidant activity; flavonoids and sterols are also present in oats. The health benefits of oat consumption are vast and include lowering cholesterol and blood pressure, slowing the absorption of glucose and stabilizing blood glucose levels, increasing satiety and bowel regularity, and aiding in cancer prevention. Oats are available in a variety of forms, including rolled groats (i.e., steamed and flattened whole oats), hulled steel cut kernels, flakes, and ground flour.

NUTRIENTS IN OATS

- The primary soluble fiber in oats is beta-glucan, which has the following benefits:

—Beta-glucan binds with water and slows the digestive process, allowing the body to better manage postprandial (i.e., after eating) glucose and insulin responses.

—It increases the volume of intestinal contents, which hinders the absorption of cholesterol. The added bulk promotes more regular bowel movements, which supports good intestinal health.

—It increases bile acid excretion into the intestines, which results in lower serum cholesterol levels.

- Oats are a rich in avenanthramides (Avn) (i.e., a beneficial phenolic compound).

—More than 20 different forms of Avns are present in oats. The 3 most notable forms are referred to as Avn-A, Avn-B, and Avn-C. Avn-C is the most abundant.

—Avns exhibit antioxidant activity that is 10–30 times greater than the other phenolic compounds found in oats.

—Avns inhibit the production of several inflammatory cytokines and chemokines, which are involved in fatty streak formation in arteries and the development of atherosclerosis.

—Avns increase nitric oxide (NO) production and endothelial NO synthase expression, which contribute to the improved blood flow and blood pressure that are associated with oat consumption.

—Avn-C has anti-proliferative (i.e. prevents spreading) effects on certain cancer cells, especially colon cancer.

—Avns appear to have antihistamine and anti-irritation activity, which explains the soothing quality of topically applied oatmeal used to treat poison ivy exposure, sunburn, eczema, and psoriasis.

DIETARY INTAKE GUIDELINES

- The United States Food and Drug Administration (FDA) recommends intake of 3 or more grams of soluble fiber per day, which is the amount provided in 1.5 cups of oatmeal.
- No adverse effects of oat consumption are reported in the literature.
- No interactions between oat consumption and medications are reported in the literature.

RESEARCH FINDINGS

- Researchers have conducted numerous studies examining the potential of oats in the prevention and treatment of metabolic syndrome and its related conditions of insulin resistance and DM, hypertension, heart disease, and obesity. These studies have consistently documented results of the ability of oat-derived beta-glucan to reduce blood cholesterol and fasting glucose levels, enhance satiety, and improve fasting lipid levels. The antioxidants found in oats, including vitamin E and Avns, are believed to protect cells from free radical damage, act as anti-inflammatory agents, and contribute to the flow-mediated vessel dilation and hypotensive effects of oats, preventing the development of atherosclerosis and providing significant cardiovascular protection. Regular consumption of oat cereal has also been shown to improve the success of weight loss, especially as assessed by smaller waist circumference, when included in a dietary program for weight loss

- Celiac disease (CD; also known as gluten-sensitive enteropathy, celiac sprue, and nontropical sprue) is a chronic, autoimmune, inflammatory disorder of the small bowel that is triggered by a hypersensitivity to gluten in genetically predisposed individuals. Persons who have CD cannot consume anything that contains or has come in contact with gluten without causing damage to the intestinal mucosa. To prevent cross-contamination, persons living in a household with a family member who has CD must prepare gluten-free foods separately from foods that contain gluten. Although current research results show that the majority of persons with CD can tolerate oats because the protein complex in oat differs from that in wheat, barley, and rye, the potential for cross-contamination in the production of oats is very high. If the oats are produced to be gluten free, they are another grain option, tolerated well by most persons on a gluten-free diet, broadening dietary possibilities.

—Some individuals with CD do not tolerate oats well. According to researchers, oat toleration by children with CD can be assessed by tracking changes (from onset to after 1 year of consuming an oat-containing, gluten-free diet) in mRNA profiles of the intestinal mucosa for the presence of activated cytotoxic lymphocytes and regulatory T cell molecules.

SUMMARY

Consumers should become knowledgeable about the physiologic benefits of oat consumption. Oats are a good source of fiber and phenolic compounds, known as avenanthramides. These nutrients help control blood sugar, reduce inflammation, improve digestion and regularity, treat skin conditions, and may help prevent heart disease and cancer. Recent research shows that individuals with Celiac disease may be able to tolerate oats specifically labeled as gluten-free.

—*Cherie Marcel, BS*

REFERENCES

Berti, C., Riso, P., Brusamolino, A., & Porrini, M. (2005). Effect on appetite control of minor cereal and pseudocereal products. *British Journal of Nutrition*, *94*(5), 850-858.

Fric, P., Gabrovaska, D., & Nevoral, J. (2011). Celiac disease, gluten-free diet, and oats. *Nutrition Reviews*, *69*(2), 107-115. doi:10.1111/j.1753-4887.2010.00368.x

Lyly, M., Ohls, N., Lahteenmaki, L., Salmenkallio-Marttila, M., Liukkonen, K., Karhunen, L., & Poutanen, K. (2010). The effect of fibre amount, energy level and viscosity of beverages containing oat fibre supplement on perceived satiety. *Food & Nutrition Research*, *54*, 1-8. doi:10.3402/fnr.v54i0.2149

Maki, K. C., Beiseigel, J. M., Jonnalagadda, S. S., Gugger, C. K., Reeves, M. S., Farmer, M. V., ... Rains, T. M. (2010). Whole-grain ready-to-eat oat cereal, as part of a dietary program for weight loss, reduces low-density lipoprotein cholesterol in adults with overweight and obesity more than a dietary program including low-fiber control foods. *Journal of the American Dietetic Association*, *110*(2), 205-214. doi:10.1016/j.jada.2009.10.037

Meydani, M. (2009). Potential health benefits of avenanthramides of oats. *Nutrition Reviews*, *67*(12), 731-735. doi:10.1111/j.1753-4887.2009.00256.x

Othman, R., Moghadasian, M. H., & Jones, P. J. H. (2011). Cholesterol-lowering effects of oat beta-glucan. *Nutrition Reviews*, *69*(6), 299-309. doi:10.1111/j.1753-4887.2011.00401.x

Reyna-Villasmil, N., Bermudez-Pirela, V., Mengual-Moreno, E., Arias, N., Cano-Ponce, C., Leal-Gonzalez, E., & Arraiz, N. (2007). Oat-derived beta-glucan significantly improves HDLS and diminishes LDLC and non-HDL cholesterol in overweight individuals with mild hypercholesterolemia. *American Journal of Therapeutics*, *14*(2), 203-212.

Richman, E. (2012). Conference on 'Malnutrition matters' symposium 1: Living with coeliac disease: The safety of oats in the dietary treatment of coeliac disease. *Proceedings of the Nutrition Society*, *71*(4), 534-537.

Ryan, D., Kendall, M., & Robards, K. (2007). Bioactivity of oats as it relates to cardiovascular disease. *Nutrition Research Reviews*, *20*(2), 147-162.

Sjoberg, V., Hollen, E., Pietz, G., Magnusson, K. E., Falth-Magnusson, K., Sundstrom, M., ... Hammarstrom, M. L. (2014). Noncontaminated dietary oats may hamper normalization of the intestinal immune status in childhood celiac disease. *Clinical and Translational Gastroenterology*, e58, 11pp. doi:10.1038/ctg.2014.9

Tapsas, D., Falth-Magnusson, K., Hogberg, L., Hammersjo, J., & Hollen, E. (2014). Swedish children with celiac disease comply well with a gluten-free diet, and most include oats without reporting any adverse effects: A long-term follow-up study. *Nutrition Research (New York, N. Y.)*, *34*(5), 436-441. doi:10.1016/j.nutres.2014.04.006

Tighe, P., Duthie, G., Vaughan, N., Brittenden, J., Simpson, W. G., Duthie, S., & Thies, F. (2010). Effect of increased consumption of whole-grain foods on blood pressure and other cardiovascular risk markers in healthy middle-aged persons: A randomized controlled trial. *American Journal of Clinical Nutrition*, *92*(4), 733-740. doi:10.3945/ ajcn.2010.29417

Wolever, T. M. S., Tosh, S. M., Gibbs, A. L., Brand-Miller, J., Duncan, A. M., Hart, V., & Wood, P. J. (2010). Physicochemical properties of oat beta-glucan influence its ability to reduce serum LDL cholesterol in humans: A randomized clinical trial. *American Journal of Clinical Nutrition*, *92*(4), 723-732.

REVIEWER(S)

Darlene Strayer, RN, MBA, Cinahl Information Systems, Glendale, CA

Nursing Executive Practice Council, Glendale Adventist Medical Center, Glendale, CA

Quinoa

WHAT WE KNOW

Quinoa, or *Chenopodium quinoa*, seeds can be ground into flour and are similar in texture to cereal grasses (e.g., oats, barley), which is why quinoa is generally categorized as a grain. Quinoa is actually a member of the *Amaranthaceae-Chenopodiaceae* family, along with beets, Swiss chard, and spinach. Quinoa is a hardy, stalk-like plant that can be cultivated in most climates. The large leaves of the quinoa plant are edible and have a palatable flavor that is consistent with Swiss chard and spinach, although the quinoa seeds are the most frequently consumed part of quinoa. Quinoa seeds are prepared in the same way as rice and can be used instead of most cooked grains. Seeds vary in color from beige to dark red and have a subtle nutty flavor. There are many culinary uses of quinoa, including as a side replacing rice with a salmon entrée, for example, as part of a stir fry, as an ingredient of soup, as a cold salad, and as ground flour for use in baking. Nutritionally, quinoa contains many phytonutrients (i.e., beneficial plant-derived chemicals), minerals, fiber, protein, and omega-3 fatty acid.

NUTRIENTS IN QUINOA

- Unlike other cereal grains (e.g., oats, barley, rice), quinoa contains all of the necessary amino acids to be considered a source of complete protein. Protein is present in every cell in the human body and is vital for the development and maintenance of skin, muscles, organs, and glands.
- Quinoa is unique among cereal grains because it contains the heart-healthy essential fatty acids (EFAs) oleic acid and alpha-linolenic acid; these omega-3 fatty acids contribute to blood clotting and are necessary for brain development, providing energy to the body, assisting the absorption of fat-soluble vitamins (i.e., A, D, E, K), and controlling inflammation.
- Quinoa is a valuable source of manganese, magnesium, folate, phosphorus, potassium, iron, and calcium.
  - Manganese is a trace mineral that is responsible for energy production, fatty acid production, cholesterol production, and protection against damage caused by free radicals.
  - Magnesium balances the action of calcium in the cells to regulate bone health and nerve and

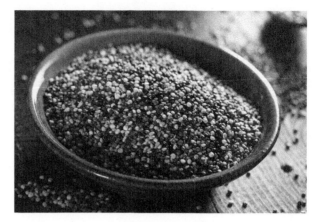

muscle tone. Magnesium maintains relaxation of the nerves and muscles, which contributes to the prevention of high blood pressure, muscle spasms, asthma, migraine headaches, general soreness, and fatigue.
  - Folate is a water-soluble B vitamin that is essential for the production and maintenance of red blood cells (RBCs). It is necessary for the production of deoxyribonucleic acid (DNA) and ribonucleic acid (RNA), and is important in the metabolism of the amino acid homocysteine.
  - Phosphorous is a mineral that combines with calcium for the formation of bones and teeth, muscle contraction, and nerve conduction. It is also essential for the structural integrity of cell membranes.
  - Calcium builds and maintains bones and teeth, regulates muscle contraction, conducts nerve impulses, activates enzymes for energy production and muscle contraction, participates in blood clotting, assists with vitamin B12 absorption, and maintains the structural integrity of intracellular membranes.
  - Iron is vital for the production of RBCs and hemoglobin, which are necessary for energy production and the transport of oxygen to the tissues. Iron supports immune function, is necessary for cognitive development, contributes to energy production, and regulates temperature.
  - Potassium is an essential element for regulating acid-base balance, maintaining fluid balance, supporting muscle contraction and cardiac function, contributing to protein

building and carbohydrate breakdown, promoting cellular growth, and promoting transmission of nerve impulses.

- The phytonutrients in quinoa include quercetin and kaempferol, which promote vascular health, inhibit tumor growth, reduce inflammation, and stimulate the production of detoxifying enzymes. Saponins (i.e., naturally occurring detergents) are also present among the phytonutrients in quinoa. Saponins have strong antimicrobial, anti-inflammatory, and antioxidant properties.

DIETARY INTAKE GUIDELINES

- Because quinoa contains oxalates, the primary component of kidney stones, there is concern that consumption of quinoa may increase risk of developing kidney stones in individuals who have a history of kidney stones. Oxalates can build up and crystallize in body fluids, causing health compromise in individuals with preexisting kidney or gallbladder dysfunction.

RESEARCH FINDINGS

- Researchers report that consumption of quinoa can reduce many of the adverse effects of fructose consumption related to lipid profile and blood glucose levels. Evidence supports the need for further research into the possibility of using quinoa and quinoa-derived supplements to prevent and treat obesity and related complications.

SUMMARY

Consumers should become knowledgeable about the physiologic benefits and risks of quinoa. Quinoa is a good source of phytonutrients, minerals, fiber, protein, and omega-3 fatty acids. These nutrients contribute to energy production, control glucose levels, improve muscle and bone health, and help fight inflammation. Recent research suggests quinoa may help improve cholesterol levels. Individuals with a history of kidney stones should know that quinoa consumption may increase the risk for developing kidney stones.

—*Cherie Marcel, BS*

REFERENCES

Bosley, E. (2011). Quinoa. *Delicious Living, 27*(4), 50.

Bowden, J., & Bessinger, J. (2011). The word's healthiest foods. Mighty, tiny quinoa: What you need to know about this mighty food in a tiny package. *Better Nutrition, 73*(3), 62.

The editorial staff at the American Institute for Cancer Research. (2013, April 10). Phytochemicals: The cancer fighters in the foods we eat. *American Institute for Cancer Research*. Retrieved June 4, 2015, from http://www.aicr.org/reduce-your-cancer-risk/diet/elements_phytochemicals.html

Foucault, A. S., Mathe, V., Lafont, R., Even, P., Dioh, W., Veillet, S., ... Quignard-Boulange, A. (2012). Quinoa extract enriched in 20-hydroxyecdysone protects mice from diet-induced obesity and modulates adipokines expression. *Obesity, 20*(2), 270-277. doi:10.1038/oby.2011.257

The George Mateljan Foundation editorial team. (n.d.). *The world's healthiest foods: Quinoa*. Retrieved July 12, 2013, from http://www.whfoods.com/genpage.php?dbid=142&tname=foodspice

Pasko, P., Barton, H., Zagrodzki, P., Izewska, A., Krosniak, M., Gawlik, M., ... Gorinstein, s. (2010). Effect of diet supplemented with quinoa seeds on oxidative status in plasma and selected tissues of high fructose-fed rats. *Plant Foods for Human Nutrition, 65*(2), 146-151. doi:10.1007/s11130-010-0164-6

Pasko, P., Zagrodzki, P., Barton, H., Chlopicka, J., & Gorinstein, S. (2010). Effect of quinoa seeds (Chenopodium quinoa) in diet on some biochemical parameters and essential elements in blood of high fructose-fed rats. *Plant Foods for Human Nutrition, 65*(4), 333-338. doi:10.1007/s11130-010-0197-x

Whole-grain boosters are keen on quinoa. (2010). *Tufts University Health & Nutrition Letter, 28*(4), 6.

REVIEWER(S)

Darlene Strayer, RN, MBA, Cinahl Information Systems, Glendale, CA

Nursing Executive Practice Council, Glendale Adventist Medical Center, Glendale, CA

Rice

WHAT WE KNOW

Rice, from the genus *Oryza* and the grass family *Poaceae*, has been a staple food in Asian and certain other countries for hundreds of years. There are 22 wild species of rice and 2 species of commonly cultivated rice (*Oryza sativa* and *Oryza glaberrima*). *Oryza sativa* is grown

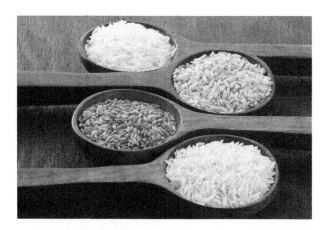

throughout the world and is currently the second largest cereal crop worldwide, feeding half of the world's population. *Oryza glaberrima* is grown primarily in West Africa. Although the majority of rice consumption occurs in Asia, its popularity within the United States has increased 3-fold since the 1930s. Rice is generally identified as either brown or white. Brown rice is the intact rice grain minus the hull. White rice is the product of a refinement process that removes all outer layers of the grain and the hull, bran, and germ, leaving the starchy, white endosperm that is called white rice. Over 70% of all rice consumed is white rice, which has lower nutritional value as a result of refinement. When compared with brown rice, white rice contains less dietary fiber, magnesium, manganese, and phytochemicals (i.e., beneficial plant-derived nutrients). White rice also produces a higher glycemic index (GI; i.e., postprandial glucose response) than brown rice, which causes elevated risk for diabetes mellitus, type 2 (DM2).

NUTRIENTS IN RICE

- Rice supplies energy that is primarily in the form of carbohydrate.
- Rice contains more protein than corn or whole wheat.
- Rice is a good source of niacin, which lowers triglycerides and low-density lipoprotein (LDL) cholesterol levels and raises high-density lipoprotein (LDL) cholesterol levels.
- Brown rice is a good source of dietary fiber and contains about twice the fiber of white rice. Some actions of fiber include the following:
  —It binds with water and slows the digestive process, allowing the body to better manage postprandial (i.e., after eating) glucose levels and insulin response.
  —It is able to increase the volume of the intestinal contents, which hinders the absorption of cholesterol. The added bulk also promotes more regular bowel movements, which supports intestinal health.
- Brown rice is a good source of manganese, a trace mineral responsible for energy production, fatty acid production, necessary cholesterol production, and protection against the damage caused by free-radicals.
- Brown rice contains magnesium, which balances the action of calcium to regulate nerve and muscle tone and bone health.
- Brown rice provides the phytochemicals known as lignans.
  —Lignans are broken down by the flora in the colon to form enterolactone and enterodiol, which have estrogen-like effects. Increasing serum levels of enterolactones may help to protect against heart disease and hormone-dependent cancers such as breast and prostate cancers.

RESEARCH FINDINGS

- Numerous study results have established the benefits of whole grain consumption in relation to the prevention or management of DM2. Because rice is a major food staple for half of the world's population, researchers have attempted to determine the effect of white rice compared with brown rice on the risk of DM2. Study results indicate that increased regular intake of white rice is associated with increased risk for DM2, cardiovascular disease, and ischemic stroke. It has been demonstrated that brown rice has a lower glycemic index (i.e., glucose response after eating) than white rice. Research results show that long-term substitution of brown rice and other whole grains for white rice can reduce risk for DM2. Despite the potential benefit of substituting brown for white rice, negative perception of brown rice remains a barrier to its acceptance. Researchers found that public awareness about the nutritional value of brown rice is weak, and discovered that, prior to tasting, many persons perceived brown rice to be inferior in taste and quality to white rice. However, after sampling brown rice and learning of its nutritional benefits, the majority of participants were willing to include brown rice in meals. Although it would take time to convince individuals to switch from white to brown rice, promotion of the health benefits of brown rice could popularize its use.

—A study conducted within the Tehran Lipid and Glucose Study, which included 1476 adults 19–70 years of age, revealed that increased white rice consumption is associated with a higher risk of developing metabolic syndrome.

- According to an analysis of the U.S. National Health and Nutrition Examination Survey (NHANES) during the period 1999–2004, individuals who consume at least 1 serving of brown or white rice each day are less likely than those who do not eat rice to exhibit risk factors associated with cardiovascular disease, DM2, and metabolic syndrome. It was also observed that these individuals are more likely to consume a diet that is higher in nutritional quality overall.

- Researchers report that rice is potential source of inorganic arsenic exposure for both children and adults in the US. Other common food sources of arsenic include grains, fruits, and juices. It is currently unknown if exposure to low levels of arsenic poses any health risks.

SUMMARY

Consumers should become knowledgeable about the physiologic effects of rice, particularly brown rice. Brown rice is a better source of dietary fiber, niacin, magnesium, manganese, and beneficial phytochemicals than white rice. These nutrients control blood sugar, facilitate energy production, reduce inflammation, and contribute to bone and muscle health. Recent research suggests brown rice may reduce risk for developing metabolic syndrome, type 2 diabetes, and cardiovascular disease.

—*Cherie Marcel, BS*

REFERENCES

Bahadoran, Z., Mirmiran, P., Delshad, H., & Azizi, F. (2014). White rice consumption is a risk factor for metabolic syndrome in Tehrani adults: A prospective approach in Tehran Lipid and Glucose Study. *Archives of Iranian Medicine (AIM)*, 17(6), 435-440. doi:014176/AIM.0011

Davis, M. A., Mackenzie, T. A., Cottingham, K. L., Gilbert-Diamond, D., Punshon, T., & Karagas, M. R. (2012). Rice consumption and urinary arsenic concentrations in U.S. children. *Environmental Health Perspectives*, 120(10), 1418-1424. doi:10.1289/ehp.1205014

Dixit, A. A., Azar, K. M. J., Gardner, C. D., & Palaniappan, L. P. (2011). Incorporation of whole, ancient grains into a modern Asian diet to reduce the burden of chronic disease. *Nutrition Reviews*, 69(8), 479-488. doi:10.1111/j.1753-4887.2011.00411.x

Fulgoni, V. L., Fulgoni, S. A., Upton, J. L., & Moon, M. (2010). Diet quality and markers for human health in rice eaters versus non-rice eaters: An analysis of the US National Health and Nutrition Examination Survey, 1999-2004. *Nutrition Today*, 45(6), 262-272. doi:10.1097/NT.0b013e3181fd4f29 Haas, R. (2010). Lower cholesterol safely. *Life Extension*, 16(3), 26-34.

Hettiaratchi, U. P. K., Ekanayake, S., & Welihinda, J. (2011). Sri Lankan rice mixed meals: Effect on glycaemic index and contribution to daily dietary fiber requirement. *Malaysian Journal of Nutrition*, 17(1), 97-104.

Khan, S. H., Butt, M. S., Anjum, F. M., & Sameen, A. (2011). Quality evaluation of rice bran protein isolate-based weaning food for preschoolers. *International Journal of Food Sciences & Nutrition*, 62(3), 280-288. doi:10.3109/09637486.2010.529802

Kumar, S., Mohanraj, R., Sudha, V., Wedick, N. M., Malik, V., Hu, F. B., & Mohan, V. (2011). Perceptions about varieties of brown rice: A qualitative study from Southern India. *Journal of the American Dietetic Association*, 111(10), 1517-1522. doi:10.1016/j.jada.2011.07.002

Liang, W., Lee, A. H., & Binns, C. W. (2010). White rice-based food consumption and ischemic stroke risk: A case-control study in southern China. *Journal of Stroke & Cerebrovascular Diseases*, 19(6), 480-484. doi:10.1016/j.jstrokecerebrovasdis.2009.09.003

Nanri, A., Mizoue, T., Noda, M., Takahashi, Y., Kato, M., Inoue, M., & Tsugane, S. (2010). Rice intake and type 2 diabetes in Japanese men and women: The Japan Public Health Center-based prospective study. *American Journal of Clinical Nutrition*, 92(6), 1468-1477. doi:10.3945/ajcn.2010.29512

Sun, Q., Spiegelman, D., van Dam, R. M., Holmes, M. D., Malik, V. S., Willett, W. C., & Hu, F. B. (2010). White rice, brown rice, and risk of type 2 diabetes in US men and women. *Archives of Internal Medicine, 170*(11), 961-969. doi:10.1001/archinternmed.2010.109

Wei, Y., Zhu, J., & Nguyen, A. (2014). Rice consumption and urinary concentrations of arsenic in US adults. *International Journal of Environmental Health Research, 24*(5), 459-470. doi:10.1080/09603123.2013.857393

Zhang, G., Malik, V. S., Pan, A., Kumar, S., Holmes, M. D., Spiegelman, D., ... Hu, F. B. (2010). Substituting brown rice for white rice to lower diabetes risk: A focus-group study in Chinese adults. *Journal of the American Dietetic Association, 110*(8), 1216-1221. doi:10.1016/j.jada.2010.05.004

Zhang, G., Pan, A., Zong, G., Yu, Z., Wu, H., Chen, X., & Lin, X. (2011). Substituting white rice with brown rice for 16 weeks does not substantially affect metabolic risk factors in middle-aged Chinese men and women with diabetes or a high risk for diabetes. *Journal of Nutrition, 141*(9), 1685-1690. doi:10.3945/jn.111.142224

REVIEWER(S)

Darlene Strayer, RN, MBA, Cinahl Information Systems, Glendale, CA

Nursing Executive Practice Council, Glendale Adventist Medical Center, Glendale, CA

Wheat

WHAT WE KNOW

Wheat, or *Triticum aestivum*, is a member of the grasses family, *Poaceae* (also known as *Gramineae*), and is classified as a grain. It is believed that wheat originated as a food source in southwest Asia over 12,000 years ago. Today, approximately a third of the world's population relies on wheat as a food staple. The nutritional value of wheat varies widely according to the degree of its refinement. In an unprocessed state, which includes the bran and germ, 100% whole wheat contains many valuable nutrients, including vitamins B1, B2, B3, and E and manganese, magnesium, calcium, phosphorus, zinc, copper, iron, and tryptophan. Although wheat is an excellent source of dietary fiber, in the United States most of the wheat used to produce breads, pastas, cookies, and cereals is processed into a 60% extraction (i.e., 40% of the original wheat, including

the bran and germ, has been removed) of bleached white flour. Because this degree of refinement strips the wheat of over half of its nutritional value, in 1941 white flour enrichment with vitamins B1, B2, B3, and iron was initiated in the U.S. Even with refortification, white flour is significantly inferior to 100% whole wheat flour in its nutritional content. Regular consumption of foods made from refined grain is associated with weight gain, increased risk for insulin resistance and diabetes mellitus, type 2 (DM2), and cardiovascular disease; consumption of whole grains is protective against these conditions. Nutritional benefits of consuming 100% whole wheat include lowering cholesterol levels and blood pressure, slowing the absorption of glucose and stabilizing blood glucose levels, and promoting bowel regularity.

- Many persons are intolerant to wheat, and wheat is identified as one of the 8 major food allergens in the U.S. in addition to peanuts, tree nuts, cow's milk, shellfish, soy, eggs, and fish. Some individuals must avoid or completely eliminate dietary wheat to prevent harmful effects of wheat intolerance, including intestinal damage that is characteristic of celiac disease (CD; also called gluten-sensitive enteropathy, celiac sprue, and nontropical sprue). Although there is speculation that following a wheat-free diet could benefit persons with autism, evidence for this is lacking.

NUTRIENTS IN WHEAT

- Whole wheat bread typically provides 2 g of dietary fiber/slice. Benefits of dietary fiber include that it:
    - —binds with water and slows the digestive process, allowing more effective physiologic management of post-prandial (i.e., after eating) glucose and insulin responses.
    - —increases the volume of the intestinal contents, which hinders the absorption of cholesterol. The added bulk also promotes more regular bowel movements, which improve intestinal health.
- Wheat contains vitamins B1, B2, and B3, which create energy by aiding the breakdown of carbohydrates, provide cardiovascular protection, maintain the nervous system, and support the production of red blood cells, hormones, and essential cholesterol.

- Whole wheat contains betaine, a metabolite of choline that reduces inflammation.
- Whole wheat has many phytonutrients (i.e., beneficial plant-derived chemicals), which serve as antioxidants, have anti-cancer properties, and reduce inflammation. One important phytonutrient in whole wheat is the lignan enterolactone, which has estrogen-like effects. Increasing serum levels of enterolactones may help protect against heart disease and hormone-dependent cancers such as breast and prostate cancers.
- Wheat germ is rich in vitamin E, a fat-soluble vitamin that functions primarily as an antioxidant, but also maintains cell membranes, assists in vitamin K absorption, and contributes to immune system function.

DIETARY INTAKE GUIDELINES

- The U.S. Food and Drug Administration (FDA) recommends 25–30 grams of dietary fiber intake per day, the amount provided in about 2 cups of 100% whole wheat flour.
- In their dietary and lifestyle recommendations, the American Heart Association (AHA) recommends at least half of all grains consumed should be whole grains.

CELIAC DISEASE

- One of the major health concerns associated with wheat consumption is CD. CD is a chronic, autoimmune, inflammatory disorder of the small bowel that is triggered by a hypersensitivity to gluten in genetically predisposed individuals.
  —Gluten is most commonly associated with wheat, but is also found on the surface layer of the cereal grains barley and rye.
  —Signs and symptoms of CD include symptoms such as chronic fatigue, iron deficiency anemia, dental enamel hypoplasia, infertility, neurologic disorders, dermatitis herpetiformis (i.e., skin rash), peripheral neuropathy, skeletal disorders (e.g., osteoporosis), and generalized pain.
    –In some cases, CD is subclinical and patients appear asymptomatic, but results of serologic tests and villi sampling are positive for CD.
  —Risk factors include a family history of CD or other autoimmune disorders, most commonly type 1 diabetes mellitus (DM1).

  —A life-long gluten-free diet (GFD) is the primary treatment for individuals diagnosed with CD.
- No information is available in the medical literature about the interaction of wheat with medications.

RESEARCH FINDINGS

- Researchers have found that the dietary fiber in wheat promotes the growth of flora (i.e., beneficial bacteria) in the intestines. This prebiotic action increases the formation of fermentation products (e.g., the short-chain fatty acids [SCFA] butyrate, propionate, and acetate) that inhibit the growth of and induce natural death of colon cancer cells. SCFA serve as an energy source to normal cells, enhancing their survival.
- Diets high in simple carbohydrates (e.g., diets containing refined wheat flour) are associated with dyslipidemia and diabetes mellitus. Even whole grains have a relatively high glycemic index, which can cause elevated blood glucose levels that lead to increased production of insulin. Diet modification for the prevention of obesity, heart disease, and diabetes mellitus should include adding sources of unsaturated fats, lean proteins, fruits, vegetables, and whole grains.
- Researchers have evaluated patients who avoid wheat and/or gluten (PWAWG) due to possible intolerance in order to identify common clinical features among them, as well as similar and differing characteristics when compared to individuals with CD. The study revealed similar characteristics among the CD and the PWAWG groups when comparing comorbidities, mean BMI, and mean hemoglobin levels. The mechanism of these similarities is not understood.
- Currently, the only treatment for CD is complete and permanent elimination of dietary gluten. Ingesting even small amounts of gluten can damage the intestinal mucosa of patients with CD, requiring that gluten-free foods be prepared separately from foods containing gluten in order to prevent cross-contamination. Gluten is also present in the ingredients of many processed foods; extensive knowledge of food products and careful reading of all food labels are vital to avoid unintentional gluten exposure.

—Common food ingredients that contain gluten include malt flavoring, dextrin, hydrolyzed plant proteins, modified food starch, dextrins, and a variety of seasonings.

—Avoiding nonfood sources of gluten that can be ingested is also important. Examples of nonfood sources of gluten include certain toothpastes, medications, dietary supplements, lipsticks, postage stamps, and envelopes.

SUMMARY

Consumers should become knowledgeable about the physiologic risks and benefits of wheat. Whole wheat is a good source of dietary fiber, vitamin E, B vitamins, and phytonutrients. These nutrients lower blood glucose, reduce inflammation, support gastrointestinal health, and may reduce the risk of developing heart disease and cancer. Individuals with Celiac disease should avoid all products containing wheat. Consuming large amounts of refined wheat is associated with obesity, type 2 diabetes, and cardiovascular disease.

—*Cherie Marcel, BS*

REFERENCES

Bodinham, C. L., Hitchen, K. L., Youngma, P. J., Frost, G. S., & Robertson, M. D. (2011). Short-term effects of whole-grain wheat on appetite and food intake in healthy adults: A pilot study. *British Journal of Nutrition*, *106*(3), 327-330. doi:10.1017/S0007114511000225

Borowicki, A., Michelmann, A., Stein, K., Scharlau, D., Scheu, K., Obst, U., & Glei, M. (2011). Fermented wheat aleurone enriched with probiotic strains IGG and Bb12 modulates markers of tumor progression in human colon cells. *Nutrition and Cancer*, *63*(1), 151-160. doi:10.1080/01635581.2010.516874

Borowicki, A., Stein, K., Scharlau, D., Scheu, K., Brenner-Weiss, G., Obst, U., & Glei, M. (2010). Fermented wheat aleurone inhibits growth and induces apoptosis in human HT29 colon adenocarcinoma cells. *British Journal of Nutrition*, *103*(3), 360-369. doi:10.1017/S0007114509991899

Costabile, A., Klinder, A., Fava, F., Napolitano, A., Fogliano, V., Leonard, C., & Tuohy, K. M. (2008). Whole-grain wheat breakfast cereal has a prebiotic effect on the human gut microbiota: A double-blind, placebo-controlled, crossover study. *British Journal of Nutrition*, *99*(1), 110-120.

Crowther, P. (2013). Wheat – staff of life or pain in the gut? *Positive Health*, *207*, 3 pp.

Evert, A. (2013). Vitamin E. *MedlinePlus*. Retrieved May 17, 2015, from http://www.nlm.nih.gov/medlineplus/ency/article/002406.htm

Fardet, A. (2010). New hypotheses for the health-protective mechanisms of whole-grain cereals: What is beyond fibre? *Nutrition Research Reviews*, *23*(1), 65-134. doi:10.1017/ S0954422410000041

The George Mateljan Foundation. (n.d.). The world's healthiest foods: Whole wheat. Retrieved March 17, 2015, fromhttp://www.whfoods.com/genpage.php?tname=foodspice&dbid=66

German, J. B., & Dillard, C. J. (2004). Saturated fats: What dietary intake? *American Journal of Clinical Nutrition*, *80*(3), 550-559.

Inomata, N. (2009). Wheat allergy. *Current Opinion in Allergy and Clinical Immunology*, *9*(3), 238-243. doi:10.1097/ACI.0b013e32832aa5bc

Johnson, L. E. (2014, November). Vitamin E. The Merck Manual for Health Care Professionals. Retrieved March 17, 2015, from http://www.merckmanuals.com/professional/ sec01/ch004/ch004l.html

Lutz, C. A., & Przytulski, K. R. (2006). In *Nutrition & diet therapy: Evidence-based applications* (4th ed., p. 484). Philadelphia, PA: F. A. Davis Company.

Saturni, L., Ferretti, G., & Bacchetti, T. (2010). The gluten-free diet: Safety and nutritional quality. *Nutrients*, *2*(1), 16-34. doi:10.3390/nu20100016

See, J., & Murray, J. A. (2006). Gluten-free diet: The medical and nutrition management of celiac disease. *Nutrition in Clinical Practice*, *21*(1), 1-15. doi:10.1177/011542650602100101

Tavakkoli, A., Lewis, S. K., Tennyson, C. A., Lebwohl, B., & Green, P. H. R. (2014). Characteristics of patients who avoid wheat and/or gluten in the absence of celiac disease. *Digestive Diseases & Sciences*, *59*(6), 1255-1261. doi:10.1007/s10620-013-2981-6

Tighe, P., Duthie, G., Vaughan, N., Brittenden, J., Simpson, W. G., Duthie, S., & Thies, F. (2010). Effect of increased consumption of whole-grain foods on blood pressure and other cardiovascular risk markers in healthy middle-aged persons: A randomized controlled trial. *American Journal of Clinical Nutrition*, *92*(4), 733-740. doi:10.3945/ ajcn.2010.29417

Youdim, A. (2014, December). Fiber. *Merck Manual*. Retrieved March 17, 2015, from http://www.merckmanuals.com/home/disorders_of_nutrition/overview_of_nutrition/ fiber.html

Lichtenstein, A. H., Appel, L. J., Brands, M., Carnethon, M., Daniels, S., Franch, H. A., ... Wylie-Rosett, J.

(2006). Summary of American Heart Association Diet and Lifestyle Recommendations revision 2006. *Arteriosclerosis, Thrombosis, and Vascular Biology*, 26(10), 2186-2191. doi:10.1161/01. ATV.0000238352.25222.5e

REVIEWER(S)

Darlene Strayer, RN, MBA, Cinahl Information Systems, Glendale, CA

Nursing Executive Practice Council, Glendale Adventist Medical Center, Glendale, CA

PROTEINS

Cashew

WHAT WE KNOW

The cashew (*Anacardium occidentale*) of the Anacardiaceae family is a kidney-shaped tree nut, or seed, that adheres to the bottom of the cashew apple, the fruit of the cashew tree, and is primarily grown in India and Brazil. Other tree nuts include almonds, pecans, and pistachios. Tree nuts contain plant sterols, which are substances that are known to reduce cholesterol absorption from the gut. Cashews also contain high amounts of potassium, magnesium, copper, vitamin A, folic acid, and, along with most nuts, are a great source of protein, fiber, and unsaturated fats. Despite the common belief that nuts are fattening, evidence supports the inclusion of nuts in weight-loss diet plans because nuts enhance satiety (i.e., a feeling of fullness) and reduce appetite. Nuts are associated with increased satisfaction with a diet plan and more efficient weight loss. Additional benefits attributed to cashews and other nuts include their association with reduced triglycerides, elevated high-density lipoprotein (HDL), reduced inflammation, and decreased risk of heart disease and diabetes mellitus, type 2 (DM2).

- Cashews are always sold without shells because the interior of their thick double shell contains a poisonous resin called urushiol (also called cashew balm), a toxin that is also found in poison ivy. The urushiol is carefully removed and used to make varnishes and insecticides. The cashew can be eaten by the handful as a healthy snack, cooked into a variety of dishes, ground and pressed to make butter or milk, chopped, roasted, blended, crumbled, and sprinkled.
- Many persons are allergic to cashews and other nuts. Because of this, it is recommended that nuts be cautiously introduced in the diets of young children after the age of 12 months, or 3 years of age in children who have a strong family history of food allergy.

NUTRIENTS IN CASHEWS

- The cashew is lower in fat than most other nuts, but is an excellent source of unsaturated fatty acids, primarily the omega-9 monounsaturated fatty acid oleic acid. Oleic acid promotes the production of antioxidants and lowers triglyceride levels, reducing the risk of arteriosclerosis, heart disease, and cancer.
- The cashew contains the amino acid arginine, which slows the formation of blood clots and reduces arterial congestion.
- The cashew is rich in soluble fiber, which reduces blood cholesterol levels and sustains colon health.
- Another notable constituent of the cashew is folic acid, a B vitamin
  —Folic acid helps to prevent high levels of the amino acid homocysteine, which is a major risk factor for heart disease.
  —Folic acid is necessary for the production of red bloods cells and genetic material vital to normal human development and maintenance of most of the body's functional systems.
- The cashew is a good source of the mineral magnesium, which has many health benefits, including the prevention of heart disease and DM2 and maintenance of healthy bones.
  —Magnesium balances calcium in the cells, which regulates tone and maintains relaxation of nerves and muscles. This action contributes to the prevention of high blood pressure, muscle spasm, asthma, migraine headache, general soreness, and fatigue.
- The cashew provides the mineral copper, which exhibits strong antioxidant activity
  —Copper is a vital component of superoxide dismutase, which is an enzyme necessary for energy production and antioxidant activity.

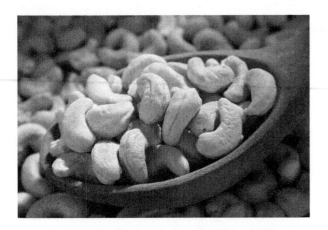

—Copper contributes to the action of lysyloxidase, which is an enzyme necessary for the cross-linking of collagen and elastin to maintain flexibility in the blood vessels, bones, and joints.

—Copper enhances the body's ability to use iron, preventing iron deficiency anemia, ruptured blood vessels, irregular heartbeat, and infection.

RECOMMENDED DIETARY INTAKE

- Although there is no standardized recommendation for the dosage of cashew, results of studies indicate that consumption of a small handful of cashew or other nut 3–5 times per week is associated with a 30–50% reduction in the risk of heart disease.
- Along with other nuts, the cashew poses high risk as a food allergen. Signs and symptoms of an allergic reaction can be severe, and can include upset stomach, pruritus, skin rash, difficulty breathing, swelling, and anaphylaxis. Because of this, it is recommended that the cashew not be added to a baby's diet until after 12 months of age or 3 years of age in children with a strong family history of food allergies.
- Consuming a whole cashew is not recommended for children under the age of 5 years due to the risk of choking.
- There is some concern that cashew intake increases the risk of kidney stones in individuals with a history of kidney stones because the cashew contains high amounts of the chemical oxalate, a primary component of kidney stones.
- Treatment for allergic reactions related to cashew consumption may include hospitalization and administration of antihistamines and epinephrine by injection.

RESEARCH FINDINGS

- Researchers report that the occurrence of cashew allergies is increasing, but is underestimated as a health risk by many.
- Metabolic syndrome is characterized by a cluster of conditions, including cardiovascular disease, dyslipidemia, abnormal glucose tolerance, hypertension, and abdominal obesity. Researchers evaluating whether the high antioxidant properties of cashew can improve the health status of individuals with metabolic syndrome had test subjects follow specific diets that included the cashew, and monitored markers such as serum antioxidant and lipid profiles, serum glucose, C-reactive protein (CRP), and blood pressure to identify results. Results indicated that while the diet plans high in cashew consumption increased antioxidant capacity, they did not improve the serum antioxidant profile or any other specified marker in the test subjects with metabolic syndrome. Further study is recommended to evaluate if longer trials or significant weight loss (most test subjects were obese) affect the results.
- Authors of a study conducted on female rats reported that extracts taken from cashew leaves inhibited laboratory-induced gastric lesions. These extracts consisted largely of phenolic compounds, including flavonoids and condensed tannins. Because the extracts were obtained using methanol, which is a poor solvent for tannins, researchers suspected that the active components of the phenolic compounds were substances other than tannins. Flavonoids are free radical scavengers, which have a protective role against ulcerative and erosive lesions of the gastrointestinal tract. Scientists hypothesize that this protection is due to the ability of flavonoids to increase mucosal prostaglandin content and decrease histamine secretion. No signs of acute toxicity were observed in flavonoid doses up to 2,000 mg/kg of body weight. Future studies are recommended to assess if the methanolic fraction of the cashew can be used as a new form of antiulcer therapy.

SUMMARY

Consumers should become knowledgeable about the physiologic risks and benefits of cashew consumption. Cashews are a good source of potassium, magnesium, copper, vitamin A, folic acid, protein, fiber, and unsaturated fats. The health benefits associated with cashew consumption (e.g., small handful of nuts, 3–5 times per week) includes; lower total cholesterol, reduced inflammation, and decreased risk of heart disease and type 2 diabetes mellitus (DM2).

Parents should be aware of the risks of nut allergies and precautions to be taken when introducing cashews and other nuts into a child's diet, as well as the high risk of choking on cashews in children under the age of 5 years. Individuals with a history of kidney stones should monitor cashew intake, as they may increase the risk of kidney stones due to high amounts of oxalate.

—Cherie Marcel, BS

REFERENCES

Berriman, M. (2007). Nuts and seeds. *Natural Health and Vegetarian Life*, 44-45.

Davis, L., Stonehouse, W., Loots, D. T., Mukuddem-Petersen, J., van der Westhuizen, F. H., Hanekom, S. M., ... Jerling, J. C. (2007). The effects of high walnut and cashew nut diets on the antioxidant status of subjects with metabolic syndrome. *European Journal of Nutrition*, 46(3), 155-164. doi:10.1007/s00394-007-0647-x

Davoren, M., & Peake, J. (2005). Cashew nut allergy is associated with a high risk of anaphylaxis. *Archives of Disease in Childhood*, 90(10), 1084-1085. doi:10.1136/ adc.2005.073817

The George Mateljan Foundation editorial team. (n.d.). The world's healthiest foods: Cashews. Retrieved February 27, 2015, fromhttp://www.whfoods.com/genpage.php? tname=foodspice&dbid=98

Grigg, A., Hanson, C., & Davis, C. M. (2009). Cashew allergy compared to peanut allergy in a U.S. tertiary care center. *Pediatric Asthma, Allergy & Immunology*, 22(3), 101-104. doi:10.1089/pai.2009.0017

Hurley, J., & Liebman, B. (2009). Going nuts sorting through the claims. *Nutrition Action Healthletter*, 36(8), 13-14.

Konan, N. A., & Bacchi, E. M. (2007). Antiulcerogenic effect and acute toxicity of a hydroethanolic extract from the cashew (Anacardium occidentale L.) leaves. *Journal of Ethnopharmacology*, 112(2), 237-242. doi:10.1016/j.jep.2007.03.003

Mukuddem-Petersen, J., Stonehouse Oosthuizen, W., Jerling, J. C., Hanekom, S. M., & White, Z. (2007). Effects of high walnut and high cashew nut diet on selected markers of the metabolic syndrome: A controlled feeding trial. *British Journal of Nutrition*, 97(6), 1144-1153.

van der Valk, J. P., Dubois, A. E., Gerth van Wijk, R., Wichers, H. J., & de Jong, N. W. (2014). Systematic review on cashew nut allergy. *Allergy*, 69(6), 692-698. doi:10.1111/ all.12401

REVIEWER(S)

Darlene Strayer, RN, MBA, Cinahl Information Systems, Glendale, CA

Nursing Executive Practice Council, Glendale Adventist Medical Center, Glendale, CA

Eggs

WHAT WE KNOW

Although many animals lay eggs, the information in this paper refers specifically to chicken eggs. Eggs contain a yellow yolk surrounded by egg white (i.e., a clear, gelatinous substance), and are encased in a protective shell that can be white or brown. The color of the shell depends on the breed of the chicken, and does not reflect nutritional quality. Every nutrient that is necessary for a developing chick is contained in an egg, making it a nutrient-dense source of food for both chicks and humans. Eggs are consumed by a variety of cultures around the world. The protein in eggs, which is about 6 g per egg, is of such high biologic value that eggs are frequently used as the standard to which other sources of protein are compared. Eggs are a rich source of the vitamins A, D, B12, riboflavin, pantothenic acid, choline, tryptophan, selenium, iodine, and phosphorous. Although egg yolks are a significant source of cholesterol, research results indicate that eating 1–2 eggs/day does not significantly affect the blood lipid profile (i.e., level of cholesterol in the blood) and does not appear to increase the risk for cardiovascular disease (CVD).

- The health benefits of eggs include promoting neurologic health, reducing inflammation, preventing blood clots, and protecting against the development of age-related macular degeneration and cataracts.

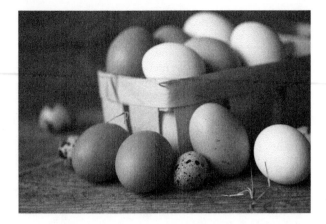

- Despite their high nutritional value, eggs are classified as a major food allergen, along with wheat, cow's milk, shellfish, tree nuts, peanuts, and soy.
- Eggs can cause salmonellosis, a food-borne illness caused by salmonella. Salmonella can be found on eggshells even if the external surface of the shell has been cleaned. Eggs should be fully cooked to destroy the salmonella bacteria. Eating soft-cooked, sunny-side up, and raw eggs increases risk for salmonellosis; eating hard-boiled, scrambled, and poached eggs is considered safe.

NUTRIENTS IN EGGS

- Eggs are a valuable source of highly bio-available (i.e., ready for the body to use) protein; eggs contain all 9 essential amino acids (i.e., amino acids that are not produced by the body). Protein is present in every cell in the human body, and is vital to the development and maintenance of skin, muscles, organs, and glands. Other important actions of protein include the following:
  —Provides oxygen to the blood
  —Involved in the formation of antibodies necessary for fighting infection
  —Contributes to the production of certain enzymes and hormones
- Eggs are a significant source of cholesterol, which is a waxy substance that is a vital part of cell membranes. Functions of cholesterol include the following:
  —Contributes to the production of vitamin D and bile acids
  —Used to make steroid hormones (e.g., estrogen, testosterone, aldosterone, cortisol)

—A vital component of cell membranes that promotes adequate permeability
—Assists in the absorption of fat and the fat-soluble vitamins A, D, E, and K
—Contributes to nerve impulse conduction
- Vitamin A, or retinol, in eggs is required for vision, maintenance of the surface linings of the eyes and other epithelial tissue, normal bone growth, immune system response, energy regulation, reproduction, embryonic development, and activation of gene expression.
- Eggs provide vitamin D, which is necessary for maintaining normal blood levels of calcium and phosphorus. Functions of vitamin D include the following:
  —Supports the absorption of calcium
  —Contributes to the formation and maintenance of bones
- Vitamin B12, or cobalamin, is a cobalt-containing member of the B complex vitamins. Vitamin B12 plays a major role in lipid, carbohydrate, and protein metabolism. Other actions of B12 include the following:
  —Required for the production of hormones, lipids and proteins
  —Contributes to nervous system function by aiding in the synthesis of neurotransmitters
  —Required for the formation of red blood cells and hemoglobin
  —Plays a significant role in deoxyribonucleic acid (DNA) and ribonucleic acid (RNA) synthesis
- Vitamin B2, or riboflavin, is an essential micronutrient that breaks down proteins for respiratory reactions to produce energy
  —The most significant biologically active forms of riboflavin are the flavocoenzymes flavin mononucleotide (FMN) and flavin adenine dinucleotide (FAD), which function as electron carriers and contribute to the formation of vitamins B6, B12, and niacin (also called vitamin B3) and their coenzymes. FAD also contributes to fatty acid oxidation and is required for the conversion of retinol to retinoic acid, making it integral to normal vision.
- Vitamin B5, or pantothenic acid, contributes to the metabolism of carbohydrates, proteins, and lipids. It plays a role in the synthesis of acetylcholine, which is a neurotransmitter in the central

and peripheral nervous system, which is necessary for the control of heart rate, respiration, and skeletal muscle function. Acetylcholine is necessary to the portions of the brain responsible for mood and memory.

- Choline is a water-soluble organic compound that is vital to normal brain development, neurotransmission, cell structure and function, and lipid transport from the liver. It is usually associated with the B vitamins, although choline is technically not a vitamin. Choline is necessary for the production of phospholipids (i.e., fatty acid and phosphate compounds), which are essential components of all cell membranes. A small amount of choline is metabolized to form acetylcholine.
  —Choline is a precursor of betaine.
  —Betaine functions as an osmolyte in the kidneys. Osmolytes are compounds that help maintain normal physiologic fluid balance.
  —Betaine is a methyl group donor that contributes to more than 50 methylation reactions, including the conversion of homocysteine (i.e., an amino acid) to methionine (i.e., an essential amino acid). Elevated levels of homocysteine are associated with cardiovascular disease and neural tube defects (NTDs); choline is vital to normal fetal brain development and neural tube closure.
  —As a methyl donor, the metabolism of betaine directly affects the metabolism of folate, vitamin B12, and methionine
- The tryptophan in eggs contributes to the synthesis of niacin and serotonin. Serotonin is thought to promote healthy sleep patterns and stabilize mood.
- Selenium is an essential trace mineral. Selenium combines with proteins to create selenoproteins, which are important antioxidant enzymes that protect cells from the damaging effects of free radicals (i.e., reactive by-products of oxygen metabolism). Other contributions of selenium include the following:
  —Regulates thyroid function
  —Provides support for immune system function
  —As a precursor to glutathione peroxidase, an antioxidant enzyme, selenium may be important to lung health
- The trace mineral iodine supports the thyroid gland, and has antifungal, antimicrobial, and antibacterial properties.

- Eggs contain phosphorous, which combines with calcium for the formation of bones and teeth, muscle contraction, and nerve conduction; phosphorous is essential to the structural integrity of cell membranes.

RESEARCH FINDINGS

- Researchers report that consuming eggs for breakfast instead of bagels, which have equivalent caloric content, results in less variation of plasma levels of glucose and insulin and reduces daily caloric intake. Research results indicate that replacing bagels with eggs at breakfast can help to promote weight loss. These benefits have no apparent detrimental effect on lipid profiles.
- According to researchers, consuming egg yolks can increase macular pigment concentrations in older adults who are receiving cholesterol-lowering statins. Results of other studies show that eggs contain highly bio-available lutein, which is a carotenoid that is believed to prevent the development of age-related macular degeneration and cataracts.

SUMMARY

Become knowledgeable about the physiologic effects of egg consumption. Along with bio-available protein, eggs are a good source of vitamins A, D, B12, riboflavin, pantothenic acid, choline, tryptophan, selenium, iodine, and phosphorous. These nutrients aid in digestion and mood stability, promote muscle, bone and organ development, support healthy immune and nervous systems, maintain thyroid function, facilitate wound healing and inhibit chronic disease. Eggs are a good source of protein for individuals who choose to follow an ovo-vegetarian diet. Although egg yolks are a significant source of cholesterol, research indicates that eating 1–2 eggs/day does not significantly increase risk of developing heart disease.

—*Cherie Marcel, BS*

REFERENCES

Ahmed, S., & Blumberg, J. (2010). Eggs and evidence-based nutrition in the Dietary Guidelines for Americans 2010. *Nutrition Close-Up, Winter/Spring,* (1), 5.

Benelam, B., Roe, M., Pinchen, H., Church, S., Buttriss, J., Gray, J., & Finglas, P. (2012). New data on the nutritional composition of UK hens' eggs. *Nutrition Bulletin, 37*(4), 344-349. doi:10.1111/j.1467-3010.2012.01993.x

The George Mateljan Foundation editorial team. (n.d.). The world's healthiest foods: Eggs. Retrieved March 24, 2015, from http://www.whfoods.com/genpage. php? tname=foodspice&dbid=92#descr

MedlinePlus editorial team. (2013). Cholesterol. *MedlinePlus.* Retrieved March 24, 2015, from http://www.nlm.nih.gov/medlineplus/cholesterol.html

Njike, V., Faridi, Z., Dutta, S., Gonzalez-Simon, A. L., & Katz, D. L. (2010). Daily egg consumption in hyperlipidemic adults—effects on endothelial function and cardio vascular risk. *Nutrition Journal, 9*(28), 9pp. doi:10.1186/1475-2891-9-28

Ratliff, J., Leite, J. O., de Ogburn, R., Puglisi, M. J., Vanheest, J., & Fernandez, M. L. (2010). Consuming eggs for breakfast influences plasma glucose and ghrelin, while reducing energy intake during the next 24 hours in adult men. *Nutrition Research, 30*(2), 96-103. doi:10.1016/j.nutres.2010.01.002

Ruxton, C. (2010). Recommendations for the use of eggs in the diet. *Nursing Standard, 24*(37), 47-56.

Vishwanathan, R., Goodrow-Kotyla, E. F., Wooten, B. R., Wilson, T. A., & Nicolosi, R. J. (2009). Consumption of 2 and 4 egg yolks/d for 5 wk increases macular pigment concentrations in older adults with low macular pigment taking cholesterol-lowering statins. *American Journal of Clinical Nutrition, 90*(5), 1272-1279. doi:10.3945/ ajcn.2009.28013

Zazpe, I., Beunza, J. J., Bes-Rastrollo, M., Warnberg, J., de la Fuente-Arrillaga, C., Benito, S., ... Martinez-Gonzalez, M. A. (2011). Egg consumption and risk of cardiovascular disease in the SUN project. *European Journal of Clinical Nutrition, 65*(6), 676-682. doi:10.1038/ejcn.2011.30

Zieve, D., Eltz, D. R., & Evert, A. (2011). Protein in diet. *MedlinePlus.* Retrieved March 24, 2015, from http://www.nlm.nih.gov/medlineplus/ency/article/002467.htm

REVIEWER(S)

Darlene Strayer, RN, MBA, Cinahl Information Systems, Glendale, CA

Nursing Executive Practice Council, Glendale Adventist Medical Center, Glendale, CA

Fish

WHAT WE KNOW

The traditional Western diet tends to include a higher percentage of red meat and poultry than fish. However, research results indicate that increasing the ratio of fish intake to other forms of meat in the diet reduces the risk for many chronic diseases that involve inflammation (e.g., cardiovascular disease [CVD], inflammatory bowel disease [IBD], cancer, rheumatoid arthritis [RA]). Fish intake is also associated with a reduction in cognitive decline. These health benefits are attributed in large part to the omega-3 fatty acids found in fatty, cold-water fish (e.g., salmon), specifically, docosahexaenoic acid (DHA) and eicosapentaenoic acid (EPA). Fish is an excellent source of protein and many other valuable nutrients, including vitamins A and D, calcium, selenium, and magnesium.

Many pregnant women do not consume enough DHA. It is probable that this inadequate intake of DHA is due to the warnings women have received regarding the high mercury content of some types of fish and seafood. Certain fish and seafood (e.g., shark, swordfish, king mackerel, tilefish) contain high levels of mercury, which can be harmful to fetal development. However, evidence suggests that there is no apparent risk of prenatal mercury exposure from ocean fish consumption alone. Low consumption of fish and other seafood during pregnancy has been associated with increased risk for preterm delivery and low birth weight infants.

NUTRIENTS IN FISH

- Fish provides omega-3 fatty acids, which have powerful anti-inflammatory and hypotensive (i.e., blood pressure lowering) properties that helps to improve lung function and prevent CVD, RA, and other chronic diseases associated with inflammation.
  —DHA is vital to the development of the brain and other parts of the central nervous system and to visual function during the first 6 months of life.
  —EPA contributes to cardiovascular health and exhibits blood pressure lowering activity
- Fish is a good source of protein, which is a necessary macronutrient for the development and maintenance of skin, muscles, organs, and

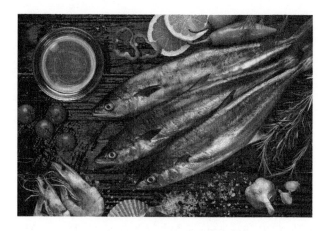

glands. Other important actions of protein include the following:
—Provides oxygen to the blood
—Involved in the formation of antibodies for fighting infection
—Contributes to the production of certain enzymes and hormones

- Vitamin A, or retinol, is a fat-soluble vitamin that is required for vision and maintenance of the surface linings of the eyes and other epithelial tissue, proper bone growth, immune system response, energy regulation, reproduction, embryonic development, and activation of gene expression.
- Vitamin D is necessary for maintaining normal blood levels of calcium and phosphorus. Functions of vitamin D include the following:
—Supports the absorption of calcium
—Contributes to the formation and maintenance of bones
- Calcium builds and maintains bones and teeth, regulates muscle contraction, conducts nerve impulses, activates enzymes for energy production and muscle contraction, participates in blood clotting, assists with vitamin B12 absorption, and maintains the structural integrity of intracellular membranes.
- Selenium is an essential trace mineral that combines with proteins to create selenoproteins
—Selenoproteins are important antioxidant enzymes that protect cells from the damaging effects of free radicals (i.e., reactive by-products of oxygen metabolism), regulate thyroid function, and support immune system function.

—As a precursor to glutathione peroxidase, an antioxidant enzyme, selenium may be important to lung health
- Magnesium balances the action of calcium in cells to regulate bone health, as well as tone in nerves and muscles. It maintains nerve and muscle relaxation, which contributes to the prevention of high blood pressure, muscle spasms, asthma, migraine headaches, general soreness, and fatigue.

DIETARY INTAKE RECOMMENDATIONS

- Recommendations for the amount of dietary fish consumed are made only for pregnant and lactating women because of the mercury-related risk to the fetus and neonate. Risk to other persons and groups is not quantified, and dietary recommendations regarding fish consumption are not made for other groups or persons.
- High levels of mercury can be harmful to fetal development and infants. Because of this, pregnant and lactating women are advised to limit their consumption of albacore tuna to no more than 6 oz/week and to avoid consuming fish that have potentially high levels of mercury, including the following:
—Shark
—Swordfish
—King mackerel
—Tilefish
- If the mercury content of locally caught fish is unknown, it is recommended that pregnant and lactating women limit their consumption of these fish to 6 oz/week.
- Other than the exceptions noted above, the United States Food and Drug Administration (FDA) suggests that women who are pregnant and lactating consume up to 12 oz/week of fish and seafood.

RESEARCH FINDINGS

- Researchers have reported that individuals who consume more fish than other forms of meat in their regular diet are more likely to make healthy dietary choices overall. For example, they tend to consume higher amounts of whole grains, fruits, and vegetables.
- The omega-3 fatty acids EPA and DHA have been shown to play a protective role against

dementia, CVD, IBD, cancer, and RA (rheumatoid arthritis), which might be attributed to their anti-inflammatory activity.

- Low fish intake during pregnancy is associated with poorer neurodevelopmental results, and more hyperactivity in children compared with children of women who consumed higher amounts of fish during pregnancy. Higher fish intake during the second trimester of pregnancy has also been shown to improve visual motor abilities in offspring.

SUMMARY

Consumers should become knowledgeable about the risks and benefits of fish consumption. Fish is an excellent source of DHA and EPA omega-3 fatty acids, as well as protein, vitamins A and D, calcium, selenium, and magnesium. These nutrients help reduce inflammation and blood pressure, maintain healthy skin, muscles, bones, eyes and organs, and support immune system and thyroid function. Pregnant women should be aware of the dietary recommendations for fish intake, especially fish with high mercury content. Research suggests regular fish consumption may help prevent dementia, CVD, IBD, cancer, and RA. Individuals with low fish consumption may consider fish oil supplementation.

—*Cherie Marcel, BS*

REFERENCES

Bloomingdale, A., Guthrie, L. B., Price, S., Wright, R. O., Platek, D., Haines, J., & Oken, E. (2010). A qualitative study of fish consumption during pregnancy. *American Journal of Clinical Nutrition*, 92(5), 1234-1240. doi:10.3945/ajcn.2010.30070

Cunningham, F. G., Leveno, K. J., Bloom, S. L., Hauth, J. C., Rouse, D. J., & Spong, C. Y. (Eds.). (2010). Prenatal care. In *Williams obstetrics* (23rd ed., p. 206). New York: McGraw-Hill Medical.

Del Gobbo, L. C., Archbold, J. A., Vanderlinden, L. D., Eckley, C. S., Diamond, M. L., & Robson, M. (2010). Risks and benefits of fish consumption for childbearing women. *Canadian Journal of Dietetic Practice & Research*, 71(1), 41-45. doi:10.3148/71.1.2010.41

Dovydaitis, T. (2008). Fish consumption during pregnancy: An overview of the risks and benefits. *Journal of Midwifery & Women's Health*, 53(4), 325-330. doi:10.1016/j.jmwh.2008.02.014

Ehrlich, S. D. (2010, September 30). Docosahexaenoic acid (DHA). *University of Maryland Medical Center*. Retrieved March 10, 2015, from http://www.umm.edu/altmed/articles/docosahexaenoic-acid-000300.htm

Ehrlich, S. D. (2010, September 30). Eicosapentaenoic acid (EPA). *University of Maryland Medical Center*. Retrieved March 10, 2015, from http://www.umm.edu/altmed/articles/eicosapentaenoic-acid-000301.htm

Evens, E. C. (2002). The FDA recommendations on fish intake during pregnancy. *Journal of Obstetric, Gynecologic & Neonatal Nursing*, 31(6), 715-720. doi:10.1177/0884217502239205

Gale, C. R., Robinson, S. M., Godfrey, K. M., Law, C. M., Schlotz, W., & O'Callaghan, F. J. (2008). Oily fish intake during pregnancy– Association with lower hyperactivity but not with higher full-scale IQ in offspring. *Journal of Child Psychology & Psychiatry*, 49(10), 1061-1068. doi:10.1111/j.1469-7610.2008.01908.x

Kesse-Guyot, E., Peneau, S., Ferry, M., Jeandel, C., Hereberg, S., & Galan, P. (2011). Thirteen-year prospective study between fish consumption, long-chain N-3 fatty acids intakes and cognitive function. *Journal of Nutrition, Health & Aging*, 15(2), 115-120. doi:10.1007/s12603-010-0318-0

Kim, J., Lim, S. Y., Shin, A., Sung, M. K., Ro, J., Kang, H. S., ... Lee, E. S. (2009). Fatty fish and fish omega-3 fatty acid intakes decrease the breast cancer risk: A case-control study. *BMC Cancer*, 9, 216. doi:10.1186/1471-2407-9-216

Lauritzen, L., & Carlson, S. E. (2011). Maternal fatty acid status during pregnancy and lactation and relation to newborn and infant status. *Maternal & Child Nutrition*, 7(Suppl 2), 41-58. doi:10.1111/j.1740-8709.2011.00303.x

Lopez, L. B., Kritz-Silverstein, D., & Barrett-Connor, E. (2011). High dietary and plasma levels of the omega-3 fatty acid docosahexaenoic acid are associated with decreased dementia risk: The Rancho Bernardo Study. *Journal of Nutrition, Health & Aging*, 15(1), 25-31. doi:10.1007/s12603-010-0114-x

Oken, E., Osterdal, M. L., Gillman, M. W., Knudsen, V. K., Halldorsson, T. I., Strom, M., ... Olsen, S. F. (2008). Associations of maternal fish intake during pregnancy and breastfeeding duration with attainment of developmental milestones in early childhood: A study from the Danish National Birth Cohort. *American Journal of Clinical Nutrition*, 88(3), 789-796.

Oken, E., Radesky, J. S., Wright, R. O., Bellinger, D. C., Amarasiriwardena, C. J., Kleinman, K. P., ... Gillman, M. W. (2008). Maternal fish intake during pregnancy, blood mercury levels, and child cognition at age 3 years in a US cohort. *American Journal of Epidemiology*, *167*(10), 1171-1181. doi:10.1093/aje/kwn034

Okubo, H., Sasaki, S., Murakami, K., & Takahashi, Y. (2008). The ratio of fish to meat in the diet is positively associated with favorable intake of food groups and nutrients among young Japanese women. *Nutrition Research*, *31*(3), 169-177. doi:10.1016/j.nutres.2011.02.005

Rogers, I., Emmett, P., Ness, A., & Golding, J. (2004). Maternal fish intake in late pregnancy and the frequency of low birth weight and intrauterine growth retardation in a cohort of British infants. *Journal of Epidemiology & Community Health*, *58*(6), 486-492. doi:10.1136/jech.2003.013565

Tremblay, L. (2011, February 1). Vitamins & minerals in fish. *Livestrong.com*. Retrieved March 10, 2015, from http://www.livestrong.com/article/371534-vitamins-minerals-in-fish/

Turunen, A. W., Mannisto, S., Suominen, A. L., Tiittanen, P., & Verkasalo, P. K. (2011). Fish consumption in relation to other foods in the diet. *British Journal of Nutrition*, *106*(10), 1570-1580. doi:10.1017/S0007114511002029

Wall, R., Ross, R. P., Fitzgerald, G. F., & Stanton, C. (2010). Fatty acids from fish: The anti-inflammatory potential of long-chain omega-3 fatty acids. *Nutrition Reviews*, *68*(5), 280-289. doi:10.1111/j.1753-4887.2010.00287.x

Wennberg, M., Bergdahl, I. A., Hallmans, G., Norberg, M., Lundh, T., Skerfving, S., ... Jansson, J. H. (2011). Fish consumption and myocardial infarction: A second prospective biomarker study from northern Sweden. *American Journal of Clinical Nutrition*, *93*(1), 27-36. doi:10.3945/ajcn.2010.29408

REVIEWER(S)

Darlene Strayer, RN, MBA, Cinahl Information Systems, Glendale, CA

Nursing Executive Practice Council, Glendale Adventist Medical Center, Glendale, CA

Legumes

WHAT WE KNOW

Legumes, plants in the Fabaceae family, are vital to agriculture, especially crop rotation, because they fix nitrogen, a natural fertilizing agent, in their roots, and thereby enrich the soil in which they grow. Legumes are grown for their seeds (also called "pulses") in many forms, including soybeans, tamarind, mesquite, carob, peanuts, lentil, beans, peas, clover, and alfalfa. Many legume seeds grow in pods.

- Farmers today use many legumes in fields that later are used for other plants. The soil-enriching qualities of legumes have been known for thousands of years. Native Americans, notably the Iroquois, used them as part of their "three sisters," corn, beans and squash, to naturally fertilize fields long before Europeans arrived. Archaeological evidence exists of 5,000-year-old gourds (squashes) in the Ohio valley.

- Legumes are symbiotic, in that they fertilize other plants in a natural cycle, fixing soil-enriching nitrogen in root nodules. The decay of legume-bearing plants also helps enrich the soil in which they lived long after they die. Following harvest, all nitrogen in the plants is released into surrounding soil. In the soil, the decaying plants' amino acids are converted to nitrate (NO_3), where it becomes available as fertilizer for new growth.

- Traces of legume production dating to more than 5,000 years ago have been discovered by archaeologists in and near the Ravi River in Punjab, a province of India, originating during the birth of the Indus River civilization. Evidence of legume production and use of similar antiquity also has been found in Egypt from the time of the pyramids' construction, as well as the Eastern Mediterranean, Mesopotamia, as well as in British and Swiss villages dating to the origins of agriculture.

- Legumes are basic to vegetarian diets around the world, and have been used in cuisine for millennia to enrich a variety of foods without use of meat. *Today, India is the world's largest producer and consumer of legumes, with significant imports from Pakistan, Canada, Burma, Australia and the United States. In 2015, the world market produced nearly 60 million tons of pulses. The United Nations in 2016 declared an International Year of

Pulses, with an emphasis on their use in sustainable agriculture, nutrition, and food security.

NUTRIENTS

- Legumes are rich in nutrition as well, including minerals, protein, carbohydrates, and fiber.
- One serving (100 grams) of chickpeas supplies a human being with nearly 1/3 of the daily recommended intake for fiber, 18% for protein, ½ the necessary manganese, and more than 40% for folate. One cup a day of various legumes helps reduce blood pressure and reduce LDL (i.e., bad) cholesterol.
- The combination of various legumes can supply complete proteins that supply human needs on par with meat or fish.
- Legumes contain insignificant amounts of fat and salt, and no cholesterol.
- Pulses supply resistant starch that aids bacteria in digestion, supplying the large intestine with fatty acids that help convert food to energy.
- Beans, especially the black and sprouted varieties, supply antioxidants. These antioxidants help protect against prostate enlargement, improve bone density, and delay dementia, including Alzheimer's disease, as well as reducing risk of breast and other types of cancer.

DIETARY INTAKE GUIDELINES

- Legumes are not popular in the United States, despite official declarations from the U.S. Department of Agriculture that any healthy diet should include at least a cup of beans a day.

RESEARCH FINDINGS

- The use of crop rotation and the natural fertilizing cycle of legumes has enjoyed a revival in recent years as traditional, pre-industrial and organic farming has become more popular. Year by year, as sales of organic food increase in grocery stores, natural crop rotation in which legumes are an essential part is being used to address an overload of artificial fertilizers that have been swept into bodies of water, including the Gulf of Mexico, to create anoxic "dead zones" where sea life has been killed by lack of oxygen.
- Alternating legumes with other plants can reduce or eliminate the need for artificial fertilizers. Organic food sales in the United States rose to

$43.3 billion in 2015, an increase of $4.2 billion from 2014. According to the United States Department of Agriculture, sales of organics have been rising an acerage of 11% a year since 2010.

- Only 3% of the calories in an average American's diet come from beans and nuts, according to the USDA.
- Only 4% of U.S. citizens eat the agency's minimum cup-a-day allowance.

SUMMARY

Consumers should become knowledgable about the physiological benefits associated with consumption of legumes. Although legumes are one of the world's oldest food sources, only a small percentage of Americans consume the one cup/day of legumes that is recommended for a healthy diet. Legumes are a good source of complete proteins, minerals, fiber and antioxidents. These nutrients may help reduce blood pressure and total cholesterol, maintain regular bowel movements and reduce the risk of heart disease and cancer.

—*Bruce E. Johansen, Ph.D.*
School of Communication,
University of Nebraska at Omaha

REFERENCES

Birt, D. F. et al. (2013). "Resistant starch: Promise for improving human health." *Advances in Nutrition* 4587–4601.

Deacon, J. (2015). "The nitrogen cycle and nitrogen fixation." Institute of Cell and Molecular Biology, The University of Edinburgh. Scotland. http://archive.bio.ed.ac.uk/jdeacon/microbes/nitrogen.htm

Ha, V. (May 13, 2014). "Effect of dietary pulse Intake on established therapeutic lipid targets for cardiovascular risk reduction: a systematic review and meta-analysis of randomized control trials." *Canadian Medical Association Journal* 186(8):586.

"The International Year of the Pulses." (2016). Food and Agriculture Organization, United Nations. http://www.fao.org/pulses-2016/en/

Jayalath V.H., de Souza R.J., Sievenpiper J. L, et al. (2014). "Effect of dietary pulses on blood pressure: A systematic review and meta-analysis of controlled feeding trials." *American Journal of Hypertension* 27(1):56-64.

Postgate, J. (1998). *Nitrogen fixation* (3rd ed.). Cambridge, U.K.: Cambridge University Press.

Sabaté, J., and Wien, M. (2015). "A perspective on vegetarian dietary patterns and risk of metabolic syndrome".

British Journal of Nutrition 113(Supplement 2):S136-143.

Varshney, R. K. and Kudapa, H. (November, 2013). "Legume biology: The basis for crop improvement." *Functional Plant Biology* 40 (12): v–viii.

REVIEWER(S)

Darlene Strayer, RN, MBA, Cinahl Information Systems, Glendale, CA

Nursing Executive Practice Council, Glendale Adventist Medical Center, Glendale, CA

Peanuts

WHAT WE KNOW

Although they are commonly thought of as nuts, peanuts are technically a type of legume (i.e., bean) called oilseeds. The soybean is also classified as an oilseed. Peanuts grow out of the flower of the *Arachis hypogaea* plant, which begins growing above ground but eventually burrows under the earth due to the weight of the peanuts. It is underground that the buttery peanut kernels mature in a woven-textured brown shell, or pod. Each shell contains two or three peanuts that are covered by a thin, reddish-brown skin. With their smooth texture and nutty flavor, peanuts have become a staple protein source in many diets. Probably best known as the childhood favorite sandwich filling, peanut butter, peanuts can also be enjoyed roasted and eaten out of the shells and processed into oil, flour, and flakes. Peanuts are rich in protein, monounsaturated fatty acids (MUFAs), biotin, niacin, folate, vitamin E, manganese, copper, molybdenum, phosphorous, and the powerful phenolic antioxidant resveratrol.

- Many persons are allergic to peanuts and tree nuts (e.g., cashews, almonds, pecans). Because of this, it is recommended that peanuts and tree nuts be cautiously introduced in the diet of young children after the age of 12 months, or at 3 years of age in children who have a strong family history of food allergy.

NUTRIENTS IN PEANUTS

- Peanuts are an excellent source of MUFAs, primarily the omega-9 monounsaturated fatty acid oleic acid. Oleic acid promotes the production of antioxidants and lowers triglyceride levels, reducing the risk of arteriosclerosis, heart disease, and cancer.

- Peanuts provide about 38 grams of protein per cup, making them a good meat-alternative protein source. Protein is present in every cell in the human body and is important to the development and maintenance of skin, muscles, organs, and glands.

- Other notable constituents of the peanut are biotin, folate, niacin, and other B-complex vitamins, which create energy by aiding the metabolism of carbohydrates, lipids, proteins, and alcohol. They also provide cardiovascular protection, maintain the nervous system, and support the production of red blood cells, hormones, and cholesterol.

    —Biotin functions as a coenzyme for carboxylases, which are enzymes required for the metabolism of fatty acids and gluconeogenesis (i.e., the conversion of protein and fat into glucose). Biotin plays a role in the formation of purines, which are important elements in DNA and RNA. The health of skin, hair, and nails is attributed to biotin.

    —Folate helps to prevent high levels of the amino acid homocysteine, which is a major risk factor for heart disease. Folate is necessary for the production of red bloods cells and genetic material that is important to normal human development and maintenance of most of the body's functional systems.

    —Niacin is involved in oxidation-reduction reactions that derive energy from carbohydrates, lipids, proteins, and alcohol and is integral to the anabolic reactions necessary to synthesize fatty acids and cholesterol.

- Peanuts are a good source of vitamin E, a fat-soluble vitamin that functions primarily as an antioxidant but also maintains cell membranes, assists in vitamin K absorption, and contributes to immune system function.

- Peanuts provide a variety of minerals, including manganese, copper, molybdenum, and phosphorous.

    —Manganese is a trace mineral that is responsible for energy production, fatty acid synthesis, cholesterol production, and protection against the damage caused by free radicals.

    —Copper is an important component of superoxide dismutase, which is an enzyme that is involved in energy production and antioxidant activity. Copper contributes to the action of lysyl oxidase, an enzyme necessary for the cross-linking of collagen and elastin, which allows flexibility in the blood vessels, bones, and joints. Copper enhances the body's ability to use iron, preventing iron-deficiency anemia, ruptured vessels, irregular heartbeat, and infection.

—Molybdenum is a cofactor for three enzymes aldehyde oxidase, xanthine oxidase, and sulfite oxidase, which are necessary for the catabolism of sulfur-containing amino acids and purines.

—Phosphorous combines with calcium for the formation of bones and teeth, muscle contraction, and nerve conduction and is essential for the structural integrity of cell membranes.

- Peanuts are a valuable source of the phytonutrient (i.e., beneficial, plant-derived chemical) resveratrol, which prevents damage to blood vessels, lowers low-density lipoprotein (LDL) cholesterol (i.e., the "bad" cholesterol), and inhibits blood clot formation.

RECOMMENDED DIETARY INTAKE

- Although there is no standardized recommendation for the dosage of peanuts, results of studies indicate that consumption of a small handful of peanuts or tree nuts 3–5 times per week is associated with a 30–50% reduction in the risk of heart disease.

- Peanuts are a substantial source of protein. The United States Food and Drug Administration (FDA) recommends the daily intake of .36 grams of protein per pound of body weight. One cup of peanuts provides 38 g of protein.

- Along with tree nuts, the peanut poses high risk as a food allergen. Because of this, it is recommended that peanuts not be added to a baby's diet until after 12 months of age or 3 years of age in children with a strong family history of food allergies. Signs and symptoms of peanut allergy include the following:
—Coughing and wheezing
—Tingling in the mouth
—Tightening of the throat and swelling of the tongue
—Difficulty breathing

—Dizziness or loss of consciousness
—Abdominal pain
—Nausea, vomiting, and diarrhea
—Nasal congestion
—Skin rash, hives, and eczema
—Migraine headache
—Anaphylactic shock; individuals with peanut allergy who are at increased risk for fatal anaphylactic shock include the following:
–Adolescents and young adults
–Persons with asthma
–Persons who do not have epinephrine available when the allergic reaction occurs
—Risk factors for peanut allergy are as follows:
–Family history of food allergies
–Having other allergies (35% of children with eczema have associated food allergies)
–Introduction of solid food before 4 months of age
—Treatment of peanut allergy:
–Complete avoidance of peanuts is the only effective method to avoid an allergic reaction.
–Persons who have peanut allergy should be educated regarding the importance of recognizing terminology that identifies hidden food allergens, reading food labels, and knowing what questions to ask when eating at restaurants.
–Food for a person with a peanut allergy must be prepared separately from food containing peanuts to prevent cross-contamination.
–Over time, oral immunotherapy (OIT) can be attempted, in which very small amounts of the allergen are introduced and gradually increased through oral feeding in a controlled environment (e.g., in a healthcare clinician's office) where immediate treatment can be provided. This process has shown promise in children with peanut allergy, increasing their reactive threshold and enabling them to eat small amounts of peanuts without reaction. This could prove to be life-saving in circumstances of accidental exposure.
–Medications are used to treat allergic reactions after known peanut exposure has occurred and/or a reaction develops.
–Antihistamines or bronchodilators can help to alleviate minor signs and

symptoms but do not relieve systemic reactions

–Intramuscular epinephrine injection is necessary for severe reactions, including anaphylactic reactions. Self-injectable EpiPens should be provided to individuals who are at high risk for anaphylaxis.

- Peanuts are susceptible to *Aspergillus flavus*, a fungus that produces the poison aflatoxin. Aflatoxin is 20 times more carcinogenic than dichlorodiphenyltrichloroethane (DDT), a powerful pesticide, and has been associated with mental retardation and reduced intelligence. The FDA requires that all food contain no more than 20 parts per billion of aflatoxin. If consuming raw peanuts, it is important to ensure that they have been stored properly (i.e., cool, dry). The fungus thrives in temperatures between 86°F and 96°F (30°C and–36°C) and in high humidity. Roasting peanuts is believed to protect against aflatoxin.

- There is some concern that peanut intake increases the risk of kidney stones in individuals with a history of kidney stones because the peanut contains a high amount of the chemical oxalate, which is a primary component of kidney stones.

RESEARCH FINDINGS

- Researchers have found that introducing solid foods prior to 4 months of age can increase the risk of food allergies in infants who are already at risk (e.g., have a family history of food allergy). However, avoiding suspected allergenic foods during pregnancy or breastfeeding does not appear to have a protective effect against peanut allergy in the child. It is recommended that a variety of solid foods with high nutritional value be introduced gradually, starting at about 6 months of age. New foods should be offered one at a time because waiting 3–5 days before adding another new food will help to identify foods that cause allergic reaction.

- Despite the widespread belief that peanuts are fattening, evidence supports the inclusion of peanuts and tree nuts in weight-loss diet plans because they enhance satiety (i.e., a feeling of fullness) and reduce appetite. Peanuts and tree nuts are associated with increased satisfaction with a diet plan and more efficient weight loss. Additional benefits attributed to peanuts include their association

with reduced triglycerides, elevated high-density lipoprotein (HDL), reduced inflammation, and decreased risk of heart disease, diabetes mellitus, type 2 (DM2), and Alzheimer's disease.

SUMMARY

Consumers should become knowledgeable about the physiologic effects of consuming peanuts. Peanuts can be beneficial to health because they contain a high amount of protein, omega-9 fatty acids, numerous vitamins and minerals, and resveratrol. These nutrients help lower total cholesterol, reduce inflammation, keep hair, skin and nails healthy, as well as potential to decrease risk of heart disease, type 2 diabetes mellitus, and Alzheimer's disease. Individuals with known a peanut allergy should always carrying an EpiPen. Consumers should be aware that raw peanuts must be stored properly to prevent the growth of aflatoxin-producing fungus. Individuals with a history of kidney stones should monitor peanut intake, as they may increase the risk of kidney stones due to high amounts of oxalate.

—*Cherie Marcel, BS*

REFERENCES

Anagnostou, K., & Clark, A. (2015). The management of peanut allergy. *Archives of Disease in Childhood, 100*(1), 68-72. doi:10.1136/archdischild-2014-306152

Emekli-Altufan, E., Kasikci, E., & Yarat, A. (2007). Peanuts improve blood glutathione, HDL-cholesterol level and change tissue factor activity in rats fed a high-cholesterol diet. *European Journal of Nutrition, 46*(8), 476-482.

Frazier, A. L., Camargo, C. A., Jr, Malspeis, S., Willett, W. C., & Young, M. C. (2014). Prospective study of peripregnancy consumption of peanuts or tree nuts by mothers and the risk of peanut or tree nut allergy in their offspring. *JAMA Pediatrics, 168*(2), 156-162. doi:10.1001/jamapediatrics.2013.4139

The George Mateljan Foundation editorial team. (n.d.). The world's healthiest foods: Peanuts. Retrieved April 4, 2015, fromhttp://www.whfoods.com/genpage.php?tname=foodspice&dbid=101#descr

King, J. C., Blumberg, J., Ingwersen, L., Jenab, M., & Tucker, K. L. (2008). Tree nuts and peanuts as components of a healthy diet. *Journal of Nutrition, 138*(9), 1736S-1740S.

Mangels, R. (2013). Scientific update. No need to avoid peanuts or tree nuts in pregnancy. *Vegetarian Journal, 32*(2), 26-27.

Mattes, R. D., Kris-Etherton, P. M., & Foster, G. D. (2008). Impact of peanuts and tree nuts on body weight and healthy weight loss in adults. *Journal of Nutrition, 138*(9), 1741S-1745S.

Nappo-Dattoma, L. (2011). Updated dietary standards: The 2010 Dietary Guidelines for Americans, MyPlate and other nutrition education resources for the oral health professional. *Access, 25*(8), 16-19.

Reis, C. E., Ribeiro, D. N., Costa, N. M., Bressan, J., Alfenas, R. C., & Mattes, R. D. (2013). Acute and second-meal effects of peanuts on glycaemic response and appetite in obese women with high type 2 diabetes risk: A randomised cross-over clinical trial. *British Journal of Nutrition, 109*(11), 2015-2023. doi:10.1017/S0007114512004217

Sales, J. M., & Resurreccion, A. V. (2014). Resveratrol in peanuts. *Critical Reviews in Food Science & Nutrition, 54*(6), 734-770. doi:10.1080/10408398.2011.606928

Schoessler, S. Z. (2005). The perils of peanuts: Creating a safe environment for the student who is allergic to peanuts and peanut products. *School Nurse News, 22*(4), 22-26.

Wien, M., Oda, K., & Sabate, J. (2014). A randomized controlled trial to evaluate the effect of incorporating peanuts into an American Diabetes Association meal plan on the nutrient profile of the total diet and cardiometabolic parameters of adults with type 2 diabetes. *Nutrition Journal, 13*(1), 10. doi:10.1186/1475-2891-13-10

REVIEWER(S)

Darlene Strayer, RN, MBA, Cinahl Information Systems, Glendale, CA

Nursing Executive Practice Council, Glendale Adventist Medical Center, Glendale, CA

Pork

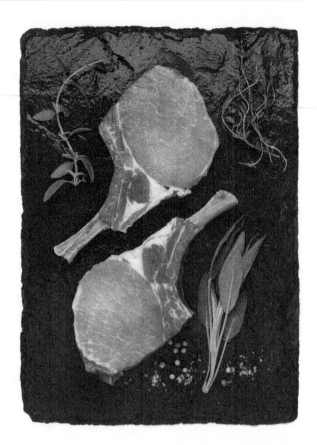

WHAT WE KNOW

The term pork refers to the fresh meat of a domesticated pig (i.e., *Sus domesticus*). Other forms of pig meat (e.g., ham, bacon, or sausage) have been processed (e.g., cured or preserved), typically resulting in high sodium content, while pork is naturally low in sodium (150 mg/4 oz serving). Pork is a nutrient-dense form of protein, providing 34 g of protein per 4 oz serving prior to preparation. The same serving size also contains 16.5 g of fat (7 g of saturated fat) and 129.5 mg of choles-terol, making pork a significant source of saturated fat and cholesterol. Lean cuts of pork (e.g., pork tenderloin) are much lower in fat and cholesterol (4 g total fat/4 oz).

- Pork can be prepared in many different ways, including sautéed, grilled, fried, or broiled. Regardless of the method used, pork must be cooked thoroughly in order to prevent contamination by the larvae of *Trichinella spiralis*, a species of roundworm.

- The United States Department of Agriculture (USDA) recommends that ground pork be cooked to reach an internal temperature of 160 °F (71°C), followed by 3 minutes of resting, and whole cuts or roasts be cooked to an internal temperature of 145 °F (63 °C), followed by a 3-minute rest.

NUTRIENTS IN PORK

- Pork is high in protein. Protein is present in every cell in the human body and is vital to the development and maintenance of skin, muscles, organs, and glands.

- Pork is an excellent source (contains more than 20% of the recommended dietary allowance [RDA]) of selenium, thiamin, niacin, vitamin B6, and phosphorus, and a good source (10–19% of the RDA) of riboflavin, zinc, and potassium.
  —Selenium is an essential trace mineral that combines with proteins to create selenoproteins.
    –Selenoproteins are important antioxidant enzymes that protect cells from the damaging effects of free radicals, regulate thyroid function, and support the immune system.
    –As a precursor to glutathione peroxidase, an antioxidant enzyme, selenium is believed to support lung health.
  —The B vitamins thiamin (B1), riboflavin (B2), and niacin (B3) create energy by aiding in the metabolism of carbohydrates, lipids, proteins, and alcohol. They provide cardiovascular protection, maintain nervous system function, and support the production of red blood cells (RBCs), hormones, and necessary cholesterol.
  —Vitamin B6, or pyridoxine, is required for the conversion of tryptophan to niacin and is involved in the conversion of homocysteine to cysteine. It supports the synthesis of serotonin and dopamine, which are neurotransmitters required for nerve cell communication. By maintaining lymphoid organs, pyridoxine contributes to proper function of the immune system.
  —Phosphorus combines with calcium to support the functions of muscle contraction, nerve conduction, and bone and teeth formation; and is essential for the structural integrity of cell membranes.
  —Zinc is an essential trace mineral that is involved in the catalytic activity of about 100 enzymes, supports the immune system and wound healing, and is essential for maintaining vision and the senses of smell and taste.
  —Potassium supports normal cellular, nerve, and muscle function, and helps to eliminate excess sodium from the body.
- Health Risks Associated with Eating Undercooked Pork

- Pork must be cooked thoroughly to prevent contamination by *T. spiralis* (see guidelines for cooking pork under *What We Know*, above).

RESEARCH FINDINGS

Researchers report that consuming lean pork in the place of other meats (e.g., beef or chicken) can significantly improve cardiometabolic health parameters such as weight, waist circumference, percent body fat, and blood lipid profile. Diets including fresh or fresh lean pork were also found to be higher in protein, selenium, thiamin, and vitamin B6 than diets that did not include fresh pork. These results indicate that lean pork can be considered a good source of protein in a healthy diet.

SUMMARY

Consumers should become knowledgeable about the physiologic effects of consuming pork. Pork can be beneficial to health because it contains a high amount of protein and numerous vitamins and minerals. Choosing healthy cooking methods (e.g., grilling, broiling, or roasting) will support a low-fat, low-cholesterol diet instead of eating high-fat cuts or pork that is battered and fried, which increases fat, cholesterol, and calorie content. Pork must be cooked thoroughly in order to prevent food contamination with *T. spiralis*. The internal temperature of ground pork should be 160°F (71°C), and whole cuts should be cooked to an internal temperature of 145°F (63 °C). Regular consumption of properly prepared pork may help maintain healthy skin, muscles, bones and organs, support immune and nervous systems, contribute to thyroid function, and reduce risk of developing heart disease. Research suggests that lean pork can be considered a good source of protein in a healthy diet.

—*Cherie Marcel, BS*

REFERENCES

Murphy, K. J., Thomson, R. L., Coates, A. M., Buckley, J. D., & Howe, P. R. C. (2012). Effects of eating fresh lean pork on cardiometabolic health parameters. *Nutrients*, 4(7), 711-723. doi:10.3390/nu4070711

Murphy, M. M., Spungen, J. H., Bi, X., & Barraj, L. M. (2011). Fresh and fresh lean pork are substantial sources of key nutrients when these products are consumed by adults in the United States. *Nutrition Research*, 31(10), 776-783.

Robinson, A. (2013). The nutritional value of pork. *Livestrong. com*. Retrieved June 3, 2015, from http://www.livestrong. com/article/271951-the-nutritional-value-of-pork/

Rubio, J. A., Rubio, M. A., Cabrerizo, L., Burdaspal, P., Carretero, R., Gomez-Gerique, J. A., ... Sanz, M. T. (2006). Effects of pork vs veal consumption on serum lipids in healthy subjects. *Nutricion Hospitalaria, 21*(1), 75-83.

USDA. (2013). Fresh pork from farm to table. Retrieved June 3, 2015, from http://www.fsis.usda.gov/wps/ portal/fsis/topics/food-safety-education/get-an- swers/food-safety-fact-sheets/meat-preparation/ fresh-pork-from-farm-to-table/CT_Index

REVIEWER(S)

Darlene Strayer, RN, MBA, Cinahl Information Systems, Glendale, CA

Nursing Executive Practice Council, Glendale Adventist Medical Center, Glendale, CA

Poultry

WHAT WE KNOW

The term poultry refers to any domesticated bird (also called fowl) that is raised for the purpose of producing eggs and/or meat for human consumption. Poultry options include chicken, turkey, duck, ostrich, and pheasant. Each type of poultry provides a unique flavor and nutrients. Because chicken and chicken eggs are the most commonly consumed poultry worldwide, the information that follows focuses on the nutritional characteristics of chicken and chicken eggs.

- Chickens (*Gallus gallus domesticus*) have been domesticated for about 5,000 years. Chickens that are raised for their meat are referred to as broiler chickens (also called roasters and fryers), and those raised for eggs are called egg-laying chickens. Prior to the 1930s, chickens were primarily raised in small family farms for the production of eggs. Chicken dinners were reserved for special occasions such as Sunday dinner. This practice changed with the introduction of "Sunday Dinner, Seven Days a Week" by Colonel Sanders and his chain of fast food restaurants, Kentucky Fried Chicken. In a relatively short time, chicken became a dietary staple in many homes, and broiler chicken production became the business of large corporate farms.

—Concern developed over the conditions in many large chicken farms in which chickens were kept in tight, unsanitary coops and frequently fed contaminated feed. In recent years, regulations have been changed to promote more humane living conditions and prevent contamination of chicken meat. Public demand has increased for organically fed chickens that are raised in outdoor pasture settings; these chickens are called pasture-raised, free-range, and cage-free chickens.

—The meat of pasture-raised chickens provides about 35 grams of protein per 4-oz serving. It is a substantial source of selenium and all of the B-complex vitamins. Other significant nutrients in chicken meat include zinc, copper, phosphorus, magnesium, and iron. The fat and cholesterol content of chicken meat varies depending on the cut of meat. Light meat (e.g., breast) contains significantly less total fat, saturated fat, and cholesterol than dark meat (e.g., thigh or leg). The method of cooking affects the fat and cholesterol content of chicken meat. For example, fried chicken has a much higher fat, cholesterol, and calorie content than grilled chicken.

—Chicken meat can be prepared in many different ways, including sautéed, grilled, fried, and broiled. Regardless of the method used, chicken must be cooked thoroughly to reach an internal temperature of 165 °F/74°C in order to prevent bacterial contamination (e.g., *Campylobacter*, *Enterococcus*, *Listeria*, and *Salmonella* organisms).

- Chicken eggs contain a round, yellow yolk that is surrounded by a clear, gelatinous substance called the egg white and encased in a protective shell. The color of the shell ranges from bright white to dark brown depending on the breed of chicken. Egg shell color is not reflective of the quality of nutrients in the egg. Eggs are equipped with every nutrient necessary for the development of a chick, making them a nutrient-dense food source for humans. The protein (about 6 grams per egg) in chicken eggs is of such high biologic value that it is frequently used as the standard to which other protein sources are compared. Eggs are rich in numerous vitamins and minerals.

—Some of the health benefits of eggs include promoting neurologic health, reducing inflammation, preventing blood clots, and protecting against age-related macular degeneration and cataracts.

—Although egg yolks are a significant source of cholesterol, research results indicate that eating one or two eggs a day does not negatively affect the blood lipid profile (i.e., cholesterol levels in blood) and does not appear to increase risk of cardiovascular disease (CVD).

—Eggs are classified as a major food allergen along with wheat, cow's milk, shellfish, tree nuts, peanuts, and soy

—*Salmonella* bacteria can be found on eggshells, even if the eggs have been cleaned. In order to destroy *Salmonella*, eggs must be fully cooked. Soft-cooked, sunny-side up, and raw eggs pose a risk for causing salmonellosis (i.e., a foodborne illness caused by *Salmonella*), and hardboiled, scrambled, and poached eggs are considered safe to eat.

NUTRIENTS IN POULTRY, SPECIFICALLY CHICKEN AND CHICKEN EGGS

- Both chicken meat and chicken eggs are a valuable source of highly bioavailable protein, meaning they contain all nine essential amino acids. Protein is present in every cell in the human body and is vital to the development and maintenance of skin, muscles, organs, and glands. Other important actions of protein include the following:
  —Oxygenating the blood
  —Forming the antibodies necessary for fighting infection
  —Contributing to the formation of enzymes and hormones
  —The amino acid tryptophan contributes to the synthesis of niacin and serotonin. Serotonin is thought to promote healthy sleep patterns and stabilize the mood
- Chicken meat and eggs contain omega-3 fatty acids, which are essential polyunsaturated fatty acids that the body requires for:
  —brain development
  —control of inflammation
  —blood clotting
  —strengthening cell membranes
  —the transport and metabolism of cholesterol

- Chicken meat and eggs are both significant sources of cholesterol, which is a waxy substance that is a vital part of cell membranes. Important functions of cholesterol include that it
  —is a vital component of cell membranes that allows for adequate permeability
  —contributes to the production of vitamin D and bile acids
  —is used in the synthesis of the steroid hormones estradiol and testosterone, the primary sex hormones, which regulate glucose metabolism
  —is used in the synthesis of the corticosteroids aldosterone and cortisol, which regulate the electrolytes concentration and hydric balance, respectively
  —assists in the absorption of fat and the fat-soluble vitamins A, D, E, and K
  —contributes to nerve impulse conduction
- Chicken meat and eggs are both rich in B-complex vitamins, which produce energy by aiding in the metabolism of carbohydrates, lipids, proteins, and alcohol. B-complex vitamins provide cardiovascular protection, maintain the nervous system, and support the production of red blood cells, hormones, and cholesterol.
- Chicken meat and eggs both contain the mineral phosphorous, which combines with calcium for the formation of bones and teeth, muscle contraction, and nerve conduction. Phosphorous is essential for the structural integrity of cell membranes.
- Chicken meat is a significant source of zinc, copper, magnesium, and iron.
  —Zinc is an essential trace mineral that is involved in the catalytic activity of about 100 enzymes, supports the immune system and wound healing, and is essential for maintaining vision and the senses of smell and taste
  —Copper is a vital component of superoxide dismutase (SOD), an enzyme involved in energy production and antioxidant activity. Copper contributes to the action of lysyl oxidase, an enzyme necessary for the cross-linking of collagen and elastin, which allows flexibility in blood vessels, bones, and joints. Copper enhances the body's ability to use iron, preventing iron-deficiency anemia, ruptured vessels, irregular heartbeat, and infection

—Magnesium balances the action of calcium in cells to regulate bone health and tone in nerves and muscles. Magnesium maintains relaxation of nerves and muscles, which contributes to the prevention of high blood pressure, muscle spasms, asthma, migraine headaches, general soreness, and fatigue

—Iron is vital for the synthesis of red blood cells and hemoglobin, which are necessary for cellular respiration and the transport of oxygen to the tissues. Iron supports immune function, is vital for mental development, contributes to energy metabolism, and regulates temperature.

- Chicken eggs are a valuable source of vitamins A and D, choline, selenium, and iodine.

  —Vitamin A, or retinol, is a fat-soluble vitamin that is required for vision, maintenance of the surface linings of the eyes and other epithelial tissue, proper bone growth, immune response, energy regulation, reproduction, embryonic development, and activation of gene expression.

  —Vitamin D is necessary for maintaining normal blood levels of calcium and phosphorous, contributing to the formation and maintenance of bones.

  —Although it is usually associated with the B vitamins, choline is technically not a vitamin. Choline is a water-soluble organic compound that is a vital component of all cells and an essential part of multiple biochemical and physiologic processes, including intracellular signaling, synthesis of numerous molecules, lipid metabolism, and regulation of gene expression.

  –As part of certain related compounds (e.g., acetylcholine, phosphatidylcholines, sphingomyelin), choline is essential to normal neural development, neurotransmission, and enterohepatic circulation of bile salts and cholesterol

  –Choline is a precursor of betaine.

    –Betaine serves as an osmolyte in the kidneys. Osmolytes are compounds that help maintain normal physiologic fluid balance.

    –Betaine functions as a methyl group donor to homocysteine, an amino acid, to form methionine, an essential amino acid.

    –Betaine participates in the metabolism of folate and vitamin B12.

—Selenium is an essential trace mineral that combines with proteins to create selenoproteins

  –Selenoproteins are important antioxidant enzymes that protect cells from the damaging effects of free radicals, regulate thyroid function, and support the immune system.

  –As a component of glutathione peroxidase, an antioxidant enzyme, selenium is believed to support lung health.

—Iodine is a trace mineral that supports the function of the thyroid gland and has antifungal, antimicrobial, and antibacterial activities.

RECOMMENDED DIETARY INTAKE

- Chicken meat contains purines, which break down to form uric acid. Uric acid can accumulate in individuals who are prone to gout or kidney stones. For this reason, persons with kidney abnormalities or gout should be advised to limit their consumption of purine-containing foods such as chicken meat.

RESEARCH FINDINGS

- There is evidence that feeding chickens high-quality feed (e.g., feed containing omega-3 fatty acid using flaxseed or fish oil) and allowing them space to peck, forage, and roam outdoors produces meat and eggs that are higher in antioxidants and omega-3 fatty acid.

  —The omega-3 fatty acids EPA and DHA have demonstrated a protective role against dementia, heart disease, inflammatory bowel disease (IBD), cancer, and rheumatoid arthritis (RA). Researchers suggest that this protective effect is attributed to the anti-inflammatory activity of EPA and DHA.

- Researchers report that the inclusion of chicken meat in a high-fiber diet that restricts total fat to 30% of total calories can lower blood pressure and levels of circulating blood triglycerides by increasing levels of anti-inflammatory omega-3 fatty acids and reducing the pro-inflammatory arachidonic acid.

- Researchers report that consuming eggs for breakfast instead of bagels, which are of equivalent caloric content, results in less variation of plasma glucose and insulin levels. Eating eggs for breakfast is associated with a reduction in total daily caloric intake. Research results indicate that replacing bagels with eggs at breakfast can help to promote weight loss. These benefits occur with no apparent detrimental impact on lipid profiles.

- According to researchers, consuming egg yolks can increase macular pigment concentrations in older adults who are receiving cholesterol-lowering statins. Results of other studies show that eggs contain highly bioavailable lutein, which is a carotenoid that is may reduce the risk of age-related macular degeneration and cataracts.

SUMMARY

Consumers should become knowledgeable about the physiologic effects of consuming poultry. Poultry can be beneficial to health because it contains a high amount of protein, omega-3 fatty acids, and numerous vitamins and minerals. Healthy cooking methods (e.g., grilling, broiling, or hard-boiling) may help support a low-fat, low-cholesterol diet instead of eating battered and fried chicken or eggs fried in butter, which are high in fat, cholesterol, and calories. It is important to cook chicken meat and eggs thoroughly in order to prevent food contamination with harmful bacteria (e.g., *Salmonella*). The internal temperature of chicken should be 165 °F/74°C and eggs should be hard-cooked. Regular consumption of properly prepared poultry may help maintain healthy skin, muscles, bones and organs, support immune and nervous systems, contribute to thyroid function, and reduce risk of developing heart disease. Individuals should be aware of possible allergies associated with poultry.

—*Cherie Marcel, BS*

REFERENCES

Ahmed, S., & Blumberg, J. (2010). Eggs and evidence-based nutrition in the Dietary Guidelines for Americans 2010. *Nutrition Close-Up, Winter/Spring,* (1), 5.

Cabré, E., Mañosa, M., & Gassull, M. A. (2012). Omega-3 fatty acids and inflammatory bowel diseases - a systematic review. *British Journal of Nutrition,* S240-S252. doi:10.1017/S0007114512001626

Castellini, C., Boggia, A., Cortina, C., Dal Bosco, A., Paolotti, L., Novelli, E., & Mugnai, C. (2012). A multicriteria approach for measuring the sustainability of different poultry production systems. *Journal of Cleaner Production,* 37, 192-201.

The George Mateljan Foundation. (n.d.). Chicken, pasture-raised. *The World's Healthiest Foods.* Retrieved July 8, 2015, from http://www.whfoods.com/genpage.php? tname=foodspice&dbid=116#safetyissues

The George Mateljan Foundation. (n.d.). Eggs, pasture-raised. Retrieved July 8, 2015, from http://www.whfoods.com/genpage.php?tname=foodspice&dbid=92#descr%20

Kartikasari, L. R., Hughes, R. J., Geier, M. S., Makrides, M., & Gibson, R. A. (2012). Dietary alpha-linolenic acid enhances omega-3 long chain polyunsaturated fatty acid levels in chicken tissues. *Prostaglandins, Leukotrienes, and Essential Fatty Acids,* 87(4-5), 103-109. doi:10.1016/j.plefa.2012.07.005

Kesse-Guyot, E., Peneau, S., Ferry, M., Jeandel, C., Hereberg, S., & Galan, P. (2011). Thirteen-year prospective study between fish consumption, long-chain N-3 fatty acids intakes and cognitive function. *Journal of Nutrition, Health & Aging,* 15(2), 115-120. doi:10.1007/s12603-010-0318-0

Lopez, L. B., Kritz-Silverstein, D., & Barrett-Connor, E. (2011). High dietary and plasma levels of the omega-3 fatty acid docosahexaenoic acid are associated with decreased dementia risk: The Rancho Bernardo Study. *Journal of Nutrition, Health & Aging,* 15(1), 25-31. doi:10.1007/s12603-010-0114-x

Melanson, K., Gootman, J., Myrdal, A., Kline, G., & Rippe, J. (2003). Weight loss and total lipid profile changes in overweight women consuming beef or chicken as the primary protein source. *Nutrition,* 19(5), 409-414.

Njike, V., Faridi, Z., Dutta, S., Gonzalez-Simon, A. L., & Katz, D. L. (2010). Daily egg consumption in hyperlipidemic adults—effects on endothelial function and cardiovascular risk. *Nutrition Journal,* 9(28). doi:10.1186/1475-2891-9-28

Ratliff, J., Leite, J. O., de Ogburn, R., Puglisi, M. J., Vanheest, J., & Fernandez, M. L. (2010). Consuming eggs for breakfast influences plasma glucose and ghrelin, while reducing energy intake during the next 24 hours in adult men. *Nutrition Research,* 30(2), 96-103. doi:10.1016/j.nutres.2010.01.002

Vishwanathan, R., Goodrow-Kotyla, E. F., Wooten, B. R., Wilson, T. A., & Nicolosi, R. J. (2009). Consumption of 2 and 4 egg yolks/d for 5 wk increases macular pigment concentrations in older adults with low macular pigment taking cholesterol-lowering statins. *American Journal of Clinical Nutrition,* 90(5), 1272-1279. doi:10.3945/ajcn.2009.28013

Wall, R., Ross, R. P., Fitzgerald, G. F., & Stanton, C. (2010). Fatty acids from fish: The anti-inflammatory potential of long-chain omega-3 fatty acids. *Nutrition Reviews, 68*(5), 280-289. doi:10.1111/j.1753-4887.2010.00287.x

Yalcin, H., & Unal, M. K. (2010). The enrichment of hen eggs with omega-3 fatty acids. *Journal of Medicinal Food, 13*(3), 610-614. doi:10.1089/jmf.2008.0024

REVIEWER(S)

Darlene Strayer, RN, MBA, Cinahl Information Systems, Glendale, CA

Nursing Executive Practice Council, Glendale Adventist Medical Center, Glendale, CA

Red Meat

WHAT WE KNOW

Red meat is defined as beef, veal, pork, or lamb from fresh, minced, or frozen sources. It is rich in protein, vitamins D and B12, zinc, iron, selenium, and omega-3 fatty acid, but it is also a significant source of saturated fat and cholesterol.

- Diets that are high in saturated fat and cholesterol have been definitively linked to coronary artery disease (CAD), obesity, and cancer.
- Overweight and obese individuals are at greater risk for cancers of the breast, colon, endometrium, gallbladder, esophagus, pancreas, and kidney.
- It is recommended that total dietary fat be limited to 30% and saturated fat to 10% of total caloric intake.
- Because red meat has nutritional risk as well as benefit, its inclusion in the diet should be limited. Leaner red meats should be chosen and their intake alternated with other sources of protein (e.g., fish, chicken, beans, and whole grains) that are lower in saturated fat and cholesterol.

NUTRIENTS IN RED MEAT

- Red meat is a valuable source of highly bioavailable (i.e., ready for the body to use) protein containing all 9 essential amino acids (i.e., amino acids that are not produced by the body). Protein is present in every cell in the human body and is vital to the development and maintenance of muscles, organs, and glands. Other important actions of protein include:

—Providing oxygen to the blood (hemoglobin)
—Aiding in the formation of antibodies necessary for fighting infection
—Contributing to the production of enzymes and hormones

- Red meat is a significant source of fat, including unsaturated omega-3 fatty acids. Fat is an essential macronutrient that provides large amounts of energy to the body. One gram of fat contains 9 calories, which is double the calories contained in 1 gm of carbohydrate or protein.
  —Physiologic functions of fat include:
    –Storing excess calories
    –Insulating the body
    –Assisting in the absorption of vitamins A, D, E, and K
    –Contributing to blood clotting
  —Fat is vital for brain development
  —Omega-3 fatty acids exhibit hypotensive (i.e., blood pressure lowering) properties and anti-inflammatory activity, which help to improve lung function and prevent cardiovascular disease (CVD), arthritis, and other chronic diseases associated with inflammation.
  —Saturated fat in red meat is responsible for raising levels of low-density lipoproteins (LDLs). When LDL levels increase beyond normal levels, cholesterol accumulates in the arteries, forming plaque. Plaque buildup results in atherosclerosis and CAD, the leading cause of mortality in the United States and other developed countries.

- Red meat provides fat-soluble vitamins, including vitamin D, which is necessary for maintaining normal blood levels of calcium and phosphorus. The functions of vitamin D include:
  —Supporting the absorption of calcium
  —Contributing to the formation and maintenance of bones

- Red meat is a good source of vitamin B12, or cobalamin, a cobalt-containing B-complex vitamin. Vitamin B12 plays a major role in lipid, carbohydrate, and protein metabolism.
  —Vitamin B12 is required for the production of hormones, lipids, and proteins.
  —By aiding in the synthesis of neurotransmitters, it contributes to nervous system function.
  —It is required for red blood cell and hemoglobin formation.

—It plays a significant role in deoxyribonucleic acid (DNA) and ribonucleic acid (RNA) synthesis.

- Red meat is rich in minerals, including zinc, iron, phosphorous, and selenium.
  —Zinc is an essential trace element that supports immune system function and wound healing and is essential for maintaining vision and the senses of smell and taste. Other functions of zinc include:
    –Maintaining endothelial cell membranes
    –Activation of approximately 100 different enzymes
    –Promoting wound healing
    –Assisting with protein and DNA synthesis and cell division
  —Iron is vital for the synthesis of red blood cells and hemoglobin, which are necessary for cellular respiration and the transport of oxygen to the tissues. Iron also supports immune function, is vital for cognitive development, contributes to energy metabolism, and regulates temperature.
  —Phosphorus, combined with calcium, promotes the formation of bones and teeth, muscle contraction, and nerve conduction and is essential for the structural integrity of cell membranes.
  —Selenium is an essential trace mineral that combines with proteins to create selenoproteins, which are important antioxidant enzymes that protect cells from the damaging effects of free radicals (i.e., reactive byproducts of oxygen metabolism). Other contributions of selenium include:
- Regulation of thyroid function
- Supporting immune system function

RECOMMENDED DIETARY INTAKE

Diets that are high in red meat tend to be high in fat and cholesterol and are associated with CAD, obesity, and cancer.

- Individuals who are overweight or obese are at an increased risk for CAD.
- Signs and symptoms of CAD include:
  —Angina, a chest pain, pressure, or tightness caused by reduced blood flow to areas of the heart
  —Shortness of breath, fatigue, and/or weakness
  —A cardiac event, including sudden cardiac death or myocardial infarction

- Individuals who are overweight and have been diagnosed with hypertension, diabetes, heart disease, liver or kidney disease, or intestinal disorders should be screened regularly for cancer.
- To reduce the risk of CAD, obesity, and cancer, it is recommended that red meat intake be minimized and replaced with lean protein options, including:
  —Plant-based proteins (e.g., beans, lentils, edamame, nuts, tempeh)
  —Fish and other seafood, particularly fish that is high in omega-3 fatty acids (e.g., albacore tuna, herring, mackerel, rainbow trout, sardines, and salmon)
  —Chicken and other poultry, prepared skinless to reduce saturated fat and cholesterol content
  —Low-fat dairy and eggs

Although it is important to limit intake of saturated fat and cholesterol, it is also important not to replace a diet high in saturated fat and cholesterol with one high in simple carbohydrates. Diets high in simple carbohydrates are associated with dyslipidemia and diabetes. A balanced diet should include unsaturated fats, lean proteins, complex carbohydrates, fruits, and vegetables.

RESEARCH FINDINGS

Red meats and saturated fats are linked to increased risk for CAD. A 10% reduction in LDL cholesterol levels could potentially save the lives of about 3,000 persons who die each year as a result of CAD and stroke.

There is also an association between red meat consumption and an increased risk of colorectal, lung, esophageal, stomach, pancreatic, prostate, and endometrial cancers.

- The exact cause for the increased cancer risk is not completely understood, but researchers believe that the saturated fat and cholesterol content of red meat is at least partly responsible. According to the American Institute for Cancer Research (AICR), more than 100,000 cases of cancer in the U.S. each year are associated with excess body fat, including 49% of endometrial cancers, 35% of esophageal cancers, 28% of pancreatic cancers, 24% of kidney cancers, 21% of gallbladder cancers, 17% of breast cancers, and 9% of colorectal cancers. Patients should be educated that trimming fat from meat and grilling meat instead of frying it can reduce the amount of fat consumed.

- The cooking method used for red meat plays a significant role in cancer risk. Cooking red meats at high temperatures by frying or broiling results in the formation of heterocyclic amines (HCAs), which are known to be carcinogenic.

SUMMARY

Consumers should become knowledgeable about the physiologic effects of red meat consumption. Red meat is rich in protein, vitamins D and B12, zinc, iron, selenium, and omega-3 fatty acid. These nutrients promote muscle, bone and organ development, support healthy immune and nervous systems, maintain thyroid function, facilitate wound healing and inhibit chronic disease. Red meat is also a significant source of saturated fat and cholesterol. Based on an individual's health and diet history, the quantity and type of red meat commonly consumed may increase risk of developing heart disease, obesity, diabetes and cancer. It is important to eat a well-balanced diet that includes appropriate fats and lean meat options along with fruits, vegetables, and complex carbohydrates.

—*Cherie Marcel, BS*

REFERENCES

Alexander, D. D., Cushing, C. A., Lowe, K. A., Sceurman, B., & Roberts, M. A. (2009). Meta-analysis of animal fat or animal protein intake and colorectal cancer. *American Journal of Clinical Nutrition*, 89(5), 1402-1409. doi:10.3945/ajcn.2008.26838

American Diabetes Association. (2014, August 26). Protein Foods. Retrieved May 7, 2015, from http://www.diabetes.org/food-and-fitness/food/what-can-i-eat/making-healthy-food-choices/meat-and-plant-based-protein.html

American Heart Association. (2014). Good vs. bad cholesterol. Retrieved May 7, 2015, from http://www.heart.org/HEARTORG/Conditions/Cholesterol/AboutCholesterol/Good-vs-Bad-Cholesterol_UCM_305561_Article.jsp

(2015). Diet and cancer. In C.A. Lutz & K.R. Przytulski (Eds.), *Nutrition & diet therapy* (6th ed., pp. 447-451). Philadelphia, PA: F. A. Davis Company.

Editorial staff of the National Cancer Institute at the National Institutes of Health. (2012). Obesity and cancer risk. *American Cancer Society*. Retrieved May 7, 2015, from http://www.cancer.gov/cancertopics/causes-prevention/risk/obesity/obesity-fact-sheet

German, J. B., & Dillard, C. J. (2004). Saturated fats: What dietary intake? *American Journal of Clinical Nutrition*, 80(3), 550-559.

Gilsing, A. M., Weijenberg, M. P., Goldbohm, R. A., den Brandt, P. A., & Schouten, L. J. (2011). Consumption of dietary fat and meat and risk of ovarian cancer in the Netherlands Cohort Study. *American Journal of Clinical Nutrition*, 93(1), 118-126. doi:10.3945/ajcn.2010.29888

Givens, D. I. (2010). Milk and meat in our diet: Good or bad for health?. *Animal: An International Journal of Animal Bioscience*, 4(12), 1941-1952.

Huxley, R., Clifton, P., Perkovic, V., Woodward, M., & Neal, B. (2009). How many Australian deaths from heart disease and stroke could be avoided by a small reduction in population cholesterol levels? *Nutrition & Dietetics*, 66(3), 158-163. doi:10.1111/j.1747-0080.2009.01360.x

Lophatananon, A., Archer, J., Easton, D., Pocock, R., Dearnaley, D., Guy, M., & Rahman, A. A. (2010). Dietary fat and early-onset prostate cancer risk. *British Journal of Nutrition*, 103(9), 1375-1380. doi:10.1017/S0007114509993291

Ruxton, C. (2011). The role of red meat in a balanced diet. *Nursing Standard*, 26(7), 41-49.

Sieri, S., Krogh, V., Ferrari, P., Berrino, F., Pala, V., Thiebut, A. C. M., ... Riboli, E. (2008). Dietary fat and breast cancer risk in the European Prospective Investigation into Cancer and Nutrition. *American Journal of Clinical Nutrition*, 88(5), 1304-1312. doi:10.3945/ajcn.2008.26090

Thiebaut, A. C., Jiao, L., Silverman, D. T., Cross, A. J., Thompson, F. E., Subar, A. F., & Stolzenberg, R. Z. (2009). Dietary fatty acids and pancreatic cancer in the NIH-AARP diet and health study. *JNCI: Journal of the National Cancer Institute*, 101(14), 1001-1011. doi:jnci/djp168

Tran, N., & Barraj, L. (2010). Contribution of specific dietary factors to CHD in US females. *Public Health Nutrition*, 13(2), 154-162. doi:10.1017/S1368980009990693

Warnica, J. W. (2013, September). Overview of coronary artery disease. *Merck manual for health care professionals*. Retrieved May 7, 2015, from http://www.merckmanuals.com/professional/sec07/ch073/ch073a.html

Wyness, L, Weichselbaum, E., O' Connor, A., Williams, E. B., Benelam, B., Riley, H., & Stanner, S. (2011). Red meat in the diet: An update.

Nutrition Bulletin, 36(1), 34-77. Retrieved from ,
doi:10.1111/j.1467-3010.2010.01871.x

REVIEWER(S)
Darlene Strayer, RN, MBA, Cinahl Information Systems,
    Glendale, CA
Nursing Executive Practice Council, Glendale Adventist
    Medical Center, Glendale, CA

Walnuts

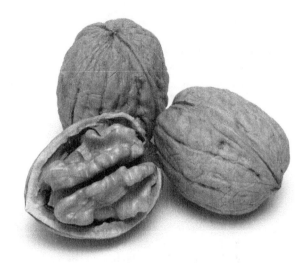

WHAT WE KNOW

Walnuts are a type of tree nut; other examples of tree
nuts are almonds and pecans. There are many species
of walnut trees, but the 3 most common are the *Juglans
regia*, which produces the English (or Persian) walnut;
the *Juglans nigra*, the producer of the black walnut; and
Juglans cinerea, the producer of the white walnut (also
called the butternut walnut). The walnut kernel (i.e., the
edible part of the walnut) has a bumpy texture that is set
into 2 lobes, covered in a thin skin, and encased in a hard,
brown, round or oblong shell. The meat of the walnut has
a subtle nutty flavor and a smooth, fatty consistency. Walnut kernels can be eaten out of hand, chopped and added
as a topping to salads, desserts, or entrees, or crushed and
blended into main dishes as a meat alternative.

- The skin of the walnut contains 90% of its phenolic compounds (i.e., beneficial plant-derived
  chemicals), including phenolic acids, tannins, flavonoids, and phytosterols, which are substances
  that are known to reduce cholesterol absorption
  from the gut. Walnuts are also a great source of
  protein, fiber, unsaturated fats, and nutrients
  such as copper, manganese, molybdenum, biotin,
  and vitamin E (in the form of gamma-tocopherol). Additional benefits attributed to walnuts
  include an association with reduced triglycerides,
  elevated high-density lipoprotein (HDL) cholesterol, reduced inflammation, and decreased risk
  of cardiovascular disease (CVD) and diabetes
  mellitus, type 2 (DM2).
- Contrary to the common belief that nuts are fattening, evidence supports the inclusion of nuts
  in weight-loss diet plans because nuts enhance
  satiety (i.e., a sense of fullness) and reduce appetite. Nuts are associated with greater dietary satisfaction and more efficient weight loss in dieters.

- Many persons are allergic to walnuts and other
  nuts. Because of this, it is recommended that
  nuts be cautiously introduced in the diets of
  young children after the age of 12 months, or 3
  years of age in children who have a strong family
  history of food allergy.

NUTRIENTS IN WALNUTS

- Walnuts are a great source of protein, fiber, and
  unsaturated fats (e.g., the omega-3 fatty acid
  alpha-linolenic acid).
  —Protein is present in every cell in the human
    body and is vital to the development and
    maintenance of skin, muscles, organs, and
    glands.
  —Dietary fiber makes many contributions to pre-
    ventive health, including reducing cholesterol
    levels and maintaining colon health.
  —Alpha-linolenic acid exhibits hypotensive (i.e.,
    blood pressure lowering) properties and anti-
    inflammatory activity, which helps to improve
    lung function and prevent cardiovascular dis-
    ease, arthritis, and other chronic diseases as-
    sociated with inflammation.
- Walnuts contain the B-complex vitamin biotin,
  which functions as a coenzyme for carboxylases, enzymes required for the metabolism of
  fatty acids and gluconeogenesis (i.e., the conversion of protein and fat into glucose). Biotin
  also plays a role in the formation of purines,
  which are vital elements in DNA and RNA. The

health of skin, hair, and nails is also attributed to biotin.

- Walnuts contain a variety of minerals, including copper, manganese, and molybdenum.
  - Copper is an important component of the antioxidant enzyme superoxide dismutase (SOD). Copper contributes to the action of lysyl oxidase, an enzyme necessary for the cross-linkingof collagen and elastin, which allows flexibility in the blood vessels, bones, and joints. Copper enhances the body's ability to use iron, preventing iron-deficiency anemia, ruptured vessels, irregular heartbeat, and infection.
  - Manganese is a trace mineral that is involved in a number of physiologic processes, including energy production, fatty acid synthesis, cholesterol production, and protection against the damage caused by free radicals.
  - Molybdenum is a cofactor for at least 3 enzymes—aldehyde oxidase, xanthine oxidase, and sulfite oxidase—which are necessary for the breakdown of sulfur-containing amino acids and purines.
- Walnuts are a good source of gamma-tocopherol, a form of vitamin E that exhibits significant heart-healthy actions.
- The skin of walnuts contains many phytonutrients, including phenolic acids, tannins, and flavonoids, which are powerful antioxidants.

DIETARY INTAKE GUIDELINES

- Although there is no standardized recommendation for the dosage of walnuts or other nuts, consumption of a small handful of nuts 3–5times per week is associated with a 30–50% reduction in the risk of heart disease.
- The U.S. FDA recommends the consumption of .36 grams of protein per pound of body weight each day. There are 3 grams of protein per ¼ cup of ground walnuts.
- Along with other tree nuts, walnuts pose high risk as a food allergen. Because of this, it is recommended that walnuts not be added to a child's diet until after 12 months of age or 3 years of age in children with a strong family history of food allergies.
  - Signs and symptoms of walnut allergy include the following:
    - Coughing and wheezing

- Tingling in the mouth
- Tightening of the throat and swelling of the tongue
- Difficulty breathing
- Dizziness or loss of consciousness
- Abdominal pain
- Nausea, vomiting, and diarrhea
- Nasal congestion
- Skin rashes, hives, and eczema
- Migraine headache

- Risk factors for walnut allergy include the following:
  - Family history of food allergies
  - Having other allergies (35% of children with eczema have associated food allergies)
  - Introduction of solid foods before 4 months of age
- Individuals with walnut allergies who are at increased risk for fatal anaphylactic shock include the following:
  - Adolescents and young adults
  - Persons with asthma
  - Those who do not have epinephrine available when the allergic reaction occurs
- Complete avoidance of walnuts is the only effective prevention strategy for allergic reactions.
  - Affected persons should be educated regarding terminology that identifies hidden food allergens, the importance of reading food labels, and what questions to ask when eating at restaurants.
  - Food for a person with food allergies must be prepared separately from food containing walnuts to prevent cross-contamination.
  - Over time, gradual allergen inclusion can be attempted. This can be done by introducing very small amounts of allergens through oral feeding in controlled environments (e.g., medical practitioner's office) where immediate treatment can be provided.
- Medications are used to treat allergic reactions after known exposure has occurred and/or a reaction develops.
  - Antihistamines or bronchodilators can help to alleviate minor signs and symptoms but do not abort systemic reactions.
  - Intramuscular epinephrine injection is necessary for severe reactions or anaphylactic reactions. Self-injectable epinephrine should

be provided to individuals who are at high risk for anaphylaxis.

–Schools should have a written action plan for providing treatment of an allergic reaction in all students with food allergies.

RESEARCH FINDINGS

Researchers who studied the association between walnut consumption and incidence of DM2 by conducting 2 large cohort studies, each spanning 10-year timeframe, found that walnut consumption is significantly inversely associated with DM2 risk.

Investigators conducting studies using mouse models have found that walnut consumption is associated with the suppression of angiogenesis and the inhibition colorectal cancer growth, as well as a reduction of prostate tumor size and growth and reduced breast cancer risk.

SUMMARY

Consumers should become knowledgeable about the physiologic effects of consuming walnuts. Walnuts can be beneficial to health because they contain a high amount of protein, omega-3 fatty acids, numerous vitamins and minerals, and phytonutrients. These nutrients are associated with reduced risk of developing iron-deficiency anemia, obesity, heart disease, type 2 diabetes and cancer. Individuals should be aware of the potential for having an allergic reaction to walnuts.

—*Cherie Marcel, BS*

REFERENCES

Cook, A. (2013). Walnut consumption and type 2 diabetes risk: The importance of associations. *Integrative Medicine Alert, 16*(5), 52-54.

Davis, P. A., Vasu, V. T., Gohil, K., Kim, H., Khan, I. H., Cross, C. E., & Yokoyama, W. (2012). A high-fat diet containing whole walnuts (Juglans regia) reduces tumour size and growth along with plasma insulin-like growth factor 1 in the transgenic adenocarcinoma of the mouse prostate model. *British Journal of Nutrition, 108*(10), 1764-1772. doi:10.1017/S0007114511007288

Frazier, A. L., Camargo, C. A., Malspeis, S., Willett, W. C., & Young, M. C. (2014). Prospective study of peripregnancy consumption of peanuts or tree nuts by mothers and the risk of peanut or tree nut allergy in their offspring. *JAMA Pediatrics, 168*(2), 156-162. doi:10.1001/jamapediatrics.2013.4139

Heuvel, J. P., Belda, B. J., Hannon, D. B., Kris-Etherton, P. M., Grieger, J. A., Zhang, J., & Thompson, J. T. (2012). Mechanistic examination of walnuts in prevention of breast cancer. *Nutrition & Cancer, 64*(7), 1078-1086. doi:10.1080/0163558 1.2012.717679

King, J. C., Blumberg, J., Ingwersen, L., Jenab, M., & Tucker, K. L. (2008). Tree nuts and peanuts as components of a healthy diet. *Journal of Nutrition, 138*(9), 1736S-1740S.

Mangels, R. (2013). Scientific update. No need to avoid peanuts or tree nuts in pregnancy. *Vegetarian Journal, 32*(2), 26-27.

Mattes, R. D., Kris-Etherton, P. M., & Foster, G. D. (2008). Impact of peanut and tree nuts on body weight and healthy weight loss in adults. *Journal of Nutrition, 138*(9), 1741S-1745S.

Nagel, J. M., Brinkoetter, M., Magkos, F., Liu, X., Chamberland, J. P., Shah, S., ... Mantzoros, C. S. (2012). Dietary walnuts inhibit colorectal cancer growth in mice by suppressing angiogenesis. *Nutrition, 28*(1), 67-75. doi:10.1016/j.nut.2011.03.004

Nappo-Dattoma, L. (2011). Updated dietary standards: The 2010 Dietary Guidelines for Americans, MyPlate and other nutrition education resources for the oral health professional. *Access, 25*(8), 16-19.

Pan, A., Sun, Q., Manson, J. E., Willett, W. C., & Hu, F. B. (2013). Walnut consumption is associated with lower risk of type 3 diabetes in women. *Journal of Nutrition, 143*(4), 512-518. doi:10.3945/jn.112.172171

Schoessler, S. Z. (2005). The perils of peanuts: Creating a safe environment for the student who is allergic to peanuts and peanut products. *School Nurse News, 22*(4), 22-26.

Weber, R. W. (2012). Allergen of the month – English walnut. *Annals of Allergy, Asthma & Immunology, 109*(3), A13. doi:10.1016/j.anai.2012.07.018

The world's healthiest foods: Walnuts. (n.d.). *The George Mateljan Foundation editorial team*. Retrieved June 4, 2015, from http://www.whfoods.com/genpage.php?tname=foodspice&dbid=99

REVIEWER(S)

Darlene Strayer, RN, MBA, Cinahl Information Systems, Glendale, CA

Nursing Executive Practice Council, Glendale Adventist Medical Center, Glendale, CA

Whey

WHAT WE KNOW

Whey and casein are the two major protein components of cow's milk. Whey is found in the watery portion of cow's milk, and casein is in the curd. Because whey contains all of the essential amino acids, it is considered to be a highly bioavailable, or complete, protein. This characteristic has led to its use as the base of protein shakes, sports drinks, and infant formulas. Whey is a highly digestible protein, and it is a common component of dietary supplements designed to improve muscle strength, prevent heart disease, assist with diabetes control, and prevent age-related bone loss. Although it has proven to be a useful protein supplement, whey is not tolerated by everyone. Some persons have allergies to cow's milk, causing them to experience adverse reactions (e.g., congestion, rash, indigestion, vomiting) to whey consumption.

NUTRIENTS IN WHEY

- Essential amino acids are amino acids that cannot be synthesized by the body and must be consumed. Whey contains all of the essential amino acids, which makes it a complete protein. Protein is present in every cell of the human body and is vital to the development and maintenance of skin, muscles, organs, and glands. Other important actions of protein include the following:
  —Provides oxygen to the blood
  —Necessary to the formation of antibodies to fight infections
  —Contributes to the production of enzymes and hormones

SOURCE(S) OF WHEY

Whey is found in cow's milk products and is added to many sports drinks, infant formulas, dietary supplements, and baked goods.

DIETARY INTAKE GUIDELINES

- Although there are no specific recommendations for daily intake of whey in the literature, the American Heart Association (AHA) dietary and lifestyle recommendations regarding the consumption of cow's milk include the following:
- Choose dairy products that are fat-free (also called skim), 1% fat, and low-fat.

- Ingest at least 1,200 mg of calcium each day to reduce risk for osteoporosis and CVD; good calcium sources are dairy products, fish with bones, broccoli, and legumes.
- According to the Institute of Medicine (IOM), protein should constitute no less than 10%, and up to 35%, of daily calorie consumption.
- Risk for Cow's Milk Protein Allergy (CMPA):
  —Cow's milk is identified as one of the 8 major food allergens in the U.S. in addition to peanuts, tree nuts, wheat, shellfish, soy, eggs, and fish. Those at risk for CMPA include:
  —infants and children under the age of 3 years
  —individuals with a family history of atopy (e.g., asthma, eczema, hay fever, food allergies)
- Signs and symptoms of CMPA include the following:
  —Colic
  —Diarrhea
  —Vomiting
  —Gastrointestinal (GI) bleeding
  —GI reflux
  —Chronic constipation
  —Sleeplessness
  —Wheezing
  —Sinus congestion
  —Bronchitis
  —Asthma
  —Sneezing
  —Coughing
  —Eczema
  —Anaphylaxis
  —Failure to thrive (FTT)

Treatment for CMPA is removal of cow's milk and all sources of cow's milk protein from the diet.

RESEARCH FINDINGS

- Researchers report that inclusion of whey in the treatment and management of diabetes and obesity can improve blood glucose control, plasma lipid profiles, and hepatic steatosis, and reduce risk for cardiovascular disease (CVD).
- Results of studies indicate that supplementation with whey protein can improve exercise tolerance, prevent age-related muscle wasting, and reduce inflammation.

SUMMARY

Consumers should become knowledgeable about the physiologic effects of consuming whey. Whey contains all of the essential amino acids, which makes it a complete protein. This rich protein source helps with the development and maintenance of skin, muscles, organs, and glands, provides oxygen to blood, helps fight infections and assists in the production of enzymes and hormones. Individuals with allergies to cow's milk, causing them to experience adverse reactions (e.g., congestion, rash, indigestion, vomiting) should avoid whey consumption.

—*Cherie Marcel, BS*

REFERENCES

Akhavan, T., Luhovyy, B. L., Brown, P. H., Cho, C. E., & Anderson, G. H. (2010). Effect of premeal consumption of whey protein and its hydrolysate on food intake and postmeal glycemia and insulin responses in young adults. *The American Journal of Clinical Nutriton*, *91*(4), 966-975. doi:10.3945/ajcn.2009.28406

Bortolotti, M., Maiolo, E., Corazza, M., Van Dijke, E., Schneiter, P., Boss, A., ... Tappy, L. (2011). Effects of a whey protein supplementation on intrahepatocellular lipids in obese female patients. *Clinical Nutrition (Edinburgh, Scotland)*, *30*(4), 494-498. doi:10.1016/j.clnu.2011.01.006

Coleman, E. (2011). Is whey healthy?. *Livestrong.com*. June 14, 2013,

Food and Nutrition Board, Institute of Medicine, National Academies. (n.d.). Dietary Reference Intakes (DRIs): Estimated Average Requirements. Food and Nutrition Board, Institute of Medicine, National Academies. Retrieved March 24, 2015, from http://iom.edu/Activities/Nutrition/SummaryDRIs/~/media/Files/Activity%20 Files/Nutrition/DRIs/New %20Material/5DRI%20 Values%20SummaryTables%2014.pdf

Gouni-Berthold, I., Schulte, D. M., Krone, W., Lapointe, J., Lemieux, P., Predel, H., & Berthold, H. K. (2012). The whey fermentation product malleable protein matrix decreases TAG concentrations in patients with metabolic syndrome: A randomized placebo-controlled trial. *British Journal of Nutrition*, *107*(11), 1694-1706. doi:10.1017/ S0007114511004843

Lichtenstein, A. H., Appel, L. J., Brands, M., Carnethon, M., Daniels, S., Franch, H. A., ... Wylie-Rosett, J. (2006). Summary of American Heart Association Diet and Lifestyle Recommendations revision 2006. *Arteriosclerosis, Thrombosis, and Vascular Biology*, *26*(10), 2186-2191. doi:10.1161/01. ATV.0000238352.25222.5e

Magne, H., Savary-Auzeloux, I., Migne, C., Peyron, M. A., Combaret, L., Remond, D., & Dardevet, D. (2012). Contrarily to whey and high protein diets, dietary free leucine supplementation cannot reverse the lack of recovery of muscle mass after prolonged immobilization during aging. *The Journal of Physiology*, *590*(Pt. 8), 2035-2049. doi:10.1113/jphysiol.2011.226266

Mayo Clinic editorial staff. (2013, November 1). Whey protein. *MayoClinic.com*. Retrieved March 17, 2015, from http://www.mayoclinic.org/drugs-supplements/ whey-protein/background/hrb-20060532

Sugawara, K., Takahashi, H., Kashiwagura, T., Yamada, K., Yanagida, S., Homma, M., ... Shioya, T. (2012). Effect of anti-inflammatory supplementation with whey peptide and exercise therapy in patients with COPD. *Respiratory Medicine*, *106*(11), 1526-1534. doi:10.1016/j.rmed.2012.07.001

Yang, Y., Breen, L., Burd, N. A., Hector, A. J., Churchward-Venne, T. A., Josse, A. R., ... Phillips, S. M. (2012). Resistance exercise enhances myofibrillar protein synthesis with graded intakes of whey protein in older men. *The British Journal of Nutrition*, *108*(10), 1780-1788. doi:10.1017/S0007114511007422

REVIEWER(S)

Darlene Strayer, RN, MBA, Cinahl Information Systems, Glendale, CA

Nursing Executive Practice Council, Glendale Adventist Medical Center, Glendale, CA

DAIRY

Cheese

WHAT WE KNOW

Cheese is a product of milk that has been fermented and aged. The process of fermentation transforms lactose, or milk sugar, into lactic acid and results in the varying degrees of textural thickening noted in cheese; depending on the type of cheese, the texture ranges from creamy to firm. Consuming 2–3 servings of dairy products each day is recommended to maintain a healthy heart and strong bones and muscles. Because cheese is made from milk and retains the calcium found in milk, cheese is a dairy product and is considered to be part of the dairy group. For decades the health benefits of cheese have been in question due to its typically high content of saturated fat, cholesterol, and sodium; however, recent studies indicate that cheese provides numerous health benefits. Cheese is a good source of calcium, phosphorus, vitamins A and D, and protein. When eaten in moderation, as part of a healthy diet, cheese contributes to strong bones and teeth, good vision, and normal function of the nervous and immune systems.

NUTRIENTS IN CHEESE

- Biologic functions of nutrients found in cheese include the following:
  - —Calcium builds and maintains bones and teeth, regulates muscle contraction, conducts nerve impulses, activates enzymes for energy production and muscle contraction, participates in blood clotting, assists with vitamin B12 absorption, and maintains the structural integrity of intracellular membranes.
  - —Phosphorous combined with calcium is important for the formation of bones and teeth, muscle contraction, and nerve conduction; phosphorous is essential for the structural integrity of cell membranes.
  - —Cheese is a source of highly bio-available protein, meaning it contains all nine essential amino acids (i.e., amino acids that are not produced by the body). Protein is present in every cell of the human body and is vital to the development and maintenance of skin, muscles, organs, and glands. Other important actions of protein include the following:
    - –Provides oxygen to the blood
    - –Important in the formation of antibodies for fighting infection
  - —Contributes to the production of enzymes and hormones
  - —Cheese contains fat. One gram of fat contains 9 calories, which is double that of carbohydrate or protein, making the fat in cheese a significant source of energy. Other vital functions of fat include the following:
    - –Stores excess calories
    - –Insulates the body
    - –Assists in the absorption of vitamins A, D, E, and K
    - –Controls inflammation
    - –Contributes to blood clotting
    - –Vital for brain development
    - –Promotes satiety (i.e., feeling of fullness)
  - —Cheese is a significant source of cholesterol, a waxy substance that is a vital part of cell membranes. Functions of cholesterol include the following:
    - –Contributes to the production of vitamin D and bile acids
    - –Used to make steroid hormones (e.g., estrogen, testosterone, aldosterone, cortisol)
    - –A vital component of cell membranes, that allows for adequate permeability
    - –Assists in the absorption of fat, and the fat-soluble vitamins A, D, E, and K
    - –Contributes to nerve impulse conduction

DIETARY INTAKE GUIDELINES

- As a dairy product, cheese is classified as a major food allergen along with wheat, eggs, shellfish, tree nuts, peanuts, and soy.

- Some individuals have an intolerance to lactose that is usually due to a deficiency in the enzyme lactase, which is required to metabolize (i.e., breakdown) lactose. Consumption of dairy products in these individuals can result in uncomfortable abdominal manifestations of cramping, diarrhea, and gas. The fermenting and aging process of cheese breaks down a significant amount of the lactose into lactic acid; because lactic acid does not require lactase for absorption, cheese is more tolerable to consume than milk for many persons with lactose intolerance. The lactose content of cheese lessens as it ages and hardens. In general, cheese should be aged at least 90 days to be considered lactose-free
  —Hard-ripened cheeses that are lower in lactose include the following:
    –Blue
    –Brick
    –Brie
    –Camembert
    –Cheddar
    –Colby
    –Edam
    –Gouda
    –Monterey
    –Muenster
    –Parmesan
    –Provolone
    –Swiss
  —Soft cheeses contain more lactose than hard cheeses, but contain less lactose than milk. These cheeses include the following:
    –Cream cheese
    –Neufchatel
    –Ricotta
    –Mozzarella
    –Cottage cheese
- Cheese contains saturated fat and cholesterol. Saturated fat is responsible for raising levels of low-density lipoproteins (LDLs; called "bad cholesterol"). When the body is supplied with more LDL than it needs, cholesterol begins to accumulate in the arteries and forms plaque. Plaque narrows the arteries and impedes blood flow, which leads to atherosclerosis and, ultimately, to coronary artery disease (CAD); which is the leading cause of mortality in the United States and other developed countries. A diet high in fat and cholesterol is also associated with obesity and cancer.
  —Signs and symptoms of CAD include the following:
    –Angina (i.e., chest pain)
    –Shortness of breath, fatigue, and/or weakness
    –A cardiac event, including sudden cardiac death
  —Recommended intake of fat and cholesterol
  —It is currently recommended that dietary fat intake should be limited as follows:
    –Total dietary fat < 30% of total caloric intake but not < 20%
    –Saturated fat < 10% of total caloric intake
    –Trans fat < 1 % of total caloric intake. Trans fats are produced during the process of hydrogenation (i.e., adding hydrogen to unsaturated fat to change it from a liquid to a solid). Trans fats increase the risk for CAD and have exhibited carcinogenic (i.e., cancer causing) properties.
    –Total cholesterol less < 200 mg of cholesterol per day

RESEARCH FINDINGS
- Cheese is a significant source of saturated fat and cholesterol, which have been associated with CAD; however, recent research findings indicate that cheese consumption is associated with lower triglycerides and increased high-density lipoproteins (HDLs; called "good cholesterol") in the blood.
- Further study revealed that cheese intake is significantly linked to a lower risk for developing metabolic syndrome (i.e., a cluster of pre-diabetic risk factors, including abdominal obesity, hyperglycemia, hypertension, and dyslipidemia).
- Researchers were able to determine that cheese appears to contain inhibitors of desaturases (i.e., components that inhibit fatty acid desaturation), preventing the formation of triglycerides, cholesterol esters, and phospholipids.
- Further study is necessary to identify the desaturase inhibitors in cheese and analyze their potential health benefits.

SUMMARY

Consumers should become knowledgeable about the risks and benefits of cheese consumption. Cheese is a good source of calcium, phosphorus, vitamins A and D, and protein. When cheese is included as part of a healthy diet, it contributes to strong bones and teeth, good vision, and normal function of the nervous and immune systems. Research suggests that cheese consumption may help reduce risk for CAD, cancer, DM2, and stroke. Individuals should be aware that as a dairy product, cheese, is classified as a major food allergen along with wheat, eggs, shellfish, tree nuts, peanuts, and soy. Individuals with lactose intolerance may need to avoid most cheese, especially soft cheese.

—Cherie Marcel, BS

REFERENCES

American Heart Association. (2015, January 12). Good vs. bad cholesterol. Retrieved February 27, 2015, from http://www.heart.org/HEARTORG/Conditions/Cholesterol/AboutCholesterol/Good-vs-Bad-Cholesterol_UCM_305561_Article.jsp

Dugdale, D. C., Chen, M. A., & Zieve, D. (2014, August 12). Coronary heart disease. *Medline Plus*. Retrieved February 27, 2015, from http://www.nlm.nih.gov/medlineplus/ ency/article/007115.htm

Hjerpsted, J., Leedo, E., & Tholstrup, T. (2011). Cheese intake in large amounts lowers LDL-cholesterol concentrations compared with butter intake of equal fat content. *American Journal of Clinical Nutrition*, 94(6), 1479-1484. doi:10.3945/ajcn.111.022426

Høstmark, A. T., & Lunde, M. S. H. (2012). Cheese can reduce indexes that estimate fatty acid desaturation. Results from the Oslo Health Study and from experiments with human hepatoma cells. *Applied Physiology, Nutrition & Metabolism*, 37(1), 31-39. doi:10.1139/h11-123

Høstmark, A. T., & Tomten, S. E. (2011). The Oslo Health Study: Cheese intake was negatively associated with the metabolic syndrome. *Journal of the American College of Nutrition*, 30(3), 182-190.

Lichtenstein, A. H., Appel, L. J., Brands, M., Carnethon, M., Daniels, S., Franch, H. A., ... Wylie-Rosett, J. (2006). Summary of American Heart Association Diet and Lifestyle Recommendations revision 2006. *Arteriosclerosis, Thrombosis, and Vascular Biology*, 26(10), 2186-2191. doi:10.1161/01.ATV.0000238352.25222.5e

Lutz, C. A., & Przytulski, K. R. (2011). Digestion, absorption, metabolism, and excretion. In *Nutrition & diet therapy* (5th ed., p. 172). Philadelphia, PA: F. A. Davis.

McAllister, C. (2011). Nutritional facts and analysis for cheese. *Livestrong.com*. Retrieved February 27, 2015, from http://www.livestrong.com/article/526222-nutritional-facts-and-analyses-for-cheese/

Roth, S. L. (2011). Diseases of the heart, blood vessels, and lungs. In E. D. Schlenker & S. L. Roth (Eds.), *Williams' essentials of nutrition and diet therapy* (10th ed., pp. 472, 480). St. Louis, MO: Elsevier Mosby.

Taylor, D. (2012). Are milk, cheese & yogurt equally healthy. *Livestrong.com*. Retrieved February 27, 2015, from http://www.livestrong.com/article/557497-are-milk-cheese-yogurt-equally-healthy/

Warnica, J. W. (2013, September). Overview of coronary artery disease. *Merck Manual*. Retrieved February 27, 2015, from http://www.merckmanuals.com/professional/ cardiovascular_disorders/coronary_artery_disease/overview_of_coronary_artery_disease.html

REVIEWER(S)

Darlene Strayer, RN, MBA, Cinahl Information Systems, Glendale, CA

Nursing Executive Practice Council, Glendale Adventist Medical Center, Glendale, CA

Milk

WHAT WE KNOW

Milk is produced from the mammary glands of mammals, including humans. Milk is a primary source of nutrition for infant mammals, before they are able to digest other foods. Children, adolescents, and adults in the United States often drink milk as a healthy beverage option. The type of milk most often consumed in the United States is cow's milk.

Cow's milk can come in pasteurized or unpasteurized form (also known as "raw milk"), although most people drink pasteurized milk. Pasteurized milk goes through a process of heating to destroy disease causing micro – organisms. Pasteurization also increases the shelf life of milk. Although raw milk is allowed to be sold on or off farm in 30 states within the United States, the U.S. Center for Disease Control and Prevention recommends only drinking pasteurized milk, as raw milk can be a breeding ground for germs such as e.coli and salmonella.

After pasteurization, milk generally undergoes homogenization to prevent the separation of milk fat and fluid milk. Homogenization allows for milk to have a smooth, uniform texture. After homogenization, milk is fortified to increase its nutritional value or to replace nutrients lost during processing. For example, in the United States, Vitamin D is added to most milk to facilitate calcium absorption. Vitamin A may also be added. Drinking milk and consuming products made from milk is associated with increased bone health in children, adolescents, and adults. This is due to the high calcium and vitamin D content in milk. Drinking low fat milk and consuming low fat milk products is also associated with a reduced risk of cardiovascular disease and blood pressure in adults.

NUTRIENTS IN MILK

- Whole milk has approximately 148 calories per (244g) cup. Skim milk has around 80 calories per (244g) cup.
- Milk is generally high in Vitamin D, Calcium, and Vitamin B12.
- Milk contains less than 10% of Vitamin A, Vitamin B6, and Magnesium.
- Vitamin D helps to absorb calcium and increase bone growth. Because milk is fortified with Vitamin D, drinking milk can help support balanced production of serotonin. Serotonin is the hormone associated with mood, appetite, and sleep.
- Calcium is important for bone health, and increases general cellular function.
- Vitamin B12 protects the heart and bones from a dangerous protein called homocysteine. High levels of homocysteine can lead to inflammation, osteoporosis, and heart disease. Vitamin B 12 also supports cellular and neural function.

DIETARY INTAKE RECOMMENDATIONS

Milk in the United States typically comes in four different forms, containing similar nutritional properties: whole milk, 2% milk, 1% milk, and skim milk. Half the calories in whole milk come from milk fat. One third of the calories in 2% milk come from fat. 1% and skim milk are considered lower fat milks. The United States

Food and Drug Administration suggest that adults and children 2 years and older generally do not need the extra fat and calories that come from whole milk or 2% milk. Therefore, drinking 1% or skim milk is generally recommended.

Products that come from milk include yogurt, butter, cheese, and ice cream. Three to five servings of low fat and fat free dairy are recommended as part of an overall healthy diet.

One of the most common food allergies in infants and young children is an allergy to cow's milk. Milk allergy symptoms can range from mild (hives) to severe (anaphylaxis). Individuals who are allergic to milk should always have access to an epinephrine auto injector, and strictly avoid milk and any products containing milk.

Lactose intolerance, unlike a milk allergy, does not effect the immune system, and is not life threatening. Those who are lactose intolerant are missing the enzyme lactase, which breaks down lactose (a sugar found in milk/dairy products). The result is that lactose intolerant individuals are have difficulty digesting milk and milk products, leading to gastrointestinal discomfort and diarrhea.

SUMMARY

Consumers should become knowledgeable about the physiological risks and benefits of milk consumption. Milk is high in Vitamin D, Calcium, and Vitamin B12. These nutrients support bone health and cellular function, and may help prevent osteoporosis and heart disease. The recommended daily intake of low fat/fat free dairy products is 3–5 servings per day. Individuals who are allergic to milk should avoid all milk products, as allergic reactions can be severe or life threatening. Lactose intolerant individuals should not drink milk to avoid GI issues.

—*Gina Riley, Ph.D.*

REFERENCES

Cornell University, College of Agriculture and Life Sciences. (2016). Dairy & milk products. Retrieved from http://foodscience.cals.cornell.edu/extension/dairy-milk-products.

Midwest Dairy Association. (2016). Milk, cheese, and yogurt pack your plate with nutrients and goodness. Retrieved from: https://www.midwestdairy.com/nutrition-and-health/dairy-nutrition/.

National Dairy Council. (2016). Milk. Retrieved from https://www.nationaldairycouncil.org/search-results?q=milk.

U.S. Food and Drug Administration. (2016). Milk Guidance Documents and Regulatory Information. Retrieved from http://www.fda.gov/food/guidance-regulation/guidancedocumentsregulatoryinformation/milk/default.htm.

United States Department of Agriculture – Economic Research Service. (2016). Milk: An overview. Retrieved from http://www.ers.usda.gov/topics/animal-products/dairy.aspx.

REVIEWER(S)

Darlene Strayer, RN, MBA, Cinahl Information Systems, Glendale, CA

Nursing Executive Practice Council, Glendale Adventist Medical Center, Glendale, CA

Yogurt

WHAT WE KNOW

Yogurt is a product of milk that has been fermented by adding live bacterial cultures such as *Lactobacillus bulgaricus* and *Streptococcus thermophilus*. The process of fermentation transforms the milk sugar and lactose into lactic acid, which results in the thick, creamy texture that is characteristic of yogurt. Although yogurt has long been a culinary staple in countries of the Middle East, Eastern Europe, and Asia (e.g., Turkey, Greece, India), only since the 20th century has yogurt grown in popularity in Western Europe and North America. With its characteristically tart flavor and pudding-like consistency, yogurt can be added as a garnish to many spicy foods, used in both sweet and savory sauces, combined with fruit for snacks or desserts, and blended into smoothies. Low-fat yogurt is considered a healthy option to include in the recommended 3–5 servings/day of dairy, because it provides calcium, phosphorus, potassium, zinc, B-complex vitamins, and protein. Probiotics, or the bacterial cultures, in yogurt provide many health benefits, including immune function support, improved cholesterol profile, and stronger bones.

- Probiotics (commonly called friendly bacteria) are live microorganisms that positively alter the flora of the intestinal tract, and provide certain health benefits when ingested. Healthcare clinicians have used probiotic supplements successfully in the treatment of *Clostridium difficile* infection, roto virus diarrhea, and traveler's diarrhea. Some researchers have also concluded that the use of the probiotics *L. acidophilus* or *L. plantarum* can reduce symptoms in persons with irritable bowel syndrome (IBS). Many manufacturers pasteurize (i.e. a treatment process using heat) yogurt in order to kill the harmful bacteria, but pasteurizing also destroys the probiotics. Because of this, some brands of pasteurized yogurts are enriched with probiotics, or they are manufactured without pasteurization in order to preserve the live cultures. Yogurt labels provide information regarding whether or not the yogurt contains live cultures. A probiotic count that is as high as possible is considered desirable.

NUTRIENTS IN YOGURT

- Health benefits attributed to the consumption of yogurt that contains probiotics include the following:
  —Improves immune system response, which increases protection against viral, yeast, and parasite infection, and aids in recovery from infection
  —Improves the blood cholesterol profile, decreasing levels of low-density lipoprotein (LDL; called "bad" cholesterol) and raising levels of high-density lipoprotein (HDL; called "good" cholesterol)
  —Provides anti-inflammatory activity, improving manifestations of inflammatory bowel disorder and arthritis
  —Promotes antioxidant activity
  —Suppresses the action of the ulcer-causing bacterium *Helicobacter pylori*
  —Promotes good dental health and fresh breath, by lowering the levels of hydrogen sulfide and other sulfide-containing compounds that cause bad breath. It wards off tongue-coating bacteria, reduces dental plaque formation, prevents cavities, and reduces the risk for gingivitis
- Biologic functions of nutrients found in yogurt include the following:
  —Calcium builds and maintains bones and teeth, regulates muscle contraction, conducts

nerve impulses, activates enzymes for energy production and muscle contraction, participates in blood clotting, assists with vitamin B12 absorption, and maintains the structural integrity of intracellular membranes.

—Phosphorus combines with calcium for the formation of bones and teeth, muscle contraction, and nerve conduction; phosphorous is essential for the structural integrity of cell membranes.

—Potassium supports normal cellular, nerve, and muscle function, and helps to eliminate excess sodium from the body.

—Zinc is an essential trace element that supports the immune system and wound healing, and is essential for maintaining vision and the senses of smell and taste. Zinc maintains endothelial cell membranes, is involved in the catalytic activity of about 100 enzymes, and assists with protein and deoxyribonucleic acid (DNA) formation and cell division.

—Riboflavin, or vitamin B2, is an essential micronutrient that builds proteins for respiratory reactions to produce energy.

—Pantothenic acid, or vitamin B5, is a water-soluble member of the B-complex vitamins that contributes to the metabolism of carbohydrates, proteins, and lipids. It also plays a role in the synthesis of acetylcholine, which is a neurotransmitter in the central and peripheral nervous system.

—Cobalamin, or vitamin B12, is a cobalt-containing B complex vitamin. Vitamin B12 plays a major role in lipid, carbohydrate, and protein metabolism. Other actions of B12 include the following:

  –It is required for the production of hormones, lipids, and proteins.

  –By aiding in the synthesis of neurotransmitters, it contributes to nervous system function.

  –It is required for the formation of red blood cells and hemoglobin.

  –It plays a significant role in DNA and ribonucleic acid (RNA) synthesis.

—Protein is present in every cell of the human body, and is vital to the development and maintenance of skin, muscles, organs, and glands. Other important actions of protein include the following:

  –Provides oxygen to the blood

  –Important in the formation of antibodies for fighting infection

  –Contributes to the production of certain enzymes and hormones

DIETARY INTAKE RECOMMENDATIONS

- Cow's milk is identified as one of the 8 major food allergens in the U.S. in addition to peanuts, tree nuts, wheat, shellfish, soy, eggs, and fish.

- Fermented dairy products, such as yogurt, are not as likely to cause adverse reactions as nonfermented dairy products.

The American Heart Association (AHA) dietary and lifestyle recommendations regarding the consumption of cow's milk include the following:

- Choose dairy products that are fat-free (also called skim), 1% fat, and low-fat.

- Ingest at least 1,200 mg of calcium each day to reduce risk for osteoporosis and CVD; good calcium sources are dairy products, fish with bones, broccoli, and legumes.

- According to the Institute of Medicine (IOM), protein should constitute no less than 10%, and up to 35%, of daily calorie consumption.

RESEARCH FINDINGS

Regular intake of yogurt that is enriched with probiotics can soothe painful gastrointestinal (GI) symptoms and boost the immune system. Probiotics have been used successfully in the treatment of C. difficile infection, rotovirus diarrhea, and traveler's diarrhea. Results of many studies show that the probiotics Saccharomyces boulardii, L. reuteri, and L. GG can reduce stool frequency and shorten the duration of infectious diarrhea by an average of 25 hours. S. boulardii and L.GG have also been shown to lower the risk for diarrhea as an adverse effect of receiving antibiotics the probiotics L. acidophilus and L. plantarum are used to promote relief of symptoms in persons with IBS.

SUMMARY

Consumers should become knowledgeable about the risks and benefits of yogurt consumption. Low-fat yogurt is considered a healthy option to include in the recommended 3–5 servings/day of dairy, because it provides calcium, phosphorus, potassium, zinc, B-complex vitamins, and protein. The probiotics in yogurt provide many health benefits, including immune function support, improved cholesterol profile, and stronger bones. Yogurt contains all of the essential amino acids, which makes it a complete protein. Protein is present in every cell of the human body and is vital to the development and maintenance of skin, muscles, organs, and glands. Individuals with allergies to cow's milk, may experience adverse reactions (e.g., congestion, rash, indigestion, vomiting) from yogurt consumption.

—*Cherie Marcel, BS*

REFERENCES

Ejtahed, H. S., Mohtadi-Nia, J., Homayouni-Rad, A., Niafar, M., Asghari-Jafarabadi, M., & Mofid, V. (2012). Probiotic yogurt improves antioxidant status in type 2 diabetic patients. *Nutrition*, 28(5), 539-543. doi:10.1016/j.nut.2011.08.013

Food and Nutrition Board, Institute of Medicine, National Academies. (n.d.). Dietary Reference Intakes (DRIs): Estimated Average Requirements. Food and Nutrition Board, Institute of Medicine, National Academies. Retrieved March 24, 2015, from http://iom.edu/Activities/Nutrition/SummaryDRIs/~/media/Files/Activity%20Files/Nutrition/DRIs/New %20Material/5DRI%20Values%20SummaryTables%2014.pdf

Irvine, S. L., Hummelen, R., & Hekmat, S. (2011). Probiotic yogurt consumption may improve gastrointestinal symptoms, productivity, and nutritional intake of people living with human immunodeficiency virus in Mwanza, Tanzania. *Nutrition Research*, 31(12), 875-881. doi:10.1016/j.nutres.2011.10.005

Lichtenstein, A. H., Appel, L. J., Brands, M., Carnethon, M., Daniels, S., Franch, H. A., ... Wylie-Rosett, J. (2006). Summary of American Heart Association Diet and Lifestyle Recommendations revision 2006. *Arteriosclerosis, Thrombosis, and Vascular Biology*, 26(10), 2186-2191. doi:10.1161/01.ATV.0000238352.25222.5e

Magee, E. (2007). The benefits of yogurt. *WebMD*. Retrieved April 20, 2015, from http://www.webmd.com/diet/features/benefits-of-yogurt

Makino, S., Ikegami, S., Kume, A., Horiuchi, H., Sasaki, H., & Orii, N. (2010). Reducing the risk of infection in the elderly by dietary intake of yoghurt fermented with Lactobacillus delbrueckii ssp. bulgaricus OLL1073R-1. *British Journal of Nutrition*, 104(7), 998-1006. doi:10.1017/S000711451000173X

McFarland, L. V. (2007). Meta-analysis of probiotics for the prevention of traveler's diarrhea. *Travel Medicine & Infectious Disease*, 5(2), 97-105. doi:10.1016/j.tmaid.2005.10.003

Morris, J. D., Diamond, K. A., & Balart, L. A. (2009). Do probiotics have a role in the management of inflammatory bowel disease?. *The Journal of the Louisiana State Medical Society: Official Organ of the Louisiana State Medical Society*, 161(3), 155-159.

Rohde, C. L., Bartolini, V., & Jones, N. (2009). The use of probiotics in the prevention and treatment of antibiotic-associated diarrhea with special interest in Clostridium difficile-associated diarrhea. *Nutrition in Clinical Practice*, 24(1), 33-40. doi:10.1177/0884533608329297

The George Mateljan Foundation editorial team. (n.d.). The world's healthiest foods: Yogurt. Retrieved April 20, 2015, from http://www.whfoods.com/genpage.php? tname=foodspice&dbid=124#descr

The George Mateljan Foundation editorial team. (n.d.). The world's healthiest foods: Can you tell me more about adverse reactions to cow's milk. Retrieved March 17, 2015, from http://www.whfoods.com/genpage.php?tname=george&dbid=52

REVIEWER(S)

Darlene Strayer, RN, MBA, Cinahl Information Systems, Glendale, CA

Nursing Executive Practice Council, Glendale Adventist Medical Center, Glendale, CA

BEVERAGES

Coffee

WHAT WE KNOW

Coffee, one of the world's most widely consumed beverages, is brewed from the seeds, or beans, found in the cherries of the coffee tree. Although there are more than 6,000 species of tropical trees and shrubs in the *Coffea* genus, from which the coffee tree descends, only two species are used by the commercial coffee industry. These are arabica and canephora (also known as robusta). *Coffea arabica* is genetically closer to the first coffee trees of Ethiopia. The arabica beans are flatter and longer than the canephora beans, and produce a smooth, aromatic flavor. Arabica trees are more expensive to cultivate because they require a climate that is not too hot or too cold, are prone to disease, and grow in steep terrain. Regardless, the aribica species makes up about 70% of the world's coffee. *Coffea canephora*, or *C. robusta*, is the more "robust" species because it is disease-resistant and easier to cultivate. The beans are rounder and smaller than the arabica beans, and produce a bold flavor. Canephora beans contain 50–60% more caffeine than arabica, and are primarily used in coffee blends or instant coffees.

- Coffee is commonly consumed for its caffeine-induced stimulant effect. Results of studies show that caffeinated coffee boosts energy, awakens and clears the mind, and wards off depression. Researchers have found that coffee provides many benefits independent of its caffeine content. Green coffee beans contain about 1,000 antioxidants, and 300 more antioxidants are added by the process of brewing. Hundreds of study results have linked coffee consumption to such benefits as a reduced risk of type 2 diabetes mellitus (DM2), prevention of certain cancers (e.g., colon and liver cancer), enhanced mental and physical performance, and protection against Parkinson's disease

- Although most research results have identified the benefits of coffee, there is some evidence that coffee consumption can aggravate certain conditions, including gastroesophageal reflux disease (GERD), migraines, arrhythmias, insomnia or other sleep disturbances, and benign fibrocystic breast disease, and can worsen anxiety in some cases. During pregnancy, consuming fewer than 3 cups of coffee per day is recommended.

NUTRIENTS IN COFFEE

- Coffee may help to prevent DM2 by lowering insulin resistance and slowing the absorption of carbohydrates from the intestines.

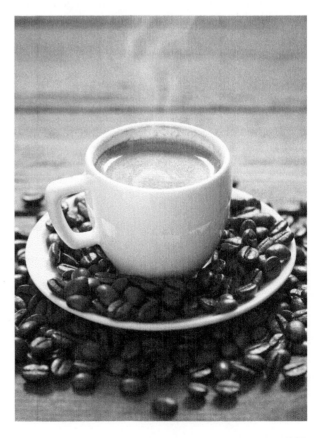

- Coffee contains the diterpenes cafestol and kahweal, which promote the anti-carcinogenic (i.e., prevent cancer causing) activities of:
    - inducing phase II enzymes involved in carcinogen detoxification
    - inhibiting phase I enzyme activity, which prevents carcinogen activation
    - stimulating intracellular antioxidant defenses
- Coffee provides valuable polyphenols (i.e., plant-derived protective chemicals) such as caffeic acid, lignan phytoestrogens, and flavonoids, which have anti-carcinogenic properties such as the inhibition of the methylation of deoxyribonucleic acid.
- Coffee is a good source of the strong antioxidant chlorogenic acid, an ester of caffeic acid. Chlorogenic acid has been shown to increase insulin sensitivity and reduce blood glucose levels.

DIETARY INTAKE RECOMMENDATIONS

- Consumption of caffeinated coffee can aggravate certain conditions such as GERD, migraines, arrhythmias, insomnia or other sleep disturbances, and benign fibrocystic breast disease.
- Caffeine consumption can amplify feelings of anxiety.
- It is recommended that women who are pregnant consume fewer than 3 cups of coffee per day to reduce risk for preterm labor or stunting of fetal growth.
- High amounts of caffeine consumption (e.g., > 300 mg/day) may interfere with normal growth and development in children and adolescents.

RESEARCH FINDINGS

- Authors of a meta-analysis of 20 cohort studies reported that there was a significant inverse relationship between coffee consumption and total mortality.
    - Results of numerous studies have reported an inverse association between coffee consumption and certain cancers, including bladder, breast, buccal, pharyngeal, colorectal, endometrial, esophageal, hepatocellular, leukemic, pancreatic, prostate, and skin cancers. Researchers suspect that moderate coffee intake may reduce total cancer incidence. This appears to be unrelated to the

caffeine content, but rather is an effect of the many phytonutrients provided by coffee.
- High intake of coffee and tea has been associated with reduced risk of DM2. This relationship exists for both caffeinated and decaffeinated coffee, suggesting that these protective effects are the result of the many chemical constituents that are present in coffee and tea. Magnesium, lignans, and chlorogenic acids appear to have a beneficial effect on glucose metabolism and insulin sensitivity, although the exact mechanisms involved have not been adequately identified. Further scientific study is warranted.
    - Although the inverse association between coffee intake and risk of DM2 is present regardless of caffeine content, authors of a meta-analysis reported that the percentage of reduced risk was higher in persons who consumed caffeinated coffee than in those who consumed decaffeinated coffee.
    - Authors of a case-control study in Sweden confirmed the inverse relationship between coffee consumption and risk for developing DM2, although the findings indicated that a positive association exists between coffee consumption the risk of developing autoimmunity, including type 1-like latent autoimmune diabetes in adults.
- Researchers report that coffee intake is associated with significantly lower risk for developing cardiovascular disease (CVD), with the lowest risk occurring with 3–5cups/day of coffee consumed. No increase in CVD risk was observed with heavy coffee consumption.
- Research results show that individuals who regularly drink coffee or hot tea are about 50% less likely to carry methicillin-resistant Staphylococcus aureus infection in their nasal passages. Scientists suggest that this is due to the antimicrobial properties of these beverages.

SUMMARY

Consumers should become knowledgeable about the physiologic risks and benefits of coffee consumption. There is the potential for caffeinated coffee consumption to exasperate the symptoms of certain conditions such as GERD, migraines, arrhythmias, sleep disturbances, anxiety, and benign fibrocystic breast disease. Women who are pregnant should consume fewer than 3 cups of coffee per day to reduce risk for preterm labor or stunting of fetal growth. High amounts of caffeine consumption (e.g., > 300 mg/day) can interfere with normal growth and development in children and adolescents. Research suggests that moderate coffee consumption may reduce the risk of heart disease and many cancers. Although further research is necessary, high intake of coffee may reduce risk of type 2 diabetes.

—*Cherie Marcel, BS*

REFERENCES

Biazevic, M. G. H., Toporcov, T. N., Antunes, J. L. F., Rotundo, L. D. B., Brasileiro, R. S., de Carvalho, M. B., & Kowalski, L. P. (2011). Cumulative coffee consumption and reduced risk of oral and oropharyngeal cancer. *Nutrition & Cancer, 63*(3), 350-356. doi:10.1080/01635581.2011.536065

Bidel, S., Hu, G., Jousilahti, P., Antikainen, R., Pukkala, E., Hakulinen, T., & Tuomilehto, J. (2010). Coffee consumption and risk of colorectal cancer. *European Journal of Clinical Nutrition, 64*(9), 917-923. doi:10.1038/ejcn.2010.103

Boggs, D. A., Rosenberg, L., Ruiz-Narvaez, E. A., & Palmer, J. R. (2010). Coffee, tea, and alcohol intake in relation to risk of type 2 diabetes in African American women. *American Journal of Clinical Nutrition, 92*(4), 960-966. doi:10.3945/ajcn.2010.29598

Boyle, A. J. (2012). Coffee consumption and mortality. *Integrative Medicine Alert, 15*(10), 119-120.

Ding, M., Bhupathiraju, S. N., Satija, A., van Dam, R. M., & Hu, F. B. (2014). Long-term coffee consumption and risk of cardiovascular disease: A systematic review and a dose-response meta-analysis of prospective cohort studies. *Circulation, 129*(6), 643-659. doi:10.1161/CIRCULSTIONAHA.113.005925

Harris, H. R., Bergkvist, L., & Wolk, A. (2012). Coffee and black tea consumption and breast cancer mortality in a cohort of Swedish women. *British Journal of Cancer, 107*(5), 874-878. doi:10.1038/bjc.2012.337

Hildebrand, J. S., Patel, A. V., McCullough, M. L., Gaudet, M. M., Chen, A. Y., Hayes, R. B., & Gapstur, S. M. (2013). Coffee, tea, and fatal oral/pharyngeal cancer in large prospective US cohort. *American Journal of Epidemiology, 177*(1), 50-58. doi:10.1093/aje/kws222

Huxley, R., Lee, C. M., Barzi, F., Timmermeister, L., Czernichow, S., Perkovic, V., ... Woodward, M. (2009). Coffee, decaffeinated coffee, and tea consumption in relation to incident type 2 diabetes mellitus: A systematic review with meta-analysis. *Archives of Internal Medicine, 169*(22), 2053-2063. doi:10.1001/archinternmed.2009.439

Je, Y., & Giovannucci, E. (2014). Coffee consumption and total mortality: A meta-analysis of twenty prospective cohort studies. *British Journal of Nutrition, 111*(7), 1162-1173. doi:10.1017/S0007114513003814

Jiang, X., Zhang, D., & Jiang, W. (2014). Coffee and caffeine intake and incidence of type 2 diabetes mellitus: A meta-analysis of prospective studies. *European Journal of Nutrition, 53*(1), 25-38. doi:10.1007/s00394-013-0603-x

Kastorini, C., Chrysohoou, C., Panagiotakos, D., Aggelopoulos, P., Liontou, C., Pitsavos, C., & Stefanadis, C. (2009). Moderate coffee consumption lowers the likelihood of developing left ventricular systolic dysfunction in post-acute coronary syndrome normotensive patients. *Journal of Medicinal Food, 12*(1), 29-36. doi:10.1089/jmf.2008.0124

Li, G., Ma, D., Zhang, Y., Zheng, W., & Wang, P. (2013). Coffee consumption and risk of colorectal cancer: A meta-analysis of observational studies. *Public Health Nutrition, 16*(2), 346-357. doi:10.1017/S1368980012002601

Lofvenborg, J. E., Andersson, T., Carlsson, P. O., Dorkhan, M., Groop, L., Martinell, M., & Carlsson, S. (2014). Coffee consumption and the risk of latent autoimmune diabetes in adults-results from a Swedish case-control study. *Diabetic Medicine, 31*(7), 799-805. doi:10.1111/dme.12469

Malerba, S., Galeone, C., Pelucchi, C., Turati, F., Hashibe, M., La Vecchia, C., & Tavani, A. (2013). A meta-analysis of coffee and tea consumption and the risk of glioma in adults. *Cancer Causes Control, 24*(2), 267-276. doi:10.1007/s10552-012-0126-4

Matheson, E. M., Mainous, A. G., Everett, C. J., & King, D. E. (2011). Tea and coffee consumption and MRSA nasal carriage. *Annals of Family Medicine, 9*(4), 299-304. doi:10.1370/afm.1262

National Coffee Association USA editorial team. (n.d.). What is coffee? Retrieved March 2, 2014, from http://www.ncausa.org/i4a/pages/index.cfm?pageid=67

Ren, J. S., Freedman, N. D., Kamangar, F., Dawsey, S. M., Hollenbeck, A. R., Schatzkin, A., & Abnet, C. C. (2010). Tea, coffee, carbonated soft drinks and upper gastrointestinal tract cancer risk in a large United States prospective cohort study. *European Journal of Cancer, 46*(10), 1873-1881. doi:1016/j.ejca.2010.03.025

Sartorelli, D. S., Fagherazzi, G., Balkau, B., Touillaud, M. S., Boutron-Ruault, M. C., de Lauzon-Guillain, B., & Clavel-Chapelon, F. (2010). Differential effects of coffee on the risk of type 2 diabetes according to meal consumption in a French cohort of women: The E3N/EPIC cohort study. *American Journal of Clinical Nutrition*, *91*(4), 1002-1012. doi:10.3945/ajcn.2009.28741

Shen, L. (2012). Beneficial effects of coffee consumption go beyond antioxidation. *Nutrition*, *28*(11/12), 1194-1195. doi:10.1016/j.nut.2012.07.001

Stokel, K. (2012). National Institutes of Health discovers protective effects of coffee. *Life Extension*, *18*(9), 54-63.

Van Dam, R., & Lane, J. D. (2011). The burning question: Should I cut back on coffee?. *Health (Time Inc.)*, *25*(7), 22.

Wilson, K. M., Kasperzyk, J. L., Rider, J. R., Kenfield, S., van Dam, R. M., Stampfer, M. J., & Mucci, L. A. (2011). Coffee consumption and prostate cancer risk and progression in the Health Professionals Follow-up study. *JNCI: Journal of the National Cancer Institute*, *103*(11), 876-884. doi:10.1093/jnci/djr151

Yu, X., Bao, Z., Zou, J., & Dong, J. (2011). Coffee consumption and risk of cancers: A meta-analysis of cohort studies. *BMC Cancer*, *11*(1), 96. doi:10.1186/1471-2407-11-96

REVIEWER(S)

Darlene Strayer, RN, MBA, Cinahl Information Systems, Glendale, CA

Rosalyn McFarland, DNP, RN, APNP, FNP-BC

Nursing Practice Council, Glendale Adventist Medical Center, Glendale, CA

Diet Soft Drinks

WHAT WE KNOW

Soft drinks (commonly called soda) are carbonated beverages that are sweetened with either a caloric sugar sweetener or a noncaloric sweetener. Many soft drinks also contain the psychoactive stimulant caffeine. Soft drinks that are sweetened with a noncaloric sweetener are referred to as diet soft drinks, which are typically sweetened with the artificial sweetener aspartame. Globally, soft drink sales have increased in recent decades, and the estimated increase in soft drink consumption is 300% in the past 20 years. The increase in soft drink consumption parallels the dramatic increase in rates of obesity over

the past two decades. Researchers believe that the high prevalence of obesity and the increased consumption of sugar-sweetened soft drinks are intimately connected. However, substituting diet soft drinks for sugar-sweetened soft drinks does not appear to prevent obesity. In fact, researchers report that consumers of diet soft drinks have a 70% larger waist circumference than persons who do not, and that intake of 1 or more diet soft drinks a day is linked to an increased risk for stroke.

- The consumption of both sugar-sweetened and diet soft drinks is associated with poor dietary and lifestyle choices, including higher intake of fast foods, unhealthy snacks, and sugary desserts; lower intake of fruits and vegetables; less time spent sleeping during the night; and engaging in exercise less regularly

- Many soft drinks (e.g., Coke, Pepsi, Dr. Pepper, Mountain Dew) contain caffeine. Studies have found that caffeine boosts energy, awakens and clears the mind, and reduces risk for depression. The primary action of caffeine is antagonism of the adenosine receptor. Adenosine dilates blood vessels and facilitates sleep. By binding with the adenosine receptor, caffeine interferes with the ability of adenosine to slow the body. The result is increased neural activity, including greater alertness and wakefulness. Caffeine is readily absorbed and its effects persist for 4–6 hours. If consumed too close to bedtime, caffeine can interfere with the ability to fall asleep and negatively affect healthy sleep patterns.

RESEARCH FINDINGS

- Diet soft drinks do not appear to be a healthy alternative to sugar-sweetened soft drinks. Although many studies have shown little or no detrimental effects associated with the intake of the artificial sweetener aspartame, results of several recent studies indicate that there are negative effects. One large study assessing the effects of aspartame intake on rats for the duration of their lifetime found that aspartame intake increased the risk for lymphoma, leukemia, and transitional cell carcinoma of the pelvis, ureter, and bladder. Another study revealed that aspartame consumption raised blood glucose levels in diabetes-prone mice. Researchers have reported that individuals who consume diet soft drinks daily have a 36% higher risk for metabolic syndrome (i.e., a condition characterized by hyperglycemia, hypertension, abdominal obesity, and high triglycerides) and a 67% higher risk for diabetes mellitus, type 2 (DM2) compared with those who do not regularly consume diet soft drinks.

SUMMARY

Consumers should become knowledgeable about the physiologic effects of consuming diet soft drinks. Reducing diet soft drink intake may reduce risk for developing certain cancers and type 2 diabetes.

—*Cherie Marcel, BS*
—*Karin Gajewski, RN, BSN*

REFERENCES

Allman-Farinelli, M. A. (2009). Do calorically sweetened soft drinks contribute to obesity and metabolic disease? *Nutrition Today, 44*(1), 17-20. doi:10.1364/OL.29.001674

Aune, D. (2012). Soft drinks, aspartame, and the risk of cancer and cardiovascular disease. *American Journal of Clinical Nutrition, 96*(6), 1249-1251. doi:10.3945/ajcn.112.051417

Bender, A. (2011). Nutritionist's notes: Are diet sodas okay? *American Institute for Cancer Research Newsletter, 2011*(112), 9.

Collison, K. S., Zaidi, M. Z., Subhani, S. N., Al-Rubeaan, K., Shoukri, M., & Al-Mohanna, F. A. (2010). Sugar-sweetened carbonated beverage consumption correlates with BMI, waist circumference, and poor dietary choices in school children. *BMC Public Health, 10,* 234. doi:10.1186/1471-2458-10-234

The editorial team of Environmental Nutrition. (2012). The diet soda-weight debate. *Environmental Nutrition, 35*(7), 7.

Evert, A., & Zieve, D. (2011). Caffeine in the diet. *MedlinePlus*. Retrieved February 12, 2013, from http://www.nlm.nih.gov/medlineplus/ency/article/002445.htm

Fiorito, L. M., Marini, M., Mitchell, D. C., Smiciklas-Wright, H., & Birch, L. L. (2010). Girls' early sweetened carbonated beverage intake predicts different patterns of beverage and nutrient intake across childhood and adolescence. *Journal of the American Dietetic Association, 110*(4), 543-550. doi:10.1016/j.jada.2009.12.027

Franz, M. (2010). Diet soft drinks: How safe are they? *Diabetes Self-Management, 27*(2), 8, 11-13.

Harrington, S. (2008). The role of sugar-sweetened beverage consumption in adolescent obesity: A review of the literature. *Journal of School Nursing, 24*(1), 3-12. doi:10.1622/1059-8405(2008)024[0003:TROSBC]2.0.CO;2

Høstmark, A. T. (2010). The Oslo health study: A dietary index estimating high intake of soft drinks and low intake of fruits and vegetables was positively associated with components of the metabolic syndrome. *Applied Physiology, Nutrition & Metabolism, 35*(6), 816-825. doi:10.1139/H10-080

Kavey, R. E. (2010). How sweet it is: Sugar-sweetened beverage consumption, obesity, and cardiovascular risk in childhood. *Journal of the American Dietetic Association, 110*(10), 1456-1460. doi:10.1016/j.jada.2010.07.028

Yamada, M., Murakami, K., Sasaki, S., Takahashi, Y., & Okubo, H. (2008). Soft drink intake is associated with diet quality even among young Japanese women with low soft drink intake. *Journal of the American Dietetic Association, 108*(12), 1997-2004. doi:10.1016/j.jada.2008.09.033

Yantis, M. A., & Hunter, K. (2010). Clinical queries. Is diet soda a healthy choice? *Nursing, 40*(11), 67. doi:10.1097/01.NURSE.0000389036.71877.61

REVIEWER(S)

Darlene Strayer, RN, MBA, Cinahl Information Systems, Glendale, CA

Nursing Executive Practice Council, Glendale Adventist Medical Center, Glendale, CA

Energy Drinks

WHAT WE KNOW

Energy drinks (e.g., Rockstar, Red Bull, Monster) are soda- or punch-like beverages that are designed to significantly increase energy. Energy drinks contain high amounts of sweetener, caffeine, and other stimulating substances (e.g., taurine, guarana, cacao, ginseng, licorice), which may or may not be strictly regulated by the United States Food and Drug Administration (FDA) depending on whether the manufacturer chooses to label the energy drink as a "beverage" or a "liquid supplement." The labeling requirements that are set by the Dietary Supplement Health and Education Act for a liquid supplement are far less rigid than those set by the Nutrition Labeling and Education Act (NLEA), which governs beverage labels.

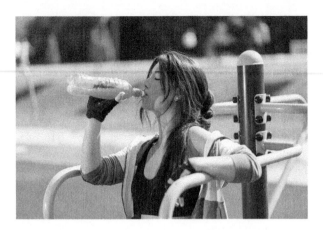

- With the inconsistency of FDA regulation and the mix of caffeine-containing ingredients, which are typically listed separately on energy drink labels, it is difficult to determine the exact caffeine content of each drink. This can be dangerous for individuals who need to limit caffeine consumption (e.g., adolescents, children, persons with cardiovascular disease [CVD], and pregnant women).
  —Energy drinks are estimated to contain 80–550 mg of caffeine per serving.
- Energy drinks are frequently sweetened with sugar, high-fructose corn syrup (HFCS), and/or aspartame (i.e., a non-caloric sweetener).

ACTION OF ENERGY DRINKS

- The primary active components of energy drinks are caffeine and sweeteners.
  —Caffeine is the world's most widely used psychoactive substance. Results of studies show that caffeine boosts energy, awakens and clears the mind, and reduces depression. The primary action of caffeine is interference of the adenosine receptor. Adenosine dilates blood vessels and facilitates sleep. By binding with the adenosine receptor, caffeine interferes with the ability of adenosine to slow the body down. The result is increased neural activity (e.g., alertness, wakefulness). Caffeine is readily absorbed and its effects usually last 4–6 hours. If consumed too close to bedtime, caffeine can interfere with the ability to fall asleep and negatively impact healthy sleep patterns.

—HFCS contains the monosaccharide (i.e., simple sugar) fructose, glucose, and processed starches that accelerate the absorption of fructose. Unlike glucose, fructose cannot be stored as glycogen for use as energy; if consumed in large amounts, fructose is likely to be converted to fat by the liver. Fat that is synthesized by the liver is released in the bloodstream as very low density lipoproteins (VLDL), which is a form of cholesterol known to contribute to coronary artery disease (CAD).

ENERGY DRINK TOXICITY AND MEDICATION INTERACTION

- The American Academy of Pediatrics recommends that young children should not consume energy drinks and that adolescents should consume no more than 100 mg of caffeine each day.
- It is recommended that adults limit caffeine consumption to 500 mg/day.
- According to the American Association of Poison Control Centers, excessive consumption of energy drinks can result in the following signs and symptoms:
  —Nausea, vomiting, and/or diarrhea
  —Agitation, anxiety, nervousness, and restlessness
  —Insomnia and/or disruption in sleep patterns
  —Delirium
  —Headache on consumption or withdrawal
  —Rapid heart rate or dysrhythmia
  —Chest pain
  —Elevated blood pressure
  —Tremors
  —Seizures
  —Dehydration
  —Kidney dysfunction
- Consumption of caffeine can worsen certain medical conditions, including gastroesophageal reflux disease (GERD), migraine, arrhythmias, insomnia or other sleep disturbances, and benign fibrocystic breast disease.
- A diet that is high in sugar is associated with CVD, dyslipidemia, and diabetes mellitus, type 2 (DM2).
- Due to the excessive caffeine and sugar/HFCS content of energy drinks, it is recommended that certain individuals minimize or

completely avoid the consumption of energy drinks. Contraindications for energy drink consumption include the following:

—Pregnant women
  –Excessive caffeine intake may increase the risk for low birth weight, small for gestational age, and preterm birth.
—Children under 18 years of age
  –High caffeine consumption (e.g., > 300 mg/day) can interfere with normal growth and development in children and adolescents.
—Individuals who have nonalcoholic fatty liver disease (NAFLD)
  –Researchers report that large amounts of fructose consumption can result in visceral fat accumulation and insulin resistance. Because fructose is converted to fat and stored by the liver, there is concern that excessive intake of HFCS-sweetened soft drinks could contribute to NAFLD.
—Individuals who have DM2
  –The consumption of energy drinks can cause a sharp increase in blood glucose levels.
—Individuals with CVD
—Individuals with an anxiety disorder
  –Caffeine consumption can amplify the symptoms of anxiety.
—Individuals who regularly drink alcohol or who have alcoholism
  –The combined consumption of energy drinks and alcohol can blunt the sensation of intoxication, leading the consumer to drink more alcohol than they normally would.
  –Researchers have observed a potential relationship between relapse in patients with a dual diagnosis of substance abuse disorder and bipolar disorder (BD) and excessive consumption of energy drins.

- Because of the high stimulatory effect of energy drinks, individuals are advised to discuss the consumption of energy drinks with the treating clinician if they are receiving medications for the treatment of a condition that can be adversely affected by energy drink consumption (e.g., CVD, NAFLD, DM2, GERD, migraine, arrhythmias, insomnia or other sleep disturbances, and benign fibrocystic breast disease).

RESEARCH FINDINGS

- Substituting aspartame-containing "diet" drinks for sugar-sweetened drinks does not appear to prevent obesity. Research results show that compared with nondrinkers of diet soft drinks, consumers of diet soft drinks have a 70% larger waist circumference, and indicate that intake of one or more diet soft drinks a day is linked to increased risk for stroke.

- Researchers report that individuals who consume aspartame-containing drinks daily have a 36% higher risk of developing metabolic syndrome (i.e., a condition characterized by the combination of hyperglycemia, hypertension, abdominal obesity, and high levels of triglycerides) and a 67% higher risk of developing DM2 compared with those who do not consume diet drinks regularly.
  —The consumption of sugar-sweetened and diet soft drinks is associated with making poor dietary and lifestyle choices such as higher intake of fast foods, eating unhealthy snacks and sugary desserts, lower intake of fruits and vegetables, getting less night-time sleep, and engaging in exercise less regularly.

- Researchers of a study on energy drinks, soft drinks, and substance abuse among secondary school students found energy drink use positively correlated with substance abuse. Researchers determined that among adolescents, consumption of energy drinks and shots is widespread, and users reported increased risk for substance abuse.

SUMMARY

Consumers should learn about the dietary considerations of energy drink consumptions. Individuals with diet-related medical conditions (e.g., CVD, DM2, GERD, NAFLD) may have increased risks associated with energy drink consumption. Healthier alternatives to increase energy include; eating small, frequent, nutrient-dense meals and snacks and getting regular exercise.

—*Cherie Marcel, BS*

REFERENCES

Aune, D. (2012). Soft drinks, aspartame, and the risk of cancer and cardiovascular disease. *American Journal of Clinical Nutrition*, 96(6), 1249-1251. doi:10.3945/ajcn.112.051417

The editorial team of Environmental Nutrition. (2012). The diet soda-weight debate. *Environmental Nutrition*, 35(7), 7.

The editorial team of the American Association of Poison Control Centers (AAPCC). (n.d.). Energy drinks. *AAPCC*. Retrieved April 6, 2015, from http://www.aapcc.org/alerts/energy-drinks/

Evert, A., & Zieve, D. (2013). Caffeine in the diet. *MedlinePlus*. Retrieved April 6, 2015, from http://www.nlm.nih.gov/medlineplus/ency/article/002445.htm

Franz, M. (2010). Diet soft drinks: How safe are they? *Diabetes Self-Management*, 27(2), 8, 11-13.

Goldfarb, M., Tellier, C., & Thanassoulis, G. (2014). Review of published cases of adverse cardiovascular events after ingestion of energy drinks. *American Journal of Cardiology*, 113(1), 168-172. doi:10.1016/j.amjcard.2013.08.058

Hellerstein, M. K. (2012). Mitigating factors and metabolic mechanisms in fructose-induced nonalcoholic fatty liver disease: The next challenge. *American Journal of Clinical Nutrition*, 96(5), 951-952. doi:10.3945/ajcn.112.049650

Howland, J., & Rohsenow, D. J. (2013). Risks of energy drinks mixed with alcohol. *Journal of the American Association*, 309(3), 245-246.

Johnson, R. J., Lanaspa, M. A., Roncal-Jimenez, C., & Sanchez-Lozada, L. G. (2012). Effects of excessive fructose intake on health. *Annals of Internal Medicine*, 156(12), 905-906. doi:10.7326/0003-4819-156-12-201206190-00024

Maslova, E., Bhattacharya, S., Lin, S. W., & Michels, K. B. (2010). Caffeine consumption during pregnancy and risk of preterm birth: A meta-analysis. *American Journal of Clinical Nutrition*, 92(5), 1120-1132. doi:10.3945/ajcn.2010.29789

Rizkallah, E., Belanger, M., Stavro, K., Dussault, M., Pampoulova, T., Chiasson, J. P., & Potvin, S. (2011). Could the use of energy drinks induce manic or depressive relapse among abstinent substance use disorder patients with comorbid bipolar spectrum disorder? *Bipolar Disorders*, 13(5-6), 578-580. doi:10.1111/j.1399-5618.2011.00951.x

Seifert, S. M., Schaechter, J. L., Hershorin, E. R., & Lipschultz, S. E. (2011). Health effects of energy drinks on children, adolescents, and young adults. *Pediatrics*, 127(3), 511-528. doi:10.1542/peds.2009-3592

Sengpiel, V., Elind, E., Bacelis, J., Nilsson, S., Grove, J., Myhre, R., ... Brantsaeter, A. (2013). Maternal caffeine intake during pregnancy is associated with birth weight but not with gestational length: Results from a large prospective observational cohort study. *BMC Medicine*, 11(1), 42. doi:10.1186/1741-7015-11-42

Seratsky, K. (2015, February 11). Can energy drinks really boost a person's energy?*Mayoclinic.org*. Retrieved September 16, 2014, from http://www.mayoclinic.org/healthy-living/nutrition-and-healthy-eating/expert-answers/energy-drinks/faq-20058349

Terry-McElrath, Y. M., O'Malley, P. M., & Johnston, L. D. (2014). Energy drinks, soft drinks, and substance use among US secondary school students. *Journal of Addiction Medicine*, 8(1), 6-13. doi:10.1097/01.ADM.0000435322.07020.53

Torpy, J. M., & Livingston, E. H. (2013). JAMA patient page. Energy drinks. *JAMA: Journal of the American Medical Association*, 309(3), 297.

Webb, D. (2013). The truth about energy drinks. *Today's Dietitian*, 15(10), 62-67.

Yantis, M. A., & Hunter, K. (2010). Clinical queries. Is diet soda a healthy choice? *Nursing*, 40(11), 67. doi:10.1097/01.NURSE.0000389036.71877.61

REVIEWER(S)

Darlene Strayer, RN, MBA, Cinahl Information Systems, Glendale, CA

Anne Danahy, MS, RDN

Nursing Executive Practice Council, Glendale Adventist Medical Center, Glendale, CA

Green Tea

WHAT WE KNOW

Tea, one of the world's most widely consumed beverages, is produced from the steamed and dried leaves of the *Camellia sinensis* plant. Depending on the preparation method used, tea can be black, green, white, or oolong. In Japan and China, green tea is the most commonly consumed tea. All 4 varieties of tea are high in polyphenols (i.e., organic chemicals containing multiple phenolic compounds), which have powerful antioxidant activity. Green tea also contains alkaloids (e.g., caffeine, theophylline, and theobromine), amino acids, carbohydrates, chlorophyll, fluoride, aluminum, and other minerals and trace elements.

- Green tea is especially high in polyphenols known as catechins, the most active of which is epigallocatechin-3-gallate (EGCG). Catechins

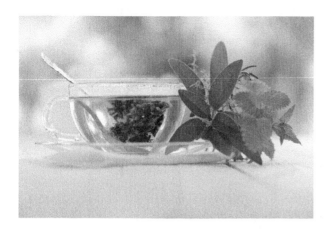

are believed to contribute most of the health benefits that are commonly attributed to tea, including the following:

—Prevention of heart disease

—Protection against many types of cancer, including esophageal, ovarian, pancreatic, and bladder cancer

—Decreased risk of developing Parkinson disease

• One of the common reasons for choosing to drink green tea is its caffeine-induced stimulant effect. Results of studies show that tea boosts energy, increases alertness and focus, and reduces risk of depression.

NUTRIENTS IN GREEN TEA

• Green tea contains phytonutrients (i.e., beneficial plant-derived nutrients) such as the polyphenols catechins and flavonoids, which promote the following anti-carcinogenic activities:

—Activation of detoxification enzymes (e.g., glutathione S-transferase, quinone reductase), which protect against tumor development.

—Inhibition of tumor cell proliferation

—Protection against damaging ultraviolet (UV) B radiation

—Enhancement of immune system function

—Stimulation of intracellular antioxidant defenses

• Evidence suggests that consuming green tea provides the following health benefits:

—Prevention of orthostatic hypotension (i.e., dizziness when arising from a lying position) and postprandial hypotension (i.e., low blood pressure after eating) by temporarily raising blood pressure

—Increased mental alertness due to the caffeine content

—Reduced risk of developing Parkinson disease

—Treatment for genital warts

–Sinecatechins (Veregen), a green tea extract ointment produced by Bradley Pharmaceuticals, is U.S. Food and Drug Administration (FDA) approved as a topical treatment for genital warts. Veregen is the first botanical agent approved for prescription in the United States. (For more information, see http:// www.veregen.com/).

ADVERSE REACTIONS

• Consumption of caffeinated tea can worsen certain medical conditions, including gastroesophageal reflux disease (GERD), migraine, arrhythmias, insomnia or other sleep disturbances, and benign fibrocystic breast disease.

• Caffeine consumption can increase anxiety.

• It is recommended that women who are pregnant consume fewer than 2 cups of tea a day to reduce risk of preterm labor and stunting of fetal growth.

• High amounts of caffeine consumption (> 300 mg/day) may interfere with normal growth and development in children and adolescents.

• Green tea can limit the absorption of non-heme iron from the diet, which poses a risk for individuals with iron-deficiency anemia; this can be mitigated by consuming foods that enhance iron absorption (e.g., foods high in vitamin C, such as lemons, oranges, and tomatoes) in the same meal or by drinking tea between meals to prevent interference with iron absorption.

RESEARCH FINDINGS

• Results of numerous in vitro and animal studies show an inverse association between certain constituents of green tea (e.g., phytonutrients) and growth of certain cancers, including bladder, esophageal, ovarian, and pancreatic. However, results of in vivo studies are mixed. Results of a systematic review of 51 studies including more than 1.6 million participants indicate that evidence to support the consumption of green tea for cancer prevention was lacking. Further in vivo research is recommended for a more definitive understanding of the effectiveness of green tea intake for cancer prevention and treatment.

- Results of a study that recorded the functional MRI of 12 healthy adults who consumed either green tea or placebo while performing a working memory task indicate that green tea extract appears to mediate working memory processing in the brain by modulating brain activity in the dorsolateral prefrontal cortex. Researchers have also stated that green tea compounds can prevent the formation of dangerous amyloid aggregates on nerve cells in the brain and can catabolize existing aggregates found in proteins that contain copper, iron, and zinc, which are associated with Alzheimer's disease (AD).

- Researchers report an inverse relationship between the regular consumption of green tea and the risk of cardiovascular disease, including stroke. Evidence also indicates that green tea consumption can significantly decrease blood pressure in mildly hypertensive individuals with type 2 diabetes.

SUMMARY

Consumers should become knowledgeable about the physiologic risks and benefits of green tea consumption. Green tea can be beneficial to health because green tea is high in polyphenols, which have powerful antioxidant activity, as well as alkaloids, amino acids, carbohydrates, chlorophyll, and fluoride, aluminum, and other minerals and trace elements. Green tea may help prevent cancer and Parkinson disease, increase blood flow and mental alertness, and treat genital warts. Research suggests that green tea may prevent Alzheimer's disease, heart disease and stroke. The caffeine in green tea can worsen certain medical conditions, including gastroesophageal reflux disease (GERD), migraine, anxiety, arrhythmias, insomnia or other sleep disturbances, and benign fibrocystic breast disease. Women who are pregnant should consume fewer than 2 cups of tea a day to reduce risk of preterm labor and stunting of fetal growth. High amounts of caffeine consumption (> 300 mg/day) may interfere with normal growth and development in children and adolescents.

—*Cherie Marcel, BS*

REFERENCES

Borgwardt, S., Hammann, F., Scheffler, K., Kreuter, M., Drewe, J., & Beglinger, C. (2012). Neural effect of green tea extract on dorsolateral prefrontal cortex. *European Journal of Clinical Nutrition*, 66(11), 1187-1192. doi:10.1038/ejcn.2012.105

Kim, Y. H., & Bowers, J. (2008). Health benefits of tea. *Alternative Therapies in Women's Health*, 10(2), 9-12.

Kokubo, Y., Iso, H., Saito, I., Yamagishi, K., Yatsuya, H., Ishihara, J., ... Tsugane, S. (2013). The impact of green tea and coffee consumption on the reduced risk of stroke incidence in Japanese population: the Japan public health center-based study cohort. *Stroke*, 44(5), 1369-1374. doi:10.1161/STROKEAHA.111.677500

Lambert, J. D., Hong, J., Yang, G. Y., Liao, J., & Yang, C. S. (2005). Inhibition of carcinogenesis by polyphenols: Evidence from laboratory investigations. *American Journal of Clinical Nutrition*, 81(1 Suppl), 284S-291S.

Miyazaki, R., Kotani, K., Ayabe, M., Tsuzaki, K., Shimada, J., Sakane, N., ... Ishii, K. (2013). Minor effects of green tea catechin supplementation on cardiovascular risk markers in active older people: A randomized controlled trial. *Geriatrics & Gerontology International*, 13(3), 622-629. doi:10.1111/j.1447-0594.2012.00952.x

Mozaffari-Khosravi, H., Ahadi, Z., & Barzegar, K. (2013). The effect of green tea and sour tea on blood pressure of patients with type 2 diabetes: A randomized clinical trial. *Journal of Dietary Supplements*, 10(2), 105-115. doi:10.3109/19390211.2013.790333

National Cancer Institute. (2010). Tea and cancer prevention: Strengths and limits of evidence. Retrieved June 2, 2015, from http://www.cancer.gov/about-cancer/causes-prevention/risk/diet/tea-fact-sheet

Natural Medicines Comprehensive Database. (2015, March 20). Green tea. *Medline Plus*. Retrieved June 2, 2015, from http://www.nlm.nih.gov/medlineplus/druginfo/ natural/960.html

Nelson, M., & Poulter, J. (2004). Impact of tea drinking on iron status in the UK: A review. *Journal of Human Nutrition and Dietetics*, 17(1), 43-54. doi:10.1046/j.1365-277X.2003.00497.x

Ren, J. S., Freedman, N. D., Kamangar, F., Dawsey, S. M., Hollenbeck, A. R., Schatzkin, A., & Abnet, C. C. (2010). Tea, coffee, carbonated soft drinks and upper gastrointestinal tract cancer risk in a large United States prospective cohort study. *European Journal of Cancer (Oxford, England: 1990)*, 46(10), 1873-1881. doi:10.1016/ j.ejca.2010.03.025

Shimizu, M., Shirakami, Y., Sakai, H., Kubota, M., Kochi, T., Ideta, T., ... Moriwaki, H. (2015). Chemopreventive potential of green tea catechins in hepatocellular carcinoma.

International Journal of Molecular Sciences, *16*(3), 6124-6139. doi:10.3390/ijms16036124

Thankachan, P., Walczyk, T., Muthayya, S., Kurpad, A. V., & Hurrell, R. F. (2008). Iron absorption in young Indian women: The interaction of iron status with the influence of tea and ascorbic acid. *American Journal of Clinical Nutrition*, *87*(4), 881-886.

Trujillo, E., & Ross, S. (2009). Tea and cancer prevention. *Oncology Nutrition Connection*, *17*(2), 10-14.

Tufts University. (2013). Green tea protects brain cells. *Tufts University Health & Nutrition Letter*, *31*(4), 7.

REVIEWER(S)

Darlene Strayer, RN, MBA, Cinahl Information Systems, Glendale, CA

Nursing Executive Practice Council, Glendale Adventist Medical Center, Glendale, CA

Herbal Tea

WHAT WE KNOW

Traditional tea is produced from the *Camellia sinensis* plant, and depending on the preparation methods used, is categorized as black, green, white, or oolong. Herbal brews, commonly called teas, are not technically considered tea but are infusions of boiled water and the flowers, seeds, or roots of various herbs. There are thousands of possible herbal tea combinations, and as many different claims of health benefits as there are warnings regarding harm. It is not possible to make a general statement about the nutritional benefits or risks of herbal tea; each variation should be separately assessed. The following summary information focuses on some of the more popular herbal brews, including peppermint, spearmint, ginger, dandelion, and chamomile.

- Peppermint (*Mentha piperita*) is a greenish-purple plant that has small purple flowers. Tea made from peppermint leaves has a fresh, strong flavor and aroma.
  - The fresh leaves of peppermint contain as much vitamin C as an orange and more beta-carotene than a carrot. Peppermint contains a high amount of manganese and trace amounts of iron, calcium, folate, potassium, magnesium, riboflavin, copper, tryptophan, and omega-3 fatty acids

  - Peppermint has been used therapeutically to resolve gastrointestinal distress and to reduce symptoms of irritable bowel syndrome (IBS)

- Spearmint (*Mentha viridis* and *Mentha spicata*) has long, spear-like leaves that can be smooth or have gray hairs and pale blue flowers. Spearmint tea has a flavor and aroma that is similar to peppermint tea, and is also rich in vitamin C and beta-carotene.
  - Historically, spearmint has been used to treat gastrointestinal distress, sinusitis, fever, the common cold, respiratory conditions, dandruff, and halitosis (i.e., bad breath). Currently, the medicinal use of spearmint is not recommended due to the lack of high-quality trials in humans

- Ginger, or *Zingiber officinale*, is a perennial, aromatic plant that has green and purple flowers. Ginger has an aromatic quality and is frequently used in aroma therapy oils. Ancient Greeks and Romans valued ginger as an antiemetic (i.e. anti-nausea) and a digestive aid, as did East Indian and Chinese civilizations. Ginger has also been used as an appetite stimulant and to treat colds, fever, arthritis, and migraine headaches.

- Dandelion, or *Taraxacum officinale*, is a perennial herb that is considered by some to be a weed. It has jagged-edged leaves and yellow flowers that become white, spherical puffballs of seeds when the flower petals die.
  - Dandelion has great nutritional value. There are approximately 1,400 international units (IU) of vitamin A in the form of beta-carotene per 100 grams of dandelion leaf. Leaves contain vitamins B, C, and D and the minerals calcium, chromium, copper, iron, magnesium, potassium, selenium, sulfur, and zinc
  - Although scientific evidence is lacking regarding the benefits of dandelion, it is frequently used as a home remedy in some populations to treat gastrointestinal distress, constipation, loss of appetite, gallstones, joint and muscle pain, hypertension, eczema, bruises, and viral infection

- The most commonly consumed chamomile teas are German chamomile (*Matricaria recutita*) and English, or Roman, chamomile (*Chamaemelum nobile*). Although the two teas are made from two different plants, they have similar properties and are used in similar ways. Both chamomile plants have very small, white flowers with yellow centers, which are used to make chamomile tea.

- —Chamomile contains small amounts of calcium, magnesium, potassium, fluoride, folate, and pro-vitamin A carotenoids
- —Chamomile is frequently used to calm or sooth anxiety and aid in sleep, and is used to treat inflammation, muscle spasms, gastrointestinal distress, and oral lesions

NUTRIENTS IN HERBAL TEAS

- Peppermint exhibits antifungal and antibacterial properties, halting the growth of numerous bacteria, including *Helicobacter pylori*, *Salmonella enteritidis*, *Escherichia coli* O157:H7, and methicillin-resistant *Staphylococcus aureus* (MRSA). The phytonutrients (i.e., beneficial plant-derived chemicals) found in peppermint have demonstrated health benefits that include the following:
  - —The menthol in peppermint soothes the smooth muscles surrounding the intestines, reducing spasms and calming indigestion
  - —Perillyl alcohol derived from the essential oils in peppermint has been shown to inhibit the growth of pancreatic, breast, and liver tumors. There is evidence that it protects against cancer of the colon, skin, and lungs
  - —Peppermint contains rosmarinic acid, which is an antioxidant and anti-inflammatory that promotes the production of prostacyclins, allowing airways to open for easier breathing
- There is some scientific evidence that spearmint exhibits antibacterial, antifungal, antidepressant, chemopreventive, antioxidant, lipid-reducing, sedative, and anti-inflammatory activities.
  - —The active components of spearmint include the phytonutrients carvone, limonene, phellandrene, and pinene. Unlike peppermint, spearmint does not contain menthol
- The most commonly used portion of the ginger plant is the rhizome, or root stem. The rhizome contains the active components gingerol and gingerdione, which have many pharmacologic properties, including the following:
  - —Antipyretic (i.e., fever reducer)
  - —Analgesic (i.e., pain reliever)
  - —Antitussive (i.e., cough suppressant)

- —Cardiac inotropic (i.e., change in force of heart contraction)
- —Sedative
- —Antibiotic
- —Mild antifungal
- —Ginger's aroma is attributed to its pungent ketones, including gingerol
- Dandelion contains many phytonutrients, some of which include the following:
  - —Sesquiterpene lactones are chemical compounds that can reduce inflammation, stimulate digestion, and relax the sympathetic nervous system
  - —Triterpenes such as the phytosterols stigmasterol and sitosterol are steroid compounds that are similar to cholesterol. It is believed that these phytosterols may inhibit tumor growth and aid regulation of blood lipids
  - —Lecithin, a fatty substance, exhibits anti-inflammatory activity
- Chamomile contains flavonoids, which are the color pigments of red, yellow, and orange. Flavonoids protect blood vessels from rupture and exhibit antioxidant, antibiotic, and anti-inflammatory activity.

DIETARY INTAKE RECOMMENDATIONS

- Although there is no recommended standardized dosage for herbal tea, some common preparations and uses include the following:
  - —Peppermint and spearmint teas are frequently consumed twice a day; preparation is by steeping 1 tablespoon of the leaves in 8 oz hot water
  - —Clinical studies on the use of ginger as an antiemetic have used 500–1,000 mg of powdered ginger or 1,000 mg of fresh ginger rhizome; preparation is by simmering the ginger in water for 10–15 minutes
  - —Dandelion tea can be made from the root or the leaves in the following ways:
    - –The root can be roasted and used as a substitute for coffee beans
    - –To prevent bitterness, the leaves are best harvested in spring before flowering. Blanching or soaking overnight can reduce the bitterness of the leaves. Preparation is by steeping 1 tablespoon of the leaves in 8 oz hot water

—Chamomile is typically consumed 3–4 times a day between meals; preparation is by steeping 2–3 heaping tablespoon of dried flower heads in 8 oz boiling water for 10–15 minutes

ADVERSE REACTIONS

- Adverse effects from the consumption of ginger are rare, but dosages higher than 5 gm/day can result in abdominal discomfort, diarrhea, and/or irritation in the mouth and throat.
  - —Extreme overdose of ginger can cause central nervous system depression and result in cardiac arrhythmias
  - —Treatment of adverse reactions is to discontinue ginger consumption
- Persons who have allergies to ragweed, daisies, chrysanthemums, marigolds, asters, or yarrow should avoid chamomile due to the possibility of an allergic reaction.
- Pregnant women are advised not to drink chamomile tea due to the potential for increased risk of miscarriage.
- Peppermint oil can slow the rate of cyclosporine breakdown in the body, potentially resulting in increased side effects of cyclosporine being received as treatment.
- There is some evidence that spearmint can inhibit iron absorption, and patients receiving iron should consider limiting spearmint consumption.
- Ginger can interact with certain medications in the following ways:
  - —Ginger can interfere with antacids by increasing stomach acid
  - —Ginger can enhance the effects of barbiturates
  - —Ginger may interfere with medications used to treat blood pressure, cardiac disease, or diabetes mellitus due to its potential to affect blood pressure, cardiac rhythm, and blood glucose levels
- Dandelion can interact with certain medications in the following ways:
  - —Consuming a large amount of dandelion may interfere with the absorption of certain antibiotics, including ciprofloxacin, enoxacin, norfloxacin, sparfloxacin, trovafloxacin, gatifloxacin, levofloxacin, lomefloxacin, moxifloxacin, ofloxacin, and grepafloxacin
  - —Dandelion can have diuretic properties that may decrease the body's efficiency in

eliminating lithium and result in excess lithium levels in persons receiving lithium as treatment

RESEARCH FINDINGS

- Researchers of several studies report that spearmint has anti-androgenic effects and could diminish sexual libido. Spearmint-induced oxidative stress in the hypothalamus leading to reduced production of luteinizing hormone (LH) and follicular stimulating hormone (FSH) is suspected to be responsible for the down-regulation of testicular testosterone production. Along with these findings, researchers report that spearmint is effective as an alternative to anti-androgenic treatment in women with hirsutism (i.e., unwanted, male-pattern hair growth). Further study is needed to test the reliability of these results.
- Many study results are promising for the use of ginger in the treatment of pregnancy-induced nausea and vomiting. Results have repeatedly indicated that ginger therapy is more effective as an antiemetic than vitamin B6 or placebo. Ginger may be a good alternative treatment option because many pharmaceutical antiemetic medications have side effects of sedation. Researchers have reported success in treating motion sickness with ginger, although ginger was not an effective treatment for individuals with vertigo. Study results are inconsistent regarding the effectiveness of ginger in treating postoperative nausea and vomiting or nausea and vomiting caused by chemotherapy.

SUMMARY

Consumers should become knowledgeable about the physiologic risks and benefits of the consumption of herbal teas. Due to the numerous varieties of herbal teas, it is difficult to make a general statement about the nutritional benefits or risks of consumption. Some of the reported benefits of herbal teas include reducing gastrointestinal distress and nausea, as well as aiding in sleep and anxiety. Pregnant women, individuals with allergies, or individuals taking medications should be aware of the possible risks and adverse effects of herbal teas. Consumers should also aim to eat a well-rounded diet that includes a variety of fruits, vegetables, whole grains, and lean proteins.

—Cherie Marcel, BS

REFERENCES

Abascal, K., & Yarnell, E. (2009). Clinical uses of Zingiber officinale (ginger). *Alternative & Complementary Therapies*, *15*(5), 231-237.

Akdogan, M., Tamer, M. N., Cure, E., Cure, M. C., Koroglu, B. K., & Delibas, N. (2007). Effect of spearmint (Mentha spicata Labiatae) teas on androgen levels in women with hirsutism. *Phytotherapy Research*, *21*(5), 444-447.

Borrelli, F., Capasso, R., Aviello, G., Pittler, M. H., & Izzo, A. A. (2005). Effectiveness and safety of ginger in the treatment of pregnancy-induced nausea and vomiting. *Obstetrics & Gynecology*, *105*(4), 849-856.

Edgar, J. (2009). Types of teas and their health benefits. *WebMD*. Retrieved June 3, 2015, from http://www.webmd.com/diet/features/tea-types-and-their-health-benefits

Ehrlich, S. D. (2011). Peppermint. *University of Maryland Medical Center*. Retrieved June 3, 2015, from http://umm.edu/health/medical/altmed/herb/peppermint

Ehrlich, S. D. (2013). Chamomile. *University of Maryland Medical Center*. Retrieved June 3, 2015, from http://umm.edu/health/medical/altmed/herb/german-chamomile

Ensiyeh, J., & Sakineh, M. C. (2009). Comparing ginger and vitamin B6 for the treatment of nausea and vomiting in pregnancy: A randomised controlled trial. *Midwifery*, *25*(6), 649-653. doi:10.1016/j.midw.2007.10.013

Ford, A. C., Talley, N. J., Spiegel, B. M. R., Foxx-Orenstein, A. E., Schiller, L., Quigley, E. M. M., & Moayyedi, P. (2010). Effect of fibre, antispasmodics, and peppermint oil in the treatment of irritable bowel syndrome: A systematic review and meta-analysis. *British Medical Journal*, *337*(7683), 1388-1392. doi:10.1136/bmj.a2313

The George Mateljan Foundation editorial staff. (n.d.). Peppermint. *The World's Healthiest Foods*. Retrieved June 3, 2015, from http://www.whfoods.com/genpage.php? tname=foodspice&dbid=102

Grant, P. (2010). Spearmint herbal tea has significant anti-androgen effects in polycystic ovarian syndrome. A randomized controlled trial. *Phytotherapy Research*, *24*(2). doi:10.1002/ptr.2900

Johnson, K. (2014, November 3). Vitamins and supplements lifestyle guide: Elderberry. *WebMD*. Retrieved June 3, 2015, from http://www.webmd.com/vitamins-and-supplements/lifestyle-guide-11/supplement-guide-elderberry

Medline Plus editorial team. (2015, February 14). Dandelion. *MedlinePlus*. Retrieved June 3, 2015, from http://www.nlm.nih.gov/medlineplus/druginfo/natural/706.html

Pillai, A. K., Sharma, K. K., Gupta, Y. K., & Bakhshi, S. (2011). Anti-emetic effect of ginger powder versus placebo as an add-on therapy in children and young adults receiving high emetogenic chemotherapy. *Pediatric Blood & Cancer*, *56*(2), 234-238. doi:10.1002/pbc.22778

Rainey, A. (2011). Nutrition & caffeine facts on chamomile tea. *Livestrong.com*. Retrieved June 3, 2015, from http://www.livestrong.com/article/517639-nutrition-caffeine-facts-on-chamomile-tea/

Schwartz, V. S. (2011). Use of ginger to relieve nausea and vomiting. *Support Line*, *33*(3), 19-24.

Ulbricht, C., Costa, D., Grimes Serrano, J. M., Guilford, J., Isaac, R., Seamon, E., & Varghese, M. (2010). An evidence-based systematic review of spearmint by the Natural Standard Research Collaboration. *Journal of Dietary Supplements*, *7*(2), 179-215. doi:10.3109/19390211.2010.486702

White, B. (2007). Ginger: An overview. *American Family Physician*, *75*(11), 1689-1691.

REVIEWER(S)

Sharon Richman, MSPT, Cinahl Information Systems, Glendale, CA

Nursing Executive Practice Council, Glendale Adventist Medical Center, Glendale, CA

Red Wine

WHAT WE KNOW

Red wine is an alcoholic beverage produced by fermenting dark colored (i.e., red, purple, black) grapes. Using fermentation to make wine out of grapes is an age-old technique that is documented as first occurring about 6,000BC in the areas of present-day Georgia and Iran. Red wine has been used in celebrations, traditions, the practice of medicine, and cooking in almost every culture, making it a highly valued commodity. In recent years scientists have researched the potential health benefits of certain constituents of red wine, particularly the phytochemical resveratrol. The skin of red grapes contains a high concentration of resveratrol, which has been reported to reduce oxidative stress and inflammation, potentially

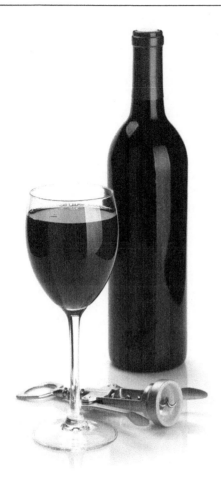

rupture. Flavonoids exhibit antioxidant, anti-biotic, and anti-inflammatory activity

DIETARY INTAKE RECOMMENDATIONS
- The American Heart Association (AHA) recommends that those who do consume alcohol do so in moderation.
  - It is recommended that men limit alcohol consumption to 2 drinks/day and women limit alcohol consumption to 1 drink/day, preferably to be consumed with meals
  - 1 alcoholic drink is equivalent to 12 oz of beer, 4 oz of wine, or 1½ oz of 80-proof liquor

ALCOHOL TOXICITY
- Alcohol is metabolized by the liver at a rate of one-half oz per hour. Alcohol is toxic to all human cells; excessive intake can have harmful effects.
- Signs and symptoms of alcohol toxicity (i.e., alcohol poisoning) include the following:
  - Confusion, stupor, loss of consciousness
  - Vomiting
  - Irregular or slowed respiration
  - Seizures
  - Hypothermia
- Treatment for alcohol toxicity includes the following:
  - Monitor breathing and provide oxygen therapy as needed
  - Provide fluids to prevent dehydration

ADVERSE REACTIONS
- Alcohol can interfere with many medications. It is important to consult the healthcare practitioner regarding the compatibility of any medications being taken with alcohol consumption.

RESEARCH FINDINGS
- Researchers report that consumption of 300 ml/day of red wine with a meal is effective in preventing the postprandial (i.e., after eating) increase in products of cholesterol oxidation in the blood (i.e., the damaging cholesterol that accumulates as plaque). Further research results reveal that red wine consumption also increases triglycerides and uric acid. High uric acid levels are indicated as a factor in nonalcoholic fatty liver disease (NAFLD); the elevated triglycerides and

reducing the risk for cardiovascular disease (CVD), cancer, and inflammatory diseases (e.g., colitis). In addition to the powerful antioxidants in red wine, researchers report that its alcohol content contributes a health benefit. However, due to the health risks associated with abuse of alcohol and alcoholism, some healthcare providers are hesitant to recommend that patients start drinking red wine.

NUTRIENTS IN RED WINE
- Red wine is a rich source of phytonutrients (i.e., beneficial plant-derived chemicals), including resveratrol and many flavonoids.
  - Resveratrol prevents damage to blood vessels, lowers low-density lipoprotein (LDL) cholesterol (i.e., the "bad" cholesterol), and inhibits blood clots from forming
  - Flavonoids are the color pigments red, yellow, and orange, which protect blood vessels from

uric acid could induce liver damage. Researchers suggest that these inconsistencies be studied to accurately determine if the consumption of red wine has more postprandial metabolic benefits or stressors.

- Results of studies indicate that moderate consumption of red wine appears to be protective against several age-related diseases (e.g., CVD, Alzheimer's disease) due to its reported favorable effects on immune function.

SUMMARY

Consumer should become knowledgeable about the physiologic effects of red wine consumption. Red wine is a rich source of phytonutrients, including resveratrol and many flavonoids, which have been reported to reduce oxidative stress and inflammation, potentially reducing the risk for heart disease, cancer, and inflammatory diseases. Red wine should be consumed in moderation due to the risks of alcohol addiction. It is recommended that men limit alcohol consumption to 2 drinks/day and women limit alcohol consumption to 1 drink/day, preferably to be consumed with meals.

—*Cherie Marcel, BS*

REFERENCES

American Heart Association staff. (2015, January 12). Alcoholic beverages and cardiovascular disease. Retrieved June 3, 2015, from http://www.heart.org/HEARTORG/GettingHealthy/NutritionCenter/HealthyEating/Alcohol-and-Heart-Health_UCM_305173_Article.jsp

Cuervo, A., Reyes-Gavilan, C. G., Ruas-Madiedo, P., Lopez, P., Suarez, A., Guerimonde, M., & Gonzalez, S. (2015). Red wine consumption is associated with fecal microbiota and malondialdehyde in human population. *Journal of the American College of Nutrition*, 34(2), 135-141. doi:10.1080/07315724.2014.904763

Magrone, T., & Jirillo, E. (2010). Polyphenols from red wine are potent modulators of innate and adaptive immune responsiveness. *Proceedings of the Nutrition Society*, 69(3), 279-285. doi:10.1017/S0029665110000121

Mayo Clinic staff. (2014, April 25). Heart Disease. Red wind and resveratrol: Good for your heart? *Mayo Clinic*. Retrieved June 3, 2015, from http://www.mayoclinic.com/health/red-wine/HB00089

Mayo Clinic staff. (2014, December 5). Alchohol poisoning. *Mayo Clinic*. Retrieved June 3, 2015, from http://www.mayoclinic.com/health/alcohol-poisoning/DS00861/DSECTION=treatments%2Dand%2Ddrugs

Mullin, G. E. (2011). Red wine, grapes, and better health – Resveratrol. *Nutrition in Clinical Practice*, 26(6), 722-723. doi:10.1177/0884533611423927

Natella, F., Macone, A., Ramberti, A., Forte, M., Mattivi, F., Matarese, R. M., & Scaccini, C. (2011). Red wine prevents the postprandial increase in plasma cholesterol oxidation products: A pilot study. *British Journal of Nutrition*, 105(12), 1718-1723. doi:10.1017/S0007114510005544

Pasinetti, G. M. (2012). Novel role of red wine-derived polyphenols in the prevention of Alzheimer's disease dementia and brain pathology: Experimental approaches and clinical implications. *Planta Medica*, 78(15), 1614-1619. doi:10.1055/s-0032-1315377

Peluso, I., Manafikhi, H., Reggi, R., & Palmery, M. (2015). Effects of red wine on postprandial stress: Potential implication in non-alcoholic fatty liver disease development. *European Journal of Nutrition*, 54(4), 497-507. doi:10.1007/s00394-015-0877-2

REVIEWER(S)

Darlene Strayer, RN, MBA, Cinahl Information Systems, Glendale, CA

Nursing Executive Practice Council, Glendale Adventist Medical Center, Glendale, CA

Sugar-Sweetened Soft Drinks

WHAT WE KNOW

Soft drinks (commonly called soda) are carbonated beverages that are sweetened with either a caloric sugar sweetener or a noncaloric sweetener. Many soft drinks also contain caffeine. The caloric sweetener that is typically used to sweeten soft drinks is high-fructose corn syrup (HFCS). Soft drinks that are sweetened with a noncaloric sweetener are commonly referred to as diet soft drinks, and are typically sweetened with the artificial sweetener aspartame. Global soft drink sales have increased in recent decades. With an estimated increase of 300% in soft drink consumption in the past 20 years, sugar-sweetened soft drinks are now considered the

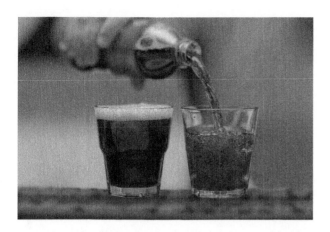

leading source of added sugar in the traditional Western diet, particularly in younger persons (i.e., persons under 40 years of age). This increase in consumption of sugar-sweetened soft drinks parallels the dramatic increase in rates of obesity over the past 2 decades. Researchers believe that the increased consumption of sugar-sweetened soft drinks and the high prevalence of obesity are intimately connected. However, drinking diet soft drinks instead of sugar-sweetened soft drinks does not appear to prevent obesity. In fact, researchers report that when compared with persons who do not consume diet soft drinks, consumers of diet soft drinks have a 70% larger waist circumference; researchers also report that intake of 1 or more diet soft drinks a day is linked to an increased risk for stroke.

- The HFCS in sugar-sweetened soft drinks contains the monosaccharide (i.e., simple sugar) fructose, glucose, and processed starches, which accelerate the absorption of fructose. Unlike glucose, fructose cannot be stored as glycogen to be used as energy; if consumed in large amounts, fructose is likely to be converted to fat by the liver. Fat that is synthesized by the liver is released into the bloodstream as very low density lipoproteins (VLDLs), which is a form of cholesterol that is known to contribute to coronary artery disease (CAD).
- Many soft drinks (e.g., Coke, Pepsi, Dr. Pepper, Mountain Dew) contain caffeine. Results of studies show that caffeine increases energy, awakens and clears the mind, and reduces the risk for depression. The primary action of caffeine is antagonism of the adenosine receptor. Adenosine dilates blood vessels and facilitates sleep. By binding with the adenosine receptor, caffeine interferes with the ability of adenosine to slow the body down. The result is increased neural activity (e.g., alertness, wakefulness). Caffeine is readily absorbed, and its effects last 4–6 hours. If consumed too close to bedtime, caffeine can interfere with the ability to fall asleep, and negatively affect sleep patterns.
- The consumption of both sugar-sweetened and diet soft drinks is associated with poor dietary and lifestyle choices, including higher intake of fast foods, unhealthy snacks, and sugary desserts; as well as lower intake of fruits and vegetables, less night-time sleep, and less regular exercise.

RESEARCH FINDINGS

- The intake of sugar-sweetened soft drinks has been shown to increase postprandial (i.e., after meals) blood glucose levels, decrease insulin sensitivity, and reduce the sensation of fullness, which results in overeating. Results of studies have linked the consumption of sugar-sweetened soft drinks to excessive weight gain, increased risk for type 2 diabetes mellitus (DM2), and increased triglycerides.
- Researchers report that large amounts of fructose consumption can result in visceral fat accumulation (i.e., in the abdominal cavity) and insulin resistance. Because fructose is converted to fat and stored in the liver, researchers are concerned that excessive intake of HFCS-sweetened soft drinks can contribute to non-alcoholic fatty liver disease (NAFLD).

SUMMARY

Consumers should become knowledgeable about the physiologic risks of sugar-sweetened soft drink consumption, specifically those with risk factors for obesity, DM2, and heart disease. Consumers should also be aware of the benefits of limiting sugar-sweetened soft drink consumption, and eating a balanced diet that includes unsaturated fats, lean proteins, complex carbohydrates, and a wide variety of fresh fruits and vegetables. Research suggests that drinking diet soft drinks instead of sugar-sweetened soft drinks does not appear to prevent obesity, and that consuming 1 or more diet soft drinks a day is associated with an increased risk for stroke.

—*Cherie Marcel, BS*

REFERENCES

Allman-Farinelli, M. A. (2009). Do calorically sweetened soft drinks contribute to obesity and metabolic disease?. *Nutrition Today, 44*(1), 17-20. doi:10.1097/NT.0b013e318195738b

Collison, K. S., Zaidi, M. Z., Subhani, S. N., Al-Rubeaan, K., Shoukri, M., & Al-Mohanna, F. A. (2010). Sugar-sweetened carbonated beverage consumption correlates with BMI, waist circumference, and poor dietary choices in school children. *BMC Public Health, 10*(234), 13. doi:10.1186/1471-2458-10-234

DeVault, N. (2014, January 29). What is the function of fructose?. *Livestrong.com*. Retrieved March 6, 2015, from http://www.livestrong.com/article/131995-what-is-function-fructose/

The editorial team of Environmental Nutrition. (2012). The diet soda-weight debate. *Environmental Nutrition, 35*(7), 7.

Evert, A., & Zieve, D. (2013, April 30). Caffeine in the diet. *MedlinePlus*. Retrieved March 6, 2015, from http://www.nlm.nih.gov/medlineplus/ency/article/002445.htm

Fiorito, L. M., Marini, M., Mitchell, D. C., Smiciklas-Wright, H., & Birch, L. L. (2010). Girls' early sweetened carbonated beverage intake predicts different patterns of beverage and nutrient intake across childhood and adolescence. *Journal of the American Dietetic Association, 110*(4), 543-550. doi:10.1016/j.jada.2009.12.027

Goodman, B. (2013). Fructose may affect hunger cues. *WebMD*. Retrieved March 6, 2015, from http://www.webmd.com/diet/news/20121231/fructose-hunger

Harrington, S. (2008). The role of sugar-sweetened beverage consumption in adolescent obesity: A review of the literature. *Journal of School Nursing, 24*(1), 3-12. doi:10.1622/1059-8405(2008)024[0003:TROSBC]2.0.CO;2

Hellerstein, M. K. (2012). Mitigating factors and metabolic mechanisms in fructose-induced nonalcoholic fatty liver disease: The next challenge. *American Journal of Clinical Nutrition, 96*(5), 951-952. doi:10.3945/ajcn.112.049650

Høstmark, A. T. (2010). The Oslo Health Study: A dietary index estimating high intake of soft drinks and low intake of fruits and vegetables was positively associated with components of the metabolic syndrome. *Applied Physiology, Nutrition & Metabolism, 35*(6), 816-825. doi:10.1139/H10-080

Jin, R., Le, N. A., Liu, S., Farkas, E. M., Ziegler, T. R., Welsh, J. A., ... Vos, M. B. (2012). Children with NAFLD are more sensitive to the adverse metabolic effects of fructose beverages than children without NAFLD. *Journal of Clinical Endocrinology & Metabolism, 97*(7), E1088-E1098. doi:10.1210/jc.2012-1370

Johnson, R.J., Lanaspa, M.A., Roncal-Jimenez, C., & Sanchez-Lozada, L.G. (2012). Effects of excessive fructose intake on health. *Annals of Internal Medicine, 156*(12), 905-906. doi:10.7326/0003-4819-156-12-201206190-00024

Kavey, R. E. (2010). How sweet it is: Sugar-sweetened beverage consumption, obesity, and cardiovascular risk in childhood. *Journal of the American Dietetic Association, 110*(10), 1456-1460. doi:10.1016/j.jada.2010.07.028

Nomura, K., & Yamanouchi, T. (2012). The role of fructose-enriched diets in mechanisms of nonalcoholic fatty liver disease. *Journal of Nutritional Biochemistry, 23*(3), 203-208. doi:10.1016/j.jnutbio.2011.09.006

Yamada, M., Murakami, K., Sasaki, S., Takahashi, Y., & Okubo, H. (2008). Soft drink intake is associated with diet quality even among young Japanese women with low soft drink intake. *Journal of the American Dietetic Association, 108*(12), 1997-2004. doi:10.1016/j.jada.2008.09.033

Yantis, M. A., & Hunter, K. (2010). Clinical queries. Is diet soda a healthy choice?. *Nursing, 40*(11), 67. doi:10.1097/01.NURSE.0000389036.71877.61

REVIEWER(S)

Sharon Richman, MSPT, Cinahl Information Systems, Glendale, CA

Nursing Executive Practice Council, Glendale Adventist Medical Center, Glendale, CA

Tea

WHAT WE KNOW

Tea, one of the world's most widely consumed beverages, is produced from the *Camellia sinensis* plant. Depending on the preparation method used, tea can be black, green, white, or oolong. Herbal brews are not technically considered tea, but are infusions of boiled water and various herbs, flowers, or fruits. Black tea is the most commonly consumed tea in the United States, United Kingdom, and Europe and accounts for nearly 75% of worldwide tea consumption. In Japan and China, green tea is the most commonly consumed tea. Of the 4 types of tea, oolong and white teas are brewed the least often.

- All 4 varieties of tea are high in polyphenols (i.e., organic chemicals containing multiple phenolic compounds), which have powerful antioxidant activity. Tea contains alkaloids (e.g., caffeine, theophylline, and theobromine), amino acids, carbohydrates, chlorophyll, fluoride, aluminum, and other minerals and trace elements. Green tea is especially high in polyphenols known as catechins, the most active of which is epigallo-catechin-3-gallate (EGCG). The catechins are believed to contribute most of the health benefits that are commonly attributed to tea consumption, including the prevention of heart disease, protection against many cancers (e.g., esophageal, ovarian, bladder), and decreased risk of developing Parkinson's disease. Tea has a caffeine-induced stimulant effect. Results of studies show that caffeinated tea boosts energy, awakens and clears the mind, and reduces risk for depression.

NUTRIENTS IN TEA

- Tea contains phytonutrients (i.e., beneficial plant-derivednutrients) such as polyphenols, including catechins and flavonoids, which promote the following anti-carcinogenic activities:
  - Activation of detoxification enzymes (e.g., glutathione S-transferase, quinone reductase) that protect against tumor development
  - Inhibition of tumor cell proliferation
  - Protective action against damaging ultraviolet (UV) B radiation
  - Enhancement of immune system function
  - Stimulation of intracellular antioxidant defenses
- Evidence suggests that consuming tea provides the following health benefits:
  - Black and green teas can prevent orthostatic hypotension (i.e., dizziness when arising from a lying position) and postprandial hypotension (i.e., low blood pressure after eating) by temporarily raising blood pressure.
  - Black and green teas increase mental alertness due to the caffeine content.

- Black and green teas are associated with reduced risk of developing Parkinson's disease.
- Black tea can reduce risk of heart attack and atherosclerosis.
- Black tea can reduce risk of developing kidney stones.
- Veregen, a green tea extract ointment produced by Bradley Pharmaceuticals, is used to treat genital warts.

ADVERSE REACTIONS

- Consumption of caffeinated tea can worsen certain medical conditions, including gastroesophageal reflux disease (GERD), migraine, arrhythmias, insomnia or other sleep disturbances, and benign fibrocystic breast disease.
- Caffeine consumption can increase anxiety.
- It is recommended that women who are pregnant consume fewer than 2 cups of tea a day to reduce risk for preterm labor and stunting of fetal growth.
- High amounts of caffeine consumption (> 300 mg/day) may interfere with normal growth and development in children and adolescents.
- Green and black teas can limit the absorption of non-heme iron from the diet, which poses a risk for individuals with iron-deficiency anemia; this can be mitigated by eating foods that enhance iron absorption (e.g., foods high in vitamin C such as lemons, oranges, and tomatoes) during the same meal or by drinking tea only between meals to prevent interference with iron absorption.

RESEARCH FINDINGS

- Results of numerous in vitro and animal studies show an inverse association between tea constituents (e.g., phytonutrients) and the cell growth of certain cancers, including bladder, esophageal, ovarian, and pancreatic cancer. This inverse association appears to be unrelated to the caffeine content, but is rather an effect of the many phytonutrients (e.g., catechins) provided by tea.
  - The catechin, epigallocatechin-3-gallate (EGCG), has demonstrated the ability to inhibit DNA methyltransferases (DNMTs) in human prostate cancer cells
  - Although the results of in vivo studies are mixed, authors of a systematic review of 51 studies that included a total of more than 1.6

million participants reported that evidence to support the consumption of green tea for cancer prevention was lacking. Further in vivo research is recommended for a more definitive understanding of the effectiveness of green tea intake for cancer prevention and treatment —Researchers report a synergistic effect between green tea and curcumin and capsium in inhibiting the growth of cancer cell lines in oral, head and neck cancers; potentially offering a preventative role against these cancers

- Recent research results show that individuals who regularly drink coffee or hot tea are about 50% less likely to have methicillin-resistant *Staphylococcus aureus* (MRSA) infection in the nasal passages. Scientists suggest that this is due to the antimicrobial properties of coffee and tea.

- High intake of coffee and tea is associated with a reduced risk of type 2 diabetes mellitus (DM2). This relationship exists with or without caffeine, suggesting that the protective effect is the result of the many chemical constituents that are present in coffee and tea, which appear to have a beneficial effect on glucose metabolism and insulin sensitivity. The exact mechanisms involved have not been identified and further scientific study is warranted.

- Researchers report an inverse relationship between the regular consumption of green tea and the risk of cardiovascular disease, including stroke. Evidence also indicates that green tea consumption can significantly decrease blood pressure in mildly hypertensive individuals with DM2.

SUMMARY

Consumers should become knowledgeable about the physiologic risks and benefits of tea consumption. Tea is high in polyphenols which have powerful antioxidant activity. Green tea is especially high in catechins, which are believed to contribute most of the health benefits commonly associated with tea consumption, including the prevention of heart disease and protection against many cancers. Caffeinated teas have a stimulant effect that has been shown to boost energy, awaken and clear the mind, and reduce the risk for depression. However, consumption of caffeinated tea can worsen certain medical conditions, including GERD, migraine,

arrhythmias, sleep disturbances, and benign fibrocystic breast disease. It is recommended that women who are pregnant consume fewer than 2 cups of tea a day to reduce risk for preterm labor and stunting of fetal growth. High amounts of caffeine consumption (> 300 mg/day) may interfere with normal growth and development in children and adolescents.

—*Cherie Marcel, BS*

REFERENCES

Boggs, D. A., Rosenberg, L., Ruiz-Narvaez, E. A., & Palmer, J. R. (2010). Coffee, tea, and alcohol intake in relation to risk of type 2 diabetes in African American women. *American Journal of Clinical Nutrition*, 92(4), 960-966. doi:10.3945/ajcn.2010.29598

The editorial staff at the American Institute for Cancer Research. (2013). Phytochemicals: The cancer fighters in the foods we eat. AICR. Retrieved March 6, 2015, from http://www.aicr.org/reduce-your-cancer-risk/diet/elements_phytochemicals.html

Fukino, Y., Ikeda, A., Maruyama, K., Aoki, N., Okubo, T., & Iso, H. (2008). Randomized controlled trial for an effect of green tea-extract powder supplementation on glucose abnormalities. *European Journal of Clinical Nutrition*, 62(8), 953-960.

Hanau, C., Morre, D. J., & Morre, D. M. (2014). Cancer prevention trial of synergistic mixture of green tea concentrate plus Capsicum (CAPSOL-T) in random population of subjects ages 40-84. *Clinical Proteomics*, 11(1), 11p. doi:10.1186/1559-0275-11-2

Huxley, R., Lee, C. M., Barzi, F., Timmermeister, L., Czernichow, S., Perkovic, V., ... Woodward, M. (2009). Coffee, decaffeinated coffee, and tea consumption in relation to incident type 2 diabetes mellitus: A systematic review with meta-analysis. *Archives of Internal Medicine*, 169(22), 2053-2063. doi:10.1001/archinternmed.2009.439

Kim, Y. H., & Bowers, J. (2008). Health benefits of tea. *Alternative Therapies in Women's Health*, 10(2), 9-12.

Kokubo, Y., Iso, H., Saito, I., Yamagishi, K., Yatsuya, H., Ishihara, J., ... Tsugane, S. (2013). The impact of green tea and coffee consumption on the reduced risk of stroke incidence in Japanese population: the Japan public health center-based study cohort. *Stroke*, 44(5), 1369-1374. doi:10.1161/STROKEAHA.111.677500

Lambert, J. D., Hong, J., Yang, G. Y., Liao, J., & Yang, C. S. (2005). Inhibition of carcinogenesis by polyphenols:

Evidence from laboratory investigations. *American Journal of Clinical Nutrition, 81*(1 Suppl), 284S-291S.

Lowenstein, K. (2011). The truth about tea. *Health, 25*(9), 88, 91-93.

Matheson, E. M., Mainous, A. G., Everett, C. J., & King, D. E. (2011). Tea and coffee consumption and MRSA nasal carriage. *Annals of Family Medicine, 9*(4), 299-304. doi:10.1370/afm.1262

Miyazaki, R., Kotani, K., Ayabe, M., Tsuzaki, K., Shimada, J., Sakane, N., ... Ishii, K. (2013). Minor effects of green tea catechin supplementation on cardiovascular risk markers in active older people: A randomized controlled trial. *Geriatrics & Gerontology International, 13*(3), 622-629. doi:10.1111/j.1447-0594.2012.00952.x

Mozaffari-Khosravi, H., Ahadi, Z., & Barzegar, K. (2013). The effect of green tea and sour tea on blood pressure of patients with type 2 diabetes: A randomized clinical trial. *Journal of Dietary Supplements, 10*(2), 105-115. doi:10.3109/19390211.2013.790333

Natural Medicines Comprehensive Database. (2013, November 11). Black tea. *Medline Plus.* Retrieved March 6, 2015, from http://www.nlm.nih.gov/medlineplus/druginfo/ natural/997.html

Natural Medicines Comprehensive Database. (2014, October 13). Green tea. *Medline Plus.* Retrieved March 6, 2015, from http://www.nlm.nih.gov/medlineplus/druginfo/ natural/960.html

Nelson, M., & Poulter, J. (2004). Impact of tea drinking on iron status in the UK: A review. *Journal of Human Nutrition and Dietetics, 17*(1), 43-54. doi:10.1046/j.1365-277X.2003.00497.x

Ramshankar, V., & Krishnamurthy, A. (2014). Chemoprevention of oral cancer: Green tea experience. *Journal of Natural Science, Biology, and Medicine, 5*(1), 7pp. doi:10.4103/0976-9668.127272

Ren, J. S., Freedman, N. D., Kamangar, F., Dawsey, S. M., Hollenbeck, A. R., Schatzkin, A., & Abnet, C. C. (2010). Tea, coffee, carbonated soft drinks and upper gastrointestinal tract cancer risk in a large United States prospective cohort study. *European Journal of Cancer (Oxford, England: 1990), 46*(10), 1873-1881. doi:10.1016/ j.ejca.2010.03.025

Song, W. O., & Chun, O. K. (2008). Tea is the major source of flavan-3-ol and flavonol in the U.S. diet. *Journal of Nutrition, 138*(8), 1543S-1547S.

Tan, A. C., Konczak, I., Sze, D. M., & Ramzan, I. (2011). Molecular pathways for cancer chemoprevention by dietary phytochemicals. *Nutrition and Cancer, 63*(4), 495-505. doi:10.1080/01635581.2011.538953

Thankachan, P., Walczyk, T., Muthayya, S., Kurpad, A. V., & Hurrell, R. F. (2008). Iron absorption in young Indian women: The interaction of iron status with the influence of tea and ascorbic acid. *American Journal of Clinical Nutrition, 87*(4), 881-886.

Trujillo, E., & Ross, S. (2009). Tea and cancer prevention. *Oncology Nutrition Connection, 17*(2), 10-14.

REVIEWER(S)

Darlene Strayer, RN, MBA, Cinahl Information Systems, Glendale, CA

Nursing Executive Practice Council, Glendale Adventist Medical Center, Glendale, CA

Herbs & Spices

Black Cohosh

WHAT WE KNOW

Black cohosh (*Actaea racemosa* or *Cimicifuga racemosa*) is an herbaceous, perennial plant from the *Ranunculaceae* (i.e., buttercup) family. Native to North America, black cohosh is a shrub that grows to be 3–8 feet tall and has large, feather-like leaves and a long plume of white flowers. The black creeping root, or rhizome, is harvested in the fall and is the portion of black cohosh that is used for medicinal preparations. With a long history of therapeutic use in both folk and traditional medicine, black cohosh is most noted for its role in the treatment of hot flashes and other symptoms of menopause. Although it was originally believed that black cohosh acted as a phytoestrogen, evidence regarding this theory is conflictive. Currently, there is no clear explanation for the mechanism of action for black cohosh.

ACTION OF BLACK COHOSH

- The active constituents in black cohosh rhizomes include triterpene glycosides, tannins, and resin (e.g., a natural plant compounds), along with fatty acids, starch, and sugar.

DOSAGE AND ADMINISTRATION

- The dosage that is most commonly used in research studies of black cohosh is 20–40 mg in tablets of standardized extract that are taken twice daily for a period of up to 6 months.

ADVERSE REACTIONS AND MEDICATION INTERACTION

- Women who are pregnant should avoid taking black cohosh due to the lack of research on its effects during pregnancy.
- Black cohosh is not recommended for persons with liver dysfunction due to the rare adverse effect of liver malfunction.
- Black cohosh is not recommended for women who have or previously had breast cancer, uterine cancer, or endometriosis due to the potential for estrogen-like activity.
- Persons at high risk for stroke or blood clots and persons with a seizure disorder should avoid taking black cohosh.
- Black cohosh should not be taken by individuals who are allergic to aspirin
- Black cohosh should not be taken with birth control pills, hormone replacement therapy, sedatives, or blood pressure medication without the close supervision of a doctor.

RESEARCH FINDINGS

- Evidence supporting the use of black cohosh extract for the treatment of menopausal symptoms is being questioned. A review of 16 studies reported that there was inadequate evidence to suggest the medicinal use of black cohosh for menopausal symptoms. However, authors of a meta-analysis of 9 randomized, placebo-controlled trials reported that in 6 of the studies, significant improvement was noted in the groups who received black cohosh compared with the groups who received placebo. Because black cohosh is one of the most commonly used herbal remedies for menopausal symptoms, researchers recommend that more research be conducted to determine if black cohosh is an effective and safe alternative to hormone replacement therapy.
- There have been claims that black cohosh can be used medicinally to treat some forms of cancer (e.g., lung), however, research does not support such claims. Additionally, there is evidence that black cohosh can interfere with some chemotherapy medications.

SUMMARY

Consumers should become knowledgeable about the physiologic effects of black cohosh. Black cohosh is rich in beneficial plant compounds making it a popular nutrition supplement. Research suggests black cohosh may aid in treating menopause symptoms and lung cancer, however further studies are needed to support claims and black cohosh may interfere with chemotherapy treatment.

—*Cherie Marcel, BS*

REFERENCES

American Cancer Society. (2011). Black Cohosh. *ACS*. Retrieved March 30, 2015, from http://www.cancer.org/treatment/treatmentsandsideeffects/complementaryandalternativemedicine/herbsvitaminsandminerals/black-cohosh

Becker, E., Letham, T., & Stoehr, J. D. (2009). Is black cohosh a safe and effective substitute for hormone replacement therapy? *Journal of the American Academy of Physician Assistants*, 22(9), 54-55.

Johnson, K. (2012). Black cohosh. *WebMD*. Retrieved March 30, 2015, from http://www.webmd.com/vitamins-and-supplements/lifestyle-guide-11/supplement-guide-black-cohosh

Johnson, T. L., & Fahey, J. W. (2012). Black cohosh: Coming full circle? *Journal of Ethnopharmacology*, 141(3), 775-779. doi:10.1016/j.jep.2012.03.050

Leach, M. J., & Moore, V. (2012). Black cohosh (Cimicifuga spp.) for menopausal symptoms. *Cochrane Database of Systematic Reviews*, 2012, 9. doi:10.1002/14651858.CD007244.pub2

McCracken, L. P., & Dunaway, A. (2011). Black cohosh. *Advance for NPs & Pas (ADV NPS PAS)*, 2(5), 41-42.

Office of dietary supplements. Black cohosh. (2008). *National institute of health*. Retrieved March 30, 2015, from http://ods.od.nih.gov/factsheets/BlackCohosh-HealthProfessional/

Ross, S. M. (2012). Menopause: A standardized isopropanolic black cohosh extract (remifemin) is found to be safe and effective for menopausal symptoms. *Holistic Nursing Practice*, 26(1), 58-61. doi:10.1097/HNP.0b013e31823d1f67

Shams, T., Setia, M. S., Hemmings, R., McCusker, J., Sewitch, M., & Ciampi, A. (2010). Efficacy of black cohosh-containing preparations on menopausal symptoms: A meta-analysis. *Alternative Therapies in Health & Medicine*, 16(1), 36-44.

Teschke, R. (2010). Black cohosh and suspected hepatotoxicity: Inconsistencies, confounding variables, and prospective use of a diagnostic causality algorithm. A critical review. *Menopause*, 17(2), 426-440. doi:10.1097/gme.0b013e3181c5159c

REVIEWER(S)

Darlene Strayer, RN, MBA, Cinahl Information Systems, Glendale, CA

Lori Porter, RD, MBA, Cinahl Information Systems, Glendale, CA

Nursing Executive Practice Council, Glendale Adventist Medical Center, Glendale, CA

Butterbur

WHAT WE KNOW

Butterbur, or *Petasites hybridus*, is an ancient, perennial, broad-leafed shrub from the sunflower, or *Asteraceae* family. Butterbur is also known as blatterdock, bog rhubarb, bogs horns, butter dock, and pestwurz. Butterbur grows throughout Europe and in Asia and North America in wet ground, and is frequently found by rivers and streams and in damp forests. As early as 65 A.D., a Greek physician named Dioscorides described the use of butterbur in medicine to treat fever, plague, chronic cough, asthma, gastrointestinal (GI) distress, and wounds. Modern science has affirmed that butterbur exhibits anti-inflammatory, antispasmodic, and antihistamine properties. Butterbur is primarily used currently to treat migraine headaches, hay fever, and asthma.

ACTION OF BUTTERBUR

- Along with a variety of phytochemicals (i.e., beneficial plant-derived chemicals; e.g., flavonoids, tannins, pyrrolizidine alkaloids), the predominant active constituents in butterbur are petasin and isopetasin:
    —Petasin has antispasmodic activity, relaxing smooth muscle and vascular walls, and reducing swollen membranes. It also acts as an antihistamine by decreasing the activation of mast cells, which interferes with the release of leukotrienes and histamine into circulation.
    —Isopetasin prevents the activation of inflammation.

RECOMMENDED DOSAGE AND ADMINISTRATION

- A dosage of 50–75mg of standardized butterbur root extract (containing 7.5 mg of isopetasin and petasin) can be taken twice daily. It is important that the extract does not contain pyrrolizidine alkaloids (PA), which can cause liver damage.

ADVERSE REACTIONS AND MEDICATION INTERACTION

- Butterbur contains PA, a plant toxin known to cause liver damage and increase the risk of developing liver cancer. Removing PA from preparations of butterbur intended for medicinal use is important.
- Women who are pregnant should not use butterbur because safety during pregnancy has not been established.
- Butterbur can interact with anticholinergic (i.e., medications that block the action of the neurotransmitter acetylcholine in the brain) such as ipratropium bromide, oxitropium bromide, and tiotropium.

RESEARCH FINDINGS

Results of many studies show significant evidence that standardized butterbur root extracts are effective in the prevention and reduction of asthma, seasonal allergies, and migraine headaches. In some cases, the effect of butterbur is equivalent to that of medications such as fexofenadine and cetirizine in the reduction of allergy symptoms. Researchers have also reported the medicinal use of butterbur to be safe, effective, and well tolerated (even among pediatric patients), with only occasional reports of belching as an adverse effect. While these results are promising, researchers suggest that more human trials be performed to confirm these findings and to determine the most effective therapeutic dosages for each condition.

SUMMARY

Consumers should become knowledgeable about the physiologic effects of butterbur ingestion. Butterbur is a good source of phytochemicals, which act as natural muscle relaxers and inflammation reducers. Research suggests that butterbur may help treat asthma symptoms, migraine headaches and allergic reactions.

—*Cherie Marcel, BS*

REFERENCES

Ackerson, A. (2006). Check out. Butterbur. *Better Nutrition*, 68(4), 16.

Brattström, A., Schapowal, A., Maillet, I., Schnyder, B., Ryffel, B., & Moser, R. (2010). Petasites extract Ze 339 (PET) inhibits allergen-induced Th2 responses, airway inflammation and airway hyperreactivity in mice. *Phytotherapy Research*, 24(5), 680-685. doi:10.1002/ptr.2972

Giles, M., Ulbricht, C., Khalsa, K. P., Kirkwood, C. D., Park, C., & Basch, E. (2005). Butterbur: An evidence-based systematic review by the Natural Standard Research Collaboration. *Journal of Herbal Pharmacotherapy*, 5(3), 119-143. doi:10.1080/J157v05n03_12

Käufeler, R., Polasek, W., Brattström, A., & Koetter, U. (2006). Efficacy and safety of butterbur herbal extract Ze 339 in seasonal allergic rhinitis: Postmarketing surveillance study. *Advances in Therapy*, 23(2), 373-384. doi:10.1007/BF02850143

Lynde, M. (2005). Herb profile: Butterbur: Help for healthy bladder control. *Alive: Canada's Natural Health and Wellness Magazine*, Jul(273), 50-51.

Martin, R. (2006). Butterbur extract: Effective, drug-free allergy relief. *Life Extension*, 12(5), 34-39.

Martin, R. (2006). What Europeans are doing to limit migraine frequency. *Life Extension*, 12(3), 30-36.

Meschino, J. P. (2010). Natural supplements for migraine prevention: Butterbur and feverfew. *Dynamic Chiropractic*, 28(19), 9p.

Oliff, H. S., & Blumenthal, M. (2005). Research reviews. Open clinical trial shows potential for butterbur root extract in asthma treatment. *HerbalGram*, Fall(68), 28.

Schapowal, A. (2005). Treating intermittent allergic rhinitis: A prospective, randomized, placebo and antihistamine-controlled study of butterbur extract Ze 339. *Phytotherapy Research*, 19(6), 530-537. doi:10.1002/ptr.1705

Smith, T. (2012). American Academy of Neurology, American Headache Society recommend special butterbur root extract for migraine prevention. *HerbalGram*, Jan(96), 19-20.

Sutherland, A., & Sweet, B. V. (2010). Butterbur: An alternative therapy for migraine prevention. *American Journal of Health-System Pharmacy*, 67(9), 705-706, 708, 710-711. doi:10.2146/ajhp090136

Utterback, G., Zacharias, R., Timraz, S., & Mershman, D. (2014). Butterbur extract: Prophylactic treatment for childhood migraines. *Complementary Therapies in Clinical Practice*, 20(1), 61-64. doi:10.1016/j.ctcp.2012.04.003

REVIEWER(S)
Rosalyn McFarland, DNP, RN, APNP, FNP-BC
Darlene Strayer, RN, MBA, Cinahl Information Systems, Glendale, CA
Nursing Executive Practice Council, Glendale Adventist Medical Center, Glendale, CA

Cacao

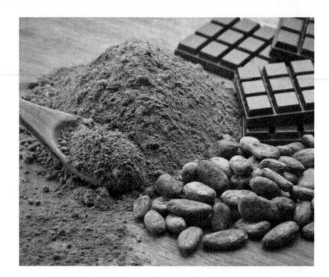

WHAT WE KNOW

The cacao tree, or *Theobroma cacao* (meaning food of god), produces the cacao bean and is more commonly known as the cocoa bean. Fermented and dried cocoa bean is the primary ingredient in chocolate. By adding varying quantities of milk solids and sweeteners to cocoa bean, its characteristic bitterness is reduced, resulting in chocolate that ranges from dark (containing a greater amount of pure cocoa) to light (containing less pure cocoa and more milk). The fat of the cocoa bean is used to make cocoa butter, which is often used as an ingredient in skin creams and fragrances. Chocolate is a well-known culinary substance that is used in baking, flavoring, cooking, and beverages. Cocoa beans have also been used medicinally for thousands of years. The ancient Mayan and Aztec civilizations are recorded as the first to use cocoa bean preparations to treat persons with ailments of the cardiovascular, gastrointestinal (GI), and nervous systems. Cocoa bean has been used to treat pain, such as toothache, rheumatism (i.e., joint pain), and abdominal discomfort. Modern research has established that the consumption of dark chocolate provides numerous health benefits, including a reduced risk for heart attack and stroke, cancer prevention, anti-inflammatory action, and improved cognitive function. These benefits are predominantly due to the polyphenolic compounds (i.e., plant-derived protective chemicals) within the cocoa bean.

ACTION OF COCOA BEANS

- Cocoa bean contains a variety of bioactive compounds, including fat, alkaloids, and polyphenolic compounds such as flavonols and procyanidins. The antioxidant properties identified in cocoa bean are primarily attributed to the polyphenols. The noted actions and benefits of these compounds include the following:
    - Polyphenols help to prevent type 2 diabetes mellitus, by decreasing insulin resistance
    - The monomeric flavonols epicatechin and catechin are thought to decrease risk of cardiovascular disease (CVD) and hypertension by preventing the oxidation of low-density lipoproteins (LDLs), enhancing endothelium-dependent relaxation, reducing inflammation, and inhibiting clot formation by the modulation of platelet function.
    - flavonols and procyanidins prevent cellular oxidation and eliminate reactive oxygen species
    - By increasing cerebral blood flow, the flavonols in cocoa bean improve sensitivity to visual contrast, spatial memory, and reaction time.
    - Other attributes of polyphenolic compounds include anti-carcinogenic activity, support of intestinal flora (i.e., "good" or "friendly" bacteria), and improvement of psychological well-being by reducing stress hormones and stimulating the release of opioids from the brain.

RECOMMENDED DOSAGE AND ADMINISTRATION

- No specific guidelines exist for therapeutic use of cocoa bean, although researchers suggest that 1 cup of dark chocolate daily is beneficial. If eating chocolate bars, a dark chocolate bar with at least 65 percent cacao that contains cocoa butter is more nutritious than a chocolate bar with a lower percent cacao that has added oils or hydrogenated or partially hydrogenated fats.
- Due to the natural caffeine content of cocoa bean, consumption of chocolate (particularly

dark chocolate) can worsen certain conditions, including gastroesophageal reflux disease (GERD) and insomnia or other sleep disturbance

RESEARCH FINDINGS

- Results of numerous studies show that moderate consumption of dark chocolate with a high cocoa content reduces the risk of heart disease and stroke. Results of one study found that 28 days of supplementation with cocoa flavonols and procyanidin significantly decreased the risk of blood clots. Researchers in a study in Germany found that adults aged 36–65 years who consumed higher amounts of dark chocolate have a lower risk for heart disease and stroke. Because chocolate has a high calorie content, excessive quantities should be avoided. Results of one study following the chocolate intake of 31,823 women aged 48–83 showed that women who consume 1–3 servings of chocolate each week are 26% less likely to experience heart failure than women who did not consume chocolate. Those who consumed 1–2 servings of chocolate each week had a 32% lower risk for heart failure. The women who consumed 3 or more servings of chocolate each week experienced no benefit compared with women who did not eat chocolate. Researchers hypothesized that this could be due to the added calories supplied by higher chocolate intake.
- Researchers report that cacao enhances the bioavailability of polyphenols (e.g., epicatechin) and that modifying cocoa powder to contain physiologically relevant concentrations of theobromine could promote human health by significantly increasing the absorption of beneficial polyphenols.

SUMMARY

Consumers should become knowledgeable about the physiologic risks and benefits of the consumption of cocoa bean.

Cocoa beans are rich in polyphenols which may help lower blood pressure and total cholesterol, and may help prevent type 2 diabetes, heart disease and cancer. Research suggests consumption of cocoa beans may improve overall health, although cocoa bean consumption from chocolate bars should be limited due to the high fat content. Cocoa beans contain caffeine which may cause GERD complications and sleep disturbances.

—*Cherie Marcel, BS*

REFERENCES

Abbey, M. J., Patil, V. V., Vause, C. V., & Durham, P. L. (2008). Repression of calcitonin gene-related peptide expression in trigeminal neurons by a Theobroma cacao extract. *Journal of Ethnopharmacology*, 115(2), 238-248. doi:10.1016/j.jep.2007.09.028

Almoosawi, S., McDougal, G. J., Fyfe, L., & Al-Dujaili, E. A. S. (2010). Investigating the inhibitory activity of green coffee and cacao bean extracts on pancreatic lipase. *Nutrition Bulletin*, 35(3), 207-212. doi:10.1111/j.1467-3010.2010.01841.x

Brill, J. B. (2011). Heal your heart with food. *Better Nutrition*, 73(2), 38-42.

Celaya, G. A. (2013). The role of the cacao bean in reducing the risk of cardiovascular disease in humans: A literature review. *Nutrition Perspectives: Journal of the Council on Nutrition*, 36(4), 5-18.

Franco, R., Onatibia-Astibia, A., & Martinez-Pinilla, E. (2013). Health benefits of methylxanthines in cacao and chocolate. *Nutrients*, 5(10), 4159-4173. doi:10.3390/nu5104159

Murphy, K. J., Chronopoulos, A. K., Singh, I., Francis, M. A., Moriarty, H., Pike, M. J., & Sinclair, A. J. (2003). Dietary flavonols and procyanidin oligomers from cocoa (Theobroma cacao) inhibit platelet function. *American Journal of Clinical Nutrition*, 77(6), 1466-1473.

Raymond, S. (2011). Longevity-promoting foods. *Alive: Canada's Natural Health & Wellness Magazine*, (348), 162-168.

Rusconi, M., & Conti, A. (2010). Theobroma cacao L., the food of the gods: A scientific approach beyond myths and claims. *Pharmacological Research: The Official Journal of the Italian Pharmacological Society*, 61(1), 5-13. doi:10.1016/j.phrs.2009.08.008

Tweed, V. (2011). Loco for cocoa. *Better Nutrition*, 18-19.

Yamamoto, T., Takahashi, H., Suzuki, K., Hirano, A., Kamei, M., Goto, T., ... Kawada, T. (2014). Theobromine enhances absorption of cacao polyphenol in rats. *Bioscience, Biotechnology, and Biochemistry*, 1, 5 pp.

REVIEWER(S)

Darlene Strayer, RN, MBA, Cinahl Information Systems, Glendale, CA

Teresa-Lynn Spears, RN, BSN, PHN, AE-C, Cinahl Information Systems, Glendale, CA

Nursing Practice Council, Glendale Adventist Medical Center, Glendale, CA

Caraway

WHAT WE KNOW

Caraway, or *Carum carvi Linn*, is an aromatic plant from the Apiaceae family that is native to Asia, Europe, and Africa. Because of its fragrant property, caraway is commonly used in perfumes, cosmetics, and as a culinary spice. It also has a long history of other uses. Medicinally, caraway has been used to treat bronchitis and gastrointestinal, rheumatic, and inflammatory disorders. Caraway exhibits antibacterial action against *Escherichia coli*, *Klebsiella* organisms, and *Enterobacter aerogenes*, and shows potential as a chemo-preventive and anti-carcinogenic agent.

ACTION OF CARAWAY

- Caraway essential oil (also called volatile oil) contains the biologically active components carvone, (+)-dihydrocarvone, limonene, and carvene.
- It has been noted for its antispasmodic, antibacterial, antimicrobial, anti-ulcerogenic, expectorant (i.e., cough suppressant), stimulant, tonic, diuretic, blood sugar lowering, anti-proliferative (i.e., cancer treating), and lipid-lowering properties.
- It is rich in petroselinic acid, an unusual monounsaturated fatty acid with a double bond at carbon 6, which provides significant antioxidant benefits.

RECOMMENDED DOSAGE AND ADMINISTRATION

- No dosage is recommended, but traditional use of caraway is 1–6 g of freshly crushed fruit (commonly referred to as seeds) ingested 2–4times daily between meals.

ADVERSE REACTIONS

- Taking very large amounts of essential caraway oil for a prolonged period of time can result in gastrointestinal (GI), liver, and/or kidney dysfunction.
- Treatment of adverse reactions is discontinuance of the use of caraway.

RESEARCH FINDING

- Researchers investigating the effectiveness of caraway in the treatment of GI disorders report that caraway oil combined with peppermint oil reduces inflammation, spasticity, and pain caused by irritable bowel syndrome (IBS) and functional dyspepsia. Scientists suspect that the spasmolytic effect is related to the calcium channel blocking activity of the two oils.
- Results of a randomized controlled trial conducted on diabetic Wistar rats showed that treatment with caraway extract can significantly lower lipids and blood glucose.
- Research results demonstrate that caraway oil has the ability to fight the pathogens E. coli, Klebsiella, Enterobacter aerogenes, and Helicobacter pylori, which are known to cause gastrointestinal dysfunction, ulcers, and cancer.
- Results of research indicate that caraway oil is chemo-preventive against colon cancer by interference with the function of phase I and II xenobiotic metabolizing enzymes in the liver.

SUMMARY

Consumers should become knowledgeable about the physiologic effects of caraway, including risks and benefits. Taking very large amounts of essential caraway oil for a prolonged period of time can result in GI, liver, and/or kidney dysfunction. Research suggests that moderate amounts of caraway may help treat inflammation and IBS pain, fight bacteria, lower blood sugar and lipid levels, and may help prevent cancer.

—*Cherie Marcel, BS*

REFERENCES

Adam, B., Liebregts, T., Best, J., Bechmann, L., Lackner, C., Neumann, J., ... Holtmann, G. (2006). A combination of peppermint oil and caraway oil attenuates the post-inflammatory visceral hyperalgesia in a rat model. *Scandinavian Journal of Gastroenterology*, 41(2), 155-160. doi:10.1080/00365520500206442

Dadkhah, A., Allameh, A., Khalafi, H., & Ashrafihelan, J. (2011). Inhibitory effects of dietary caraway essential oils on 1,2-dimethylhydrazine-induced colon carcinogenesis is mediated by liver xenobiotic metabolizing enzymes. *Nutrition & Cancer*, 63(1), 46-54. doi:10.1 080/01635581.2010.516473

Deeptha, K., Kamaleeswari, M., Sengottuvelan, M., & Nalini, N. (2006). Dose dependent inhibitory effect of dietary caraway on 1, 2-dimethylhydrazine induced colonic aberrant crypt foci and bacterial enzyme activity in rats. *Investigational New Drugs*, 24(6), 479-488. doi:10.1007/s10637-006-6801-0

Editorial team of Health-Care-Tips.org. (2013). Caraway herb description -- drug interactions, dosage, and some of its useful properties. *Health-Care-Tips. org.* Retrieved February 27, 2015, from http://www. health-care-tips.org/herbal-medicines/caraway.htm

Goerg, K. J., & Spilker, T. (2003). Effect of peppermint oil and caraway oil on gastrointestinal motility in healthy volunteers: A pharmacodynamic study using simultaneous determination of gastric and gall-bladder emptying and orocaecal transit time. *Alimentary Pharmacology & Therapeutics, 17*(3), 445-451. doi:10.1046/j.1365-2036.2003.01421.x

Holtmann, G., Haag, S., Adam, B., Funk, P., Wieland, V., & Heydenreich, C. J. (2003). Effects of a fixed combination of peppermint oil and caraway oil on symptoms and quality of life in patients suffering from functional dyspepsia. *Phytomedicine, 10*(Suppl 4), 56-57. doi:10.1078/1433-187X-00310

Jalali-Heravi, M., Zekavat, B., & Sereshti, H. (2007). Use of gas chromatography-mass spectrometry combined with resolution methods to characterize essential oil components of Iranian cumin and caraway. *Journal of Chromatography. A, 1143*(1-2), 215-226. doi:10.1016/j.chroma.2007.01.042

Koppula, S., Kopalli, S. R., & Sreemantula, S. (2009). Adaptogenic and nootropic activities of aqueous extracts of Carum carvi Linn (caraway) fruit: An experimental study in Wistar rats. *Australian Journal of Medical Herbalism, 21*(3), 72-78.

Laribi, B., Kouki, K., Mougou, A., & Marzouk, B. (2010). Fatty acid and essential oil composition of three Tunisian caraway (Carum carvi L.) seed ecotypes. *Journal of the Science of Food and Agriculture, 90*(3), 391-396. doi:10.1002/jsfa.3827

May, B., Funk, P., & Schneider, B. (2003). Peppermint oil and caraway oil in functional dyspepsia—efficacy unaffected by H. pylori. *Alimentary Pharmacology & Therapeutics, 17*(7), 975-976. doi:10.1046/j.1365-2036.2003.01522.x

Micklefield, G., Greving, I., & May, B. (2000). Effects of peppermint oil and caraway oil on gastroduodenal motility. *Phytotherapy Research, 14*(1), 20-23. doi:10.1002/(SICI)1099-1573(200002)14:1<20::AID-PTR542>3.0.CO;2-Z

Micklefield, G., Jung, O., Greving, I., & May, B. (2003). Effects of intraduodenal application of peppermint oil (WS(R) 1340) and caraway oil (WS(R) 1520) on gastroduodenal motility in healthy volunteers. *Phytotherapy Research: PTR, 17*(2), 135-140. doi:10.1002/ptr.1089

Sadeghian, S., Neyestani, T. R., Shirazi, M. H., & Ranjabarian, P. (2005). Bacteriostatic effect of dill, fennel, caraway and cinnamon extracts against Helicobacter pylori. *Journal of Nutritional & Environmental Medicine, 15*(2-3), 47-55. doi:10.1080/13590840500535313

Sadjadi, N. S., Shahi, M. M., Jalali, M. T., & Haidari, F. (2014). Short-term caraway extract administration imporves cardiovascular disease risk markers in streptozotocin-induced diabetic rats: A dose-response study. *Journal of Dietary Supplements, 11*(1), 30-39. doi:10.3109/19390211.2013.859214

Seidler-Lozykowska, K., Baranska, M., Baranski, R., & Krol, D. (2010). Raman analysis of caraway (Carum carvi L.) single fruits. Evaluation of essential oil content and its composition. *Journal of Agriculture and Food Chemistry, 58*(9), 5271-5275. doi:10.1021/jf100298z

REVIEWER(S)

Darlene Strayer, RN, MBA, Cinahl Information Systems, Glendale, CA

Nursing Practice Council, Glendale Adventist Medical Center, Glendale, CA

Cayenne Pepper

WHAT WE KNOW

Cayenne pepper (CP) is a member of the genus Capsicum from the Solanaceae family, which also includes bell pepper and jalapeño pepper. There are two species of CP: *Capsicum annuum*, which is native to Europe and the US, and *Capiscum frutescens*, which is native to South America and warmer regions of the US. Native Americans have used CP for medicinal and culinary purposes for thousands of years. As a spicy food additive, CP can be eaten raw, dried, or ground into a powder. Dietary consumption of CP has been shown to ease stomach ache and cramps, and may also help to protect the stomach lining from irritation by aspirin. Topically, elements derived from CP are used to treat the pain of arthritis, shingles, muscle spasm, and neuropathy. Other benefits of CP consumption include lowering of low-density lipoprotein cholesterol and triglycerides, and protection from free radicals. There is also evidence that it increases thermogenesis (i.e., calorie burning) and suppresses appetite, making it a potential dietary aid in weight control efforts.

ACTION OF CAYENNE PEPPER

- The active component of CP is capsaicin, which is predominantly found in the white membrane of the pepper. Capsaicin is known to reduce pain by lowering substance P, a chemical in the brain that transmits pain signals.
- CP has been used to treat sore throat, cough, gastric and intestinal discomfort, toothache, rheumatism, and parasitic infection.

RECOMMENDED DOSAGE AND ADMINISTRATION

- Capsaicin is sold over-the-counter in the form of topical creams. Each brand has specified instructions for use.
- For treatment of stomach ache, a few drops of hot sauce made with CP can be mixed with food twice a day, and increased up to 1 teaspoon per meal.
  - —Persons with stomach ache should avoid black pepper because it can irritate the stomach.

ADVERSE REACTIONS

- Individuals who have an ulcer or gastritis should use CP with caution because it can exacerbate those conditions.
- Topical capsaicin should not be applied to open wounds because it can irritate the wound and increase pain.

RESEARCH FINDINGS

- Authors of several studies report that capsaicin suppresses appetite and energy intake, increases the burning of calories, and enhances satiety, making capsaicin a useful strategy in managing weight loss. Researchers also report increased fat oxidation, noting that test subjects treated with capsinoids 6 mg/day experienced loss of abdominal fat.
  - —Capsinoids are a group of compounds in CP that are structurally similar to capsaicin.

SUMMARY

Consumers should become knowledgeable about the physiologic effects of CP, including its risks and benefits. CP is used to treat pain and infections, lowers total cholesterol and assists with weight loss efforts. Individuals who have an ulcer or gastritis should use CP with caution because it can exacerbate those conditions.

—*Cherie Marcel, BS*

REFERENCES

Cayenne (Capsicum spp.): An evidence-based systematic review by the Natural Standard Research Collaboration. (2014). *Alternative & Complementary Therapies*, *20*(3), 154-156. doi:10.1089/act.2014.20306

Galgani, J. E., & Ravussin, E. (2010). Effect of dihydrocapsiate on resting metabolic rate in humans. *American Journal of Clinical Nutrition*, *92*(5), 1089-1093. doi:10.3945/ ajcn.2010.30036

Goldstein, L. (2003). Fight fire with fire. *Prevention*, *55*(6), 2.

Ravishankar, G. (2008). Healing with the herb pepper - A plant with immense medicinal value. *Positive Health*, *143*, 28-29.

Reinbach, H. C., Smeets, A., Martinussen, T., Moller, P., & Westerterp-Plantenga, M. S. (2009). Effects of capsaicin, green tea and CH-19 sweet pepper on appetite and energy intake in humans in negative and positive energy balance. *Clinical Nutrition*, *28*(3), 260-265. doi:10.1016/j.clnu.2009.01.010

Singletary, K. (2011). Red pepper: Overview of potential health benefits. *Nutrition Today*, *46*(1), 33-47. doi:10.1097/NT.0b013e3182076ff2

Snitker, S., Fujishima, Y., Shen, H., Ott, S., Pi-Sunyer, X., Furuhata, Y., ... Takahashi, M. (2009). Effects of novel capsinoid treatment on fatness and energy metabolism in humans: Possible pharmacogenetic implications. *American Journal of Clinical Nutrition*, *89*(1), 45-50. doi:10.3945/ajcn.2008.26561

Toews, V. D. (2007). Hot news about cayenne. *Better Nutrition*, *69*(12), 22.

REVIEWER(S)

Darlene Strayer, RN, MBA, Cinahl Information Systems, Glendale, CA

Nursing Practice Council, Glendale Adventist Medical Center, Glendale, CA

Chive

WHAT WE KNOW

Chive (also known as Allium schoenoprasum and Allium tuberosum) is a hardy, bulb-forming herbaceous perennial plant from the Alliaceae family, which is native to Europe, Asia, and North America.

- Chive is appreciated for its savory, aromatic quality and is popular as a culinary herb. Chive has a long history of medicinal use for pain relief and antimicrobial activity. Planting chive in a garden is useful because it repels most insects but attracts bees.

- In addition to chive, the *Allium* genus includes many vegetables (e.g., garlic, onion, leeks, scallions) that are commonly referred to as allium vegetables.

ACTION OF CHIVE

- Chive is rich in folate, iron, magnesium, potassium, calcium, fiber, vitamins K, C, and B6, and the phytonutrient beta-carotene (i.e., provitamin-A, the precursor to vitamin A).
- Most of the active constituents of chive are found in the seeds and the grass-like hollow leaves that sprout from the bulb.
- Some reported actions of chive include pain relief, stimulant, diuretic, antiseptic, antimicrobial, antibacterial, and lowers blood pressure.
- The chive plant has been noted to have aphrodisiac properties.

ADVERSE REACTIONS

- Adverse reactions are rare.
- Very large amounts of chive can cause intestinal gas and discomfort.
- Adverse reactions are treated by discontinuing the use of chive.

RESEARCH FINDINGS

- Results of a study on allium vegetables and prostate cancer risk found that men who consumed > 10 g/day of allium vegetables were less prone to prostate cancer than men whose intake was < 2.2 g/day. This reduced risk was independent of other dietary variables. Other research results show that the chive extracts thiosulfinates inhibit cell growth and induce apoptosis (i.e., programmed cell death) in human prostate and colon cancer cells.
- When chive seed extracts were fed to normal rats to determine if it affected their sexual behavior, researchers found an overall increase in the sexual behavior of rats that received the extract, and reported that chive seed extract appears to have aphrodisiac activity.
- Results of a study regarding the antimicrobial activity of chive oil against food-born pathogenic bacteria show that chive oil inhibits several strains

of food-borne pathogens, including *Escherichia coli*.

SUMMARY

Consumers should become knowledgeable about the physiologic effects of chive consumption, including its risks and benefits. Chive is rich in vitamins, minerals, fiber and beta-carotene. Chive is used to treat pain and infections, and has been noted to have aphrodisiac properties. Research suggests chive may help prevent prostate cancer and may inhibit bacterial food borne illnesses.

—*Cherie Marcel, BS*

REFERENCES

Chung, D. M., Choi, N. S., Chun, H. K., Maeng, P. J., Park, S. B., & Kim, S. (2010). A new fibrinolytic enzyme (55 kDa) from Allium tuberosum: Purification, characterization, and comparison. *Journal of Medicinal Food*, 13(6), 1532-1536. doi:10.1089/jmf.2010.1144

Guohua, H., Yanhua, L., Rengang, M., Donghzi, W., Zhengzhi, M., & Hua, Z. (2009). Aphrodisiac properties of Allium tuberosum seeds extract. *Journal of Ethnopharmacology*, 122(3), 579-582. doi:10.1016/j.jep.2009.01.018

Hsing, A. W., Chokkalingam, A. P., Gao, Y. T., Madigan, M. P., Deng, J., Gridley, G., & Fraumeni, J. F., Jr. (2002). Allium vegetables and risk of prostate cancer: A population-based study. *Journal of the National Cancer Institute*, 94(21), 1648-1651. doi:10.1093/jnci/94.21.1648

Kim, S. Y., Park, K. W., Kim, J. Y., Jeong, I. Y., Byun, M. W., Park, J. E., ... Seo, K. I. (2008). Thiosulfinates from Allium tuberosum L. induce apoptosis via caspase-dependent and -independent pathways in PC-3 human prostate cancer cells. *Bioorganic & Medicinal Chemistry Letters*, 18(1), 199-204. doi:10.1016/j.bmcl.2007.10.099.

Lam, Y. W., Wang, H. X., & Ng, T. B. (2000). A robust cysteine-deficient chitinase-like antifungal protein from inner shoots of the edible chive Allium tuberosum. *Biochemical and Biophysical Research Communications*, 279(1), 74-80. doi:10.1006/bbrc.2000.3821.

Lee, J. H., Yang, H. S., Park, K. W., Kim, J. Y., Lee, M. K., Jeong, I. Y., ... Seo, K. I. (2009). Mechanisms of thiosulfinates from Allium tuberosum L.-induced apoptosis in HT-29 human colon cancer cells. *Toxicology Letters*, 188(2), 142-147. doi:10.1016/j.toxlet.2009.03.025.

McMillan, W. (2009). Health matters. In season: Chives. *Natural Solutions*, (120), 25.

Rattanachaikunsopon, P., & Phumkhachorn, P. (2008). Diallyl sulfide content and antimicrobial activity against food-borne pathogenic bacteria of chives (Allium schoenoprasum). *Bioscience, Biotechnology, and Biochemistry*, 72(11), 2987-2991. doi:10.1271/bbb.80482.

REVIEWER(S)

Darlene Strayer, RN, MBA, Cinahl Information Systems, Glendale, CA

Nursing Practice Council, Glendale Adventist Medical Center, Glendale, CA

Cinnamon

WHAT WE KNOW

Cinnamon (*Cinnamomum verum*; also known as Ceylon and "true cinnamon") is harvested from the bark of the cinnamon tree (*Cinnamomum zeylanicum*), which belongs to the laurel family. Although cinnamon is native to Sri Lanka, it is now cultivated worldwide in warmer climates such as the West Indies and East Asia.

- Cinnamon is appreciated for its aromatic quality and is commonly used as a culinary spice. It has a long history of other uses. Medicinally, cinnamon has been used to treat indigestion, cramps, colds, influenza, and yeast and fungal infections. It has been used as an antiseptic mouthwash, and some individuals believe it prevents cancer.

ACTION OF CINNAMON

- Cinnamon bark oils contain cinnamaldehyde, the organic compound that gives cinnamon it's flavor and odor and contributes to the antimicrobial and anti-inflammatory properties of cinnamon.

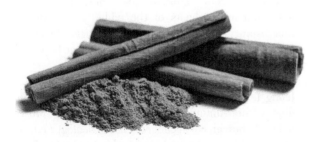

- Cinnamon has high levels of broadly bioactive compounds known as procyanidins, which have strong antioxidant properties and help regulate blood glucose levels.
- The polyphenols in cinnamon enhance insulin sensitivity, lower blood glucose levels, and minimize damage by glycation (i.e., process of protein or fat combining with a sugar molecule) end products.
- Cinnamon induces the sense of fullness when eating.

RECOMMENDED DOSAGE AND ADMINISTRATION

- Clinician researchers in studies have used 250 mg of cinnamon administered twice daily, or ¼ to 1 tsp of cinnamon daily for the management of blood glucose levels.

ADVERSE REACTIONS

- Adverse reactions to cinnamon are rare, although ingesting very large amounts can result in increased heart rate, increased intestinal motility, sleepiness, and depression.
- Treatment of adverse reactions is discontinuing the use of cinnamon.

RESEARCH FINDINGS

- Many studies have shown promising results for the use of cinnamon to help regulate blood glucose levels in individuals at risk for type 2 diabetes mellitus (DM2) and those with poorly controlled DM2. There is evidence that cinnamon may contribute to the prevention of metabolic syndrome and cardiovascular diseases, and study results demonstrate beneficial effects of cinnamon on lipids, antioxidant status, blood pressure, lean body mass, and gastric emptying.
  —Findings of a meta-analysis showed a statistically significant reduction of fasting blood glucose levels in individuals with DM2 and individuals with prediabetes after receiving cinnamon supplementation, although authors of a separate research review reported that cinnamon had no more of an effect on DM2 than placebo. Researchers suggest that further studies are necessary to determine the long-term benefits or risks associated with cinnamon use for persons with DM2.

- Researchers have investigated the effectiveness of cinnamon as a chemo-preventive agent. The results of one study showed that cinnamon extract was able to induce apoptosis (i.e., natural cell death) in cervical cancer cells by increasing intracellular calcium signaling. Results of another study indicated that cinnamon extract enhanced apoptosis, strongly inhibiting tumor cell proliferation and inducing active tumor cell death.

- Results of a study on the effect of cinnamon on multiple sclerosis (MS) showed that sodium benzoate, which is a metabolite of cinnamon, can inhibit the action of pro-inflammatory molecules in brain cells, which blocks the disease process of MS in mice.

SUMMARY

Consumers should become knowledgeable about the physiologic effects of cinnamon, including its risks and benefits. Cinnamon is used to lower blood sugars and research supports it may reduce the risk of developing type 2 diabetes. Cinnamon may also help treat infections and cancer.

—*Cherie Marcel, BS*

REFERENCES

Abascal, K., & Yarnell, E. (2010). The medicinal uses of cinnamon. *Integrative Medicine: A Clinician's Journal*, 9(1), 29-32.

Akilen, R., Tsiami, A., Devendra, D., & Robinson, N. (2010). Glycated haemoglobin and blood pressure-lowering effect of cinnamon in mulit-ethnic type 2 diabetic patients in the UK: A randomized, placebo-controlled, double-blind clinical trial. *Diabetic Medicine*, 27(10), 1159-1167.

Allen, R. W., Schwartzman, E., Baker, W. L., Coleman, C. I., & Phung, O. J. (2013). Cinnamon use in type 2 diabetes: An updated systematic review and meta-analysis. *Annals of Family Medicine*, 11(5), 452-459.

Andrews, L. (2013). Cochrane review brief: Cinnamon for diabetes mellitus. *Online Journal of Issues in Nursing*, 18(2), 12.

Chezem, J., Fernandes, N., Holden, J., & Bollinger, L. (2012). Efficacy and safety of 'true' cinnamon (Cinnamomum zeylanicum) as a pharmaceutical agent in diabetes: A systematic review and meta-analysis. *Journal of the Academy of Nutrition & Dietetics*, 112(Supplement A43).

Davis, P. A., & Yokoyama, W. (2011). Cinnamon intake lowers fasting blood glucose: Meta-analysis. *Journal of Medicinal Food*, 14(9), 884-889.

Gruenwald, J., Freder, J., & Armbruester, N. (2010). Cinnamon and health. *Critical Reviews in Food Science and Nutrition*, 50(9), 822-834.

Koppikar, S. J., Choudhari, A. S., Suryavanshi, S. A., Kumari, S., Chattopadhyay, S., & Kaul-Ghanekar, R. (2010). Aqueous cinnamon extract (ACE-c) from the bark of Cinnamomum cassia causes apoptosis in human cervical cancer cell line (SiHa) through loss of mitochondrial membrane potential. *BMC Cancer*, 10, 210.

Kwon, H. K., Hwang, J. S., So, J. S., Lee, C. G., Sahoo, A., Ryu, J. H., ... Im, S. H. (2010). Cinnamon extract induces tumor cell death through inhibition of NFKappaB and AP1. *BMC Cancer*, 10, 392. doi:10.1186/1471-2407-10-392

Lu, Z., Jia, Q., Wang, R., Wu, X., Wu, Y., Huang, C., & Li, Y. (2011). Hypoglycemic activities of A- and B-type procyanidin oligomer-rich extracts from different cinnamon barks.

Phytomedicine, 18(4), 298-302.

Magistrelli, A., & Chezem, J. C. (2012). Effect of ground cinnamon on postprandial blood glucose concentration in normal-weight and obese adults. *Journal of the Academy of Nutrition & Dietetics*, 112(11), 1806-1809.

Potential impact of cinnamon on multiple sclerosis studied. (2011). *News-Line for Speech-Language Pathologists & Audiologists*, 10(7-8), 4-5.

Qin, B., Panickar, K. S., & Anderson, R. A. (2010). Cinnamon: Potential role in the prevention of insulin resistance, metabolic syndrome, and type 2 diabetes. *Journal of Diabetes Science and Technology*, 4(3), 685-693.

Roth, S. L. (2011). Diabetes mellitus. In E. D. Schlenker & S. L. Roth (Eds.), *Williams' essentials of nutrition and diet therapy* (10th ed., p. 507). St. Louis, MO: Elsevier Mosby.

Zanteson, L. (2010). Celebrate the season with cinnamon for health. *Environmental Nutrition*, 33(12), 8.

Akilen, R., Tsiami, A., Devendra, D., & Robinson, N. (2012). Cinnamon in glycaemic control: Systematic review and meta analysis. *Clinical Nutrition*, 31(5), 609-615.

REVIEWER(S)

Darlene Strayer, RN, MBA, Cinahl Information Systems, Glendale, CA

Nursing Practice Council, Glendale Adventist Medical Center, Glendale, CA

Curcumin

WHAT WE KNOW

Curcumin, sometimes referred to as the curcumin complex, is a group of phytochemicals derived from the rhizome of the turmeric plant. The tall, tropical shrub turmeric, or *Curcuma longa*, is a member of the Zingiberaceae family, as is ginger. Curcumin gives turmeric a bright yellow color, as is apparent in yellow curry; curcumin is also used as a dye for clothes, foods, and cosmetics. It has long been appreciated for its vast medicinal qualities; for centuries, proponents of folk medicine have claimed that curcumin aids in digestion, heals wounds, reduces inflammation, reduces arthritic pain, soothes eye discomfort, promotes good health of ears and skin, treats liver disorders, controls blood glucose levels, resolves lung abnormalities, and has antiseptic properties. With over 1,875 articles on research results published during the period 1996–2005, modern science has substantiated many of these claims. Curcumin has proven to be a powerful antioxidant that has antitoxic, anti-inflammatory, and many other beneficial properties.

ACTION OF CURCUMIN

- Curcumin is a potent antioxidant that protects body cells and tissues by blocking free radical attacks by toxins in food; in the environment, including in water and air; and those produced internally, such as superoxide, hydrogen peroxide, and nitric oxide.
  —Curcumin protects deoxyribonucleic acid (DNA) from oxidation, reducing the risk of mutations, and protects the liver from solvent toxicity. It protects the brain from alcohol-induced damage and preserves the heart and kidneys from damage caused by pharmaceutical drugs.
  —By binding with key proteins, curcumin helps maintain gene integrity, supports hormonal regulation, and encourages detoxification, and is fundamental to homeostasis processes.
- Curcumin supports the health and vitality of the digestive system, including the stomach, intestines, gall bladder, liver, and pancreas.
- Curcumin supports memory and mental adaptability by supporting growth factors necessary for the formation of replacements for damaged circuits in the brain. In addition, curcumin reduces stress on the brain and protects it from metabolic toxins such as homocysteine
- Curcumin reduces lipid peroxide levels in the blood, lowering low-density lipoprotein (LDL) cholesterol and raising high-density lipoprotein (HDL) cholesterol levels
- Topically, curcumin protects the skin cells from radiation and free radical attack
- Curcumin supports immunity by inhibiting the proliferation of damaging cells and toxins, and by boosting macrophage and antibody activity.

RECOMMENDED DOSAGE AND ADMINISTRATION

- A commonly used dosage is 500 mg to 3 g daily taken on an empty stomach.
- Combining curcumin with phospholipid (e.g., lecithin) supplementation increases their absorption.

ADVERSE REACTIONS

- When taken with ginkgo or garlic, curcumin can increase the risk of bleeding.

RESEARCH FINDINGS

- A great deal of research has been conducted on the potential of curcumin as an anticancer and chemo-preventive agent. There is evidence that curcumin increases the chemo-sensitivity and radio-sensitivity of tumors, decreases cancer-causing inflammation, and promotes apoptosis (i.e., programmed cell death) in rapidly reproducing cancer cells, while providing protection for other tissues and the internal organs. Curcumin prevents and combats cancers of the breast, cervix, uterus, prostate, colon and other parts of the gastrointestinal system, blood, brain, lung, and bladder.
- Curcumin decreases alcohol-induced oxidative liver damage in rats, and exhibits therapeutic and protective effects against organ dysfunction due to sepsis, shock, and diseases associated with inflammation (e. g., inflammatory bowel disease). Curcumin was shown to especially enhance antioxidant defense, protecting against liver damage, when administered as a pretreatment, demonstrating its potential as a preventative therapy.
- Researchers report evidence of the role of curcumin in regulating lipid metabolism and reducing obesity and related conditions, including

diabetes mellitus. Curcumin interacts with adipocytes, pancreatic cells, hepatic stellate cells, macrophages, and muscle cells, suppressing inflammatory factors and reversing insulin resistance, hyperglycemia, hyperlipidemia, and other abnormalities.

- Curcumin treatment has shown potential for improving spatial memory disorders such as Alzheimer's Disease (AD). Researchers report that curcumin inhibits the activation of astrocytes and regulates the expression of glial fibrillary acidic protein, which are key factors in the early pathology of AD. This evidence supports the theory that curcumin could serve to prevent AD.

- In a six week, randomized controlled trial, which studied 60 patients diagnosed with major depressive disorder (MDD), curcumin was demonstrated to be an effective and safe treatment of patients with MDD, who do not also have suicidal ideation or other psychotic disorders.

WHAT WE CAN DO

Consumers should become knowledgeable about the physiologic effects of curcumin, including its risks and benefits. Curcumin is a rich group of phytochemicals that contribute to the health of the digestive system, support memory and mental adaptability, lower LDL cholesterol and raise HDL cholesterol levels, promote immune function, and protect the skin cells from radiation and free radical attack. Individuals with bleeding disorders that, when taken with ginkgo or garlic, curcumin can increase the risk of bleeding. Research suggests curcumin may help prevent cancer and treat Alzheimer's Disease and depression.

—*Cherie Marcel, BS*

REFERENCES

Aggarwal, B. B. (2010). Targeting inflammation-induced obesity and metabolic diseases by curcumin and other nutraceuticals. *Annual Review of Nutrition, 30,* 173-199. doi:10.1146/annurev.nutr.012809.104755

Alappat, L., & Awad, A. B. (2010). Curcumin and obesity: Evidence and mechanisms. *Nutrition Reviews, 68*(12), 729-738. doi:10.1111/j.1753-4887.2010.00341.x

Bao, W., Li, K., Rong, S., Yao, P., Hao, L., Ying, C., ... Liu, L. (2010). Curcumin alleviates ethanol-induced hepatocytes oxidative damage involving hem oxygenase-1 induction. *Journal of Ethnopharmacology, 128*(2), 549-553. doi:10.1016/j.jep.2010.01.029

Borger, J. E. (2011). How curcumin protects against cancer. *Life Extension, 17*(3), 1-9.

Cabrespine-Faugeras, A., Bayet-Robert, M., Bay, J., Chollet, P., & Barthomeuf, C. (2010). Possible benefits of curcumin regimen in combination with taxane chemotherapy for hormone-refractory prostate cancer treatment. *Nutrition & Cancer, 62*(2), 148-153. doi:10.1080/01635580903305383

Chuengsamarn, S., Rattanamongkolgul, S., Luechapudiporn, R., Phisalaphong, C., & Jirawatnotai, S. (2012). Curcumin extract for prevention of type 2 diabetes. *Diabetes Care, 35*(11), 2121-2127. doi:10.2337/dc12-0116

Epelbaum, R., Schaffer, M., Vizel, B., Badmaev, V., & Bar-Sela, G. (2010). Curcumin and gemcitabine in patients with advanced pancreatic cancer. *Nutrition & Cancer, 62*(8), 1137-1141. doi:10.1080/01635581.2010.513802

Finkle, J. (2011). Curcumin could prevent liver damage. *Life Extension, 17*(2), 4.

Goel, A., & Aggarwal, B. B. (2010). Curcumin, the golden spice from Indian Saffron, is a chemosensitizer and radiosensitizer for tumors and chemoprotector and radioprotector for normal organs. *Nutrition & Cancer, 62*(7), 919-930. doi:10.1080/01635581.2010.509835

Gutierres, V. O., Pinheiro, C. M., Assis, R. P., Vendramini, R. C., Pepato, M. T., & Brunetti, I. L. (2012). Curcumin-supplemented yoghurt improves physiological and biochemical markers of experimental diabetes. *British Journal of Nutrition, 108*(3), 440-448. doi:10.1017/S0007114511005769

Hilchie, A. L., Furlong, S. J., Sutton, K., Richardson, A., Robichaud, M. R. J., Giacomantonio, C. A., ... Hoskin, D. W. (2010). Curcumin-induced apoptosis in PC3 prostate carcinoma cell is caspase-independent and involves cellular ceramide accumulation and damage to mitochondria. *Nutrition & Cancer, 62*(3), 379-389. doi:10.1080/01635580903441238

Kiefer, D. (2008). Soy isoflavones, curcumin synergize to thwart pancreatic cancer. *Life Extension, 14*(11), 24.

Kumar, S., Ahuja, V., Sankar, M. J., Kumar, A., & Moss, A. C. (2012). Curcumin for maintenance of remission in ulcerative colitis. *Cochrane Database of Systematic Reviews, 10.* Art. No.: CD008424. doi:10.1002/14651858.CD008424

Majumdar, A. P. N., Banerjee, S., Nautiyal, J., Patel, B. B., Patel, V., Du, J., ... Sarkar, F. H. (2009). Curcumin synergizes with resveratrol to inhibit colon cancer. *Nutrition & Cancer*, *61*(4), 544-553. doi:10.1080/01635580902752262

Memis, D., Hekimoglu, S., Sezer, A., Altaner, S., Sut, N., & Usta, U. (2008). Curcumin attenuates the organ dysfunction caused by endotoxemia in the rat. *Nutrition*, *24*(11-12), 1133-1138. doi:10.1016/j.nut.2008.06.008

Nam, S. M., Choi, J. H., Yoo, D. Y., Kim, W., Jung, H. Y., Kim, J. W., ... Hwang, I. K. (2014). Effects of curcumin (Curcuma longa) on learning and spatial memory as well as cell proliferation and neuroblast differentiation in adult and aged mice by upregulating brain-derived neurotrophic factor and CREB signaling. *Journal of Medicinal Food*, *17*(6), 641-649. doi:10.1089/jmf.2013.2965

National Institutes of Health. (2012, December 11). Turmeric. *MedlinePlus*. Retrieved October 9, 2014, from http://www.nlm.nih.gov/medlineplus/druginfo/natural/662.html

Nayak, S., & Sashidhar, R. B. (2010). Metabolic intervention of aflatoxin B1 toxicity by curcumin. *Journal of Ethnopharmacology*, *127*(3), 641-644. doi:10.1016/j.jep.2009.12.010

Pan, Y., Zhu, G., Wang, Y., Cai, L., Cai, Y., Hu, J., ... Liang, G. (2013). Attentuation of high-glucose-induced inflammatory response by a novel curcumin derivative B06 contributes to its protection from diabetic pathogenic changes in rat kidney and heart. *Journal of Nutritional Biochemistry*, *24*(1), 146-155. doi:10.1016/j.jnutbio.2012.03.012

Patel, V. B., Misra, S., Patel, B. B., & Majumdar, A. P. N. (2010). Colorectal cancer: Chemopreventive role of curcumin and resveratrol. *Nutrition & Cancer*, *62*(7), 958-967. doi:10.1080/01635581.2010.510259

Randomized trial finds curcumin helps prevent diabetes. (2012). *Tufts University Health & Nutrition Letter*, *30*(9), 3.

Samuhasaneeto, S., Thong-Ngam, D., Kulaputana, O., Suyasunanont, O. K. D., & Klaikeaw, N. (2009). Curcumin decreased oxidative stress, inhibited NF-kappaB activation, and improved liver pathology in ethanol-induced liver injury in rats. *Journal of Biomedicine & Biotechnology*, 981963. doi:10.1155/2009/981963

Sanmukhani, J., Satodia, V., Trivedi, J., Patel, T., Tiwari, D., Panchal, B., ... Tripathi, C. B. (2014). Efficacy and safety of curcumin in major depressive disorder: A randomized controlled trial. *Phytotherapy Research*, *28*(4), 579-585. doi:10.1002/ptr.5025

Shehzad, A., Ha, T., Subhan, F., & Lee, Y. (2011). New mechanisms and the anti-inflammatory role of curcumin in obesity and obesity-related metabolic diseases. *European Journal of Nutrition*, *50*(3), 151-161. doi:10.1007/s00394-011-0188-1

Taylor, R. A., & Leonard, M. C. (2011). Curcumin for inflammatory bowel disease: A review of human studies. *Alternative Medicine Review*, *16*(2), 152-156.

Wang, Y., Yin, H., Wang, L., Shuboy, A., Lou, J., Han, B., ... Li, J. (2013). Curcumin as a potential treatment for Alzheimer's disease: A study of the effects of curcumin on hippocampal expression of glial fibrillary acidic protein. *American Journal of Chinese Medicine*, *41*(1), 59-70. doi:10.1142/S0192415X13500055

Zhang, J., Xu, L., Zhang, L., Ying, Z., Su, W., & Wang, T. (2014). Curcumin attenuates d-Galactosamine/Lipopolysaccharide-induced liver injury and mitochondrial dysfunction in mice. *Journal of Nutrition*, *144*(8), 1211-1218. doi:10.3945/jn.114.193573

REVIEWER(S)

Darlene Strayer, RN, MBA, Cinahl Information Systems, Glendale, CA

Helle Heering, RN, CRRN, Cinahl Information Systems, Glendale, CA

Nursing Practice Council, Glendale Adventist Medical Center, Glendale, CA

Dandelion

WHAT WE KNOW

Dandelion, or *Taraxacum officinale*, is a member of the Asteraceae/Compositae family and the Cichorioideae subfamily, along with chicory. Dandelion is a perennial herb that is considered by some to be a weed. It grows abundantly throughout areas of warmer climate in the Northern hemisphere. The jagged-edged leaves of dandelion are the inspiration for its name, which is derived from the French term "dent de lion" (i.e., tooth of the lion). Dandelion has yellow flowers that become white, spherical puffballs when the flower petals die (called "going to seed").

- Since ancient times, the roots, leaves, and flowers of the dandelion plant have been believed to have medicinal value. Although science has not substantiated the medicinal benefits of dandelion, many persons use it for treatment of gastrointestinal distress, constipation, loss of appetite, gallstones, joint and muscle pain, hypertension, eczema, bruises, viral infection, and cancer.

- Dandelion is appreciated as an ingredient in salad, soup, wine, and tea. The root can be roasted and used as a substitute for coffee. To prevent bitterness, the leaves are best harvested in the spring before flowering of the dandelion. Blanching or soaking overnight can reduce the bitterness of leaves. It is important not to cut or tear the leaves until they are ready for use because doing so triggers the oxidation of vitamin C.

ACTION OF DANDELION

- Dandelion has great nutritional value. There are approximately 1,400 international units (IU) of vitamin A per 100 grams of dandelion leaf. Leaves also contain vitamins B, C, and D, and the minerals calcium, chromium, copper, iron, magnesium, potassium, selenium, sulfur, and zinc.
- Dandelion contains the following compounds:
  —Sesquiterpene lactones are chemical compounds that can reduce inflammation, stimulate digestion, and relax the sympathetic nervous system.
   –Triterpenes such as the phytosterols stigmasterol and sitosterol, are plant-based steroid compounds that are similar to cholesterol. Theoretically, it is believed that these phytosterols could inhibit tumor growth and aid in regulation of blood lipids.
  —Lecithin, a fatty substance derived from plants, exhibits anti-inflammatory activity.

ADVERSE REACTIONS AND MEDICATION INTERACTION

- Dandelion is considered to be safe when eaten in amounts that are normally found in food or beverages
- Consuming a large amount of dandelion can interfere with the absorption of certain antibiotics, including ciprofloxacin, enoxacin, norfloxacin, sparfloxacin, trovafloxacin, gatifloxacin, levofloxacin, lomefloxacin, moxifloxacin, ofloxacin, and grepafloxacin.
- Dandelion has diuretic properties, which can decrease the body's efficiency in eliminating lithium and result in abnormally increased lithium levels in persons receiving lithium as a prescribed medication.

RESEARCH FINDINGS

- Results of a study of the potential anti-carcinogenic property of dandelion root extract (DRE) showed that DRE contains components that induce apoptosis of human leukemia cells. Researchers suggested further study on DRE as a nontoxic alternative to traditional therapy for leukemia.
- Due to the increase in antimicrobial resistance to treatment of urinary tract infections caused by *Escherichia coli*, researchers are seeking alternative treatment options. Results of a recent study indicated that, although no direct antibacterial activity was exhibited, dandelion helped to protect against *E. coli* infection by decreasing bacterial colonization of bladder epithelial cells.

SUMMARY

Consumers should become knowledgeable about the physiologic effects of consuming dandelion. Dandelion is rich in vitamins, minerals and phytosterols. Dandelion is used to reduce inflammation, stimulate digestion, and relax the sympathetic nervous system. Dandelion should be avoided when individuals are taking certain antibiotics and lithium. Research suggests that dandelion may help treat cancer and bacterial infections.

—*Cherie Marcel, BS*

REFERENCES

Altshul, S. (2007). Dandelion: The answer to tummy troubles?. *Prevention*, 59(9), 38.

Burnett, B. (2007). More nutritious than spinach! Dandelion – the amazing weed. *Alive: Canada's Natural Health & Wellness Magazine*, Mar, 60.

Burnett, B. (2009). The top 10 healing herbs. *Alive: Canada's Natural Health & Wellness Magazine*, (325), 18-19.

Luthje, P., Dzung, D. N., & Brauner, A. (2011). Lactuca indica extract interferes with uroepithelial infection by Escherichia coli. *Journal of Ethnopharmacology*, 135(3), 672-677. doi:10.1016/j.jep.2011.03.069

Medline Plus editorial team. (2014, March 4). Dandelion. *MedlinePlus*. Retrieved March 5, 2015, from http://www.nlm.nih.gov/medlineplus/druginfo/natural/706.html

Ovadje, P., Chatterjee, S., Griffin, C., Tran, C., Hamm, C., & Pandey, S. (2011). Selective induction of apoptosis through activation of caspase-8 in human leukemia cells (Jurkat) by dandelion root extract. *Journal of Ethnopharmacology*, 133(1), 86-91. doi:10.1016/j.jep.2010.09.005

Poulette, A. (2008). Dandelions. *Organic Gardening*, 55(3), 80.

Schutz, K., Carle, R., & Schieber, A. (2006). Taraxacum – A review on its phytochemical and pharmacological profile. *Journal of Ethnopharmacology*, 107(3), 313-323. doi:10.1016/j.jep.2006.07.021

Sweeny, B., Vora, M., Ulbricht, C., & Basch, E. (2005). Evidence-based systematic review of dandelion (Taraxacum officinale) by Natural Standard Research Collaboration. *Journal of Herbal Pharmacotherapy*, 5(1), 79-93. doi:10.1300/J157v05n01_09

Yarnell, E., & Abascal, K. (2009). Dandelion (Taraxacum officinale and T. mongolicum). *Integrative Medicine: A Clinician's Journal*, 8(2), 34-38.

REVIEWER(S)

Darlene Strayer, RN, MBA, Cinahl Information Systems, Glendale, CA

Nursing Practice Council, Glendale Adventist Medical Center, Glendale, CA

Dong Quai

WHAT WE KNOW

Dong quai, or *Angelica sinensis*, is an herb from the Apiaceae, or Umbelliferae, family, which includes anise, celery, dill, fennel, and parsley. Other names for dong quai are Chinese Angelica, dang qui (Chinese), toki (Japanese), tang wei (Korean), and kinesisk kvan (Danish). While it is best known for its therapeutic use in the treatment of menstrual pain and menopause, the dried root of dong quai has a long history of medicinal use in support of heart, lung, liver, and intestinal health.

ACTION OF DONG QUAI

- Dong quai is a substantial source of many nutrients, including vitamins A (along with carotenoids), E, C, and B12, as well as folic acid, biotin, magnesium, and calcium. Dong quai also contains many valuable and active phytochemicals (i.e., plant-derived chemicals) such as adenine and myristic acid
- One of the most frequent uses for dong quai is for the treatment of menopause and menstrual cramps. It is reported to reduce the vasomotor symptoms associated with menopause by 70% when used in combination with other herbs, including *Paeonia lactiflora* (Chinese peony) root, *Ligusticum* rhizome, and *Atractylodes* rhizome.

- Dong quai exhibits cardio-protective activity by dilating the coronary vessels, increasing coronary blood flow, and reducing the respiratory rate.
- Preparations that include dong quai have been used to retard the progression of renal fibrosis and treat nephrotic syndrome.
- The volatile oil found in the root of dong quai contains several active components, including n-butylidenephthalide, ligustilide, n-butylphthalide, and ferulic, nicotinic, and succinic acids.
  —Ferulic acid inhibits blood clotting and release of serotonin.
  —n-Butylidenephthalide, ligustilide, and n-butylphthalide exhibit antispasmodic activity in uterine and other smooth muscles.
  –The coumarin derivatives are natural anticoagulants (i.e., blood thinners).
  –The polysaccharide in dong quai has a molecular weight of about 3,000 and has demonstrated immune system support, due to the presence of vitamin B12, folic acid, and biotin in dong quai.

RECOMMENDED DOSAGE AND ADMINISTRATION

- Tea: 1 cup of freshly brewed tea taken 1–3 times daily is prepared by steeping 1 g of dried root in 250 mL of boiling water for 10–15minutes
- Dried root: 3–15 g daily of dried root is prepared by decoction, which is a method of mashing and temperature-related treatment
- Powdered root: 1–2 g is taken 1–3 times daily
- Capsules/tablets: 500 mg can be taken up to 6 times daily

ADVERSE REACTIONS AND MEDICATION INTERACTION

- Women who are pregnant should avoid dong quai root because it can cause uterine stimulation and relaxation.
- Dong quai can increase bleeding risk. People who have bleeding disorders or who are taking medications that increase bleeding (e.g., warfarin) should avoid taking dong quai.
- Persons who are taking warfarin should consult with their treating clinician before consuming

dong quai because it can amplify both the therapeutic and adverse effects of warfarin treatment.

RESEARCH FINDINGS

- The effect of alcohol extract from dong quai root on β-amyloidpeptide (i.e., a pathologic marker for Alzheimer's disease) was found to protect against β-amyloid peptide-induced neurotoxicity. Researchers suggest that dong quai could be useful in preventing Alzheimer's disease.
- Results of a recent study revealed that dong quai-derived components stimulate osteoblasts involved in periodontal and bone regeneration and enhanced the deposition of hyaluronic acid. This indicates that dong quai may have strong potential as a treatment for periodontal disease and other bone diseases.

SUMMARY

Consumers should become knowledgeable about the physiologic effects of dong quai, including its risks and benefits. Dong quai is a good source of vitamins, minerals and phytochemicals. Dong quai is used to ease menstrual pain and menopause symptoms, as well as supportive treatment of heart, lung, liver, and intestinal health. Pregnant women and individuals taking blood thinner medications should avoid dong quai. Researchers suggest that dong quai may be useful in preventing Alzheimer's disease and bone diseases.

—*Cherie Marcel, BS*

REFERENCES

Bass, S. (2007). Dong quai. A great team player. *Alive*, (297), 66-67.

Editorial staff at MayoClinic.org. (2013). Dong quai (Angelica sinensis). *Mayo Clinic*. Retrieved March 12, 2015, from http://www.mayoclinic.org/drugs-supplements/dong-quai/background/hrb-20059206

Head, K. (2004). Angelica sinensis (Dong quai). *Alternative Medicine Review*, 9(4), 429-433.

Huang, S., Lin, C., & Chiang, B. (2008). Protective effects of Angelica sinensis extract on amyloid beta-peptide-induced neurotoxicity. *Phytomedicine*, 15(9), 710-721. doi:10.1016/j.phymed.008.02.022.

Liu, C., Li, J., Meng, F. Y., Liang, S. X., Deng, R., Li, C. K., ... Yang, M. (2010). Polysaccharides from the root of Angelica sinensis promotes hematopoiesis and thrombopoiesis through the P13K/AKT pathway.

BMC Complementary & Alternative Medicine, 10, 79. doi:10.1186/1472-6882-10-79.

Willard, T. (2003). Herb profile: Dong quai. *Alive*, (249), 58-59.

Zampieron, E., & Kamhi, E. (2000). Natural medicine chest: Treat PMS with dong quai. *Healthy & Natural Journal*, 7(33), 32.

Zhao, H., Alexeev, A., Sharma, V., Guzman, L. D., & Bojanowski, K. (2008). Effect of SBD.4A--A defined multicomponent preparation of Angelica sinensis--in periodontal regeneration models. *Phytotherapy Research*, 22(7), 923-928. doi:10.1002/ptr.2421.

REVIEWER(S)

Darlene Strayer, RN, MBA, Cinahl Information Systems, Glendale, CA

Anne Danahy, MS, RDN

Nursing Practice Council, Glendale Adventist Medical Center, Glendale, CA

Eucalyptus

WHAT WE KNOW

Eucalyptus represents over 700 species from the Australian native, Eucalyptus, or Myrtaceae, family. Eucalyptus trees and shrubs (also called gum trees because of the large amount of resin they produce when damaged) tend to be aromatic, supplying essential oils that are commonly considered medicinal. For example, essential oils derived from the *Eucalyptus* species *tereticornis* and *globulus* are used to treat respiratory conditions, such as cough, cold, and sore throat. Other biologic actions associated with the Eucalyptus family include antibacterial, antifungal, anti-hyperglycemic, analgesic (i.e., pain reliever), and anti-inflammatory properties. Although most frequently applied topically or used as an inhalant, eucalyptus has historically also been administered orally in encapsulated form for intestinal release, and small amounts of eucalyptus oil have been added to food as a flavoring agent. Eucalyptus is not considered safe for consumption in large amounts; ingesting more than 3.5 mL at one time of undiluted oil can be fatal.

ACTION OF EUCALYPTUS

- Some of the active constituents of eucalyptus, which are found in varying quantities, depending on the species, include the following:

—1,8-Cineole has antiseptic properties known to kill halitosis-causing bacteria (i.e., the bacteria causing bad breath). It also controls airway mucus hyper secretion, which can reduce symptoms of asthma, sinusitis, and chronic obstructive pulmonary disease (COPD).

—Aromadendrene has strong antimicrobial properties.

—Tannins found in eucalyptus leaves exhibit anti-inflammatory properties.

—Flavonoids act as antioxidants.

RECOMMENDED DOSAGE AND ADMINISTRATION

- Eucalyptus is generally used topically or as an inhalant, although its use is not recommended for children under the age of 2 years.

ADVERSE REACTIONS AND MEDICATION INTERACTION

- Undiluted eucalyptus oil is toxic if ingested and should only be consumed under the supervision of a physician.
- Topical application of eucalyptus should not be used in combination with other topical treatments without medical supervision because its use can interfere with the effectiveness of other topical medications.

RESEARCH FINDINGS

- Oral administration of ethanolic extracts from eucalyptus leaves significantly reduces serum triglyceride and cholesterol levels in diabetic rats. The exact mechanisms of this result are not fully understood, although a study of the effect of eucalyptus leaf extract on the pancreatic islets of rats showed that the extract treatment partially restores pancreatic beta cells and repairs damage. Researchers suggest that eucalyptus would be beneficial in the treatment of diabetes.
- Eucalyptus oil exhibits strong antimicrobial activity against a wide range of microorganisms. The major constituents of eucalyptus oil—1,8-cineole and aromadendrene—were examined for potential antibacterial activity against multidrug-resistant bacteria. Results indicated that all gram-positive bacteria were susceptible to the eucalyptus oil, particularly the methicillin-resistant *Staphylococcus aureus* (MRSA) and vancomycin-resistant

Enterococcus faecalis. Researchers also found the oil of *Eucalyptus* species *robusta* to significantly inhibit the growth of MRSA, *Escherichia coli*, *Helicobacter pylori*, and *Candida albicans*.

SUMMARY

Consumers should become knowledgeable about the physiologic effects of eucalyptus. Essential oils extracted from eucalyptus are used to treat respiratory conditions, and have been reported to also contain antibacterial, antifungal, anti-hyperglycemic, analgesic and anti-inflammatory properties. Consumers should be aware that undiluted eucalyptus oil is toxic if ingested and should only be consumed under the supervision of a physician. Eucalyptus is not recommended for children under the age of 2 years.

—*Cherie Marcel, BS*

REFERENCES

Almeida, I. F., Fernandes, E., Lima, J. L. F., Valentão, P., Andrade, P. B., Seabra, R. M., & Bahia, M. F. (2009). Oxygen and nitrogen reactive species are effectively scavenged by Eucalyptus globulus leaf water extract. *Journal of Medicinal Food, 12*(1), 175-183. doi:10.1089/jmf.2008.0046

Dey, B., Mitra, A., Katakam, P., & Singla, R. K. (2014). Exploration of natural enzyme inhibitors with hypoglycemic potentials amongst Eucalyptus Spp. by in vitro assays. *World Journal of Diabetes, 5*(2), 209-218. doi:10.4239/wjd.v5.i2.209

Eidi, A., Eidi, M., Givianrad, M. H., & Abaspour, N. (2009). Hypolipidemic effects of alcoholic extract of eucalyptus (Eucalyptus globulus Labill.) leaves on diabetic and non-diabetic rats. *Iranian Journal of Diabetes and Lipid Disorders, 8*, 105-112.

Hendry, E. R., Worthington, T., Conway, B. R., & Lambert, P. A. (2009). Antimicrobial efficacy of eucalyptus oil and 1,8-cineole alone and in combination with chlorhexidine digluconate against microorganisms grown in planktonic and biofilm cultures. *Journal of Antimicrobial Chemotherapy, 64*(6), 1219-1225. doi:10.1093/jac/dkp362

Lawal, T. O., Adeniyi, B. A., Moody, J. O., & Mahady, G. B. (2012). Combination studies of Eucalyptus torelliana F. Muell. Leaf extracts and clarithromycin on Helicobacter pylori. *Phytotherapy Research, 26*(9), 1393-1398. doi:10.1002/ptr.3719

Lima, F. J., Brito, T. S., Freire, W. B., Costa, R. C., Linhares, M. I., Sousa, F. C., ... Magalhães, P. J. (2010). The essential oil of Eucalyptus tereticornis, and its constituents alpha- and beta-pinene, potentiate acetylcholine-induced contractions in isolated rat trachea. *Fitoterapia, 81*(6), 649-655. doi:10.1016/j.fitote.2010.03.012

Mahmoudzadeh-Sagheb, H., Heidari, Z., Bokaeian, M., & Moudi, B. (2010). Antidiabetic effects of Eucalyptus globulus on pancreatic islets: A stereological study. *Folia Morphologica, 69*(2), 112-118.

Mulyaningsih, S., Sporer, F., Zimmermann, S., Reichling, J., & Wink, M. (2010). Synergistic properties of the terpenoids aromadendrene and 1,8-cineole from the essential oil of Eucalyptus globulus against antibiotic-susceptible and antibiotic-resistant pathogens. *Phytomedicine, 17*(13), 1061-1066. doi:10.1016/j.phymed.2010.06.018

Olsen, S. (2009). Eucalyptus. *Similia: Journal of the Australian Homoeopathic Association, 21*(1), 8-11.

Sadlon, A. E., & Lamson, D. W. (2010). Immune-modifying and antimicrobial effects of eucalyptus oil and simple inhalation devices. *Alternative Medicine Review, 15*(1), 33-47.

Sartorelli, P., Marquioreto, A. D., Amaral-Baroli, A., Lima, M. E. L., & Moreno, P. R. H. (2007). Chemical composition and antimicrobial activity of the essential oils from two species of eucalyptus. *Phytotherapy Research, 21*(3), 231-233. doi:10.1002/ptr.2051

Sego, S. (2012). Alternative meds update. Medicinal uses of eucalyptus oil. *The Clinical Advisor*. Retrieved March 5, 2015, from http://www.clinicaladvisor.com/medicinal-uses-of-eucalyptus-oil/article/267119/

REVIEWER(S)

Darlene Strayer, RN, MBA, Cinahl Information Systems, Glendale, CA

Nursing Executive Practice Council, Glendale Adventist Medical Center, Glendale, CA

Ginger

WHAT WE KNOW

Ginger, or *Zingiber officinale*, is a perennial, aromatic herb that has green and purple flowers, that grow from an underground rhizome, or root stem. The rhizome can be white, yellow, or red and is covered in a brown skin. The rhizome is the portion of the ginger plant that is used for culinary and medicinal purposes. Ginger grows in India, Jamaica, and China and is a member of the Zingiberaceae family, along with cardamom and turmer-

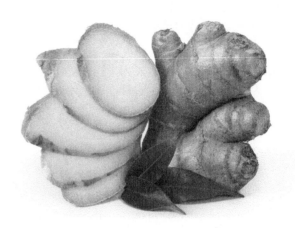

ic. Other names for ginger include African ginger, black ginger, cochin ginger, gingembre, ginger root, imber, Jamaica ginger, race ginger, and zingiberis rhizome.

- Ginger is appreciated for its aromatic quality and is frequently used as the fragrance component in soaps and cosmetics. It is also commonly used as a culinary flavoring agent. The ancient Greeks and Romans valued ginger as an antiemetic (i.e., anti-nausea) and a digestive aid, as did Ancient East Indian and Chinese civilizations. Ginger has also been used as an appetite stimulant and to treat colds, fever, arthritis, and migraine headaches. Modern research has supported the use of ginger as an antioxidant and anti-inflammatory agent, most notably for the relief of gastrointestinal (GI) distress (e.g., from motion sickness and pregnancy).

ACTION OF GINGER

- The rhizome contains the active components gingerol and gingerdione, which have many pharmacologic properties, including the following:
    - Antipyretic (i.e., fever reducer)
    - Analgesic
    - Antitussive (i.e., cough suppressant)
    - Cardiac inotropic (i.e., change in force of heart contraction)
    - Sedative
    - Antibiotic
    - Mild antifungal
- Ginger has anti-carcinogenic properties. Ginger has been shown to inhibit the growth of colorectal tumors in mice and has exhibited antioxidant, anti-inflammatory, and antitumor effects in ovarian cancer cell lines.

- Ginger's aroma is attributed to its pungent ketones, including gingerol.

RECOMMENDED DOSAGE AND ADMINISTRATION

- Clinical studies on the use of ginger as an antiemetic have used 500–1,000 mg of powdered ginger or 1,000 mg of fresh ginger rhizome.

ADVERSE REACTIONS AND MEDICATION INTERACTION

- Adverse effects are rare, but dosages higher than 5 gm/day can result in abdominal discomfort, diarrhea, or irritation in the mouth and throat.
- Extreme overdose can depress the central nervous system and result in cardiac arrhythmias.
- Treatment of adverse reactions is achieved by discontinuing ginger use.
- Ginger may interfere with antacids by increasing stomach acid.
- Ginger may enhance the effects of barbiturates.
- Theoretically, ginger could interfere with medications used to treat blood pressure, heart disease, or diabetes mellitus (DM) due to its potential to affect blood sugar, blood pressure, and cardiac rhythm.

RESEARCH FINDINGS

- Many study results are promising for the use of ginger in the treatment of pregnancy-induced nausea and vomiting. Results have repeatedly indicated that ginger therapy is more effective as an antiemetic than vitamin B or placebo. Ginger may be a good alternative treatment option because many pharmaceutical antiemetic medications have side effects of sedation. Researchers have also reported success in treating motion sickness with ginger, although ginger was not effective in individuals with vertigo. Study results are inconsistent regarding the effectiveness of ginger in treating postoperative or chemotherapy-related nausea and vomiting.
- Researchers are investigating the effectiveness of ginger for pain management and report mixed results. Results from a recent study on the treatment of migraine demonstrate that sublingual fever few and ginger are effective as first-line abortive treatment for individuals who experience mild headache prior to developing more severe headache. Ginger was also found to be as useful in relieving pain for women with primary dysmenorrhea (i.e., pelvic pain around the time of menstruation) as ibuprofen or mefenamic acid. Although evidence is conflicting, there is some evidence that the use of ginger is effective in treatment of exercise-induced muscle pain. Results of one study showed that daily consumption of raw and heat-treated ginger is effective in reducing muscle pain following exercise-induced muscle injury. Similar anti-inflammatory properties were reported in studies on the use of ginger to treat osteoarthritis and rheumatoid arthritis, although evidence is conflicting.

SUMMARY

Consumers should become knowledgeable about the physiologic effects of ginger, including its risks and benefits. Ginger is an antioxidant and anti-inflammatory agent, commonly used for the relief of GI distress and treatment for the common cold and migraines. Consumers should be aware of ginger's potential to interfere with antacids, barbiturates, and medications used to treat blood pressure, heart disease and DM.

—*Cherie Marcel, BS*

REFERENCES

Abascal, K., & Yarnell, E. (2009). Clinical uses of Zingiber officinale (ginger). *Alternative & Complementary Therapies, 15*(5), 231-237.

Black, C. D., Herring, M. P., Hurley, D. J., & O'Connor, P. J. (2010). Ginger (Zingiber officinale) reduces muscle pain caused by eccentric exercise. *Journal of Pain, 11*(9), 894-903. doi:10.1016/j.jpain.2009.12.013

Black, C. D., & O'Connor, P. J. (2008). Acute effects of dietary ginger on quadriceps muscle pain duringmoderate-intensity cycling exercise. *International Journal of Sport Nutrition & Exercise Metabolism, 18*(6), 653-664.

Borrelli, F., Capasso, R., Aviello, G., Pittler, M. H., & Izzo, A. A. (2005). Effectiveness and safety of ginger in the treatment of pregnancy-induced nausea and vomiting. *Obstetrics & Gynecology, 105*(4), 849-856.

Byrne, K. (2011). Cancer. In E. D. Schlenker & S. L. Roth (Eds.), *Williams' essentials of nutrition and diet therapy* (10th ed., pp. 563-567). St. Louis, MO: Mosby, Inc, an affiliate of Elsevier Inc.

Cady, R. K., Goldstein, J., Nett, R., Mitchell, R., Beach, M. E., & Browning, R. (2011). A double-blind placebo-controlled pilot study of sublingual feverfew and ginger in the treatment of migraine. *Headache:*

The Journal of Head & Face Pain, 51(7), 1078-1086. doi:10.1111/j.1526-4610.2011.01910.x

Chaiyakunapruk, N., Kitikannakorn, N., Nathisuwan, S., Leeprakobboon, K., & Leelasettagool, C. (2006). The efficacy of ginger for the prevention of postoperative nausea and vomiting: A meta-analysis. *American Journal of Obstetrics & Gynecology*, 194(1), 95-99.

Ensiyeh, J., & Sakineh, M. C. (2009). Comparing ginger and vitamin B6 for the treatment of nausea and vomiting in pregnancy: A randomised controlled trial. *Midwifery*, 25(6), 649-653. doi:10.1016/j.midw.2007.10.013

Fetrow, C. W., & Avila, J. R. (Eds.). (2004). Ginger. In *Professional's handbook of complementary & alternative medicines* (3rd ed., pp. 352-357). Philadelphia, PA: Lippincott, Williams & Wilkins.

George Mateljan Foundation. (n.d.). Ginger. *World's Healthiest Foods*. Retrieved June 23, 2015, from http://www.whfoods.com/genpage.php?tname=foodspice&dbid=72

Gordon, D. (2006). Review of ginger for cancer patients. *Oncology Nutrition Connection*, 14(3), 26.

Ginger. (2003). In J. M. Jellin, P. J. Gregory, F. Batz, & K. Hitchens (Eds.), *Pharmacist's letter/prescriber's letter natural medicines comprehensive database* (5th ed., pp. 605-608). Stockton, CA: Therapeutic Research Faculty.

Keegan, G. T., & Keegan, L. (2006). The use of ginger to alleviate nausea. *Alternative Therapies in Women's Health*, 8(8), 57-61.

Keller, A. C. (2012). Effect of ginger on acute and delayed chemotherapy-induced nausea and vomiting. *HerbalGram*, (95), 36-37.

Kubra, I. R., & Rao, L. J. (2012). An impression on current developments in the technology, chemistry, and biological activities of ginger (Zingiber officinale Roscoe). *Critical Reviews in Food Science & Nutrition*, 52(8), 651-688.

Leach, M. J., & Kumar, S. (2008). The clinical effectiveness of ginger (Zingiber officinale) in adults with osteoarthritis. *International Journal of Evidence-Based Healthcare*, 6(3), 311-320.

Lutz, C. A., & Przytulski, K. R. (Eds.). (2006). Complementary medicine: Nutritional aspects. In *Nutrition & diet therapy: Evidence-based applications* (4th ed., pp. 333-335). Philadelphia, PA: F. A. Davis Company.

National Institutes of Health. (2015, February 14). Ginger. *MedlinePlus*. Retrieved June 23, 2015, from http://www.nlm.nih.gov/medlineplus/druginfo/natural/961.html

Ozgoli, G., Goli, M., & Moattar, F. (2009). Comparison of effects of ginger, mefenamic acid, and ibuprofen on pain in women with primary dysmenorrhea. *Journal of Alternative and Complementary Medicine*, 15(2), 129-132. doi:10.1089/acm.2008.0311

Ozgoli, G., Goli, M., & Simbar, M. (2009). Effects of ginger capsules on pregnancy, nausea, and vomiting. *Journal of Alternative & Complementary Medicine*, 15(3), 243-246. doi:10.1089/acm.2008.0406

Pillai, A. K., Sharma, K. K., Gupta, Y. K., & Bakhshi, S. (2011). Anti-emetic effect of ginger powder versus placebo as an add-on therapy in children and young adults receiving high emetogenic chemotherapy. *Pediatric Blood & Cancer*, 56(2), 234-238. doi:10.1002/pbc.22778

Rhode, J., Fogoros, S., Zick, S., Wahl, H., Giffith, K. A., Huang, J., & Liu, J. R. (2007). Ginger inhibits cell growth and modulates angiogenic factors in ovarian cancer cells.

BMC Complement Altern Med, 7:44.

Schwartz, V. S. (2011). Use of ginger to relieve nausea and vomiting. *Support Line*, 33(3), 19-24.

Therkleson, T. (2010). Ginger compress therapy for adults with osteoarthritis. *Journal of Advanced Nursing*, 66(10), 2225-2233. doi:10.1111/j.1365-2648.2010.05355.x

Thomson, M., Corbin, R., & Leung, L. (2014). Effects of ginger for nausea and vomiting in early pregnancy: A meta-analysis. *JABFM*, 27(1), 115-122. doi:10.3122/jabfm.2014.01.130167

White, B. (2007). Ginger: An overview. *American Family Physician*, 75(11), 1689-1691.

REVIEWER(S)

Darlene Strayer, RN, MBA, Cinahl Information Systems, Glendale, CA

Nursing Practice Council, Glendale Adventist Medical Center, Glendale, CA

Horseradish

WHAT WE KNOW

Horseradish (*Armoracia rusticana*; also known as mountain radish, pepperrot, and red cole) is a member of the Brassicaceae, or Cruciferae, family, which is more commonly referred to as the cruciferous vegetable family. Other cruciferous vegetables include cabbage, cauliflower, kale, and mustard. With its pungent taste and aroma, horseradish has been ground into a spice, prepared as a condiment, and used medicinally for centuries. Historically known as a cure for scurvy due to its high vitamin C content, horseradish has also been used to treat urinary tract infections (UTIs), kidney stones, fluid retention, respiratory distress, rheumatism, gallbladder dysfunction, sciatic nerve pain, and gout. It has also been applied as a topical ointment to soothe headaches and pain in muscles and joints. Horseradish contains calcium, iron, valuable secondary metabolites referred to as glucosinolates, and other bioactive components (e.g., flavonoids). These nutrients regulate enzymes, control apoptosis (i.e., programmed cell death) and the cell cycle, and prevent oxidation, making horseradish and its relatives useful in reducing risk for cancer and heart disease.

ACTION OF HORSERADISH

- Horseradish is a source of the sulfur-containing phytochemicals glucosinolates (specifically, sinigrin and gluconasturtiin), whose degradation products isothiocyanates and indoles appear to have chemo-preventive and therapeutic activity.
  —Glucosinolates enhance the liver's ability to detoxify carcinogens. They also inhibit the growth and kill multiple strains of *Helicobacter pylori*, a bacterium known to cause stomach ulcers and increase the risk for gastric cancer.
- Horseradish contains flavonoids, which protect blood vessels from rupture and exhibit antioxidant, antibiotic, and anti-inflammatory activity.
- The water-soluble vitamin C in horseradish neutralizes free radicals, protecting against inflammation and cellular damage. Adequate vitamin C intake is vital for proper immune system function and has been associated with the prevention of heart disease, stroke, and cancer.
- Horseradish is a source of calcium, which builds and maintains bones and teeth, promotes conduction of nerve impulses, activates enzymes for energy production and muscle contraction, participates in blood clotting, assists with vitamin B12 absorption, and maintains the structural integrity of intracellular membranes.
- The iron in horseradish is vital for the synthesis of red blood cells and hemoglobin, which are necessary for cellular respiration and the transport of oxygen to the tissues. Iron also supports immune function, is vital for brain development, contributes to energy metabolism, and regulates temperature.

ADVERSE REACTIONS AND MEDICATION INTERACTION

- Horseradish contains mustard oil, which can irritate the lining of the mouth, throat, nose, digestive system, and urinary tract.
- Horseradish can decrease the effects of levothyroxine, a medication that is prescribed to treat low thyroid function.

RESEARCH FINDINGS

- Scientists have demonstrated that horseradish roots exhibit antioxidant, radical scavenging, and anti-mutagenic activity (i.e., prevention of a mutation).

SUMMARY

Consumers should become knowledgeable about the physiologic effects of horseradish. Horseradish contains calcium, iron, glucosinolates, and flavonoids which may reduce risk for cancer and heart disease. Consumers should be aware that horseradish contains mustard oil which may cause irritation to the digestive and urinary tract, and can also interfere with thyroid medication.

—*Cherie Marcel, BS*

REFERENCES

The editorial team of WebMD. (2009). Horseradish. *WebMD*. Retrieved June 18, 2015, from http://www.webmd.com/vitamins-supplements/ingredientmono-257-horseradish.aspx?activeIngredientId=257&activeIngredientName=horseradish&source=1

Goodman, S. (2009). Super foods. Horseradish: Protection against cancer and more. *Life Extension*, *15*(11), 89-92.

Kinae, N., Masuda, H., Shin, I. S., Furugori, M., & Shimoi, K. (2000). Functional properties of wasabi and horseradish. *Biofactors*, *13*(1-4), 265-269.

Tremblay, L. (2013). Horseradish nutrition. *Livestrong.com*. Retrieved June 18, 2015, from http://www.livestrong.com/article/366608-horseradish-nutrition/

Wedelsback, B., & Olsson, K. M. (2011). Introduction and use of horseradish (Armoracia rusticana) as food and medicine from antiquity to the present: Emphasis on the Nordic countries. *Journal of Herbs, Spices & Medicinal Plants*, 17(3), 197-213. doi:10.10 80/10496475.2011.595055

REVIEWER(S)

Darlene Strayer, RN, MBA, Cinahl Information Systems, Glendale, CA

Nursing Executive Practice Council, Glendale Adventist Medical Center, Glendale, CA

Kava Kava

WHAT WE KNOW

Kava kava, or *Piper methysticum*, is an herb from the pepper (Piperaceae) family. Other names for kava kava include ava, ava pepper, awa, intoxicating pepper, kew, kawa, rauschpfeffer, sakau, tonga, wurzelstock, and yagona. Native to the South Pacific, kava kava has been used medicinally and ceremonially by Pacific Islanders for over 2,000 years. Kava kava is best known for its ability to decrease anxiety and cause relaxation, and has been used to treat urinary tract infections (UTIs), asthma, and topical pain. The active constituents of kava kava are found in its rootstalk and rhizome, which are the parts most frequently used to make a tea or beverage. Kava roots contain fiber, protein, potassium, and fat-soluble kava lactones (also called kavalactones and kavapyrones). Kava lactones are thought to be the most active ingredient of kava kava, responsible for reducing anxiety by influencing the activity of the brain's limbic system. As an antianxiety treatment in the clinical setting, kava kava has higher patient tolerability and is not associated with physiologic dependence and withdrawal compared to conventional pharmacologic agents such as oxazepam, a benzodiazepine. However, there have been some reports that kava kava may be linked to liver damage, which has led to controversy and hesitation regarding its therapeutic use. These reports prompted the U.S. Food and Drug Administration (FDA) to issue an advisory stating that persons with a liver condition should consult their treating clinician prior to taking kava kava. Many believe that the FDA acted hastily, as the reports that kava kava was directly responsible for the liver damage were not conclusive.

ACTION OF KAVA KAVA

- The kava lactones methysticin, dihydromethysticin, kavain, dihydrodrokavain, and desmethoxyyangonin are considered the most active components and are found in the root and stem of the kava kava plant. The kava lactones are believed to have antianxiety, analgesic (i.e., pain reducer), muscle-relaxing, anesthetic (i.e., numbing), and anticonvulsant properties.

RECOMMENDED DOSAGE AND ADMINISTRATION

- Tea: 1 cup of freshly brewed tea taken 1–3 times daily; prepared by simmering 2–4 g of ground root in 5 oz of boiling water for 5–10minutes, then straining and cooling.
- Standardized extract: 50–70 mg of purified kava-lactones taken 3 times daily.
- Tincture (i.e., liquid alcohol extract of fresh kava kava root): 1–3ml taken 3 times daily.

ADVERSE REACTIONS AND MEDICATION INTERACTION

- Potential adverse effects of kava kava consumption include the following:
  —An initial numbing sensation on contact with the skin or mouth
  —Reports have linked products containing kava kava with hepatitis, cirrhosis, and liver failure. Signs and symptoms of liver dysfunction are jaundice, brown urine, light-colored stool, nausea, vomiting, fatigue, weakness, stomach and/or abdominal pain, and loss of appetite.
- Persons with impaired liver function should consult their treating clinician prior to taking kava kava.
- Women who are pregnant or nursing should avoid intake of kava kava.
- Persons under 18 years of age should not take kava kava.
- Kava kava can interact with other drugs or substances that are metabolized by the liver, including alcohol, barbiturates, benzodiazepines, levodopa, monoamine oxidase (MAO) type B inhibitors, and antidepressant medications.

RESEARCH FINDINGS

- Since reports of potential kava kava–induced hepatotoxicity emerged and the FDA advisory was published, researchers have been attempting to identify the relationship between kava kava and liver injury. Critics argue that many of the reported cases involve individuals already affected by liver conditions such as hepatitis and cirrhosis, and suggest that the blame has wrongfully been placed on kava kava but is more likely to be a result of drug interactions, alcohol abuse, or viral infection. Another explanation could be the type of kava kava extract used. Traditionally kava kava beverages were prepared as water extracts of the root, although many European companies use kava kava stem with its higher concentration of lactones, which are metabolized in the liver. Additionally, alcohol and acetone are frequently used to develop standardized kava kava extracts, which results in a product that is different from the traditional aqueous preparations with the potential for additional and/or stronger effects.

- Kava kava, used as an aqueous root extract, has demonstrated effectiveness similar to anxiolytic medications. Without the adverse effects (e.g., impaired sexual function, withdrawal issues) associated with benzodiazepines, kava kava could serve as a substitute for such anxiolytic medications. Further long-term safety studies are recommended to confirm these findings.
- Researchers report that use of water-based kava kava in medicinal doses (180 mg of kava lactones) does not adversely affect a person's ability to drive.
- Researchers report that the hepatic adverse effects associated with kava kava use may be a result of depleted glutathione levels. Glutathione is a vital contributor to the phase II conversion of kava lactones. Insufficient glutathione levels could result in increased adverse effects from high levels of kava lactones. It has been suggested that clinicians consider glutathione supplementation when treating patients with standardized kava kava extracts.
- Researchers have investigated the apoptosis-inducing (i.e., natural cell death) and antimetastatic possibilities (i.e. prevention of secondary cancer cells) of kava kava–derived flavokawains A and B (FKA and FKB). Further in vivo research is needed.

SUMMARY

Consumers should become knowledgeable about the physiologic effects of kava kava. Kava kava contains lactones that may help reduce anxiety, and has been reported to have higher tolerability without the risk of dependence or withdrawal as compared to conventional agents. Consumers with impaired liver function should consult their doctor prior to taking kava kava. Women who are pregnant or nursing, as well as individuals under 18 years of age, should avoid taking kava kava.

—*Cherie Marcel, BS*

REFERENCES

Abu, N., Mohamed, N. E., Yeap, S. K., Lim, K. L., Akhtar, M. N., Zulfadli, A. J., ... Alitheen, N. B. (2015). vivo antitumor and antimetastatic effects of flavokawain B in 4T1 breast cancer cell-challenged mice. *Drug Design, Development and Therapy*, 9, 1401-1417. doi:10.2147/DDDT.S67976

Abu, N., Akhtar, M. N., Yeap, S. K., Lim, K. L., Ho, W. Y., Zulfadli, A. J., ... Alitheen, N. B. (2014). Flavokawain A induces apoptosis in MCF-7 and MDA-MB231 and inhibits the metastatic process in vitro. *PLoS One9*, 9(10), e105244. Retrieved from , doi:10.1371/journal.0105244

Ackerson, A. D. (2005). Kava. *Better Nutrition*, 67(9), 18.

Fu, P. P., Xia, Q., Guo, L., Yu, H., & Chan, P. C. (2008). Toxicity of kava kava. *Journal of Environmental Science and Health. Part C*, 26(1), 89-112. doi:10.1080/10590500801907407.

Habib, C., & Roberts, C. (2014). Common supplements for anxiety. *Naturopathic Doctor News & Review*, 10(3), 1-3.

Li, X. Z., & Ramzan, I. (2010). Role of ethanol in kava hepatotoxicity. *Phytotherapy Research*, 24(4), 475-480. doi:10.1002/ptr.3046

McBride, K. (2005). Herbs to change your mood. *Share Guide*, 23.

National Institutes of Health (NIH). (2015). Kava. *MedlinePlus*. Retrieved June 15, 2015, from http://www.nlm.nih.gov/medlineplus/druginfo/natural/872.html

Provino, R. (2009). Toxicology: Piper methysticum, kava kava. *Australian Journal of Medical Herbalism*, 21(4), 104-105.

Ross, S. M. (2014). Psychophytomedicine. *Holistic Nursing Practice*, 28(4), 275-280. doi:10.1097/HNP.0000000000000040

Sarris, J., Laporte, E., Scholey, A., King, R., Pipingas, A., Schwietzer, I., & Stough, C. (2013). Does a medicinal dose of kava impair driving? A randomized, placebo-controlled, double-blind study. *Traffic Injury Prevention*, 14(1), 13-17. doi:10.1080/15389588.2012.682233

Sarris, J., LaPorte, E., & Schweitzer, I. (2011). Kava: A comprehensive review of efficacy, safety, and psychopharmacology. *The Australian and New Zealand College of Psychiatry*, 45(1), 27-35. doi:10.3109/0004 8674.2010.522554

Sarris, J., Stough, C., Teschke, R., Wahid, Z. T., Bousman, C. A., Murray, G., ... Schweitzer, I. (2013). Kava for the treatment of generalized anxiety disorder RCT: Analysis of adverse reactions, liver function, addiction, and sexual effects. *Phytotherapy Research*, 27. doi:10.1002/ptr.4916

Teschke, R., Fuchs, J., Bahre, R., Genthner, A., & Wolff, A. (2010). Kava hepatotoxicity: Comparative study of two structured quantitative methods for causality assessment. *Journal of Clinical Pharmacy & Therapeutics*, 35(5), 545-563. doi:10.1111/j.1365-2710.2009.01131.x

Teschke, R., Schwarzenboeck, A., & Hennermann, K. (2008). Kava hepatotoxicity: A clinical survey and critical analysis of 26 suspected cases. *European Journal of Gastroenterology & Hepatology*, 20(12), 1182-1193. doi:10.1097/MEG.0b013e3283036768

REVIEWER(S)

Darlene Strayer, RN, MBA, Cinahl Information Systems, Glendale, CA

Nursing Practice Council, Glendale Adventist Medical Center, Glendale, CA

Licorice

WHAT WE KNOW

Licorice (also spelled liquorice; also called sweet root), or *Glycyrrhiza glabra*, is a perennial plant that grows wild in parts of Europe and Asia. The licorice plant grows 3–7 feet high and has an elaborate root system. Licorice root has been used medicinally for thousands of years to treat conditions such as upset stomach, asthma, cough, and halitosis (i.e., chronic bad breathe). It continues to be used today to treat canker sores, peptic ulcers, eczema, indigestion, and respiratory distress. Although licorice contains the compound glycyrrhizin, which is 50 times sweeter than sugar, the most commonly eaten licorice candy is actually flavored with the herbs anise or fennel because they are similar in taste and aroma to licorice. The reason for substituting anise or fennel as flavoring is that consuming a large amount of licorice can cause severe side effects, toxicities, and interactions with certain medications. Long-term high intake of licorice can cause hypokalemia (i.e., low potassium), hypertension, and an adrenal imbalance similar to Cushing's syndrome. Licorice root has many potential medicinal uses, and its medicinal use should be closely monitored by an experienced healthcare clinician.

ACTION OF LICORICE

* Licorice exhibits anti-inflammatory properties and provides liver cell protection, respiratory support, adrenal support, and relief of gastrointestinal distress. Most of the medicinal activity of licorice can be attributed to glycyrrhizin, or glycyrrhetinic acid (i.e., plant extract).
    —The glycyrrhetinic acid in licorice blocks the breakdown of cortisol, which can help to restore normal adrenal function in individuals experiencing adrenal fatigue.
    —Licorice is a demulcent to the upper digestive tract, meaning it provides a soothing coating. This can help to relieve heartburn, gastric reflux, and gastric and intestinal ulcers.

RECOMMENDED DOSAGE AND ADMINISTRATION

* A dosage of no more than 100 mg/day is recommended for chronic use. Doses should be taken with breakfast and lunch; taking at dinner should be avoided so that normal cortisol patterns can be restored.

ADVERSE REACTIONS AND MEDICATION INTERACTIONS

* Women who are pregnant should not use licorice in medicinal doses because of the potential for harm to the fetus.
    —Licorice inhibits the enzyme that normally protects the fetus from high cortisol levels in the mother's blood.
    —Although licorice appears to lower testosterone in both male and female fetuses, more research is needed to confirm this effect. This adverse reaction could be particularly harmful for a male fetus because large amounts of testosterone are necessary for sexual differentiation in males.
* Licorice contains glycyrrhetinic acid, which, in large amounts, can prevent cortisol breakdown, resulting in pseudoaldosteronism (i.e., excessive

levels of aldosterone). Pseudoaldosteronism can cause hypertension, buildup of sodium and fluid, and loss of potassium. Close follow-up care is necessary when licorice is prescribed for use as an herbal medication.

- Licorice components can have adverse interactions with oral contraceptives, nonsteroidal anti-inflammatory drugs (NSAIDs), potassium chloride, thiazide diuretics, corticosteroids, and blood thinning agents.

RECENT FINDINGS

- Results of studies show that the active components of licorice have antimicrobial and anti-inflammatory properties, which provide therapeutic benefits in the treatment of oro-dental diseases (e.g., dental caries, periodontitis, candidiasis, and recurrent canker sores). Clinical studies are needed to validate these results, which have primarily been observed in in vitro assays. Safe application techniques also need to be devised to prevent the toxicity and adverse reactions associated with the chronic use of licorice.
- A clinical trial was conducted involving 60 patients with peptic ulcer disease (PUD) to compare the effectiveness of licorice versus bismuth in therapeutic regimens against *Helicobacter pylori*. Both groups (i.e., case and control) of patients responded well to treatment. Researchers concluded that for cases in which bismuth is contraindicated, licorice can be safely substituted.
- Researchers suggest that licorice may be useful for preventing hyperkalemia (i.e., high potassium levels) and related cardiac events in dialysis patients due to the action of glycyrrhetinic acid against cortisol breakdown and the resulting depletion of potassium in the blood. Further research is necessary to determine if licorice treatment can help prevent hyperkalemia and resulting cardiac events in patients undergoing hemodialysis.

SUMMARY

Consumers should become knowledgeable about the physiologic risks and benefits of licorice. Licorice is used to treat conditions such as upset stomach, asthma, cough, bad breathe, canker sores, stomach ulcers, eczema, indigestion, and respiratory distress. Licorice components can have adverse interactions with oral contraceptives,

nonsteroidal anti-inflammatory drugs (NSAIDs), potassium chloride, thiazide diuretics, corticosteroids, and blood thinning agent. Research suggests that licorice may be helpful in treating ulcers, as well as reducing cardiac events common in hemodialysis patients.

—*Cherie Marcel, BS*

REFERENCES

Challem, J. (2011). Shop smart. Licorice twist. *Better Nutrition, 73*(10), 22-23.

Choi, J., Han, J., Ahn, H., Ryu, H., Kim, M., Chung, J., ... Koren, G. (2013). Fetal and neonatal outcomes in women reporting ingestion of licorice (Glycyrrhiza uralensis) during pregnancy. *Planta Medica, 79*(2), 97-101. doi:10.3109/01443615.2012.734871

Eid, T. J., Morris, A. A., & Shah, S. A. (2011). Hypertension secondary to ingestion of licorice root tea. *Journal of Pharmacy Technology, 27*(6), 266-268.

Ferrari, P. (2009). Licorice: A sweet alternative to prevent hyperkalemia in dialysis patients? *Kidney International, 76*(8), 811-812. doi:10.1038/ki.2009.282

Liao, H. L., Ma, T. C., Li, Y. C., Chen, J. T., & Chang, Y. S. (2010). Concurrent use of corticosteroids with licorice-containing TCM preparations in Taiwan: A National Health Insurance Database study. *Journal of Alternative and Complementary Medicine (New York, N.Y.), 16*(5), 539-544. doi:10.1089/acm.2009.0267

Mentes, J. C., Kang, S., Spackman, S., & Bauer, J. (2012). Can licorice lollipop decrease cariogenic bacteria in nursing home residents? *Research in Gerontological Nursing, 5*(4), 233-237. doi:10.3928/19404921-20120906-07

Messier, C., Epifano, F., Genovese, S., & Grenier, D. (2012). Licorice and its potential beneficial effects in common oro-dental diseases. *Oral Diseases, 18*(1), 32-39. doi:10.1111/j.1601-0825.2011.01842.x

Momeni, A., Rahimian, G., Kiasi, A., Amiri, M., & Kheiri, S. (2014). Effect of licorice versus bismuth on eradication of Helicobacter pylori in patients with peptic uler disease. *Pharmacognosy Research, 6*(4), 341-344. doi:10.4103/0974-8490.138289

Raikkonen, K., Pesonen, A. K., Heinonen, K., Lahti, J., Komsi, N., Eriksson, J. G., & Strandberg, T. E. (2009). Maternal licorice consumption and detrimental cognitive and psychiatric outcomes in children. *American Journal of Epidemiology, 170*(9), 1137-1146. doi:10.1093/aje/kwp272

Sego, S. (2011). Alternative meds update. Licorice. *Clinical Advisor for Nurse Practitioners, 14*(4), 156, 158.

Tu, J. H., He, Y. J., Chen, Y., Fan, L., Zhang, W., Tan, Z. R., & Zhou, H. -H. (2010). Effect of glycyrrhizin on the activity of CYP3A enzyme in humans. *European Journal of Clinical Pharmacology, 66*(8), 805-810.

Yorgun, H., Aksoy, H., Sendur, M. A., Ates, A. H., Kaya, E. B., Aytemir, K., & Oto, A. (2010). Brugada syndrome with aborted sudden cardiac death related to liquorice-induced hypokalemia. *Medical Principles and Practice, 19*(6), 485-489.

Yoshino, T., Yanagawa, T., & Watanabe, K. (2014). Risk factors for pseudoaldosteronism with rhabdomyolosis caused by consumption of drugs containing licorice and differences between incidence of these conditions in Japan and other countries: Case report and literature review. *Journal of Alternative & Complementary Medicine, 20*(6), 516-520. doi:10.1089/acm.2013.0454

REVIEWER(S)

Darlene Strayer, RN, MBA, Cinahl Information Systems, Glendale, CA

Nursing Executive Practice Council, Glendale Adventist Medical Center, Glendale, CA

Mint

WHAT WE KNOW

Mint, or *mentha*, is an evergreen plant of the Lamiaceae family, which is native to Europe. Although there are about 200 species in the mint family, peppermint and spearmint are the most commonly used cultivations and are used as flavoring agents, inhalants, liquid extracts, oils, and teas. Peppermint oil, a volatile (i.e., rapidly evaporating) oil, is primarily composed of menthol, which is used in many topical analgesics, anesthetics, itch relievers, antitussive ointments, lozenges, creams, lotions, and throat sprays.

ACTION OF MINT

- The active components of mint are found in the leaves and flowering tops of the plant.
- The fresh leaves of peppermint contain as much vitamin C as an orange and more provitamin A carotenoids (i.e., any of the group of carotenoids [e.g., beta-carotene] that are precursors of vitamin A) than a carrot. Additionally, peppermint provides a high amount of manganese and trace amounts of iron, calcium, folate, potassium, magnesium, tryptophan, omega-3 fatty acids, riboflavin, copper, and fiber. Other valuable phytonutrients (i.e., beneficial plant-derived chemicals) found in peppermint include menthol, perillyl alcohol, and rosmarinic acid. Peppermint's medicinal qualities are primarily attributed to menthol. The actions of peppermint include the following:
  - —Peppermint oil exhibits antifungal, antiviral, and antibacterial properties, halting the growth of numerous bacteria, including *Helicobacter pylori*, *Salmonella enteritidis*, *Escherichia coli* O157:H7, and methicillin-resistant *Staphylococcus aureus* (MRSA).
  - —It serves as an anesthetic, antiemetic, antiflatulent, antiseptic, aromatic, diaphoretic, digestive aid, flavoring agent, and stimulant.
  - —It has been used in treatment of headache, neuralgia, rheumatism, throat infection, and toothache.
  - —As an inhalant, menthol in peppermint improves bronchitis, chest congestion, laryngitis, and nasal congestion.
  - —As aromatherapy, peppermint appears to increase concentration and stimulate the mind.
  - —In animal studies, peppermint has been found to relax the sphincter of Oddi and stimulate bile flow.
  - —It depresses sensory cutaneous receptors, which reduces itch and irritation.
  - —Peppermint has relieves spasms in the smooth muscles within the digestive tract.
  - —Azulene, an extract of peppermint oil, has anti-inflammatory and anti-ulcerative effects in animals.
- Spearmint is primarily used as a flavoring agent. Although the action of spearmint is not well documented, its action is suspected to be more subtle than but similar to peppermint's.
  - —Along with vitamin C and provitamin A carotenoids, active components of spearmint include carvone, limonene, phellandrene, and pinene. Unlike peppermint, spearmint does not contain a significant amount of menthol.
  - —There is some scientific evidence that spearmint exhibits antibacterial, antifungal, antidepressant, chemo-preventive, antioxidant, lipid-reducing, sedative, and anti-inflammatory activities.
  - —Spearmint is thought to whiten teeth, heal mouth sores, resolve nausea, and resolve signs and symptoms of bites and stings.

RECOMMENDED DOSAGE AND ADMINISTRATION

- There are no defined or recommended therapeutic dosages for mint. Suggestions for the use of peppermint are as follows:
  —Oral
  —Enteric-coated capsules: 1 or 2 capsules can be taken 3 times daily between meals
  —1 mL of peppermint spirits (i.e., composed of 10% oil and 1% leaf extract) combined with water can be taken 3 times daily
  —Oil 0.2–0.4 mL in dilute preparations can be taken 2–3 times daily
  —1 tablespoon of dried leaves in a tea with 160 mL of boiling water can be taken 2–3 times daily
  —Tincture of 1% mint preparation to 45% ethanol can be taken 2–3 times daily
  —Topical: Essential mint oil can be prepared as an ointment and applied externally, as appropriate

ADVERSE REACTIONS

- Menthol is thought to be fatal at dosages of about 1,000 mg/kg of body weight.
- Individuals who are pregnant or breastfeeding should not use mint in medicinal dosages.
- Individuals who are hypersensitive or allergic to plants such as grass should not use mint medicinally.
- Mint should not be used on infants or young children; applying menthol to an infant's nostrils to relieve congestion can cause syncope.
- Topical agents should not be applied to broken skin, and use of topical mint preparations in combination with a heating pad can cause skin damage.
- Individuals with acid reflux should not ingest mint or mint-containing products.
- Treatment is generally discontinuing mint administration and managing signs and symptoms.

RESEARCH FINDINGS

- Study results have identified potentially protective qualities of mint against radioactivity, possibly through free radical, antioxidant, and anti-inflammatory actions. Researchers suggest that pretreatment with mint could reduce damage inflicted by radioactive treatments (e.g., radiation therapy). Results show that mint exhibits neuroprotective qualities, suggesting the potential for preventing radiation-induced behavioral changes related to neurologic system damage.
- Researchers report that spearmint oil allergy is a possible cause of some cases of oral lichen planus (OLP), a chronic inflammatory condition of the oral mucous membranes.
- With the availability of newer and more expensive medications, peppermint oil is frequently overlooked as a treatment option. Authors of several studies and reviews have reported that peppermint oil is a safe and effective therapeutic agent for the treatment of irritable bowel syndrome (IBS), functional indigestion, and postoperative nausea.

SUMMARY

Consumers should become knowledgeable about the physiologic effects of mint, including its risks and benefits. Fresh mint leaves can contribute to health as a rich source of vitamin C, provitamin A carotenoids, numerous phytonutrients, and menthol (primarily found in peppermint). Mint can be used to treat headache, congestion and nausea. Mint also acts as an antibacterial, antifungal, antidepressant, chemo-preventive, antioxidant, lipid-reducing, sedative, and anti-inflammatory agent. Individuals should be aware the potential for adverse reactions when using mint medicinally, especially that menthol may be fatal at dosages of about 1,000 mg/kg of body weight. Research suggests that mint may be helpful in treating patients undergoing radiation therapy.

—*Cherie Marcel, BS*

REFERENCES

Baliga, M. S., & Rao, S. (2010). Radioprotective potential of mint: A brief review. *Journal of Cancer Research and Therapeutics*, 6(3), 255-262. doi:10.4103/0973-1482.73336

Burnett, B. (2011). Versatile mint: From garden to table. *Alive: Canada's Natural Health & Wellness Magazine*, (344), 34-38.

Ehrlich, S.D. (2013, May 7). Peppermint. *University of Maryland Medical Center*. Retrieved June 18, 2015, from http://www.umm.edu/altmed/articles/peppermint-000269.htm

Fetrow, C. W., & Avila, J. R. (2004). Mint. In *Professional's handbook of complementary & alternative medicines* (3rd ed., pp. 563-566). Springhouse, PA: Lippincott Williams & Wilkins A Wolters Kluwer Company.

The George Mateljan Foundation editorial team. (n.d.). Peppermint. *The World's Healthiest Foods*. Retrieved June 18, 2015, from http://www.whfoods.com/genpage.php? tname=foodspice&dbid=102

Gunatheesan, S., Tam, M. M., Tate, B., Tvresky, J., & Nixon, R. (2012). Retrospective study of oral lichen planus and allergy to spearmint oil. *The Australasian Journal of Dermatology*, 53(3), 224-228. doi:10.1111/j.1440-0960.2012.00908.x

Haksar, A., Sharma, A., Chawla, R., Kumar, R., Lahiri, S. S., Islam, F., & Arora, R. (2009). Mint oil (Mentha spicata Linn.) offers behavioral radioprotection: A radiation-induced conditioned taste aversion study. *Phytotherapy Research: PTR*, 23(2), 293-296. doi:10.1002/ptr.2604

Lane, B., Cannella, K., Bowen, C., Copelan, D., Nteff, G., Barnes, K., ... Lawson, J. (2012). Examination of the effectiveness of peppermint aromatherapy on nausea in women post C-section. *Journal of Holistic Nursing*, 30(2), 90-104. doi:10.1177/0898010111423419

Lopez, V., Martin, S., Gomez-Serranillos, M. P., Carretero, M. E., Jager, A. K., & Calvo, M. I. (2010). Neuroprotective and neurochemical properties of mint extracts. *Phytotherapy Research*, 24(6), 869-874. doi:10.1002/ptr.3037

Mann, N. S., & Sandhu, K. S. (2012). Peppermint oil in irritable bowel syndrome: Systematic evaluation of 1634 cases with meta-analysis. *International Medical Journal*, 19(1), 5-6.

Smith, G. D. (2011). Peppermint oil in gastrointestinal medicine. *Gastrointestinal Nursing*, 9(8), 13-14.

Spearmint nutrition facts. (n.d.). *Nutrition-and-you.com*. Retrieved June 18, 2015, from http://www.nutrition-and-you.com/spearmint.html

Tourney, A. (2013, August 16). Teas to drink for irritable bowel syndrome. *Livestrong.com*. Retrieved June 18, 2015, from http://www.livestrong.com/article/342990-teas-to-drink-for-irritable-bowel-syndrome/

Ware, M. (2015, June 4). Mint: Health benefits, uses and risks. *Medicalnewstoday.com*. Retrieved June 18, 2015, from http://www.medicalnewstoday.com/articles/275944.php

REVIEWER(S)

Darlene Strayer, RN, MBA, Cinahl Information Systems, Glendale, CA

Nursing Executive Practice Council, Glendale Adventist Medical Center, Glendale, CA

Mustard

WHAT WE KNOW

Mustard (*Synapis alba*) is a member of the Brassicaceae, or Cruciferae, family. Members of the Brassicaceae family are commonly referred to as cruciferous vegetables; other cruciferous vegetables include cabbage; cauliflower, kale, and horseradish. The dried ripe seeds of white mustard (*Brassica alba*) and black mustard (*Brassica nigra*) are ground into a powder for use as a spice, made into a condiment, or prepared as a medicinal agent. Mustard has been used to treat upper respiratory tract conditions (e.g., bronchitis, sinusitis), fever, colds, gastric ulcers, constipation, and inflammation of the mouth and pharynx. It has been applied as a topical ointment to soothe pulmonary congestion, rheumatism, and arthritis. The active components of mustard are the valuable secondary metabolites referred to as glucosinolates, which are responsible for the pungent odor associated with mustard and have bacteriostatic and anti-carcinogenic activities. Glucosinolates are also potent skin irritants.

ACTION OF MUSTARD

- Mustard is a source of the sulfur-containing phytochemicals sinigrin and sinalbin, which are glucosinolates, whose degradation products isothiocyanates and p-hydroxybenzyl appear to have chemo-preventive and anti-bacterial activity.
  —Glucosinolates enhance the liver's ability to detoxify carcinogens. They also inhibit the growth of and kill multiple strains of *Helicobacter pylori*, a bacteria known to cause stomach ulcers and increase risk for stomach cancer.
- Mustard is also a good source of provitamin A carotenoids (e.g., beta-carotene), which are converted into vitamin A in the human body. Vitamin A, or retinol, is a fat-soluble vitamin that is required for vision, maintenance of the surface lining of the eyes and other epithelial tissue, bone growth, immune response, energy regulation, reproduction, embryonic development, and activation of gene expression.
- Mustard greens are a good source of vitamins C, E, and K and provide minerals, such as copper, manganese, and calcium.
  —Vitamin C is a water-soluble vitamin that neutralizes free radicals, protecting against

inflammation and cellular damage. Adequate vitamin C intake is vital for proper function of the immune system and has been associated with prevention of heart disease, stroke, and cancer.

—Vitamin E is a fat-soluble vitamin that functions primarily as an antioxidant but also maintains cell membranes, assists in vitamin K absorption, and contributes to immune system function.

—Vitamin K acts as a coenzyme involved in maintaining normal levels of blood-clotting proteins and contributes to bone metabolism.

—Copper is a vital component of superoxide dismutase (SOD), which is an enzyme involved in energy production and antioxidant activity. Copper contributes to the action of lysyl oxidase, an enzyme necessary for the cross-linking of collagen and elastin to allow flexibility in blood vessels, bones, and joints. Copper enhances the body's ability to use iron, preventing iron-deficiency anemia, ruptured vessels, irregular heartbeat, and infection.

—Manganese is a trace mineral that is responsible for energy production, fatty acid synthesis, cholesterol production, and protection against damage caused by free radicals.

—Calcium builds and maintains bones and teeth, regulates muscle contraction, conducts nerve impulses, activates enzymes for energy production and muscle contraction, participates in blood clotting, assists with vitamin B12 absorption, and maintains the structural integrity of intracellular membranes.

ADVERSE REACTIONS AND MEDICATION INTERACTIONS

- Mustard oil can irritate the lining of the nose; the mouth, throat, and other parts of the digestive system; and the urinary tract.
- Mustard can increase stomach acid production, which can decrease the effects of antacids, H2 blockers, proton pump inhibitors, and sucralfate.

RESEARCH FINDINGS

- Scientists have demonstrated that *Brassica*-derived isothiocyanates exhibit properties inhibiting tumor growth and reducing risk of cancer.

SUMMARY

Consumers should become knowledgeable about the physiologic effects of mustard. Mustard is a good source of calcium, manganese, copper, sulfur-containing phytonutrients, provitamin A carotenoids, and vitamins C, E, and K. These nutrients contribute to bone, muscle and eye health, as well as digestion and immune system support. Mustard intake may reduce the risk of developing iron-deficiency anemia, heart disease, cancer and stroke. Mustard oil can irritate the lining of the nose; the mouth, throat, and other parts of the digestive system; and the urinary tract. Research suggests that mustard may help reduce the spread cancer.

—*Cherie Marcel, BS*

REFERENCES

Caballero, T., San-Martín, M. S., Padial, M. A., Contreras, J., Cabañas, R., Barranco, P., & López-Serrano, M. C. (2002). Clinical characteristics of patients with mustard hypersensitivity. *Annals of Allergy, Asthma & Immunology*, 89(2), 166-171. doi:10.1016/S1081-1206(10)61933-3

Evert, A. (2013). Vitamin E. *MedlinePlus*. Retrieved June 5, 2015, from http://www.nlm.nih.gov/medlineplus/ency/article/002406.htm

Johnson, L. E. (2014). Vitamin E. The Merck Manual for Health Care Professionals. Retrieved June 5, 2015, from http://www.merckmanuals.com/professional/sec01/ch004/ch004l.html

Kumar, A., D'Souza, S. S., Tickoo, S., Salimath, B. P., & Singh, H. B. (2009). Antiangiogenic and proapoptotic activities of allyl isothiocyanate inhibit ascites tumor growth in vivo. *Integrative Cancer Therapies*, 8(1), 75-87. doi:10.1177/1534735408330716

Lamy, E., Garcia-Käufer, M., Prinzhorn, J., & Mersch-Sundermann, V. (2012). Antigenotoxic action of isothiocyanate-containing mustard as determined by two cancer biomarkers in a human intervention trial. *European Journal of Cancer Prevention: The Official Journal of the European Cancer Prevention Organisation*, 21(4), 400-406. doi:10.1097/CEJ.0b013e32834ef140

Lutz, C. A., Mazur, E. E., & Litch, N. A. (Eds.). (2015). Vitamins. In *Nutrition & diet therapy* (6th ed., pp. 98-103). Philadelphia, PA: F. A. Davis Company.

Oregon State University. Linus Pauling Institute. (2014). Copper. *Micronutrient Information Center*. Retrieved June 5, 2015, from http://lpi.oregonstate.edu/infocenter/minerals/ copper/

The George Mateljan Foundation. (n.d.). Manganese. *The World's Healthiest Foods*. Retrieved June 5, 2015, from http://www.whfoods.com/genpage.php?tname=nutrient&dbid=77

The George Mateljan Foundation editorial team. (n.d.). Mustard seeds. *The World's Healthiest Foods*. Retrieved June 5, 2015, from http://www.whfoods.com/genpage.php? tname=foodspice&dbid=106

The George Mateljan Foundation editorial team. (n.d.). The World's Healthiest Foods. Retrieved June 5, 2015, from http://www.whfoods.com/genpage.php?tname=foodspice&dbid=93

USDA National Nutrient Database for Standard Reference, Release 24. (2012). Vitamin A, IU content of selected foods per common measure, sorted by nutrient content. Retrieved June 5, 2015, from http://www.docstoc.com/docs/30903437/USDA-National-Nutrient-Database-for-Standard-Reference_-Release-22

Wanasundara, J. P. (2011). Proteins of Brassicaceae oilseeds and their potential as a plant protein source. *Critical Reviews in Food Science & Nutrition*, 51(7), 635-677. doi:10.1080/10408391003749942

Zieve, D., & Eltz, D. R. (2013, February 18). Vitamin C. *MedlinePlus*. Retrieved June 5, 2015, from http://www.nlm.nih.gov/medlineplus/ency/article/002404.htm

Calcium. (2015). *MedlinePlus*. Retrieved June 5, 2015, from http://www.nlm.nih.gov/medlineplus/calcium.html

REVIEWER(S)

Darlene Strayer, RN, MBA, Cinahl Information Systems, Glendale, CA

Helle Heering, RN, CRRN, Cinahl Information Systems, Glendale, CA

Nursing Executive Practice Council, Glendale Adventist Medical Center, Glendale, CA

Nutmeg

WHAT WE KNOW

Nutmeg is harvested from *Myristica fragrans*, an aromatic evergreen tree that is indigenous to Banda, the largest of the Molucca Islands (commonly called Spice Islands) of Indonesia. The tree produces a yellow fruit that contains a nut, or seed, with a scarlet aril (i.e., a bright red, fleshy covering). Nutmeg is the actual nut, and the scarlet aril is known as mace.

- Nutmeg has long been coveted and even fought over. In the 17th century, the Dutch gained control of the Spice Islands and nutmeg production, a monopoly they maintained until World War II.

- Although nutmeg has a long history of use in folk medicine, modern science has not proven its medicinal value. Raw, freshly ground nutmeg contains myristicin, a monoamine oxidase inhibitor (MAOI) that induces psychoactive effects (e.g., hallucinations). Myristicin poisoning, with signs and symptoms of nausea, pain, and hallucinations, can result if large quantities of nutmeg are ingested. Culinary quantities are safe for human consumption but may be harmful to pets and livestock.

ACTION OF NUTMEG

- Culinary use of nutmeg as a seasoning in various recipes and food preparations is common.

- Nutmeg is well known for its hallucinogenic effects, which are attributed to myristicin, and nutmeg is used by some individuals as an alternative intoxicant to induce hallucinations and euphoria.

- Evidence is insufficient to support the use of nutmeg clinically, but many claim to have used it successfully for the treatment of diarrhea, nausea and vomiting, arthritic pain, insomnia, and anxiety. It has also been used to lower blood pressure and to treat male impotence.

ADVERSE REACTIONS

- Nutmeg toxicity
  —Raw, freshly ground nutmeg contains myristicin, which has psychoactive effects and can cause toxicity when large amounts are consumed. Signs and symptoms of myristicin poisoning include the following:
    –Convulsions
    –Palpitations
    –Nausea
    –Dehydration
    –Generalized body pain, including headache
    –Hallucinations and euphoria
  —Toxicity can develop over a period of several hours and can produce signs and symptoms for several days.

- Historically, nutmeg was believed to induce abortion, but evidence is lacking. Culinary use of nutmeg is generally considered safe during pregnancy.

RESEARCH FINDINGS

- Myristicin poisoning can cause serious manifestations, including delusions, muscle weakness, ataxia, and convulsions. Many persons are not aware of the dangerous effects of myristicin poisoning, and abuse of nutmeg as a recreational hallucinogenic is increasing. This is probably due to its low cost, ease of acquisition, and perceived holistic quality. Because the effects of poisoning can take hours to manifest, users may not attribute the negative effects to the consumption of nutmeg.

- Results of a study conducted on the pharmacologic properties of nutmeg oil showed that nutmeg oil exhibited an anti-inflammatory effect in rats and mice similar to that of anti-inflammatory medications. Researchers also reported that nutmeg had antidiarrheal effects.

- Researchers investigating the impact of nutmeg on male sexual function found that nutmeg possesses aphrodisiac activity and increases libido and potency. This may be due to nutmeg's ability to stimulate the nervous system.

SUMMARY

Consumers should become knowledgeable about the physiologic effects of nutmeg, including its risks and benefits. Excessive intake of nutmeg may result in myristicin poisoning which causes nausea, pain, and hallucinations. Regular culinary amounts of nutmeg may help treat diarrhea, nausea and vomiting, arthritic pain, insomnia, and anxiety. It has also been used to lower blood pressure and to treat male impotence.

—*Cherie Marcel, BS*

REFERENCES

Barceloux, D. G. (2009). Nutmeg (Myristica fragrans Houtt.). *Disease-A-Month*, 55(6), 373-379. doi:10.1016/j.disamonth.2009.03.007.

Carstairs, S. D., & Cantrell, F. L. (2011). The spice of life: An analysis of nutmeg exposures in California. *Clinical Toxicology*, 49(3), 177-180. doi:10.3109/15563650.2011.561210.

Demetriades, A. K., Wallman, P. D., McGuiness, A., & Gavalas, M. C. (2005). Low cost, high risk: Accidental nutmeg intoxication. *Emergency Medicine Journal*, 22(3), 223-225. doi:10.1136/emj.2002.004168

Kelly, B. D., Gavin, B. E., Clarke, M., Lane, A., & Larkin, C. (2003). Nutmeg and psychosis. *Schizophrenia Research*, 60(1), 95-96.

Landis, R. (1997). The baker's trio: Therapeutic uses of cloves, cinnamon, nutmeg. *Vegetarian Times*, (244), 6.

McKenna, A., Nordt, S. P., & Ryan, J. (2004). Acute nutmeg poisoning. *European Journal of Emergency Medicine: Official Journal of the European Society for Emergency Medicine*, 11(4), 240-241.

Olajide, O. A., Makinde, J. M., & Awe, S. O. (2000). Evaluation of the pharmacological properties of nutmeg oil in rats and mice. *Pharmaceutical Biology*, 38(5), 385-390. doi:10.1076/phbi.38.5.385.5976.

Sangalli, B. C., Sangalli, B., & Chiang, W. (2000). Toxicology of nutmeg abuse. *Journal of Toxicology. Clinical Toxicology*, 38(6), 671-678. doi:10.1081/CLT-100102020

Shepherd, L. (2007). There's more to Chai than meets the eye. *Natural Health and Vegetarian Life*, 42.

Stein, U., Greyer, H., & Hentschel, H. (2001). Nutmeg (myristicin) poisoning-report on a fatal case and a series of cases recorded by a poison information centre. *Forensic Science International*, 118(1), 87-90.

Tajuddin, A. S., Ahmad, S., Latif, A., Qasmi, I. A., & Amin, K. M. (2005). An experimental study of sexual function improving effect of Myristica fragrans Houtt (nutmeg). *BMC Complementary and Alternative Medicine*, 5, 16. doi:10.1186/1472-6882-5-16

Takikawa, A., Abe, K., Yamamoto, M., Ishimaru, S., Yasui, M., Okubo, Y., & Yokoigawa, K. (2002). Antimicrobial activity of nutmeg against Escherichia coli O157. *Journal of Bioscience and Bioengineering*, 94(4), 315-320. doi:10.1016/S1389-1723(02)80170-0.

REVIEWER(S)

Darlene Strayer, RN, MBA, Cinahl Information Systems, Glendale, CA

Nursing Executive Practice Council, Glendale Adventist Medical Center, Glendale, CA

Oregano

WHAT WE KNOW

Oregano, or *Origanum vulgare*, is a sprawling, aromatic plant with pink or white flowers. It is a member of the mint (Lamiaceae or Labiatae) family. Other names for oregano include carvacrol, dostenkraut, European oregano, Mediterranean oregano, mountain mint, oil of oregano,

oregano oil, organy, Origani vulgaris herba, origano, origanum, phytoprogestin, wild marjoram, winter marjoram, and winterswee.

- Oregano is well known as an herb used in culinary seasoning and as a preservative, but is also used medicinally. Research regarding the medicinal use of oregano in humans is inadequate to support its recommendation for any indication, but because of its antibacterial and antioxidant properties oregano has been used to treat a variety of infections and other conditions. These include respiratory tract infections, cough, asthma, croup, bronchitis, indigestion, bloating, urinary tract infections, sinusitis, colds, influenza, menstrual cramps, rheumatoid arthritis, headache, heart conditions, allergies, earache, fatigue, and intestinal parasites.
- Topical oregano is applied to treat acne, athlete's foot, dandruff, insect and spider bites, canker sores, gum disease, toothache, psoriasis, seborrhea, ringworm, rosacea, muscle pain, varicose veins, and warts.

ACTION OF OREGANO

- The active components of oregano are found in the leaves and include carvacrol and thymol, which have anthelmintic (i.e., kills parasites and worms), fungicidal, antibacterial, antioxidant, and antiseptic properties.

RECOMMENDED DOSAGE AND ADMINISTRATION

- A typical dose of oregano is 1 cup of freshly brewed tea prepared by steeping a heaping teaspoon of oregano leaf in 250 ml of boiling water for 10–15 minutes and then straining.

ADVERSE REACTIONS AND MEDICATION INTERACTION

- Concentrated, non-emulsified oil of oregano and large quantities of oregano can cause gastrointestinal upset and localized irritation of the gastrointestinal tract.
- Oregano should be avoided by individuals who are hypersensitive to oregano or to other plants in the mint family.
- Treatment of adverse reactions to oregano is discontinuation of its use.
- Oregano can reduce iron absorption. Medicinal doses of oregano should be taken 2 hours before or 2 hours after ingestion of iron supplements.

RESEARCH FINDINGS

- Researchers studying the effects of oregano on the behavior of rats determined that oregano elevated extracellular serotonin levels in the brain. They suggested that further studies be conducted to investigate if such an extract would exhibit mood-enhancing benefits in humans.
- Oregano extract may contribute to weight reduction and improve diabetes-related vascular complications (e.g., atherosclerosis) by activating endothelial nitric oxide synthase. Further research is merited to investigate the potential of oregano extract to prevent and improve metabolic syndrome (i.e., the coexistence of obesity, hyperglycemia, hypertension, and hyper/dyslipidemia) and its complications.
- Researchers have reported that oregano-based ointments show broad antimicrobial activity, which could offer alternatives for treating methicillin-resistant Staphylococcus aureus (MRSA) infections. They found that an ointment containing 1–10% oregano could inhibit most microorganisms. Investigating tissue toxicity and potential adverse reactions is necessary before testing on humans. Oregano also shows strong potential for assisting wound healing. Results of a study of oregano-containing ointments used in traditional Turkish medicine revealed that a cream formulated from olive oil extract, oregano extract, and Salvia triloba essential oil demonstrated significant wound healing activity. Such an ointment could be used for rapid healing of acute and chronic wounds.
- Researchers evaluated the anti-inflammatory and antiulcer activities of carvacrol, an active constituent of the essential oil of oregano. They determined from the results of the study that carvacrol most likely interferes with the synthesis and release of inflammatory mediators (e.g., prostanoids), an action which supports the healing process of gastric ulcers.

SUMMARY

Consumers should become knowledgeable about the physiologic effects of oregano, including its risks and benefits. Oregano is used to treat respiratory tract infections, cough, asthma, croup, bronchitis, indigestion, bloating, urinary tract infections, sinusitis, colds, influenza, menstrual cramps, rheumatoid arthritis, headache, heart conditions, allergies, earache, fatigue, and intestinal parasites. Topical oregano is applied to treat acne, athlete's foot, dandruff, insect and spider bites, canker sores, gum disease, toothache, psoriasis, seborrhea, ringworm, rosacea, muscle pain, varicose veins, and warts. Large quantities of non-emulsified oil of oregano can cause GI issues and oregano may inhibit iron absorption. Research suggests that oregano may improve mood, assist with wound healing, help with weight control and reduce risk for type 2 diabetes.

—*Cherie Marcel, BS*

REFERENCES

Eng, W., & Norman, R. (2010). Development of an oregano-based ointment with anti-microbial activity including activity against methicillin-resistant Staphlococcus aureus. *Journal of Drugs in Dermatology*, 9(4), 377-380.

Oregano. (2004). In C. W. Fetrow, & J. R. Avila (Eds.), *Professional's handbook of complementary & alternative medicines* (3rd ed., pp. 613-614). Springhouse, PA: Lippincott Williams & Wilkins A Wolters Kluwer Company.

Oregano. (2003). In J. M. Jellin, P. J. Gregory, F. Batz, & K. Hitchens (Eds.), *Pharmacist's letter/prescriber's letter natural medicines comprehensive database* (5th ed., pp. 982-983). Stockton, CA: Therapeutic Research Faculty.

Mechan, A. O., Fowler, A., Seifert, N., Rieger, H., Wohrle, T., Etheve, S., & Mohajeri, M. H. (2011). Monoamine reuptake inhibition and mood-enhancing potential of a specified oregano extract. *The British Journal of Nutrition*, 105(8), 1150-1163. doi:10.1017/S0007114510004940

Mueller, M., Lukas, B., Novak, J., Simoncini, T., Genazzani, A. R., & Jungbauer, A. (2008). Oregano: A source for peroxisome proliferator-activated receptor gamma antagonists. *Journal of Agricultural and Food Chemistry*, 56(24), 11621-11630.

Silva, F. V., Guimaraes, A. G., Silva, E. R. S., Sousa-Neto, B. P., Machado, F. D. F., Quintans-Junior, L. J., & Oliveira, R. C. M. (2012). Anti-inflammatory and anti-ulcer activities of carvacrol, a monoterpene present in the essential oil of oregano. *Journal of Medicinal Food*, 15(1), 984-991. doi:10.1089/jmf.2012.0102

Singletary, K. (2010). Oregano: Overview of the literature on health benefits. *Nutrition Today*, 45(3), 129-138.

Suntar, I., Akkol, E. K., Keles, H., Oktem, A., Baser, K. H., & Yesilada, E. (2011). A novel wound healing ointment: A formulation of Hypericum perforatum oil and sage and oregano essential oils based on traditional Turkish knowledge. *Journal of Ethnopharmacology*, 134(1), 89-96. doi:10.1016/j.jep.2010.11.061

REVIEWER(S)

Darlene Strayer, RN, MBA, Cinahl Information Systems, Glendale, CA

Nursing Practice Council, Glendale Adventist Medical Center, Glendale, CA

Parsley

WHAT WE KNOW

Parsley, or *Petroselinum crispum*, is a member of the Apiaceae (or Umbelliferae) family, which includes anise, celery, dill, and fennel. Italian flat leaf parsley (fragrant and mild flavored) and curly parsley (more bitter than Italian flat leaf) are the most commonly used forms of parsley. Turnip-rooted (also known as Hamburg) parsley is a lesser known variety of parsley that is cultivated for its roots. Although parsley is best known as an herb used in culinary seasoning and garnishment, it also has a long history of medicinal use. It is a substantial source of many nutrients, including minerals, phytonutrients (i.e., beneficial plant-derived substances), and fiber. Because of its ample flavonoid content, parsley has very strong antioxidant properties. The leaves, seeds, and dried root have been used for a variety of therapeutic indications. Parsley has been administered in treatment of gastrointestinal disorders, urinary tract infections, hypertension, painful menstruation, gallstones, colds, and influenza. It has also been used as a diuretic, mild laxative, antimicrobial agent, and breath freshener. Parsley may play a role in the prevention of certain cancers, tumor growth, cardiac damage, and arthritis.

ACTION OF PARSLEY

- The active components of parsley are found in the leaves, seeds, and roots and include vitamins (e.g., C, K, folate), minerals (e.g., calcium, potassium, iron), volatile oil compounds (e.g., myristicin, apiol, limonene, eugenol, alpha-thujene), flavonoids (e.g., apiin, apigenin, chrysoeriol, luteolin), and carotenoids (e.g., beta-carotene, zeaxanthin, lutein, cryptoxanthin),which have powerful antibacterial, antimicrobial, anti-inflammatory, and antioxidant properties.

—Vitamin K acts as a coenzyme and is involved in maintaining normal levels of blood clotting proteins and contributing to bone metabolism.

—Vitamin C neutralizes free radicals, protecting against inflammation and cellular damage. Adequate intake of vitamin C is vital for immune system function and has been associated with prevention of heart disease, stroke, and cancer.

—Folate is a water-soluble, B vitamin that is essential for the production and maintenance of red blood cells (RBCs). Folate is vital for the synthesis of deoxyribonucleic acid (DNA) and ribonucleic acid (RNA), the genetic code for the cells, and is important in the metabolism of homocysteine, an amino acid.

—Calcium builds and maintains bones and teeth, promotes conduction of nerve impulses, activates enzymes for energy production and muscle contraction, participates in blood clotting, assists with vitamin B12 absorption, and maintains the structural integrity of intracellular membranes.

—Potassium supports normal cellular, nerve, and muscle function and helps to eliminate excess sodium from the body.

—Iron is vital for the synthesis of RBCs and hemoglobin, which are necessary for cellular respiration and the transport of oxygen to the tissues. Iron also supports immune function, is vital for cognitive development, contributes to energy metabolism, and regulates temperature.

—Volatile oils are bioactive compounds that produce powerful effects in extremely small amounts. The volatile oils in parsley have exhibited antioxidant, anti-inflammatory, antibacterial, antimicrobial, and anticancer activities.

—Flavonoids inhibit tumor growth, reduce inflammation, and stimulate the production of detoxifying enzymes.

—Carotenoids are powerful antioxidants with anticancer activity. Carotenoids protect the eyes from age-related macular degeneration (AMD).

—Provitamin A carotenoids (e.g., beta-carotene, cryptoxanthin) are precursors of vitamin A, or retinol, a fat-soluble vitamin that is required for vision, maintenance of the surface lining of the eyes and other epithelial tissue, bone growth, immune response, energy regulation, reproduction, embryonic development, and activation of gene expression.

RECOMMENDED DOSAGE AND ADMINISTRATION

- A typical dosage is 1 cup of freshly brewed parsley tea 3 times daily that includes up to 6 g of prepared parsley per day. The tea is prepared by steeping 2 g of crushed parsley or its root in 250 mL of boiling water for 10–15 minutes.

ADVERSE REACTIONS AND MEDICATION INTERACTION

- Parsley seeds and root can cause uterine contractions, which may lead to abortion.

- Individuals with renal or liver disease should avoid parsley consumption due to the potential for certain components (e.g., myristicin and apiol) in parsley to cause kidney or liver dysfunction.

- There is some concern that parsley can increase the risk of kidney stones in individuals with a history of kidney stones because parsley contains a measurable amount of the chemical oxalate, which is a primary component of kidney stones. Oxalates can build up and crystallize in body fluids and cause health problems in individuals with preexisting kidney or gallbladder dysfunction.

- Treatment of adverse reactions is discontinuing parsley use.

- Persons who are taking lithium should consult with their treating practitioner before consuming parsley, as the combination can result in lithium toxicity.

RESEARCH FINDINGS

- Results of a crossover trial investigating the effect of parsley intake on urinary excretion of flavones and biomarkers for oxidative stress indicated that dietary parsley intake reduces oxidative damage to plasma proteins.

- Results of a recent study of the impact of parsley intake on urinary stones were that no significant relationship was found between parsley leaf tea consumption and the risk of urinary stone formation in healthy individuals.

SUMMARY

Consumers should become knowledgeable about the physiologic effects of parsley consumption, including its risks and benefits. Parsley can contribute to health because it is a good source of vitamins C and K, folate, calcium, potassium, iron, volatile oils, flavonoids, carotenoids, and fiber. Parsley contains strong antioxidant and anti-inflammatory properties and can be used to treat gastrointestinal disorders, urinary tract infections, hypertension, painful menstruation, gallstones, colds, and influenza. It has also been used as a diuretic, mild laxative, antimicrobial agent, and breath freshener. Parsley may play a role in the prevention and treatment of certain cancers, heart disease, and arthritis. Individuals with kidney or liver disease should avoid parsley consumption due to the potential for certain components (e.g., myristicin and apiol) in parsley to cause kidney or liver dysfunction. Individuals with a history of kidney stones may want to avoid parsley because it can increase the risk of kidney stones due to its high oxalate content. Pregnant women should avoid parsley seeds and root which can cause uterine contractions, which may lead to abortion.

—*Cherie Marcel, BS*

REFERENCES

Alyami, F. A., & Rabah, D. M. (2011). Effect of drinking parsley leaf tea on urinary composition and urinary stones' risk factors. *Saudi Journal of Kidney Diseases and Transplantation: An Official Publication of the Saudi Center for Organ Transplantation, Saudi Arabia, 22*(3), 511-514.

Craig, W. J. (2006). Herb watch. Please pass the parsley. *Vibrant Life, 22*(5), 20-21.

Dorman, H. J., Lantto, T. A., Raasmaja, A., & Hiltunen, R. (2011). Antioxidant, pro-oxidant and cytotoxic properties of parsley. *Food & Function, 2*(6), 328-337. doi:10.1039/ C1FO10027K.

Downey, M. (2015). Parsley more than a decorative garnish. *Life Extension*, 91-93.

George Mateljan Foundation. (n.d.). Parsley. *The World's Healthiest Foods*. Retrieved June 18, 2015, from http://www.whfoods.com/genpage. php?tname=foodspice&dbid=100

Higdon, J., & Drake, V. J. (2008). Flavonoids. Linus Pauling Institute Micronutrient Information Center, Oregon State University. Retrieved June 18, 2015, from http://lpi.oregonstate.edu/mic/dietary-factors/phytochemicals/flavonoids

Higdon, J., & Drake, V. J. (2009). Carotenoids. *Linus Pauling Institute Micronutrient Information Center, Oregon State University*. Retrieved June 18, 2015, from http://lpi.oregonstate.edu/mic/dietary-factors/phytochemicals/carotenoids

Nielsen, S. E., Young, J. F., Daneshvar, B., Lauridsen, S. T., Knuthsen, P., Sandstrom, B., & Dragsted, L. O. (1999). Effect of parsley (Petroselinum crispum) intake on urinary apigenin excretion, blood antioxidant enzymes and biomarkers for oxidative stress in human subjects. *British Journal of Nutrition, 81*(6), 447-455. doi:10.1017/ S000711459900080X

Raymond, S. (2010). Parsley more than just garnish. *Alive*, 130-131.

Premkumar, L. S. (2014). Ingredients in spices that produce health benefits. In Fascinating facts about phytonutrients in spices and healthy food: Scientifically proven facts. Xlibris, LLC, p. 138. Retrieved June 18, 2015, from https://books.google.com/books?id=gNtIA wAAQBAJ&pg=PA138&lpg=PA138&dq=myristicin+ phytonutrient&source=bl&ots=7jknkx2rAv&sig=rCo qrY6GrFAmFyV7_ZQCANoH0RQ&hl=e

Tanaka, T., Shnimizu, M., & Moriwaki, H. (2012). Cancer chemoprevention by carotenoids. *Molecules, 17*(3), 3202-3242. doi:10.3390/molecules17033202

The editorial staff at the American Institute for Cancer Research. (2013). Phytochemicals: The cancer fighters in the foods we eat. *AICR*. Retrieved June 18, 2015, from http://www.aicr.org/reduce-your-cancer-risk/diet/elements_phytochemicals.html

The George Mateljan Foundation. (n.d.). Can you tell me what oxalates are and in which foods they can be found?. *The World's Healthiest Foods*. Retrieved June 18, 2015, from http://www.whfoods.com/genpage. php?tname=george&dbid=48

REVIEWER(S)

Darlene Strayer, RN, MBA, Cinahl Information Systems, Glendale, CA

Nursing Practice Council, Glendale Adventist Medical Center, Glendale, CA

Passionflower

WHAT WE KNOW

Passionflower (*Passiflora incarnata*; also known as apricot vine, passion vine, and maypop) is an herb of the Passifloraceae family. Native to North America, Asia, and Europe, passionflower has been used medicinally for hundreds of years. The Aztecs and Native Americans appreciated it for its ability to soothe anxiety and relax the body. These calming properties lead to its therapeutic use for insomnia, gastrointestinal (GI) upset, seizures, asthma, attention deficit hyperactivity disorder (ADHD), hypertension, fibromyalgia, and narcotic drug withdrawal. The active constituents of passionflower are found in its flowers, fruits, leaves, and stems, which are used to make teas, infusions, liquid extracts, and tinctures.

ACTION OF PASSIONFLOWER

- Passionflower is rich in phytonutrients (i.e., beneficial plant-derived chemicals) such as flavonoids, maltol, and the indole alkaloids harmaline and harmalol. These phytonutrients are considered to have sedative, anti-anxiety, antispasmodic, analgesic, muscle-relaxing, and hypnotic qualities.
  —Flavonoids are the color pigments red, yellow, and orange that protect blood vessels from rupture and exhibit antioxidant, antibiotic, and anti-inflammatory activity.
  —Maltol acts as a sedative and anticonvulsant and potentiates the activity of hexobarbital, a barbiturate medication.
  —Indole alkaloids (e.g., harmaline, harmalol) form the basis for serotonin and tryptophan and increase levels of the amino acid that acts as a calming neurotransmitter, called gamma-aminobutyric acid (GABA).

RECOMMENDED DOSAGE AND ADMINISTRATION

- Tea: 1 cup of freshly brewed tea taken 1–4 times daily; prepared by simmering 0.5–2 g of dried passionflower in 1 cup of boiling water for 10 minutes, then straining and cooling.
- Standardized extract of 1:1 in 25% alcohol: 10–20 drops taken 3 times daily.
- Tincture of 1:5 in 45% alcohol: 10–45 drops taken 3 times daily.

ADVERSE REACTIONS AND MEDICATION INTERACTIONS

- Passionflower is generally considered to be safe if taken in recommended doses.
- Women who are pregnant or nursing should not take passionflower.

- Passionflower can increase the effects of sedative medications (e.g., phenytoin, barbiturates, benzodiazepines, sleep aids, tricyclic anti-depressants)
- Passionflower can enhance the effects of blood-thinning medications such as clopidogrel (Plavix), warfarin (Coumadin), and aspirin.

RESEARCH FINDINGS

- Although the passionflower seeds are usually discarded during processing, researchers discovered that the seed actually contains high-quality oil that is a novel source of the essential fatty acids linoleic and linolenic acid.
- Results of a study of the effect of purple passion fruit peel extract consumption and symptoms of osteoarthritis indicated that passion fruit peel extract significantly alleviated pain and stiffness, and improved physical function, and the general symptoms of osteoarthritis of the knee. Researchers suggested that this is due to the high antioxidant and anti-inflammatory properties of the extract.
- Although researchers believe that passionflower has potential as an herbal therapeutic option for the treatment of anxiety disorders, there is currently no evidence to definitively recommend its medicinal use for anxiety disorders.

SUMMARY

Consumers should become knowledgeable about the physiologic effects of passionflower. Passionflower is rich in phytonutrients, which are considered to have sedative, anti-anxiety, antispasmodic, analgesic, muscle-relaxing, and hypnotic qualities. Passionflower is used to treat insomnia, gastrointestinal (GI) upset, seizures, asthma, attention deficit hyperactivity disorder (ADHD), hypertension, fibromyalgia, and narcotic drug withdrawal. Women who are pregnant or nursing should avoid taking passionflower. Individuals taking sedative or blood-thinning medications that passionflower can enhance the effects of such medications. Research suggests that the seeds of passionflower may be a good source of essential fatty acids and the peel of passionflower may help elevate osteoarthritis symptoms.

—*Cherie Marcel, BS*

REFERENCES

Ehrlich, S. D. (2013, May 7). Passionflower. *University of Maryland Medical Center*. Retrieved April 7, 2015, from http://www.umm.edu/altmed/articles/passion-flower-000267.htm

Farid, R., Rezaieyazdi, Z., Mirfeizi, Z., Hatef, M. R., Mirhcidari, M., Mansouri, H., ... Watson, R. R. (2010). Oral intake of purple passion fruit peel extract reduces pain and stiffness and improves physical function in adult patients with knee osteoarthritis. *Nutrition Research, 30*(9), 601-606.

Liu, S., Yang, F., Li, J., Zhang, C., Ji, H., & Hong, P. (2008). Physical and chemical analysis of Passiflora seeds and seed oil from China. *International Journal of Food Sciences & Nutrition, 59*(7-8), 706-715.

Moore, S. (2013, August 16). Uses of passion flower. *Livestrong.com.* Retrieved January 7, 2015, from http://www.livestrong.com/article/408532-uses-of-passion-flower/

Miyasaka, L. S., Atallah, I. N., & Soares, B. (2007). Passiflora for anxiety disorder. *Cochrane Database of Systematic Reviews, 2007,* 1.

Ulbricht, C., Basch, E., Boon, H., Karpa, K. D., Gianutsos, G., Nummy, K., ... Woods, J. (2008). An evidence-based systematic review of passion flower (Passiflora incarnata L.) by the Natural Standard Research Collaboration. *Journal of Dietary Supplements, 5*(3), 310-340.

REVIEWER(S)

Darlene Strayer, RN, MBA, Cinahl Information Systems, Glendale, CA

Nursing Executive Practice Council, Glendale Adventist Medical Center, Glendale, CA

Peppermint

WHAT WE KNOW

Peppermint (*Mentha piperita*), a hybrid of water mint and spearmint, is a member of the Labiatae (or Lamiaceae) family along with basil, rosemary, sage, thyme, oregano, perilla, marjoram, and mint. Peppermint is native to Europe and Asia, but it grows well in most climates. The peppermint plant has greenish-purple leaves and small purple flowers. The fresh, vibrant flavor and aroma of peppermint make it a desirable ingredient in many foods, drinks, teas, candies, toothpastes, mouthwashes, shampoos, and soaps. Peppermint leaves can be eaten whole, chopped, dried, ground, or preserved in salt, sugar, alcohol, or oil. Unlike spearmint, peppermint oil is made primarily of menthol. The fresh leaves of peppermint contain as much vitamin C as an orange and more provitamin A, or beta-carotene, than a carrot. Additionally, peppermint provides a high amount of manganese and trace amounts of iron, calcium, folate, potassium, magnesium, tryptophan, omega-3 fatty acids, riboflavin, copper, and fiber. Peppermint has been used therapeutically for at least 10,000 years. It calms GI distress and has been used effectively to reduce the symptoms of irritable bowel syndrome (IBS). Topically applied peppermint oil soothes myalgia, pruritus, and tension headaches. Peppermint has also been used to treat sinusitis, fever, the common cold, respiratory problems, and halitosis.

ACTION OF PEPPERMINT

- Peppermint oil exhibits antifungal and antibacterial properties, halting the growth of numerous bacteria, including *Helicobacter pylori, Salmonella enteritidis, Escherichia coli* O157:H7, and methicillin-resistant *Staphylococcus aureus* (MRSA).
- Peppermint contains valuable phytonutrients (i.e., beneficial plant-derived chemicals), including menthol, perillyl alcohol, and rosmarinic acid.
  - —Menthol soothes the smooth muscles surrounding the intestines, reducing spasm and the indigestion that results from spasm.
  - —Perillyl alcohol has been shown to inhibit the growth of pancreatic, breast, and liver tumors. There is also evidence that it protects against cancers of the colon, skin, and lungs.
  - —Rosmarinic acid is an antioxidant and anti-inflammatory that promotes the production of prostacyclins, which allow airways to open for easier breathing.
- Provitamin A is a precursor of vitamin A, or retinol. Vitamin A is a fat-soluble vitamin that is required for vision, maintenance of the surface linings of the eyes and other epithelial tissue, proper bone growth, healthy immune response, energy regulation, reproduction, embryonic development, and activation of gene expression.
- The water-soluble vitamin C in peppermint neutralizes free radicals, protecting against inflammation and cellular damage. Adequate vitamin C intake is vital for healthy immune system function and has been associated with the prevention of heart disease, stroke, and cancer.
- Manganese is a trace mineral responsible for energy production, fatty acid synthesis, cholesterol

production, and protection against the damage caused by free radicals.

RECOMMENDED DOSAGE AND ADMINISTRATION

- There is no standardized dosage recommendation for peppermint. Peppermint is commonly used as a tea and often taken twice a day; the tea is prepared by steeping 1 tablespoon of peppermint leaves in hot water.
- Topically, 10% peppermint oil in an ethanol solution can be applied to the forehead and temples for the treatment of tension headaches.

ADVERSE REACTIONS AND MEDICATION INTERACTION

- Peppermint is considered to be safe when eaten in amounts normally found in food or beverages.
- Peppermint oil can slow the rate that cyclosporine, a medication used to suppress the immune system post organ transplant surgery, is broken down in the body, potentially resulting in increased incidence of adverse effects from cyclosporine treatment.

RESEARCH FINDINGS

- With the availability of newer and more expensive medications, peppermint oil is frequently overlooked as a treatment option. Authors of several studies and reviews have reported that peppermint oil is a safe and effective therapeutic agent for the treatment of IBS, functional dyspepsia, and postoperative nausea.
- A recent study investigated the efficacy and safety of topical application of menthol 10% solution as a treatment for migraine. Researchers reported that the menthol solution was significantly effective in aborting migraine attacks as well as in alleviating migraine-induced nausea, vomiting, phonophobia, and photophobia when compared with placebo.

SUMMARY

Consumers should become knowledgeable about the physiologic effects of peppermint. The fresh leaves of peppermint are a rich source of vitamin C and provitamin A carotenoids and also contains manganese and trace amounts of iron, calcium, folate, potassium, magnesium, tryptophan, omega-3 fatty acids, riboflavin,

copper, and fiber. Peppermint has antifungal and anti-inflammatory properties, and may be used to treat GI distress, as well as help prevent cancer, heart disease and stroke. Individuals taking cyclosporine should be aware that peppermint oil can interfere with treatment. Research suggests that peppermint is often overlooked as an effective, inexpensive treatment for IBS, functional dyspepsia, and postoperative nausea.

—*Cherie Marcel, BS*

REFERENCES

Ehrlich, S. D. (2013). Peppermint. University of Maryland Medical Center. Retrieved June 18, 2015, from http://www.umm.edu/altmed/articles/peppermint-000269.htm

Ford, A. C., Talley, N. J., Spiegel, B. M. R., Foxx-Orenstein, A. E., Schiller, L., Quigley, E. M. M., & Moayyedi, P. (2010). Effect of fibre, antispasmodics, and peppermint oil in the treatment of irritable bowel syndrome: A systematic review and meta-analysis. *British Medical Journal*, 337(7683), 1388-1392. doi:10.1136/bmj.a2313

The George Mateljan Foundation editorial team. (n.d.). World's healthiest foods: Peppermint. The World's Healthiest Foods. Retrieved June 18, 2015, fromhttp:// www.whfoods.com/genpage. php?tname=foodspice&dbid=102

Grigoleit, H. G., & Grigoleit, P. (2005). Peppermint oil in irritable bowel syndrome. *Phytomedicine*, 12(8), 601-606. doi:10.1016/j.phymed.2004.10.005

Haghighi, A. B., Motazedian, S., Rezaii, R., Mohammadi, F., Salarian, L., Pourmokhtari, M., ... Miri, R. (2010). Cutaneous application of menthol 10% solution as an abortive treatment of migraine without aura: A randomised, double-blind, placebo-controlled, crossed-over study. *International Journal of Clinical Practice*, 64(4), 451-456. doi:10.1111/j.1742-1241.2009.02215.x

Keifer, D., Ulbricht, C., Abrams, T. R., Basch, E., Giese, N., Giles, M., & Woods, J. (2007). Peppermint (Mentha xpiperita): An evidence-based systematic review by the National Standard Research Collaboration. *Journal of Herbal Pharmacotherapy*, 7(2), 91-143. doi:10.1080/J157v07n02_07

Khvorova, Y., & Neill, J. (2008). A review of the effect of peppermint oil in various gastrointestinal conditions. *J.GENCA*, 18(3), 6-15.

Lane, B., Cannella, K., Bowen, C., Copelan, D., Nteff, G., Barnes, K., ... Lawson, J. (2012). Examination of the effectiveness of peppermint aromatherapy on nausea in women post C-section. *Journal of Holistic Nursing, 30*(2), 90-104. doi:10.1177/0898010111423419

Mann, N. S., & Sandhu, K. S. (2012). Peppermint oil in irritable bowel syndrome: Systematic evaluation of 1634 cases with meta-analysis. *International Medical Journal, 19*(1), 5-6.

Sego, S. (2008). Alternative meds update. Peppermint. *Clinical Advisor for Nurse Practitioners, 11*(6), 111-112.

Smith, G. D. (2011). Peppermint oil in gastrointestinal medicine. *Gastrointestinal Nursing, 9*(8), 13-14.

Sridhar, S., & Rakel, D. (2010). Peppermint oil as a therapeutic agent for irritable bowel syndrome. *Evidence-Based Practice, 13*(2), 1-2.

Tourney, A. (2013). Teas to drink for irritable bowel syndrome. *Livestrong.com*. Retrieved June 18, 2015, from http://www.livestrong.com/article/342990-teas-to-drink-for-irritable-bowel-syndrome/

REVIEWER(S)

Darlene Strayer, RN, MBA, Cinahl Information Systems, Glendale, CA

Nursing Executive Practice Council, Glendale Adventist Medical Center, Glendale, CA

Rosemary

WHAT WE KNOW

Rosemary is an evergreen plant of the mint (Lamiaceae or Labiatae) family, which is native to Mediterranean regions. Other names for rosemary include its scientific name, *Rosmarinus officinalis*, as well as compass plant, compass weed, old man, and polar plant.

- Although rosemary is widely known as a culinary spice, it is also used medicinally because of its antioxidant and antibacterial activity, both orally and topically. Some of the conditions that are commonly treated with rosemary include dyspepsia, flatulence, gout, cough, headache, liver and gallbladder dysfunction, cardiovascular conditions, alopecia areata, circulatory disturbances, toothache, myalgia, and neuralgia.

ACTION OF ROSEMARY

- The active components of rosemary are found in the dried leaves, twigs, and flowering tops of the plant.
  - Rosemary leaves supply a volatile oil that contains multiple compounds, including

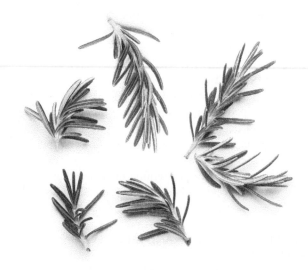

monoterpene hydrocarbons, camphor, borneol, carnosol, ursol, cineole, and caffeic acid and its derivative, rosmarinic acid. Rosemary oil has antibacterial, antifungal, and antioxidant properties.
  - The flavonoid pigments diosmin, diosmetin, and genkwanin are found in the leaves. Diosmin reduces capillary permeability and fragility.
- Rosmarinic acid inhibits HIV integration into the DNA of infected cell.
- Rosemary appears to have anti-carcinogenic properties, showing potential to decrease activation and detoxify carcinogens.
- Although substantial evidence is lacking, there are claims that rosemary exhibits anti-flatulent, antispasmodic, astringent, diaphoretic, and tonic (i.e., capable of both increasing and decreasing the activity of certain body processes) properties.

RECOMMENDED DOSAGE AND ADMINISTRATION

- There are no defined or recommended therapeutic dosages; suggested dosages are as follows:
  - Oral: 1–4 g dried leaves/flowers in tea or 1–4 mL fluid extract 3 times daily.
  - Topical: Essential rosemary oil can be prepared as an ointment and used externally as needed.

ADVERSE REACTIONS AND MEDICATION INTERACTION

- Individuals who are pregnant or breastfeeding should not use rosemary in medicinal dosages.

- Individuals who are hypersensitive or allergic to plants such as grass should not use rosemary in medicinal dosages.
- Undiluted rosemary oil should not be taken internally because safety is not confirmed.
- Potential adverse reactions can occur and include the following signs and symptoms:
  —Intake of large quantities of volatile oil can result in renal damage, coma, uterine bleeding, and pulmonary edema.
  —Topical rosemary can result in dermatitis, erythema, and photosensitivity.
  —Rosemary can inhibit fertility by preventing implantation.
  —Diarrhea, nausea, or vomiting
  —Seizures
  —Asthma
- Treatment is generally discontinuing rosemary administration and managing the signs and symptoms.
- Rosemary can interfere with the absorption of iron.

RESEARCH FINDINGS

- A study was conducted on mice, which were fed a Western-style diet high in fat containing 5% rosemary or thyme over a period of 12 weeks. Researchers concluded that long-term, daily consumption of either rosemary or thyme has an antithrombotic effect without prolonging bleeding time, unlike many anti-platelet agents that often have bleeding as a side effect. The researchers suspected that the antithrombotic activity might be the result of platelet reactivity suppression and stimulation of the vascular endothelium.
- Researchers report that the rosemary extract carnosic acid shows high anti-proliferative, cytotoxic effects against cancerous cells and suggest that carnosic acid, alone or combined with pharmaceuticals, should be considered as a strategy for treating a variety of chemotherapy-resistant cancers. Other research results show that rosemary has strong inhibitive activity against breast cancer.
- When used as aromatherapy, rosemary and lavender essential oils have anti-anxiety effects. A study of the effects of lavender and rosemary on anxiety of nursing students regarding taking a test revealed that, while lavender promoted relaxation, it also decreased the ability to focus

on test questions. Rosemary, however, increased focus and provided a sense of clarity, while still reducing anxiety.

SUMMARY

Consumers should become knowledgeable about the physiologic effects of rosemary. Rosemary oil has antibacterial, antifungal, and antioxidant properties; and that the leaves of rosemary contain diosmin, which reduces capillary permeability and fragility. Rosemary is used to treat GI distress, gout, cough, headache, liver and gallbladder dysfunction and cardiovascular conditions. Women who are pregnant or breastfeeding should not to use rosemary in medicinal dosages. Rosemary may interfere with iron absorption. Research suggests that rosemary may reduce blood clotting and anxiety, and help treat certain cancers.

—*Cherie Marcel, BS*

REFERENCES

Abascal, K., & Yarnell, E. (2001). Herbs and breast cancer: Research review of seaweed, rosemary, and ginseng. *Alternative & Complementary Therapies*, 7(1), 32-36. doi:10.1089/107628001300000705

Fetrow, C. W., & Avila, J. R. (Eds.). (2004). Rosemary. In *Professional's handbook of complementary & alternative medicines* (3rd ed., pp. 715-717). Springhouse, PA: Wolters Kluwer Health/Lippincott Williams & Wilkins.

Lopez-Jimenez, A., Garcia-Cabellero, M., Medina, M., & Quesada, A. (2013). Anti-angiogenic properties of carnosol and carnosic acid, two major dietary compounds from rosemary. *European Journal of Nutrition*, 52(1), 85-95. doi:10.1007/s00394-011-0289-x

Luqman, S., Dwivedi, G. R., Darokar, M. P., Kalra, A., & Khanuja, S. P. S. (2007). Potential of rosemary oil to be used in drug-resistant infections. *Alternative Therapies in Health & Medicine*, 13(5), 54-59.

McCaffrey, R., Thomas, D. J., & Kinselman, A. O. (2009). The effects of lavender and rosemary essential oils on test-taking among graduate nursing students. *Holistic Nursing Practice*, 23(2), 88-93. doi:10.1097/HNP.0b013e3181a110aa

Naemura, A., Ura, M., Yamashita, T., Arai, R., & Yamamoto, J. (2008). Long-term intake of rosemary and common thyme herbs inhibits experimental thrombosis without prolongation of bleeding time. *Thrombosis Research*, 122(4), 517-522. doi:10.1016/j.thromres.2008.01.014

Rosemary. (2003). In J. M. Jellin, P. J. Gregory, F. Batz, & K. Hitchens (Eds.), *Pharmacist's letter/prescriber's letter natural medicines comprehensive database* (5th ed., pp. 1134-1136). Stockton, CA: Therapeutic Research Faculty.

Sego, S. (2012). Rosemary. *Clinical Advisor for Nurse Practitioners, 15*(12), 75-76.

Ulbricht, C., Abrams, T. R., Brigham, A., Ceurvels, J., Clubb, J., Curtiss, W., ... Windsor, R. C. (2010). An evidence-based systematic review of rosemary (rosmarinus officinalis) by the Natural Standard Research Collaboration. *Journal of Dietary Supplements, 7*(4), 351-413. doi:10.3109/19390211.2010.525049

Yesil-Celiktas, O., Sevimli, C., Bedir, E., & Vardar-Sukan, F. (2010). Inhibitory effects of rosemary extracts, carnosic acid and rosmarinic acid on the growth of various human cancer cell lines. *Plant Foods for Human Nutrition, 65*(2), 158-163. doi:10.1007/s11130-010-0166-4

REVIEWER

Nursing Executive Practice Council, Glendale Adventist Medical Center, Glendale, CA

Sage

WHAT WE KNOW

Sage, or *Salvia officinalis* and *Salvia lavandulaefolia*, is a perennial plant with violet-blue flowers that is native to southern Europe. It is a member of the mint (Lamiaceae or Labiatae) family. Other names for sage include common sage, Dalmatian sage, garden sage, meadow sage, sauge, scarlet sage, Spanish sage, and true sage. Sage is rich in beta-carotene and is commonly known as an herb used in culinary seasoning.

- Sage is also used medicinally. Although evidence is lacking to support its benefits, sage has been claimed as an antispasmodic, astringent, and antioxidant. It has been used to treat diarrhea, dysmenorrhea, galactorrhea (i.e., excessive production of maternal milk), gastritis, gingivitis, and sore throat and as an inhalant to calm asthma.

ACTION OF SAGE

- The active components of sage are in the volatile oil, which is found in the leaves. Sage oil contains camphor and thujone, which are potentially toxic.

- Sage may act as an antiflatulent, antispasmodic, astringent, fungistatic (i.e., inhibits the growth of fungus), antibacterial, virustatic (i.e., inhibits the growth or reproduction of viruses), and antiperspirant agent.
- There is limited evidence that sage may lower blood sugar levels.

RECOMMENDED DOSAGE AND ADMINISTRATION

- A typical dosage of sage is 1 cup of freshly brewed tea given 3 times a day. The tea is prepared by steeping 1–2 g of sage leaf in 150 mL of boiling water for 10–15 minutes and then straining it. This preparation is not intended for long-term use due to the potential for adverse reactions.

ADVERSE REACTIONS AND MEDICATION INTERACTION

- Prolonged use or use of large quantities of sage can cause stomatitis, cheilitis (i.e., lip inflammation), dry mouth, restlessness, vomiting, vertigo, tachycardia (i.e., abnormally rapid heart rate), tremors, seizures, mental and physical deterioration, and kidney damage.
- Medicinal dosages of sage should be avoided by individuals who have diabetes mellitus, as sage may interfere with blood glucose control.
- Medicinal doses of sage should be avoided by persons with seizure disorders due to the potential that sage will cause tremors or seizures.
- Intake of sage should be limited during pregnancy and lactation due to its potential to stimulate menstruation and reduce maternal milk supply.
- Treatment of adverse reactions is to discontinue sage use and treat signs and symptoms as necessary.
- Theoretically, sage could interfere with anticonvulsant drug therapy.
- Sage might interfere with hypoglycemic drugs (i.e., medications used to lower blood sugar) due to the potential hypoglycemic effects of sage.
- Sage could potentially increase the effects and side effects of drugs with sedative properties.

RESEARCH FINDINGS

- Researchers studying the effects of sage leaf extract on mental well-being found that sage significantly improved test subjects' self-ratings of mood. Lower dosages reduced anxiety, while higher dosages enhanced alertness, calmness, and contentment. This and other studies have been conducted in an effort to find alternative forms of treatment to improve mood and cognitive function in persons with Alzheimer's disease. Preliminary results are promising and warrant further investigation of sage and its potential to improve mental health.

- Researchers have been studying the potential hypoglycemic effects of sage extract and its implications in the treatment of patients with diabetes mellitus. Results of one study indicate that sage tea is effective as a food supplement for the prevention of type 2 diabetes mellitus because it lowers plasma glucose in persons at risk. Results of another study found sage tea to improve the lipid profile and lower cholesterol levels without adverse effects.

- Sage shows strong potential for its antioxidant activity and its assistance in wound healing. Results of a study of oregano-containing ointments used in traditional Turkish medicine revealed that a cream formulated from olive oil extract, oregano extract, and sage essential oil demonstrates significant wound healing activity. Such an ointment could be used for rapid healing of acute and chronic wounds.

SUMMARY

Consumers should become knowledgeable about the physiologic effects of sage, including its risks and benefits. Sage is rich in beta-carotene, the precursor to vitamin A, which contributes to vision, growth, cell division, and immune function. Sage is used medicinally to treat diarrhea, dysmenorrhea, galactorrhea, gastritis, gingivitis, and sore throat. Consumers should be aware that long-term treatment with sage is not recommended due to the potential for adverse reactions. Women who are pregnant should limit their intake of sage due to its potential to decrease maternal milk supply. Individuals taking anticonvulsant drug therapy or hypoglycemic drugs should also avoid taking sage.

—*Cherie Marcel, BS*

REFERENCES

Fetrow, C. W., & Avila, J. R. (2004). Sage. In *Professional's handbook of complementary & alternative medicines*

(3rd ed., pp. 728-730). Springhouse, PA: Lippincott Williams & Wilkins A Wolters Kluwer Company.

Houghton, P. J. (2004). Activity and constituents of sage: Relevant to the potential treatment of symptoms of Alzheimer's disease. *HerbalGram*, *61*, 38-53.

Kennedy, D. O., Dodd, F. L., Robertson, B. C., Okello, E. J., Reay, J. L., Scholey, A. B., & Haskell, C. F. (2010). Monoterpenoid extract of sage (Salvia lavandulaefolia) with cholinesterase inhibiting properties improves cognitive performance and mood in healthy adults. *Journal of Psychopharmacology*, *25*(8), 1088-1100. doi:10.1177/0269881110385594

Kim, J. Y., Kim, H. S., Kang, H. S., Choi, J. S., Yokozawa, T., & Chung, H. Y. (2008). Antioxidant potential of dimethyl lithospermate isolated from Salvia miltiorrhiza (red sage) against peroxynitrite. *Journal of Medicinal Food*, *11*(1), 21-28. doi:10.1089/jmf.2007.040

Lima, C. F., Azevedo, M. F., Araujo, R., Fernandes-Ferreira, M., & Pereira-Wilson, C. (2006). Metformin-like effect of Salvia officinalis (common sage): Is it useful in diabetes prevention? *British Journal of Nutrition*, *96*(2), 326-333. doi:10.1079/BJN20061832

Oliff, H. S. (2006). Research reviews. Sage leaf extract reduces anxiety in clinical trial. *HerbalGram*, (72), 24-25.

Rau, O., Wurglics, M., Paulke, A., Zitzkowski, J., Meindl, N., Bock, A., & Schubert-Zsilavecz, M. (2006). Carnosic acid and carnosol, phenolic diterpene compounds of the labiate herbs rosemary and sage, are activators of the human peroxisome proliferator-activated receptor gamma. *Planta Medica*, *72*(10), 881-887. doi:10.1055/s-2006-946680

Sa, C. M., Ramos, A. A., Azevedo, M. F., Lima, C. F., Fernandes-Ferreira, M., & Pereira-Wilson, C. (2009). Sage tea drinking improves lipid profile and antioxidant defences in humans. *International Journal of Molecular Sciences*, *10*(9), 3937-3950. doi:10.3390/ijms10093937.

Sage. (2003). In J. M. Jellin, P. J. Gregory, F. Batz, & K. Hitchens (Eds.), *Pharmacist's letter/prescriber's letter natural medicines comprehensive database* (5th ed., pp. 1150-1151). Stockton, CA: Therapeutic Research Faculty.

Suntar, I., Akkol, E. K., Keles, H., Oktem, A., Baser, K. H., & Yesilada, E. (2011). A novel wound healing ointment: A formulation of Hypericum perforatum oil and sage and oregano essential oils based on traditional Turkish knowledge. *Journal of Ethnopharmacology*, *134*(1), 89-96. doi:10.1016/j.jep.2010.11.061 (R)

REVIEWER(S)
Sharon Richman, MSPT, Cinahl Information Systems, Glendale, CA
Nursing Executive Practice Council, Glendale Adventist Medical Center, Glendale, CA

Spearmint

WHAT WE KNOW

Spearmint (*Mentha viridis* or *Mentha spicata*) is a member of the Labiatae, or Lamiaceae, family together with basil, rosemary, sage, thyme, oregano, perilla, marjoram, and mint. It is native to Europe and Asia, but grows well in most climates. The spearmint plant has long spear-like, smooth or gray-haired leaves and pale blue flowers. The fresh, vibrant flavor and aroma of spearmint make it a desirable ingredient in many foods, drinks, teas, toothpastes, mouthwashes, shampoos, and soaps. Spearmint leaves can be eaten whole, chopped, dried, ground, or preserved in salt, sugar, alcohol, or oil. The fresh leaves of spearmint contain as much vitamin C as an orange and more provitamin A (i.e., any of the group of carotenoids that are precursors to vitamin A and have the biologic activity of beta-carotene; found in milk products, fish-liver oils, egg yolk, and leafy green and yellow vegetables) than a carrot.

- Historically, spearmint has been used to treat gastrointestinal distress, sinusitis, fever, the common cold, respiratory conditions, dandruff, and halitosis (i.e., bad breath). Currently, the medicinal use of spearmint for any condition is not recommended due to the lack of high-quality human trials.

ACTION OF SPEARMINT

- The active components of spearmint include carvone, limonene, phellandrene, and pinene. Unlike peppermint, spearmint does not contain menthol.
- There is some scientific evidence that spearmint exhibits antibacterial, antifungal, antidepressant, chemo-preventive, antioxidant, lipid-reducing, sedative, and anti-inflammatory activities.

RECOMMENDED DOSAGE AND ADMINISTRATION

- There is no standardized dosage recommended for spearmint, although it is commonly used as a tea and consumed twice a day; preparation is by steeping 1 tablespoon of spearmint leaves in hot water.

ADVERSE REACTIONS

- Spearmint is considered to be safe when eaten in amounts normally found in food or beverages.
- There is some evidence that spearmint can inhibit iron absorption, so patients receiving iron should consider limiting spearmint consumption.

RESEARCH FINDINGS

- Researchers of several studies report that spearmint has antiandrogenic effects and could diminish sexual libido. Spearmint-induced oxidative stress in the hypothalamus leading to reduced production of luteinizing hormone (LH) and follicular stimulating hormone (FSH) is suspected to be responsible for the down-regulation of testicular testosterone production. Along with these findings, researchers report that spearmint is effective as an alternative to antiandrogenic treatment in women with hirsutism (i.e., unwanted male-pattern hair growth). Further study is needed to test the reliability of these results.
- Results of a study conducted on rats with chronic obstructive pulmonary disease (COPD) showed that spearmint plays a protective role against lung injury by reducing pulmonary inflammation and oxidative stress.
- Researchers report that spearmint oil allergy is a possible cause of some cases of oral lichen planus (OLP), a chronic inflammatory condition of the mouth.

SUMMARY

Consumers should become knowledgeable about the properties and physiologic effects of spearmint. The fresh leaves of spearmint are a rich source of vitamin C and provitamin A, and may exhibit antioxidant, antibacterial, and anti-inflammatory activities. Individuals that are taking iron supplements should consider limiting spearmint consumption since spearmint might inhibit iron absorption.

—*Cherie Marcel, BS*

REFERENCES

Akdogan, M., Tamer, M. N., Cure, E., Cure, M. C., Koroglu, B. K., & Delibas, N. (2007). Effect of spearmint (Mentha spicata Labiatae) teas on androgen levels in women with hirsutism. *Phytotherapy Research*, *21*(5), 444-447.

Fetrow, C. W., & Avila, J. R. (2004). Mint. In K. C. Comerford (Ed.), *Professional's handbook of complementary & alternative medicines* (3rd ed., pp. 563-567). Springhouse, PA: Lippincott, Williams & Wilkins, a Wolters Kluwer company.

Grant, P. (2010). Spearmint herbal tea has significant anti-androgen effects in polycystic ovarian syndrome. A randomized controlled trial. *Phytotherapy Research*, *24*(2). doi:10.1002/ptr.2900

Gunatheesan, S., Tam, M. M., Tate, B., Tvresky, J., & Nixon, R. (2012). Retrospective study of oral lichen planus and allergy to spearmint oil. *The Australasian Journal of Dermatology*, *53*(3), 224-228. doi:10.1111/j.1440-0960.2012.00908.x

Ulbricht, C., Costa, D., Grimes Serrano, J. M., Guilford, J., Isaac, R., Seamon, E., & Varghese, M. (2010). An evidence-based systematic review of spearmint by the Natural Standard Research Collaboration. *Journal of Dietary Supplements*, *7*(2), 179-215. doi:10.3109/19390211.2010.486702

REVIEWER

Nursing Executive Practice Council, Glendale Adventist Medical Center, Glendale, CA

Thyme

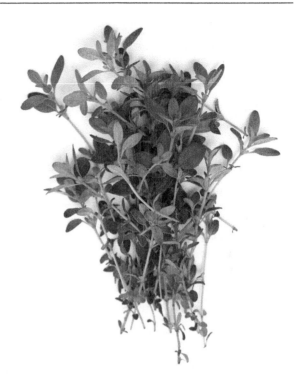

WHAT WE KNOW

Thyme is an evergreen plant of the mint (Lamiaceae or Labiatae) family, which is native to Mediterranean regions. Other names for thyme include *Thymus vulgaris*, *Thymus zygis*, common thyme, French thyme, garden thyme, Spanish thyme, and thymi herba. Thyme is rich in iron.

- Although thyme is most commonly known as a culinary spice/herb, because of its antioxidant and antimicrobial effects it is also used medicinally in oral and topical preparations. Thyme has been used to treat various conditions, including bronchitis, pertussis (i.e., whooping cough), sore throat, colic, dyspnea (i.e., difficulty breathing), laryngitis, tonsillitis, stomatitis (i.e., sores in the mouth), and halitosis (i.e., bad breath).

ACTION OF THYME

- The active components of thyme are found in the dried leaves and flowering tops of the plant.

- Thyme contains flavonoids such as thymol and carvacrol, which act as antispasmodic, antitussive (i.e., cough suppressant), and expectorant (i.e., clearance of mucus) agents.
- Thyme has been shown to have antifungal activity, exhibiting inhibitory effects on protozoa and certain bacteria.
- Liquid extracts of thyme have spasmolytic action (i.e., relieves muscle spasms), antioxidant effects, and antiplatelet effects (i.e., prevents blood clotting).

RECOMMENDED DOSAGE AND ADMINISTRATION

- Oral: 1–2 g dried leaves/flowers or fluid extract several times daily not to exceed 10 g/ day of dried preparation or 6 g/day of the fluid extract.
  —Thyme tea is made by steeping 1–2 g in 150 mL of boiling water for 10 minutes
- Topical: steep 5 g dried leaves/flowers per 100 mL boiling water for 10 minutes and strain for use as a compress, or for gargling.

ADVERSE REACTIONS

- Individuals with gastritis, intestinal disorders, or cardiac insufficiency and pregnant women should not use thyme in medicinal doses.

- Individuals who are hypersensitive or allergic to thyme or to plants such as grass should not use thyme medicinally.
- Although rare, adverse reactions can occur. Potential signs and symptoms include the following:
  —Dizziness
  —Headache
  —Bradycardia (i.e., abnormally slow heart beat)
  —Cheilitis or glossitis (i.e., inflammation of the mouth or tongue)
  —Diarrhea, nausea, and/or vomiting
  —Muscle weakness
  —Slowed respiration
  —Dermatitis
- Treatment is generally discontinuing thyme administration.

RESEARCH FINDINGS
- A study was conducted on mice, which were fed a Western-style diet high in fat containing 5% rosemary or thyme over a period of 12 weeks. Researchers concluded that long-term, daily consumption of either rosemary or thyme has an antithrombotic effect (i.e., preventing blood clotting) without prolonging bleeding time, unlike many antiplatelet agents for which bleeding is often a side effect. The researchers suspected that the antithrombotic activity might be the result of platelet reactivity suppression and stimulation of the vascular endothelium.
- The antifungal activity of thyme essential oil and thymol was studied on mold samples obtained from damp dwellings. Findings revealed that the vaporous phase of thyme essential oil is effective in long-term suppression of these molds. It is possible that thyme essential oils and thymol could be used as a disinfectant for molds in damp living spaces, potentially preventing physical impairment of the inhabitants.
- Researchers have recently reported new evidence of antispasmodic activity in thyme extracts, which they believe is due to the flavone luteolin.

SUMMARY
Consumers should become knowledgeable about the physiologic effects of thyme, including its risks and benefits. Thyme contains flavonoids which act as antispasmodic, antitussive and expectorant agents. Thyme has also been shown to have antifungal activity, antioxidant effects, and can aid in preventing blood clots. Women who are pregnant and individuals with gastritis, intestinal disorders, or cardiac insufficiency should not use thyme in medicinal doses.

—*Cherie Marcel, BS*

REFERENCES
Basch, E., Ulbricht, C., Hammerness, P., Bevins, A., & Sollars, D. (2004). Thyme (Thymus vulgaris L.), thymol. *Journal of Herbal Pharmacotherapy, 4*(1), 49-67. doi:10.1300/ J157v04n01_07

Thyme. (2004). In C. W. Fetrow, & J. R. Avila (Eds.), *Professional's handbook of complementary & alternative medicines* (3rd ed., pp. 820-822). Springhouse, PA: Lippincott Williams & Wilkins A Wolters Kluwer Company.

Thyme. (2003). In J. M. Jellin, P. J. Gregory, F. Batz, & K. Hitchens (Eds.), *Pharmacist's letter/prescriber's letter natural medicines comprehensive database* (5th ed., pp. 1280-1281). Stockton, CA: Therapeutic Research Faculty.

Martinez-Gonzalez, M. C., Goday Bujan, J. J., Martinez Gomez, W., & Fonseca Capdevila, E. (2007). Concomitant allergic contact dermatitis due to Rosmarinus officinalis (rosemary) and Thymus vulgaris (thyme). *Contact Dermatitis, 56*(1), 49-50. doi:10.1111/j.1600-0536.2007.00951.x

Naemura, A., Ura, M., Yamashita, T., Arai, R., & Yamamoto, J. (2008). Long-term intake of rosemary and common thyme herbs inhibits experimental thrombosis without prolongation of bleeding time. *Thrombosis Research, 122*(4), 517-522. doi:10.1016/j.thromres.2008.01.014

Segvic Klaric, M., Kosalec, I., Mastelic, J., Pieckova, E., & Pepeljnak, S. (2007). Antifungal activity of thyme (Thymus vulgaris, L.) essential oil and thymol against moulds from damp dwellings. *Letters in Applied Microbiology, 44*(1), 36-42. doi:10.1111/j.1472-765X.2006.02032.x

Engelbertz, J., Lechtenberg, M., Studt, L., Hansel, A., & Verspohl, E. J. (2012). Bioassay-guided fractionation of a thymol-deprived hydrophilic thyme extract and its antispasmodic effect. *Journal of Ethnopharmacology, 141*(3), 848-853. doi:10.1016/j.jep.2012.03.025

REVIEWER(S)
Darlene Strayer, RN, MBA, Cinahl Information Systems, Glendale, CA
Nursing Practice Council, Glendale Adventist Medical Center, Glendale, CA

Turmeric

WHAT WE KNOW

Turmeric, also known as Indian saffron, is a peppery spice derived from the rhizome of the *Curcuma longa* plant. Along with ginger, the tall, tropical *Curcuma longa* shrub is a member of the Zingiberacaea family. Curcumin, the biologically active component of turmeric, is responsible for its deep yellow-orange color (e.g., as seen in yellow curry) and is used to flavor or color clothes, foods (e.g., curry powders, cheeses, mustards, butters), and cosmetics. Curcumin has long been appreciated for its many medicinal qualities. For nearly 4,000 years, folk medicine practitioners have claimed that curcumin aids in digestion; heals wounds; reduces inflammation; reduces arthritic pain; sooths eyes, ears, and skin; treats liver disorders; controls blood sugar; treats lung conditions; eases menstrual difficulties; and has antiseptic properties. With more than 3,000 research articles on turmeric published over the last 25 years, many of these claims have been substantiated using modern scientific methods. Curcumin has proven to be a powerful antioxidant and to have antitoxic, anti-inflammatory, and many other beneficial properties.

ACTION OF TURMERIC

- The polyphenol curcumin is a potent antioxidant that protects cells and tissues by blocking free radical attacks from toxins in food, water, air, and the environment as well as toxins produced internally such as superoxide, hydrogen peroxide, and nitric oxide.
  - Curcumin protects deoxyribonucleic acid (DNA) from oxidation, reducing the risk for mutations.
  - It has anti-inflammatory and antimicrobial properties.
  - It protects the liver from solvent toxicity.
  - It protects the brain from alcohol-induced damage.
  - It preserves the heart and kidneys from damage caused by pharmaceutical drugs.
  - By binding with key proteins, curcumin helps to maintain gene integrity, support hormonal regulation, promote detoxification, and is fundamental to processes involved in homeostasis (i.e., the body's self-maintenance of equilibrium in response to external stimuli).
- Turmeric supports the vitality of the digestive system, including the stomach, intestines, gall bladder, liver, and pancreas.
- Turmeric promotes memory and mental adaptability by supporting growth factors necessary for the formation of replacements for damage circuits in the brain. In addition, it reduces stress on the brain and protects it from metabolic toxins such as homocysteine.
- Turmeric reduces lipid peroxide levels in the blood, lowering low-density lipoprotein (LDL) cholesterol levels and raising high-density lipoprotein (HDL) cholesterol levels.
- Topically, turmeric protects the skin cells against radiation and free radical attack.
- Turmeric supports immunity by inhibiting the proliferation of damaging cells and toxins and by boosting macrophage and antibody activity.

RECOMMENDED DOSAGE AND ADMINISTRATION

- Standard dosage is 450 mg to 3 g/day of curcumin, which should be taken on an empty stomach.
- Combining curcumin with phospholipid (e.g., lecithin) supplementation increases its absorption.
- Ingestion of turmeric in higher doses may be unsafe during pregnancy due to the potential for it to stimulate the uterus; there is insufficient evidence to determine whether turmeric use is safe during breastfeeding.
- Turmeric should be avoided by patients with gallstones or bile duct obstruction and can worsen gastroesophageal reflux disease (GERD).

ADVERSE REACTIONS

- Because curcumin can slow blood clotting, taking turmeric while receiving anticoagulant or antiplatelet medications increases risk for bruising and bleeding.

- Curcumin increases risk for bleeding when taken with ginkgo, garlic, angelica, clove, danshen, red clover, and willow.

RESEARCH FINDINGS

- Turmeric has been shown to have significant antidepressant activity. Researchers report that turmeric treatment in the form of a water-soluble preparation produces effects similar to St. John's wort and the antidepressant medication fluoxetine. It also exhibited the action of boosting neurotransmitter levels.
- A great deal of research has been conducted on the potential use of curcumin as an anti-cancer and chemopreventive agent. There is evidence that curcumin increases the chemosensitivity and radiosensitivity of tumors, blunts cancer-causing inflammation, and promotes apoptosis (i.e., cell death) in rapidly reproducing cancer cells while providing protection for the internal organs. Curcumin prevents and combats cancers of the breast, cervix, uterus, prostate, colon and other parts of the gastrointestinal system, blood, brain, lung, and bladder.
- Curcumin decreases alcohol-induced oxidative liver damage in rats. It exhibits therapeutic and protective effects against organ dysfunction due to sepsis (i.e., life-threatening complication of infection), shock, and diseases associated with inflammation (e. g., inflammatory bowel disease).
- Researchers report that there is evidence of a role for curcumin in regulating lipid metabolism and reducing obesity and related conditions, including type 2 diabetes mellitus (DM2). Curcumin interacts with adipocytes, pancreatic cells, liver stellate cells, macrophages, and muscle cells in suppressing inflammatory factors and reversing insulin resistance, hyperglycemia, hyperlipidemia, and other abnormalities.

SUMMARY

Consumers should become knowledgeable about the physiologic effects of turmeric. Turmeric contains the polyphenol curcumin, a powerful antioxidant that has demonstrated antitoxic, anti-inflammatory, and many other beneficial properties. Consumers should be aware of the risk for bleeding and related complications when turmeric is taken with anticoagulant or antiplatelet medications, as well as certain herbs and supplements, including ginkgo or garlic.

—*Cherie Marcel, BS*

REFERENCES

Aggarwal, B. B. (2010). Targeting inflammation-induced obesity and metabolic diseases by curcumin and other nutraceuticals. *Annual Review of Nutrition*, 30, 173-199. doi:10.1146/annurev.nutr.012809.104755

Alappat, L., & Awad, A. B. (2010). Curcumin and obesity: Evidence and mechanisms. *Nutrition Reviews*, 68(12), 729-738. doi:10.1111/j.1753-4887.2010.00341.x

The American Herb Association editorial team. (2012). Herbal clippings: Stay happy with turmeric. *The American Herb Association*, 27(3), 12.

Bao, W., Li, K., Rong, S., Yao, P., Hao, L., Ying, C., & Liu, L. (2010). Curcumin alleviates ethanol-induced hepatocytes oxidative damage involving heme oxygenase-1 induction. *Journal of Ethnopharmacology*, 128(2), 549-553. doi:10.1016/j.jep.2010.01.029

Bharaj, B. (2013). Turmeric -- From tradition to research. *Positive Health*, 1, 5 pp.

Borger, J. E. (2011). How curcumin protects against cancer. *Life Extension*, 17(3), 1-9.

Cabrespine-Faugeras, A., Bayet-Robert, M., Bay, J., Chollet, P., & Barthomeuf, C. (2010). Possible benefits of curcumin regimen in combination with taxane chemotherapy for hormone-refractory prostate cancer treatment. *Nutrition & Cancer*, 62(2), 148-153. doi:10.1080/01635580903305383

Curtin, K. (2009). Fresh. Herbs & supplements 101: Curcumin. *Delicious Living*, 25(1), 16.

Dye, D. (2008). Curcumin may offer protection against diabetes. *Life Extension*, 14(10), 16.

Epelbaum, R., Schaffer, M., Vizel, B., Badmaev, V., & Bar-Sela, G. (2010). Curcumin and gemcitabine in patients with advanced pancreatic cancer. *Nutrition & Cancer*, 62(8), 1137-1141. doi:10.1080/01635581.2010.513802

Finkle, J. (2011). Curumin could prevent liver damage. *Life Extension*, 17(2), 4.

Goel, A., & Aggarwal, B. B. (2010). Curcumin, the golden spice from Indian Saffron, is a chemosensitizer and radiosensitizer for tumors and chemoprotector and radioprotector for normal organs. *Nutrition & Cancer*, 62(7), 919-930. doi:10.1080/01635581.2010.509835

Hilchie, A. L., Furlong, S. J., Sutton, K., Richardson, A., Robichaud, M. R., Giacomantonio, C. A., ... Hoskin, D. W. (2010). Curcumin-induced apoptosis in PC3 prostate carcinoma cells is caspase-independent and involves cellular ceramide accumulation and damage to mitochondria. *Nutrition & Cancer*, 62(3), 379-389. doi:10.1080/01635580903441238

Kidd, P. M., & Prakash, L. (2009). The curcumin complex: At the interface of nutrition and medicine. *Total Health*, 30(4), 30-31.

Kiefer, D. (2008). Soy isoflavones, curcumin synergize to thwart pancreatic cancer. *Life Extension*, 14(11), 24.

Majumdar, A. P. N., Banerjee, S., Nautiyal, J., Patel, B. B., Patel, V., Du, J., ... Sarkar, F. H. (2009). Curcumin synergizes with resveratrol to inhibit colon cancer. *Nutrition & Cancer*, 61(4), 544-553. doi:10.1080/01635580902752262

Memis, D., Hekimoglu, S., Sezer, A., Altaner, S., Sut, N., & Usta, U. (2008). Curcumin attenuates the organ dysfunction caused by endotoxemia in the rat. *Nutrition*, 24(11-12), 1133-1138. doi:10.1016/j.nut.2008.06.008

Nayak, S., & Sashidhar, R. B. (2010). Metabolic intervention of aflatoxin B1 toxicity by curcumin. *Journal of Ethnopharmacology*, 127(3), 641-644. doi:10.1016/j.jep.2009.12.010

Patel, B. B., & Majumdar, A. P. (2009). Synergistic role of curcumin with current therapeutics in colorectal cancer: Minireview. *Nutrition & Cancer*, 61(6), 843-846. doi:10.1080/01635580903285106

Patel, V. B., Misra, S., Patel, B. B., & Majumdar, A. P. N. (2010). Colorectal cancer: Chemopreventive role of curcumin and resveratrol. *Nutrition & Cancer*, 62(7), 958-967. doi:10.1080/01635581.2010.510259

Pesakhov, S., Khanin, M., Studzinski, G. P., & Danilenko, M. (2010). Distinct combinatorial effects of the plant polyphenols curcumin, carnosic acid, and silibinin on prolifertion and apoptosis in acute myeloid leukemia cells. *Nutrition & Cancer*, 62(6), 811-824. doi:10.1080/01635581003693082

Prasad, S., & Aggarwal, B. B. (2011). Turmeric, the golden spice. I. F. F. Benzie & S. Wachtel-Galor (Eds.), *Herbal medicine: Biomolecular and clinical aspects* (2nd ed.). Boca Raton, FL: CRC Press.

Samuhasaneeto, S., Thong-Ngam, D., Kulaputana, O., Suyasunanont, O. K. D., & Klaikeaw, N. (2009). Curcumin decreased oxidative stress, inhibited NF-kappaB activation, and improved liver pathology in ethanol-induced liver injury in rats. *Journal of Biomedicine & Biotechnology*, 981963. doi:10.1155/2009/981963

Schulz, O. (2008). The biological activity of curcumin. *Wellness Foods Europe*, (2), 10-14.

Shehzad, A., Ha, T., Subhan, F., & Lee, Y. (2011). New mechanisms and the anti-inflammatory role of curcumin in obesity and obesity-related metabolic diseases. *European Journal of Nutrition*, 50(3), 151-161. doi:10.1007/s00394-011-0188-1

Singletary, K. (2010). Turmeric: An overview of potential health benefits. *Nutrition Today*, 45(5), 216-225. doi:10.1097/NT.0b013e3181f1d72c

Taylor, R. A., & Leonard, M. C. (2011). Curcumin for inflammatory bowel disease: A review of human studies. *Alternative Medicine Review*, 16(2), 152-156.

Turmeric. (2014, October 9). *Medline Plus*. Retrieved March 12, 2015, from http://www.nlm.nih.gov/medlineplus/druginfo/natural/662.html

Ulbricht, C., Basch, E., Barrette, E., Boon, H., Chao, W., Costa, D., & Woods, J. (2011). Turmeric (Curcuma longa): An evidence-based systematic review by the Natural Standard Research Collaboration. *Alternative & Complementary Therapies*, 17(4), 225-236. doi:10.1089/act.2011.17409

Wickenberg, J., Ingemansson, S. L., & Hlebowicz, J. (2010). Effects of Curcuma longa (turmeric) on postprandial plasma glucose and insulin in healthy subjects. *Nutrition Journal*, 9, 43. doi:10.1186/1475-2891-9-43

REVIEWER(S)

Darlene Strayer, RN, MBA, Cinahl Information Systems, Glendale, CA

Nursing Executive Practice Council, Glendale Adventist Medical Center, Glendale, CA

Vinegar

WHAT WE KNOW

Vinegar is a product of the fermentation of alcohol and sugar. It is an acidic liquid primarily consisting of acetic acid and water. Vinegar can be made from many different sources such as wine, cider, beer, fruit, and maple syrup; each results in a different flavor and other properties. Vinegar can be used as a preservative, cleanser, and culinary flavoring. Some of the more popular vinegars include apple cider, balsamic, white wine, and red wine vinegar. These vinegars can be used as a flavoring agent in sautés and marinades, boiled into tasty reductions, or mixed with oils and seasonings to make vinaigrette dressings. Each vinegar contains unique nutrients and health benefits.

ACTION OF VINEGAR

- Apple cider vinegar is a common home remedy for a variety of conditions such as indigestion, sore throat, fungal infection, and influenza. Although vinegar essentially contains no vitamins and contains only a trace of minerals, the phytonutrients, enzymes, and beneficial bacteria provided by apple cider appear to have immune modulating activities (i.e., enhancing immune function). Results of studies also indicate that including apple cider vinegar in a meal reduces postprandial (i.e., after a meal) blood glucose spikes by slowing the release of sugar into the bloodstream.
- Balsamic vinegar, made from the balsam plant, has an intensely tart and subtly sweet flavor and dark color. It contains small amounts of calcium, magnesium, phosphorous, potassium, and sodium.
- White wine vinegar is clear in color and contains no notable nutrients. It has a tart flavor, making it a useful, low-calorie addition to salad dressing mixes.
- Red wine vinegar contains a trace of vitamin C, calcium, iron, magnesium, phosphorous, and potassium. With its tart and slightly sweet flavor, red wine vinegar is commonly used in dressings, marinades, sautés and sauces.

RESEARCH FINDINGS

- Results of several studies indicate that consuming apple cider vinegar with meals reduces postprandial spike in blood glucose. Researchers suggest that consuming it with meals could help to protect against diabetes and facilitate weight loss.

SUMMARY

Consumers should become knowledgeable about the physiologic effects of consuming vinegar. Vinegar contains phytonutrients, enzymes, and beneficial bacteria that appear to have immune modulating activities.

Incorporating apple cider vinegar in a meal may reduce postprandial blood glucose spikes.

—*Cherie Marcel, BS*

REFERENCES

Challem, J. (2008). Medical journal watch: Context and applications. Apple-cider vinegar reduces fasting blood sugar. *Alternative & Complementary Therapies*, *14*(2), 102-104.

Colemna, E. (2014, February 15). What is the nutritional value of vinegar. *Livestrong.com*. Retrieved March 16, 2015, from http://www.livestrong.com/article/21611-nutritional-value-vinegar/

Johnston, C. S., Steplewska, I., Long, C. A., Harris, L. N., & Ryals, R. H. (2010). Examination of the antiglycemic properties of vinegar in healthy adults. *Annals of Nutrition & Metabolism*, *56*(1), 74-79.

Kadley, M. G., & Chappell, M. M. (2010). Apple cider vinegar: Pucker up for a dose of healthfulness. *Vegetarian Times*, 22-23.

White, A. M., & Johnston, C. S. (2007). Vinegar ingestion at bedtime moderates waking glucose concentrations in adults with well-controlled type 2 diabetes. *Diabetes Care*, *30*(11), 2814-2815. doi:10.2337/dc07-1062

REVIEWER(S)

Darlene Strayer, RN, MBA, Cinahl Information Systems, Glendale, CA

Nursing Executive Practice Council, Glendale Adventist Medical Center, Glendale, CA

Yarrow

WHAT WE KNOW

Yarrow (*Achillea millefolium*) is an ancient fern-like herb from the sunflower, or *Asteraceae* family, along with chrysanthemums and chamomile. Considered to be a sacred plant by ancient civilizations, the genus for yarrow, *Achillea*, is believed to have been named after the mythical Greek hero Achilles, who treated his warriors' wounds with the nutmeg-scented yarrow leaves. Yarrow is a perennial herb that grows to about 2 1/2 feet tall. It has fuzzy, fern-like leaves and flat-topped clusters of white, pink, fuchsia, red, or yellow flowers at the tops of its stems. Yarrow is used in European folk medicine to treat gastrointestinal distress, anxiety, insomnia, and wounds. Today, yarrow is commonly used for the treatment of menstrual cramps, muscle spasms, inflammation, fever, infection, poor appetite, pneumonia, and bleeding. Evidence for these uses is lacking, but research is growing; scientists have identified over 100 biologically active compounds in the yarrow plant, including flavonoids, phenolic acids, coumarins, terpenoids, and sterols.

ACTION OF YARROW

- The many phytonutrients (i.e., beneficial plant chemicals) in yarrow include the following:
  —Menthol soothes the smooth muscles surrounding the intestines, reducing spasm and indigestion.
  —Apigenin has anti-mutagenic activity (i.e., preventing cell mutation) and has been shown to reduce the size of prostate tumors and prevent the development of progestin-induced breast cancer.
  —Luteolin is a potent antioxidant and an anti-carcinogenic compound
  —Rutin provides strong antioxidant and anti-inflammatory protection. It also has antihistamine, antimicrobial, antidiabetic, and anti-carcinogenic properties.
  —Limonene increases liver enzymes involved in detoxifying carcinogens
- Yarrow contains inulin, which is a soluble fiber that is not absorbed by the human digestive tract. Inulin is sometimes used to increase the fiber content in processed foods or as a substitute for cane sugar.
- Salicylic acid, which is the primary metabolite of aspirin, is found in yarrow leaves and is commonly used as a topical treatment for acne.
- The calcium in yarrow builds and maintains bones and teeth, regulates muscle contraction, conducts nerve impulses, activates enzymes for energy production and muscle contraction, participates in blood clotting, assists with vitamin B12 absorption, and maintains the structural integrity of intracellular membranes.

RECOMMENDED DOSAGE AND ADMINISTRATION

- A dosage of 4 g or 1 tsp of dried yarrow or 300–600 mg of yarrow in a capsule daily is commonly recommended.
- Yarrow is available as a tea and should be used as directed on the packaging.

ADVERSE REACTIONS AND MEDICATION INTERACTION

- Persons with allergies to ragweed or daisies should avoid yarrow.
- Women who are pregnant should not use yarrow because results of animal studies indicate that yarrow can increase the risk of having a low-birth-weight baby.
- Yarrow can increase sensitivity to sunlight.
- Yarrow can slow blood clotting and should not be taken in combination with medications that also slow blood clotting, such as aspirin, clopidogrel (Plavix), diclofenac (Voltaren, Cataflam), ibuprofen (Advil, Motrin), naproxen (Anaprox, Naprosyn), and dalteparin (Fragmin).
- Yarrow can increase the effects of sedating medications (e.g., barbiturates).

RESEARCH FINDINGS

Results of current research are beginning to substantiate claims regarding many of the traditional medicinal uses of yarrow. Researchers have reported that yarrow extract exhibits vasoprotective (i.e., alleviating conditions of the blood vessels) and hypotensive activity (i.e., lowering blood pressure) through estrogenic and anti-inflammatory mechanisms. Yarrow also produces bronchodilatory effects, supporting its potential use in the treatment of asthma. Additionally, scientists have demonstrated that yarrow possesses potent antioxidant and cytoprotective (i.e., providing protection to cells against harmful agents) properties.

SUMMARY

Consumers should become knowledgeable about the physiologic effects of yarrow. Yarrow is rich in calcium; the soluble fiber, inulin; and in many phytonutrients which contain antioxidant, anti-mutagenic, antihistamine, antimicrobial, antidiabetic, and anti-carcinogenic properties. Women who are pregnant should not to use yarrow because results of animal studies indicate that yarrow can increase the risk of having a low-birth-weight baby.

Yarrow may also increase the effects of sedating medications and can slow blood clotting and should not be taken in combination with medications that also slow blood clotting.

—*Cherie Marcel, BS*

REFERENCES

Conis, E. (2006). Supplements. Modern uses for mythical herb. Los Angeles Times-Southern California Edition. Jan 30 Health: F3.

Dall'Acqua, S., Bolego, C., Cignarella, A., Gaion, R. M., & Innocenti, G. (2011). Vasoprotective activity of standardized Achillea millefolium extract. *Phytomedicine*, *18*(12), 1031-1036. doi:10.1016/j.phymed.2011.05.005

De Souza, P., Gasparotto, A., Jr, Crestani, S., Stefanello, M. E., Marques, M. C., da Silva-Santos, J. E., & Kassuya, C. A. (2011). Hypotensive mechanism of the extracts and artemetin isolated from Achillea millefolium L. *Phytomedicine*, *18*(10), 819-825. doi:10.1016/j.phymed.2011.02.005

The editorial team of WebMD. (2009). Yarrow. *WebMD*. Retrieved March 17, 2015, from http://www.webmd.com/vitamins-supplements/ingredientmono-151-YARROW.aspx?activeIngredientId=151&activeIngredientName=YARROW

Ehrlich, S. D. (2013). Yarrow. *University of Maryland Medical Center*. Retrieved March 17, 2015, from http://www.umm.edu/altmed/articles/yarrow-000282.htm

Giorgi, A., Bombelli, R., Luini, A., Speranza, G., Cosentino, M., Lecchini, S., & Cocucci, M. (2009). Antioxidant and cytoprotective properties of infusions from leaves and inflorescences of Achillea collina Becker ex Rchb. *Phytotherapy Research*, *23*(4), 540-545. doi:10.1002/ptr.2679

Khan, A. U., & Gilani, A. H. (2011). Blood pressure lowering, cardiovascular inhibitory and bronchodilatory actions of Achillea millefolium. *Phytotherapy Research*, *25*(4), 577-583. doi:10.1002/ptr.3303

Saeidnia, S., Gohari, A. R., Mokhber-Dezfuli, N., & Kiuchi, F. (2011). A review on phytochemistry and medicinal properties of the genus Achillea. *DARU*, *19*(3), 173-186.

Stone, A. B. (2007). Say yes to yarrow. *Herb Quarterly*, (111), 42-45.

Yazdanparast, R., Ardestani, A., & Jamshidi, S. (2007). Experimental diabetes treated with Achillea santolina: Effect on pancreatic oxidative parameters. *Journal of Ethnopharmacology*, *112*(1), 13-18. doi:10.1016/j.jep.2007.01.030

REVIEWER(S)

Darlene Strayer, RN, MBA, Cinahl Information Systems, Glendale, CA

Nursing Executive Practice Council, Glendale Adventist Medical Center, Glendale, CA

Fats & Oils

Butter

KEY TERMS

Butter: pale yellow or white edible fatty substance made by churning fresh or fermented milk or cream.

Sweet butter: traditional butter without salt used in cooking and baking.

Salted butter: most common butter with salt used as a spread on bread or to favor vegetables.

Clarified butter/Ghee: paste-like butter used primarily for frying or sauteeing.

Saturated fat: solid at room temperature and contains only saturated fatty acids. Found primarily in animal food products.

WHAT WE KNOW

Butter is a pale yellow or white edible fatty substance made by churning fresh or fermented milk or cream that remains soft but solid at room temperature. This process separates the butter fat from the remaining buttermilk. Although often seen alone as a spread for bread, butter can be used in baking and frying. Many sauces use butter as a base. Butter can be added to foods like vegetables or meat for additional flavor

Butter has been valued as a dietary mainstay for thousands of years in diverse global cultures. However, butter fell from grace in the American diet in the 1960s and 1970s with the low-fat diet movement and its avoidance of saturated fat to minimize heart disease. However, recent studies have elevated the status of butter so it is no longer considered a health villain. Butter may be useful in the diet when eaten in moderation.

SOME COMMON TYPES OF BUTTER INCLUDE THE FOLLOWING:
- sweet or unsalted butter- traditional 80% butter fat, unsalted, for use in cooking or baking. Allows control of the amount of salt in a recipe.
- salted butter- traditional 80% butter fat, salted, used as a spread on bread or vegetables.

- organic butter- made from milk of range-fed cows allowed to graze in a pasture over time unlike stall feed cows. Free of antibiotics, hormones, or pesticides.
- European style butter- slow churned and creamy with a butterfat of 85%. Used to create rich desserts and sauces. May be more expensive.
- whipped butter- mixed with air to be more spreadable. May be salted or unsalted. Not useful for baking.
- light butter- may be labeled "reduced fat butter" with 50% fewer calories. Spreadable. Usually not used for baking.
- butter blends- mixed with some form of oil like olive oil or canola oil. Spreadable. Usually not used in baking.
- raw butter- unpasteurized, unprocessed, and made from raw cream. Safety is debated and tends to be expensive.
- clarified butter/ Ghee- heated to separate milk solid and moisture can evaporate. Paste-like consistency, used for frying or sauteeing. Commonly used in South Asian cuisine. Available in U.S. markets.
- flavored butter- mixed with herbs or spices like garlic and chives for additional flavoring. Used on vegetables or meat.

NUTRIENTS/ACTION OF BUTTER

Besides adding flavor to food, butter has many health benefits.
- Butter is rich with fat soluble vitamins such as A, E, and K2. Vitamin A is important for vision, the immune system, and cell health. Vitamin E, an antioxidant, needs fat to be absorbed which is provided in butter. Vitamin K2, a lesser known K vitamin, is thought to play a key role in calcium metabolism. This action could be useful in preventing the buildup of vascular calcium for better heart health and supporting dental and bone health with lowered risk of osteoporosis.

- Butter contains protein necessary for the building and repair of body tissue as well as calcium and phosphorous to support bone health.
- Butter contains saturated fat and monounsaturated fat which may have health benefits. Some studies have linked saturated fat to heart disease, but other research has found that butter may be unrelated to health disease. Ingesting saturated fat can provide the feeling of satiety and may reduce the risk of obesity from overeating.
- Butter is a good source of butyrate, a 4-carbon fatty acid, which supports colon health and may prevent weight gain. Some studies have shown that butyrate may improve the function of mitochondria to help lower insulin and fasting triglycerides. It also has anti-carcinogenic and anti-inflammatory properties.
- Butter contains conjugated linoleic acid (CLA), a fatty acid, that impacts metabolism for weight loss, can lower body fat, and protect against weight gain.

RESEARCH FINDINGS

Research on butter and its benefits are conflictive. For several decades now, butter has held minimum respect in the American diet due to its saturated fat content and the relationship of saturated fat to heart disease. Older studies have been questioned as more is known now about diet and the impact of the various components of butter.

For example, the meta-analysis of over seventy separate studies were published in the Annals of Internal Medicine in March 2014. Dr. Chowdhury and his research associates found that evidence from the aggregate studies did not support current cardiovascular health guidelines that encourage increased use of polyunsaturated fats and low consumption of total saturated fats.

In response, Dr. Walter Willett, chair of the Department of Nutrition at Harvard School of Public Health, stated that the results of the meta-analysis were misleading for the public. He contends that the issue is what replaces saturated fat in the diet, and that use of polyunsaturated fat or monounsaturated fat, as in olive oil, nuts, and plant oils, is preferred to reduce cardiovascular risk.

In the November 2014 issue of *Today's Dietitian*, Marsha McCulloch provided an excellent overview of key studies addressing the relationship of saturated fat

and cardiovascular disease and the notion that butter may be a better choice than once thought. Along with her summaries of the research, McCulloch demonstrated that the answers and issues are not as simple as once thought. She closed with a thought from the Chowdhury et al. study that one should look at the overall dietary pattern as no one nutrient is the responsible for or the answer to one's health issues.

SUMMARY

Butter has been a cultural favorite over thousands of years. There are many types of butter to choose from in the marketplace. Besides adding flavor to food, butter has many health benefits and may be useful when ingested in moderation. However, one's overall dietary pattern is the key to good health rather than individual nutrients.

—*Marylane Wade Koch, RN, MSN*

REFERENCES

Chowdberry et al. "Association of Dietary, Circulating, and Supplement Fatty Acids With Coronary Risk: A Systematic Review and Meta-analysis." *Annuls of Internal Medicine*. March 18, 2014. Web 10 July 2016. http://wphna.org/wp-content/uploads/2014/08/2014-03_Annals_of_Int_Med_Chowdhury_et_al_Fat_and_CHD_+_responses.pdf

"Dietary fat and heart disease study is seriously misleading" *Harvard School of Public Health: The Nutrition Source*. n.d. Web 8 July 2016. https://www.hsph.harvard.edu/nutritionsource/2014/03/19/dietary-fat-and-heart-disease-study-is-seriously-misleading/

"Different Types of Butter." *The Dairy Dish*. n.d. Web 1 July 2016. http://thedairydish.com/types-butter/

Gunnars, Kris. "7 Reasons Why Butter is Healthy in Moderation" *Authority Nutrition*. n. d. Web 9 July 2016. https://authoritynutrition.com/7-reasons-why-butter-is-good-for-you/

Leech, Joe. "Vitamin K2: Everything You Need to Know." *Authority Nutrition*. n.d. Web 4 July 2016. https://authoritynutrition.com/vitamin-k2/

McCulloch, Marsha. "Saturated Fat: Not So Bad or Just Bad Science?" *Today's Dietitian*. November 2014, Vol. 16 No. 11 P. 32. Web 11 July 2016. http://www.todaysdietitian.com/newarchives/111114p32.shtml

"Nutrients in Butter." *The Daily Council*. n.d. Web 1 July 2016. http://www.milk.co.uk/page.aspx?intPageID=375

Sifferlin, Alexandra "The Case for Eating Butter Just Got Stronger" *Time Magazine* June 29, 2016. Web 1 July 2016 http://time.com/4386248/fat-butter-nutrition-health/?xid=newsletter-brief

Teicholz, Nina. (2014) *The Big Fat Surprise: Why Butter, Meat and Cheese Belong in a Healthy Diet.* 1st ed. New York: Simon & Schuster.

"What is butter?" *WebExhibits* n.d.Web 4 July 2016. http://www.webexhibits.org/butter/composition.html

REVIEWER(S)

Darlene Strayer, RN, MBA, Cinahl Information Systems, Glendale, CA

Nursing Executive Practice Council, Glendale Adventist Medical Center, Glendale, CA

Canola Oil

WHAT WE KNOW

Canola oil is derived from the crushed seeds of the canola plant. The canola plant is a yellow, flowering member of the *Brassicaceae* family and a variation of the rapeseed plant. Canadian scientists bred the first canola plant in 1976 in an attempt to develop a rapeseed plant that was low in uric acid. Today, canola (created from combining "Canada" and "ola," or oil) is one of the most highly consumed oilseed crops in the world. With a relatively high smoking point and a neutral flavor, canola oil is a versatile cooking oil that can be used in salad dressings, sautéing, baking, and frying. Canola oil is considered one of the healthiest cooking oils; it contains only 7% saturated fat content and ample amounts of the cardioprotective unsaturated fatty acids oleic acid (71%), linoleic acid (21%), and alpha-linolenic acid (11%).

- Although it has been believed by some that canola oil is developed through genetic engineering, this is not the case. Canola plants were bred from the rapeseed plant nearly a decade before the first genetically modified plant cell was reported. While modern day canola oil can be genetically modified in the same way that other crops (e.g., corn, wheat) are genetically modified, organic canola brands are available that are guaranteed to not be genetically engineered.

ACTION OF CANOLA OIL

- Canola oil is a rich source of monounsaturated fatty acids (MUFAs) and polyunsaturated fatty acids (PUFAs).

—The MUFA oleic acid promotes the production of antioxidants and lowers triglyceride levels, reducing the risk of atherosclerosis, heart disease, and cancer.

—Linoleic acid (i.e., omega-6 PUFA) and alpha-linolenic acid (i.e., omega-3 PUFA) are essential fatty acids (EFAs), which are polyunsaturated fatty acids that the body requires for:
  –brain development
  –control of inflammation
  –blood clotting
  –strengthening of cell membranes
  –the transport and production of cholesterol

—Canola oil is rich in tocopherols, which maintain cell membranes, support the immune system, and protect fats from oxidation.

RECOMMENDED INTAKE OF CANOLA OIL

- There is no established recommendation for intake of canola oil. Recommendations regarding fat intake include the following:
  —The established adequate intake (AI) for linoleic acid is 17g/day for men and 12 g/day for women 19–50 years of age, and 14 g/day for men and 11 g/day for women > 51 years of age
  —The AI for alpha-linolenic acid is 1.6 g/day and 1.1 g/day for adult men and women, respectively
  —It is currently recommended that dietary fat intake be limited as follows:
    –Total dietary fat should be 20–30% of total caloric intake
    –Saturated fat should be < 10% of total caloric intake
    –Trans fat should be < 1% of total caloric intake

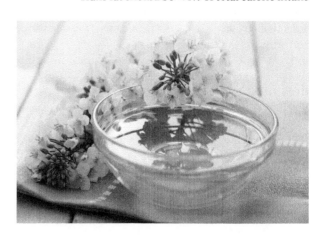

RESEARCH FINDINGS

- Researchers conducted a study on mice, which compared the effects of maternal consumption of canola oil verses maternal consumption of corn oil on the development of mammary gland tumors in respective offspring. Results indicated that the offspring of mothers that consumed canola oil experienced a delayed appearance of mammary gland tumors and slower growth of the tumors that developed compared with the offspring of corn oil-fed mothers. Researchers suggest that substituting canola oil for corn oil in maternal diets could reduce the risk for developing breast cancer in daughters.

- Researchers report that consumption of canola oil appears to exhibit chemo-preventive action against colon tumor development in Fischer rats compared with colon tumor development in rats who consumed corn oil. Researchers suggest that this is likely due to the increase in alpha-linolenic (i.e. omega-3) fatty acid levels.

  —The alpha-linolenic components eicosapentaenoic acid (EPA) and docosahexaenoic acid (DHA) have demonstrated a protective effect against dementia, heart disease, inflammatory bowel disease, cancer, and rheumatoid arthritis (RA). Researchers suggest that this protective activity is attributed to the anti-inflammatory activity of EPA and DHA.

SUMMARY

Consumers should become knowledgeable about the physiologic effects of consuming canola oil. Canola oil contains monounsaturated and polyunsaturated fatty acids that are essential for brain development, blood clotting, and fighting inflammation. Recent research suggests that canola oil may help fight cancer, heart disease, and arthritis.

—*Cherie Marcel, BS*

REFERENCES

Bairstow, I. S. (2009). Is canola bad for you? *Delicious Living, 24*(15), 15.

Bhatia, E., Doddivenaka, C., Zhang, X., Bommareddy, A., Krishman, P., Matthees, D. P., & Dwivedi, C. (2011). Chemopreventive effects of dietary canola oil on colon cancer development. *Nutrition and Cancer, 63*(2), 242-247. doi:10.1080/01635581.2011.523498

Cabré, E., Mañosa, M., & Gassull, M. A. (2012). Omega-3 fatty acids and inflammatory bowel diseases - a systematic review. *British Journal of Nutrition,* S240-S252. doi:10.1017/S0007114512001626

Food and Nutrition Board, Institute of Medicine, National Academies. (n.d.). Dietary Reference Intakes (DRIs): Estimated Average Requirements. Food and Nutrition Board, Institute of Medicine, National Academies. Retrieved March 30, 2015, from http://fnic.nal.usda.gov/dietary-guidance/dietary-reference-intakes

Ion, G., Akinsete, J. A., & Hardman, W. E. (2010). Maternal consumption of canola oil suppressed mammary gland tumorigenesis in C3(1) TAg mice offspring. *BMC Cancer, 10*, 81. doi:10.1186/1471-2407-10-81

Kesse-Guyot, E., Peneau, S., Ferry, M., Jeandel, C., Hereberg, S., & Galan, P. (2011). Thirteen-year prospective study between fish consumption, long-chain N-3 fatty acids intakes and cognitive function. *Journal of Nutrition, Health & Aging, 15*(2), 115-120. doi:10.1007/s12603-010-0318-0

Lin, L., Allemekinders, H., Dansby, A., Campbell, L., Durance-Tod, S., Berger, A., & Jones, P. J. H. (2013). Evidence of health benefits of canola oil. *Nutrition Reviews, 71*(6), 370-385. doi:10.1111/nure.12033

Lopez, L. B., Kritz-Silverstein, D., & Barrett-Connor, E. (2011). High dietary and plasma levels of the omega-3 fatty acid docosahexaenoic acid are associated with decreased dementia risk: The Rancho Bernardo Study. *Journal of Nutrition, Health & Aging, 15*(1), 25-31. doi:10.1007/s12603-010-0114-x

Lutz, C. A., & Przytulski, K. R. (2011). Fats. In *Nutrition & diet therapy* (5th ed., pp. 46-62). Philadelphia, PA: F. A. Davis Company.

Nation Health and Medical Research Council. (2013). Australian Dietary Guidelines. In *Canberra: National Health and Medical Research Council* (pp. 48-58).

Wall, R., Ross, R. P., Fitzgerald, G. F., & Stanton, C. (2010). Fatty acids from fish: The anti-inflammatory potential of long-chain omega-3 fatty acids. *Nutrition Reviews, 68*(5), 280-289. doi:10.1111/j.1753-4887.2010.00287.x

REVIEWER(S)

Darlene Strayer, RN, MBA, Cinahl Information Systems, Glendale, CA

Amy Hurst, RN, MSN, Cinahl Information Systems, Glendale, CA

Nursing Executive Practice Council, Glendale Adventist Medical Center, Glendale, CA

Lard

WHAT WE KNOW

Lard is composed primarily of fat from the pig's abdomen or any other part of the animal with a high proportion of adipose tissue. It may be rendered by boiling, steaming, or with dry heat. After it had been used in cooking around the world for many hundreds of years, during the late twentieth century lard acquired a reputation as nutritional suicide on par with bacon for its high proportion of saturated fat. Vegetable oils often were preferred because they contain less saturated fat, until research established that the way in which vegetable oils are manufactured can make them dangerous.

*The content of lard can vary widely, reflecting the diet of any given pig, which leads to a great deal of variation because pigs are among the most omnivorous animals on Earth. They will eat nearly anything offered to them. In some parts of the world, pigs are fed acorns, or peanuts. In the United States, they often eat corn.

*Lard has been used as a spread for more than 200 years in the United States and Europe; during times of war (one example was World War I) it was used nearly universally in areas where butter was scarce (and thus expensive) or unavailable. Before the Industrial Revolution, lard was widely available wherever pigs were slaughtered, and thus usually less expensive than butter.

NUTRIENTS

- By late in the twentieth century, oils were largely separated into two classes: animal and vegetable, with the former disparaged as unhealthy. More detailed studies revealed that some vegetable fats actually contain more saturated fats than lard. Even margarine can be unhealthy if it is manufactured with trans-fats.
- Lard is classified as a triglyceride that is composed of three fatty acids.
- Lard also supplies an omega 6 fatty acid called linoleic acid, which helps to govern the body's inflammatory response.
- Lard contains a relatively high oleic acid content, an essential fatty acid, also found in canola and olive oil. Oleic acid helps reduces LDLs, lowering "bad" cholesterol and helping to prevent heart disease. Lard's oleic acid content is roughly twice that of butter.

DIETARY INTAKE GUIDELINES

- While overconsumption of lard can be dangerous to one's health, in moderate amounts, this long-standing cooking oil poses little harm. Shortly after the year 2000, lard developed a following among bakers and chefs in many countries. In some countries (such as Britain in 2004) it became so popular so quickly that shortages developed. In recent years, lard has re-assumed its position as a favored fat among many pastry chefs.
- Lard's high "smoke point" (190 degrees F. or 375 C.) makes it less likely than other fats to burn and become carcinogenic during cooking. Properly rendered, lard has no odor or taste.

RESEARCH FINDINGS

- Recent research has found that lard may be less unhealthy than previously believed, notably because it lacks trans-fats, which are such a threat to heart health that several countries have banned their use. Lard is not used in cultures that prohibit consumption of pigs or products derived from them, such as those where most of the population is comprised of Muslims and Jews. In cultures where pigs are an acceptable food (most of the Americas, Europe, and China, for example), lard is often used as a cooking fat or a spread, similar to butter. It also may be used in pates and sausages, as well as pastries.
- Lard began to pass out of favor shortly after the year 1900, as Upton Sinclair, in *The Jungle* (a novel based on abuse of people and animals in Chicago's stockyards) gave it a bad name in a story that described working men falling into rendering vats and later being sold as bricks of it. The book sold so many copies that it reduced lard demand for years.
- During the swing toward plant-based oils, lard was sometimes removed from grocery-store

shelves in the United States. It has returned, but with health-conscious shoppers seeking a pure form that has not been treated with hydrogenated fats and chemicals that contribute to clogging of the arteries and heart disease. Such forms of lard are often sold in block form as a commercial product.

SUMMARY

Consumers should become knowledgeable about the health risks and benefits of lard consumption. Overall, consumption of lard in small amounts is now considered part of a healthy diet. Lard contains 15% more monounsaturated fats than butter, decreasing risk for inflammation and heart disease. Lard does not contain trans fats making it a healthier alternative to some vegetable oils, such as margarine.

—*Bruce E. Johansen, Ph.D.*

REFERENCES

Alfred T. (2002). "Fats and fatty oils". *Ullmann's encyclopedia of industrial chemistry*. Weinheim, U.K.: Wiley-VCH.

Davidson, A. (2002). *The Penguin companion to food*. New York: Penguin Books, 175-177, 530-531.

Kaminsky, P. (2005). *Pig perfect: Encounters with remarkable swine and some great ways to cook them*. New York: Hyperion.

Katragadda, H. R.; Fullana, A. S.; Sidhu, S.; Carbonell-Barrachina, Á. A. (2010). "Emissions of volatile aldehydes from heated cooking oils". *Food Chemistry* 120: 59.

Lee, M. and Lee, T. "Light, fluffy – believe It, It's not butter." *New York Times*, October 11, 2000, n.p.

National Research Council. (1976). *Fat content and composition of animal products*. Washington, DC: Printing and Publishing Office, National Academy of Sciences, 203.

Ockerman, H. W. and Basu, L. (2006). Edible rendering – rendered products for human use. In: Meeker D.L. (ed). *Essential rendering: All about the animal by-products industry*. Arlington, VA: National Renderers Association, 95–110.

Rombaur, I. S, et al. (1997).*Joy of cooking*, revised ed. New York: Scribner, 1069.

"Why Lard's Healthier Than You Think." The Star.com. United Kingdom. May 14, 2013. https://www.thestar.com/life/health_wellness/nutrition/2013/05/14/why_lards_healthier_than_you_think.html

REVIEWER(S)

Darlene Strayer, RN, MBA, Cinahl Information Systems, Glendale, CA

Nursing Executive Practice Council, Glendale Adventist Medical Center, Glendale, CA

Linseed Oil

WHAT WE KNOW

Linseed oil (also called flaxseed oil) is derived from the seeds of linseed (also called flax), a common garden flower with the Latin name *Linum usitatissimum*. The brown, sometimes golden linseed seeds are ground and pressed to produce linseed oil, which is rich in the essential omega-3 fatty acid alpha-linolenic acid. Linseed oil has been shown to promote the health of the nervous and immune systems with its anti-inflammatory, anti-proliferative, and anti-thrombotic effects, which have been linked to the prevention of kidney disease, heart disease, and certain cancers (e.g., colon, breast, and prostate cancer). Although research continues and scientific evidence is not yet conclusive, linseed oil has been suggested as treatment for colitis, asthma, skin and vision conditions, migraine headaches, infertility, varicose veins, enlarged prostate, depression, and attention deficit disorder (ADD). As a culinary agent, linseed oil has a subtle nutty flavor and can be used for making salad dressings or as a topping on rice or vegetables.

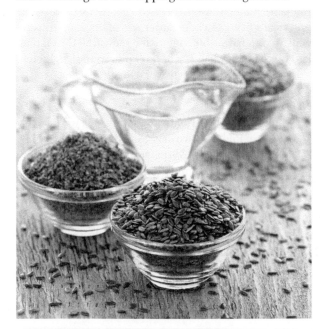

ACTION OF LINSEED OIL

- Linseed oil is an excellent source of alpha-linolenic acid.
  —Alpha-linolenic acid exhibits hypotensive (i.e., blood pressure lowering) properties and anti-inflammatory activity, which helps to improve lung function and prevent cardiovascular disease (CVD), arthritis, and other chronic diseases associated with inflammation.

RECOMMENDED INTAKE OF LINSEED OIL

- Approximately 1 tablespoon of linseed oil per 100 pounds of body weight is recommended daily to supply adequate alpha-linolenic acid (e.g., about 1.1 g/day for females and 1.6 g/day for males).

MEDICATION INTERACTIONS

- Pregnant women should be cautioned against taking supplemental linseed oil due to its lignan content, which is thought to potentially induce menstruation and increase bleeding time.
- Persons with hemophilia or those receiving blood thinners should consult the treating clinician before taking supplemental linseed oil because linseed oil has blood thinning effects.

RESEARCH FINDINGS.

Results of a study analyzing the effects of dietary linseed oil on colon tumors in rats showed that dietary linseed oil increased the circulating omega-3 fatty acid levels and significantly inhibited colon tumor development compared with dietary corn oil. Researchers suggest that this protective action is due to the omega-3 fatty acid alpha-linolenic acid.

SUMMARY

Consumers should become knowledgeable about the physiologic effects of linseed oil. Linseed oil contains alpha-linoleic acid, which helps lower blood pressure and fights inflammation. Individuals should be aware of potential interactions between linseed oil and blood thinners. Recent research suggests that linseed oil may help fight cancer.

—*Cherie Marcel, BS*

REFERENCES

Banks, D. (2011). Your body loves linseed oil. *Positive Health*, (180), 5p.

Dwivedi, C., Natarajan, K., & Matthees, D. P. (2005). Chemopreventive effects of dietary flaxseed oil on colon tumor development. *Nutrition & Cancer*, 51(1), 52-58.

Fernandes, F. S., de Souza, A. S., do Carmo, M. D., & Boaventura, G. T. (2011). Maternal intake of flaxseed-based diet (Linum usitatissimum) on hippocampus fatty acid profile: Implications for growth, locomotor activity and spatial memory. *Nutrition*, 27(10), 1040-1047. doi:10.1016/j.nut.2010.11.001

Fischer, W. L. (1990). The linseed oil diet according to Dr. Johanna Budwig. *Townsend Letter for Doctors & Patients*, (89), 5p.

Forster, G. A. (2004). Holistic health Q & A. *New Times Naturally*, 10-12.

Wood, R. (2002). Flax seed. *Sentient Times*, 21. doi:10.1016/j.jand.2012.06.221

REVIEWER(S)

Darlene Strayer, RN, MBA, Cinahl Information Systems, Glendale, CA

Nursing Executive Practice Council, Glendale Adventist Medical Center, Glendale, CA

Olive Oil

WHAT WE KNOW

Unlike most oils, which are derived from nuts or seeds, olive oil is extracted from the fruit of the olive tree (*Olea europaea*). Depending on the stage of extraction, olive oil is categorized as extra-virgin, which is obtained from the first pressing of olives and is considered highest quality; virgin, which is obtained with later pressings; refined, which is considered lower quality olive oil that is refined to remove flavor defects; and the most commonly consumed category, which is referred to simply as olive oil, which consists of a mixture of refined and virgin olive oils.

- Some of the powerful nutrients found in olive oil include many phytonutrients (i.e., beneficial plant-derived chemicals), the monounsaturated fat oleic acid, and vitamin E. Olive oil has been shown to have antioxidant, anti-inflammatory, anti-carcinogenic, anti-blood clotting, antihypertensive, and antibacterial properties. Among the many health benefits associated with olive oil consumption are prevention of heart disease, cancer (e.g., breast, skin, intestinal), diabetes mellitus, type 2 (DM2), obesity, rheumatoid arthritis, osteoporosis, stroke, and depression. Results of ongoing studies show the prevention

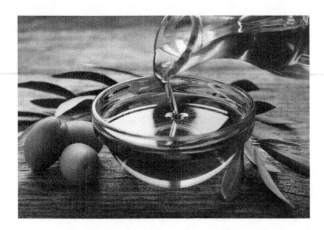

of Alzheimer's disease as a potential benefit of olive oil consumption. Olive oil is recognized as being one of the most significant protective components of the famed Mediterranean diet, which is a diet based on the dietary patterns of persons living in the Mediterranean basin during the 1960s because of the notably low rates of heart disease in Cretan men.

- As a culinary agent, olive oil can be used for low-heat sautéing, making salad dressings and sauces, or drizzling over entrees.

ACTION OF OLIVE OIL

- Olive oil is an excellent source of the monounsaturated fatty acid oleic acid, which lowers triglyceride levels, reducing the risk of atherosclerosis, heart disease, and cancer.
- Olive oil provides vitamin E, which protects lipids from oxidation.
- Olive oil contains squalene, a steroidal precursor that helps to regulate sebum, an oil barrier that inhibits bacterial growth on skin and lubricates skin and hair.
- Olive oil contains many valuable phytonutrients, including phenols, terpenes, anthocyanidins, flavones, and lignans, that exhibit powerful antioxidant, blood thinning, anti-inflammatory, and anti-carcinogenic properties.

RESEARCH FINDINGS

- Numerous studies have analyzed the cardioprotective properties demonstrated by olive oil and its various constituents. Many of these studies have focused on the antioxidant effects of olive oil–derived phytonutrients, but evidence also shows that olive oil consumption is associated with anti-inflammatory and antihypertensive (i.e., blood pressure lowering) properties, protection against blood clotting, and enhanced cardiac energy production. Researchers suggest that inclusion of dietary olive oil can be advised to persons with dyslipidemia, hypertension, or a family history of heart disease.
  - —In the Prevencion con DietaMediterranea (PREDIMED) trial, researchers demonstrated that inclusion of extra-virgin olive oil or mixed nuts in a Mediterranean dietary pattern lowers the incidence of stroke, heart attack, and cardiovascular-related death. Further findings from a post hoc analysis of the PREDIMED trial revealed that the inclusion of extra-virgin olive oil (but not mixed nuts) in a Mediterranean diet can also reduce the risk of atrial fibrillation.
- Researchers who conducted a recent study in France analyzing the dietary intake data of 7,625 participants reported an association between consumption of olive oil and lower risk of stroke. Participants who consumed regular quantities of olive oil were shown to have a 41% lower likelihood of stroke. A follow-up study revealed that participants with the highest plasma levels of oleic acid had a reduction in stroke risk of 73% compared with participants whose levels were the lowest. Researchers suggest that further randomized trials should be conducted to confirm these results.

SUMMARY

Consumers should become knowledgeable about the physiologic effects of olive oil consumption. Olive oil contains unsaturated fats, phytochemicals and vitamin E, which fight inflammation and reduce the risk of cancer and heart disease. Recent research suggests that olive oil can help prevent heart attacks and stroke.

—*Cherie Marcel, BS*

REFERENCES

Bendinelli, B., Masala, G., Saieva, C., Salvini, S., Calonico, C., Sacerdote, C., & Panico, S. (2011). Fruit, vegetables, and olive oil and risk of coronary heart disease in Italian women: The EPICOR study. *American Journal of Clinical Nutrition, 93*(2), 275-283.

Bester, D., Esterhuyse, A. J., Truter, E. J., & van Rooyen, J. (2010). Cardiovascular effects of edible oils: A comparison between four popular edible oils. *Nutrition Research Reviews, 23*(2), 334-348. doi:10.1017/S0954422410000223

Buckland, G., Mayen, A. L., Agudo, A., Travier, N., Navarro, C., Huerta, J. M., ... Gonzalez, C. (2012). Olive oil intake and mortality within the Spanish population (EPIC-Spain). *American Journal of Clinical Nutrition, 96*(1), 142-149. doi:10.3945/ajcn.111.024216

Buckland, G., Travier, N., Barricarte, A., Ardanaz, E., Moreno-Iribas, C., Sanchez, M., ... Gonzalez, C. A. (2012). Olive oil intake and CHD in the European Prospective Investigation into Cancer and Nutrition Spanish cohort. *British Journal of Nutrition, 108*(11), 2075-2082. doi:10.1017/S000711451200298X

Chrysohoou, C., Kastorini, C., Panagiotakos, D., Aggelopoulos, P., Tsiachris, D., Pitsavos, C., & Stefanadis, C. (2010). Exclusive olive oil consumption is associated with lower likelihood of developing left ventricular systolic dysfunction in acute coronary syndrome patients: The Hellenic Heart Failure Study. *Annals of Nutrition & Metabolism, 56*(1), 9-15. doi:10.1159/000261898

Covas, M., Ruiz-Gutierrez, V., la Torre, R., Kafatos, A., Lamuela-Raventos, R. M., Osada, J., & Visioli, F. (2006). Minor components of olive oil: Evidence to date of health benefits in humans. *Nutrition Reviews, 64*(10 Part 2), S20-S30.

de Roos, B., Zhang, X., Rodriguez Gutierrez, G., Wood, S., Rucklidge, G., Reid, M., & O'Kennedy, N. (2011).Anti-platelet effects of olive oil extract: In vitro functional and proteomic studies. *European Journal of Nutrition, 50*(7), 553-562. doi:10.1007/s00394-010-0162-3

Dye, D. (2011). In the news: Olive oil use linked with lower risk of stroke. *Life Extension, 15*.

Finkle, J. (2011). In the news: Cardiac fat oxidation aided by olive oil compounds. *Life Extension, 1*.

The George Mateljan Foundation editorial team. (n.d.). The world's healthiest foods: Olive oil, extra virgin. Retrieved June 23, 2015, fromhttp://whfoods.org/genpage.php? tname=foodspice&dbid=132

Gonzalez Correa, J. A., Lopez-Villodres, J. A., Asensi, R., Espartero, J. L., Gutierrez, G., & De La Cruz, J. P. (2009). Virgin olive oil polyphenol hydroxytyrosol acetate inhibits in vitro platelet aggregation in human whole blood: Comparison with hydroxytyrosol and acetylsalicylic acid. *British Journal of Nutrition, 101*(8), 1157-1164. doi:10.1017/ S0007114508061539

Martinez-Gonzalez, M. A., Toledo, E., Aros, F., Fiol, M., Corella, D., Salas-Salvado, J., ... Alonso, A. (2014). Extravirgin olive oil consumption reduces risk of atrial fibrillation: The PREDIMED (Prevencion con Dieta Mediterranea) Trial. *Circulation, 130*(1), 18-26. doi:10.1161/CIRCULATIONAHA.113.006921

Petty, L. (2011). Botanical balms: Plant oils for beautiful skin. *Alive: Canada's Natural Health and Wellness Magazine,* (343), 35-38.

Rodriguez-Rodriguez, R., Herrera, M. D., de Sotomayor, M. A., & Ruiz-Gutierrez, V. (2009). Effects of pomace olive oil-enriched diets on endothelial function of small mesenteric arteries from spontaneously hypertensive rats. *British Journal of Nutrition, 102*(10), 1435-1444. doi:10.1017/S0007114509990754

Ros, E. (2012). Olive oil and CVD: Accruing evidence of a protective effect. *British Journal of Nutrition, 108*(11), 1931-1933. doi:10.1017/S0007114512003844

REVIEWER(S)

Darlene Strayer, RN, MBA, Cinahl Information Systems, Glendale, CA

Nursing Executive Practice Council, Glendale Adventist Medical Center, Glendale, CA

Sesame Oil

WHAT WE KNOW

Sesame oil, or *Sesamum indicum*, is derived from sesame seeds. Golden sesame oil pressed from raw sesame seeds and roasted sesame oil pressed from roasted sesame seeds are the two types of sesame oil that are commonly used in cooking. Sesame oil adds a nutty flavor to sauces and dressings and can be used for roasting, broiling, and sautéing. Refined sesame oil is recommended for stir-frying over high heat because it has a higher smoke point than unrefined oil. In addition to its culinary uses, sesame oil has certain health benefits. Because sesame oil

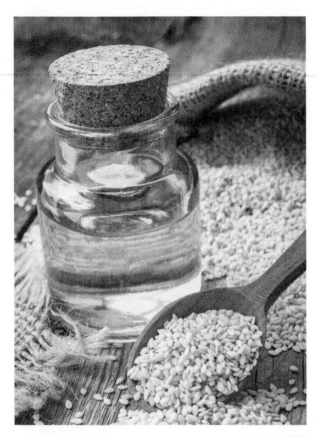

is rich in unsaturated fats and vitamins E and K, its use promotes heart health by lowering cholesterol, facilitating blood clotting, and providing protection from damaging free radicals.

ACTION OF SESAME OIL

- Sesame oil is a good source of the unsaturated fatty acids linoleic acid and oleic acid.
  —Oleic acid promotes the production of antioxidants and lowers triglyceride levels, reducing risk for arteriosclerosis, heart disease, and cancer.
  —Linoleic acid is vital to the production and maintenance of skin, hair, and bones and regulates the reproductive system and energy production.
- Sesame oil is rich in vitamins E and K.
  —Vitamin E is a fat-soluble vitamin that functions primarily as an antioxidant but also maintains cell membranes, assists in vitamin K absorption, and contributes to the functioning of the immune system.

—Alpha-tocopherol, the predominate form of vitamin E, protects lipids from oxidation.
—Vitamin K maintains normal levels of blood clotting proteins and contributes to bone building.
- Sesame oil contains the lignan (i.e., a phytonutrient) called sesamin.
  —Lignans are broken down by the normal flora in the colon to form enterolactone and enterodiol, which have estrogen-like effects. Increasing serum levels of enterolactones may help to protect against heart disease and hormone-dependent cancers such as breast and prostate cancers.

RECOMMENDED INTAKE OF SESAME OIL

- Sesame oil is a significant source of dietary fat. It is currently recommended that dietary fat and cholesterol intake should be limited as follows:
  —Total dietary fat < 35% of total caloric intake but not < 20%
  —Saturated fat < 7% of total caloric intake
  —Trans fat < 1% of total caloric intake
  —Cholesterol < 300 mg/day

RESEARCH FINDINGS

- Researchers have reported that the combination of sesame oil and rice bran is nearly as effective as the use of a calcium-channel blocker for lowering blood pressure (BP). Individuals who received both the sesame oil/rice bran mixture and their prescribed medication(s) experienced more than twice the drop in BP of those who took prescribed medication alone. Sesame oil was found to enhance the effectiveness of the glucose-lowering agent glibenclamide in the treatment of hyperglycemia in patients with diabetes mellitus, type 2 (DM2). The results of another study indicated that in persons with hypertension and DM2 the substitution of sesame oil for all other oils in the diet resulted in lowered plasma levels of glucose and lowered BP levels. Similarly, sesame oil-containing diets in mice were shown to significantly reduce atherosclerosis and plasma levels of cholesterol and triglyceride.
- Researchers report that a topical application of a compound of sesame and rose geranium oils can significantly improve the severity of nose-bleeds in patients with hereditary hemorrhagic telangiectasia (HHT), also known as Osler-Weber-Rendu syndrome (i.e., an inherited disorder characterized by recurrent nose-bleeds, and visceral

arteriovenous malformations [AVM's]). Further study is necessary to determine the effectiveness of this treatment in comparison to other therapies.

SUMMARY

Consumers should become knowledgeable about the physiologic effects of sesame oil consumption. Sesame oil contains unsaturated fats, phytonutrients and vitamins E and K, which fight inflammation, build bone, and helps fight cancer. Recent research suggests that sesame oil can help prevent heart disease and treat diabetes.

—*Cherie Marcel, BS*

REFERENCES

Bhaskaran, S., Santanam, N., Penumetcha, M., & Parthasarathy, S. (2006). Inhibition of atherosclerosis in low-density lipoprotein receptor-negative mice by sesame oil. *Journal of Medicinal Food, 9*(4), 487-490.

Monteiro, E. M., Chibli, L. A., Yamamoto, C. H., Pereira, M. C., Vilela, F. M., Rodarte, M. P., ... de Sousa, O. V. (2014). Antinociceptive and anti-inflammatory activities of the sesame oil and sesamin. *Nutrients, 6*(5), 10 pp. doi:10.3390/nu6051931

Namiki, M. (2007). Nutraceutical functions of sesame: A review. *Critical Reviews in Food Science and Nutrition, 47*(7), 651-673.

Reh, D. D., Hur, K., & Merlo, C. A. (2013). Efficacy of a topical sesame/rose geranium oil compound in patients with hereditary hemorrhagic telangiectasia associated epistaxis. *Laryngoscope, 123*(4), 820-822. doi:10.1002/lary.23736

Sankar, D., Ali, A., Sambandam, G., & Rao, R. (2011). Sesame oil exhibits synergistic effect with anti-diabetic medication in patients with type 2 diabetes mellitus. *Clinical Nutrition, 30*(3), 351-358. doi:10.1016/j.clnu.2010.11.005

Sankar, D., Rao, M. R., Sambandam, G., & Pugalendi, K. V. (2006). A pilot study of open label sesame oil in hypertensive diabetics. *Journal of Medicinal Food, 9*(3), 408-412.

Sankar, D., Sambandam, G., Rao, M. R., & Pugalendi, K. (2004). Sesame oil exhibits additive effect on nifedipine and modulates oxidative stress and electrolytes in hypertensive patients. *Journal of Nutraceuticals, Functional & Medical Foods, 4*(3/4), 133-145. doi:10.1300/J133v04n0309

Turner, L. (2010). Off the shelf: Food/Oil change. *Better Nutrition, 72*(10), 48-49.

REVIEWER

Nursing Executive Practice Council, Glendale Adventist Medical Center, Glendale, CA

Soybean Oil

WHAT WE KNOW

Soybean oil is a pale yellow oil derived from the seed of the nutrient-rich soybean plant. The soybean is high in protein; iron; calcium; E and B-complex vitamins; and phytonutrients (i.e., beneficial plant-derived chemicals), including beta-carotene, a precursor to vitamin A. Soybean oil is well known as a source of the unsaturated fat lecithin, which contains linoleic, oleic, linolenic, and palmitic acids. Among its health benefits, lecithin has been shown to boost immunity against infection, prevent gallstones, and promote CNS health. As a culinary agent, soybean oil is used for frying, baking, and making salad dressings. It is also used topically as a skin moisturizer, and for protecting the skin from free-radical damage. There is some evidence that soybean oil has the potential to protect against alopecia areata, an autoimmune skin condition that results in hair loss.

ACTION OF SOYBEAN OIL

- Soybean oil is the best-known source of lecithin. Some of the benefits of lecithin include that it:
  —emulsifies fats, preventing atherosclerosis (i.e., hardening of arteries) and reducing the concentration of cholesterol and fats in the blood
  —improves utilization of vitamins A and E
  —is rich in the B vitamins inositol and choline, which support liver function

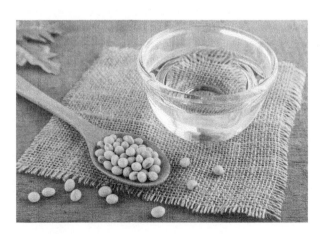

—is an excellent source of linoleic, oleic, linolenic, and palmitic acids

- –Linoleic acid is vital to the production and maintenance of skin, hair, and bones and regulates the reproductive system and energy production.
- –Oleic acid promotes the production of antioxidants and lowers triglyceride levels, reducing risk for arteriosclerosis, heart disease, and cancer.
- –Linolenic acid exhibits hypotensive (i.e., blood pressure lowering) properties and anti-inflammatory activity, which helps to improve lung function and prevent cardiovascular disease, arthritis, and other chronic diseases associated with inflammation.
- –Palmitic acid is primarily used as a moisturizing agent in soaps and cosmetics.

RECOMMENDED INTAKE OF SOYBEAN OIL

- Soybean oil used for the purpose of treating osteoarthritis: 300 mg/day by mouth, to be combined with avocado oil.

MEDICATION INTERACTIONS

- Individuals who are allergic to members of the Fabaceae/Leguminosea family (e.g. peanuts, soybeans) may also be allergic to soybean oil.
- No information is available on soybean oil interactions with medications.

RESEARCH FINDINGS

- In the United States, a study was conducted to analyze the effect of fatty acid intake when commonly used commercial frying oil is replaced with the newly developed low-saturated, high-oleic, low-linolenic (LSHO) soybean oil. LSHO soybean oil was developed through genetic modification and traditional breeding to improve the acceptability of using soybean oil for frying. The oil substitution was used in preparing fried meat, poultry, and fish dishes as well as French fries, potato chips, and puffs. Results clearly indicated that use of the LSHO soybean oil decreases total dietary intake of saturated fat and increases intake of oleic acid. Intake of the essential fatty acids linoleic and linolenic acid also decreased but remained within the recommended intake ranges. Researchers concluded that substitution with LSHO soybean oil encourages fatty acid consumption that is more consistent with current dietary recommendations for lower saturated fat intake, thereby contributing to the prevention of cardiovascular disease.

SUMMARY

Consumers should become knowledgeable about the physiologic effects of soybean oil consumption. Soybean oil contains lecithin and unsaturated fatty acids that help prevent heart disease, lower blood pressure, and support skin, hair, and bone health. Individuals with food allergies should be aware that soybean oil may trigger an allergic reaction. Recent research suggests that using genetically modified soybean oil may decrease intake of saturated fats.

—*Cherie Marcel, BS*

REFERENCES

Crawford, A. W., Wang, C., Jenkins, D. J., & Lemke, S. L. (2011). Estimated effect on fatty acid intake of substituting a low-saturated, high-oleic, low-linolenic soybean oil for liquid oils. *Nutrition Today*, 46(4), 189-196. doi:10.1097/NT.0b013e3182261d97

The George Mateljan Foundation editorial team. (n.d.). Soybeans. *The World's Healthiest Foods*. Retrieved March 5, 2015, from http://www.whfoods.com/genpage.php? tname=foodspice&dbid=79

Goulart, F. S. (1992). Soy foods for fitness: More than a hill of beans. *Total Health*, 14(3), 33.

Lichtenstein, A. H., Matthan, N. R., Jalbert, S. M., Resteghini, N. A., Schaefer, E. J., & Ausman, L. M. (2006). Novel soybean oils with different fatty acid profiles alter cardiovascular disease risk factors in moderately hyperlipidemic subjects. *American Journal of Clinical Nutrition*, 84(3), 497-504.

Petty, L. (2011). Botanical balms. *Alive: Canada's Natural Health and Wellness Magazine*, (343), 35-38.

WebMD. (n.d.). Soybean oi. *WebMD*. Retrieved March 5, 2015, from http://www.webmd.com/vitamins-supplements/ingredientmono-196-soybean%20oil.aspx?activeingredientid=196&activeingredientname=soybean%20oil

REVIEWER(S)

Sharon Richman, MSPT, Cinahl Information Systems, Glendale, CA

Nursing Executive Practice Council, Glendale Adventist Medical Center, Glendale, CA

NUTRITION INFORMATION FROM THE USDA

TABLE OF CONTENTS

The Guidelines

1 **Follow a healthy eating pattern across the lifespan.** All food and beverage choices matter. Choose a healthy eating pattern at an appropriate calorie level to help achieve and maintain a healthy body weight, support nutrient adequacy, and reduce the risk of chronic disease.

2 **Focus on variety, nutrient density, and amount.** To meet nutrient needs within calorie limits, choose a variety of nutrient-dense foods across and within all food groups in recommended amounts.

3 **Limit calories from added sugars and saturated fats and reduce sodium intake.** Consume an eating pattern low in added sugars, saturated fats, and sodium. Cut back on foods and beverages higher in these components to amounts that fit within healthy eating patterns.

4 **Shift to healthier food and beverage choices.** Choose nutrient-dense foods and beverages across and within all food groups in place of less healthy choices. Consider cultural and personal preferences to make these shifts easier to accomplish and maintain.

5 **Support healthy eating patterns for all.** Everyone has a role in helping to create and support healthy eating patterns in multiple settings nationwide, from home to school to work to communities.

Figure ES-1.
2015-2020 Dietary Guidelines for Americans at a Glance

The *2015-2020 Dietary Guidelines* focuses on the big picture with recommendations to help Americans make choices that add up to an overall healthy eating pattern. To build a healthy eating pattern, combine healthy choices from across all food groups—while paying attention to calorie limits, too. Check out the 5 Guidelines that encourage healthy eating patterns:

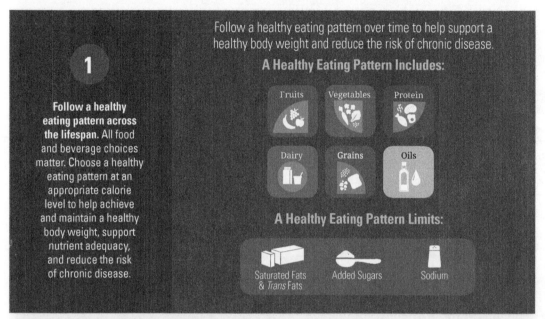

1

Follow a healthy eating pattern across the lifespan. All food and beverage choices matter. Choose a healthy eating pattern at an appropriate calorie level to help achieve and maintain a healthy body weight, support nutrient adequacy, and reduce the risk of chronic disease.

Follow a healthy eating pattern over time to help support a healthy body weight and reduce the risk of chronic disease.

A Healthy Eating Pattern Includes:

Fruits　Vegetables　Protein

Dairy　Grains　Oils

A Healthy Eating Pattern Limits:

Saturated Fats & *Trans* Fats　Added Sugars　Sodium

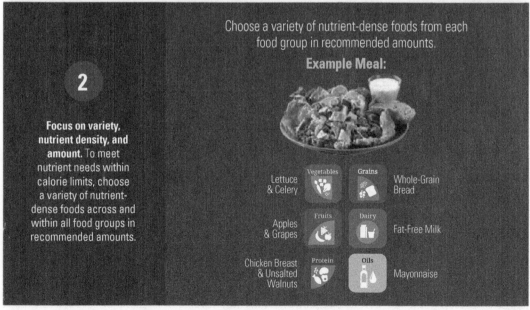

2

Focus on variety, nutrient density, and amount. To meet nutrient needs within calorie limits, choose a variety of nutrient-dense foods across and within all food groups in recommended amounts.

Choose a variety of nutrient-dense foods from each food group in recommended amounts.

Example Meal:

Lettuce & Celery　Vegetables　Grains　Whole-Grain Bread

Apples & Grapes　Fruits　Dairy　Fat-Free Milk

Chicken Breast & Unsalted Walnuts　Protein　Oils　Mayonnaise

Figure ES-1. *(continued...)*

2015-2020 Dietary Guidelines for Americans at a Glance

The *2015-2020 Dietary Guidelines* focuses on the big picture with recommendations to help Americans make choices that add up to an overall healthy eating pattern. To build a healthy eating pattern, combine healthy choices from across all food groups—while paying attention to calorie limits, too. Check out the 5 Guidelines that encourage healthy eating patterns:

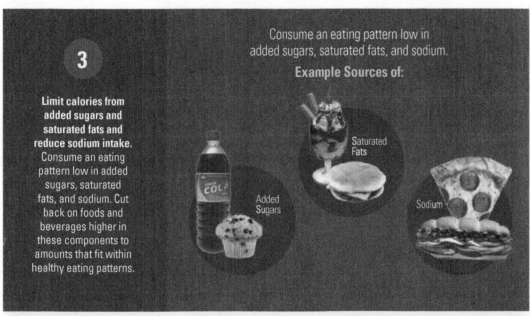

3

Limit calories from added sugars and saturated fats and reduce sodium intake. Consume an eating pattern low in added sugars, saturated fats, and sodium. Cut back on foods and beverages higher in these components to amounts that fit within healthy eating patterns.

Consume an eating pattern low in added sugars, saturated fats, and sodium.

Example Sources of:

Added Sugars

Saturated Fats

Sodium

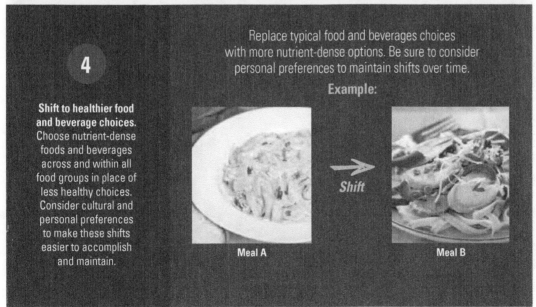

4

Shift to healthier food and beverage choices. Choose nutrient-dense foods and beverages across and within all food groups in place of less healthy choices. Consider cultural and personal preferences to make these shifts easier to accomplish and maintain.

Replace typical food and beverages choices with more nutrient-dense options. Be sure to consider personal preferences to maintain shifts over time.

Example:

Meal A

Shift

Meal B

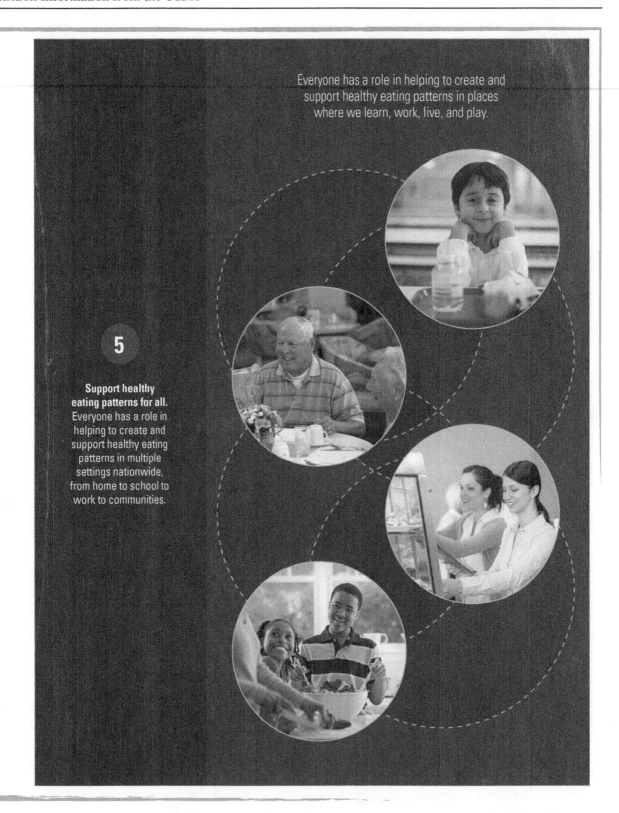

Everyone has a role in helping to create and
support healthy eating patterns in places
where we learn, work, live, and play.

5

**Support healthy
eating patterns for all.**
Everyone has a role in
helping to create and
support healthy eating
patterns in multiple
settings nationwide,
from home to school to
work to communities.

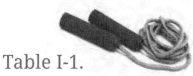

Table I-1.

Facts About Nutrition & Physical Activity-Related Health Conditions in the United States

Health Condition	Facts
Overweight & Obesity	<ul><li>For more than 25 years, more than half of the adult population has been overweight or obese.</li><li>Obesity is most prevalent in those ages 40 years and older and in African American adults, and is least prevalent in adults with highest incomes.</li><li>Since the early 2000s, abdominal obesity[a] has been present in about half of U.S. adults of all ages. Prevalence is higher with increasing age and varies by sex and race/ethnicity.</li><li>In 2009-2012, 65% of adult females and 73% of adult males were overweight or obese.</li><li>In 2009-2012, nearly one in three youth ages 2 to 19 years were overweight or obese.</li></ul>

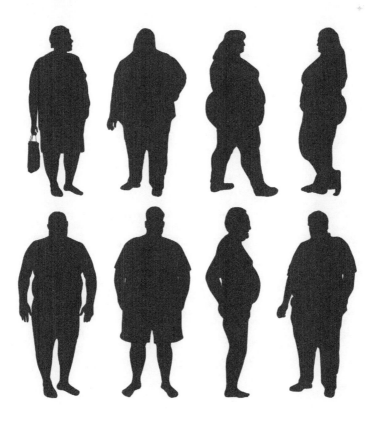

Table I-1. *(continued...)*

Facts About Nutrition & Physical Activity-Related Health Conditions in the United States

Health Condition	Facts
Cardiovascular Disease (CVD) & Risk Factors: Coronary Heart Disease Stroke Hypertension High Total Blood Cholesterol	• In 2010, CVD affected about 84 million men and women ages 20 years and older (35% of the population). • In 2007-2010, about 50% of adults who were normal weight, and nearly three-fourths of those who were overweight or obese, had at least one cardiometabolic risk factor (i.e., high blood pressure, abnormal blood lipids, smoking, or diabetes). • Rates of hypertension, abnormal blood lipid profiles, and diabetes are higher in adults with abdominal obesity. • In 2009-2012, almost 56% of adults ages 18 years and older had either prehypertension (27%) or hypertension (29%).[b] • In 2009-2012, rates of hypertension among adults were highest in African Americans (41%) and in adults ages 65 years and older (69%). • In 2009-2012, 10% of children ages 8 to 17 years had either borderline hypertension (8%) or hypertension (2%).[c] • In 2009-2012, 100 million adults ages 20 years or older (53%) had total cholesterol levels ≥200 mg/dL; almost 31 million had levels ≥240 mg/dL. • In 2011-2012, 8% of children ages 8 to 17 years had total cholesterol levels ≥200 mg/dL.
Diabetes	• In 2012, the prevalence of diabetes (type 1 plus type 2) was 14% for men and 11% for women ages 20 years and older (more than 90% of total diabetes in adults is type 2). • Among children with type 2 diabetes, about 80% were obese.
Cancer[d]: Breast Cancer Colorectal Cancer	• Breast cancer is the third leading cause of cancer death in the United States. • In 2012, an estimated 3 million women had a history of breast cancer. • Colorectal cancer is the second leading cause of cancer death in the United States. • In 2012, an estimated 1.2 million adult men and women had a history of colorectal cancer.
Bone Health	• A higher percent of women are affected by osteoporosis (15%) and low bone mass (51%) than men (about 4% and 35%, respectively). • In 2005-2010, approximately 10 million (10%) adults ages 50 years and older had osteoporosis and 43 million (44%) had low bone mass.

[a] Abdominal obesity, as measured by waist circumference, is defined as a waist circumference of >102 centimeters in men and >88 centimeters in women.

[b] For adults, prehypertension was defined as a systolic blood pressure of 120-139 mm mercury (Hg) or diastolic blood pressure of 80-89 mm Hg among those who were not currently being treated for hypertension. Hypertension was defined as systolic blood pressure (SBP) >140 mm Hg, diastolic blood pressure (DBP) >90 mm Hg, or taking antihypertensive medication.

[c] For children, borderline hypertension was defined as systolic or diastolic blood pressure at the 90th percentile or higher but lower than the 95th percentile or as blood pressure levels of 120/80 mm Hg or higher (but less than the 95th percentile). Hypertension was defined as a systolic or diastolic blood pressure at the 95th percentile or higher.

[d] The types of cancer included here are not a complete list of all diet- and physical activity-related cancers.

Figure I-1.
Adherence of the U.S. Population Ages 2 Years and Older to the *2010 Dietary Guidelines*, as Measured by Average Total Healthy Eating Index-2010 (HEI-2010) Scores

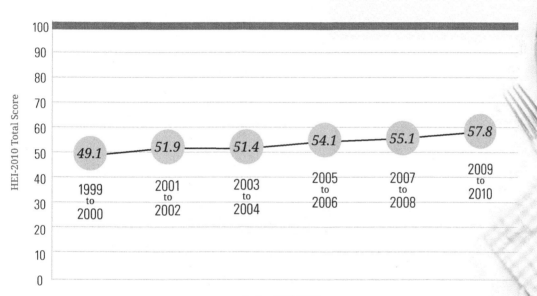

Maximum Total Score

Cycle of NHANES

DATA SOURCES: Analyses of What We Eat in America, National Health and Nutrition Examination Survey (NHANES) data from 1999-2000 through 2009-2010.

NOTE: HEI-2010 total scores are out of 100 possible points. A score of 100 indicates that recommendations on average were met or exceeded. A higher total score indicates a higher quality diet.

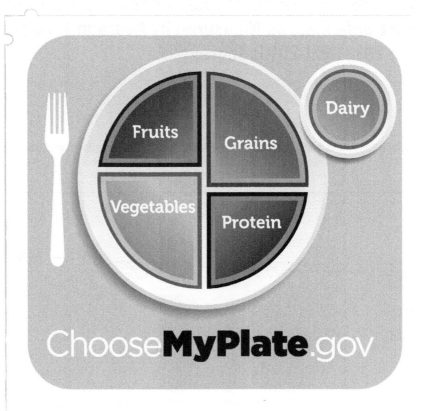

Implementation of the *Dietary Guidelines* Through MyPlate

MyPlate is a Federal symbol that serves as a reminder to build healthy eating patterns by making healthy choices across the food groups. For more information about *Dietary Guidelines* implementation for the public through MyPlate, see Chapter 3 and **Figure 3-2.**

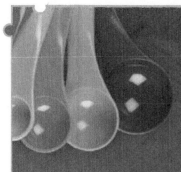

Figure 1-1.
Cup- & Ounce-Equivalents

Within a food group, foods can come in many forms and are not created equal in terms of what counts as a cup or an ounce. Some foods are more concentrated, and some are more airy or contain more water. Cup- and ounce-equivalents identify the amounts of foods from each food group with similar nutritional content. In addition, portion sizes do not always align with one cup-equivalent or one ounce-equivalent. See examples below for variability.

Vegetables	Fruits	Grains	Dairy	Protein

1 large egg is equal to 1 ounce-equivalent protein foods

1/2 cup portion of green beans is equal to 1/2 cup-equivalent vegetables

1/2 cup portion of strawberries is equal to 1/2 cup-equivalent fruit

1 slice of bread is equal to 1 ounce-equivalent grains

6 ounce portion of fat-free yogurt is equal to 3/4 cup-equivalent dairy

2 tablespoons of peanut butter is equal to 2 ounce-equivalents protein foods

1 cup portion of raw spinach is equal to 1/2 cup-equivalent vegetables

3/4 cup portion of 100% orange juice is equal to 3/4 cup-equivalent fruit

1/2 cup portion of cooked brown rice is equal to 1 ounce-equivalent grains

1 1/2 ounces portion of cheddar cheese is equal to 1 cup-equivalent dairy

1 ounce portion of walnuts is equal to 2 ounce-equivalents protein foods

1/2 cup portion of black beans is equal to 2 ounce-equivalents protein foods

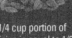

1/4 cup portion of raisins is equal to 1/2 cup-equivalent fruit

4 ounce portion of pork is equal to 4 ounce-equivalents protein foods

Figure 1-3.

Hidden Components in Eating Patterns

Many of the foods and beverages we eat contain sodium, saturated fats, and added sugars. Making careful choices, as in this example, keeps amounts of these components within their limits while meeting nutrient needs to achieve a healthy eating pattern.

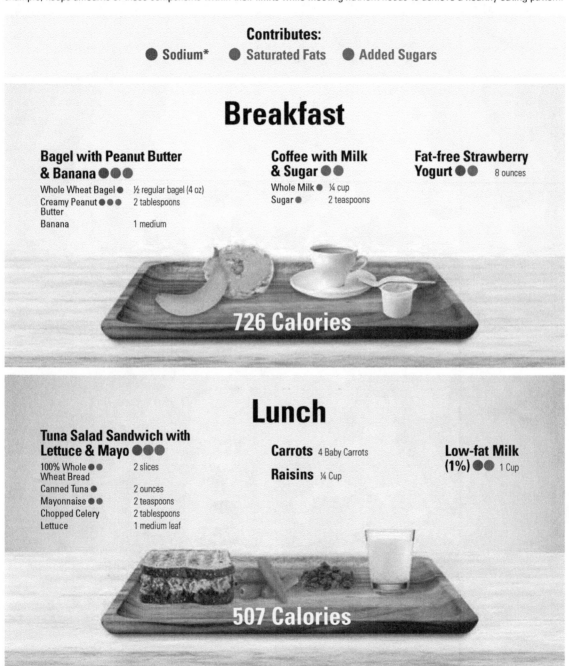

Contributes:

● Sodium*   ● Saturated Fats   ● Added Sugars

Breakfast

Bagel with Peanut Butter & Banana ●●●

Whole Wheat Bagel ●	½ regular bagel (4 oz)
Creamy Peanut ●●● Butter	2 tablespoons
Banana	1 medium

Coffee with Milk & Sugar ●●

Whole Milk ●	¼ cup
Sugar ●	2 teaspoons

Fat-free Strawberry Yogurt ●●   8 ounces

726 Calories

Lunch

Tuna Salad Sandwich with Lettuce & Mayo ●●●

100% Whole ●● Wheat Bread	2 slices
Canned Tuna ●	2 ounces
Mayonnaise ●●	2 teaspoons
Chopped Celery	2 tablespoons
Lettuce	1 medium leaf

Carrots 4 Baby Carrots

Raisins ¼ Cup

Low-fat Milk (1%) ●● 1 Cup

507 Calories

Foods very low in sodium not marked

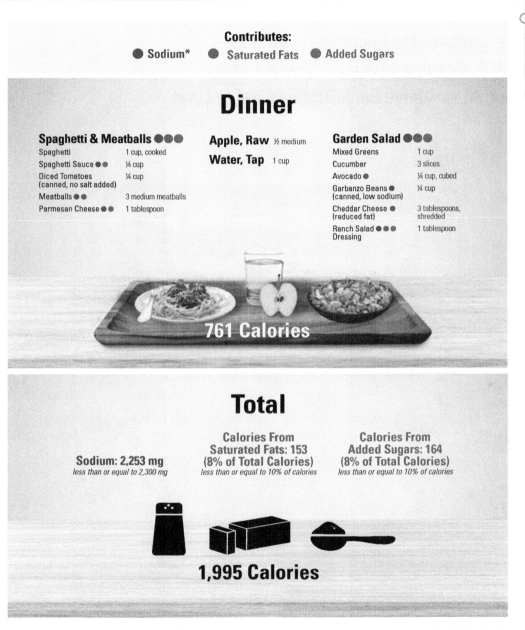

Contributes:

● Sodium*   ● Saturated Fats   ● Added Sugars

Dinner

Spaghetti & Meatballs ●●●

Spaghetti	1 cup, cooked
Spaghetti Sauce ●●	¼ cup
Diced Tomatoes (canned, no salt added)	¼ cup
Meatballs ●●	3 medium meatballs
Parmesan Cheese ●●	1 tablespoon

Apple, Raw ½ medium

Water, Tap 1 cup

Garden Salad ●●●

Mixed Greens	1 cup
Cucumber	3 slices
Avocado ●	¼ cup, cubed
Garbanzo Beans ● (canned, low sodium)	¼ cup
Cheddar Cheese ● (reduced fat)	3 tablespoons, shredded
Ranch Salad Dressing ●●●	1 tablespoon

761 Calories

Total

Sodium: 2,253 mg	Calories From Saturated Fats: 153 (8% of Total Calories)	Calories From Added Sugars: 164 (8% of Total Calories)
less than or equal to 2,300 mg	*less than or equal to 10% of calories*	*less than or equal to 10% of calories*

1,995 Calories

* Foods very low in sodium not marked

Figure 2-1.
Dietary Intakes Compared to Recommendations.
Percent of the U.S. Population Ages 1 Year & Older
Who Are Below, At, or Above Each Dietary Goal or Limit

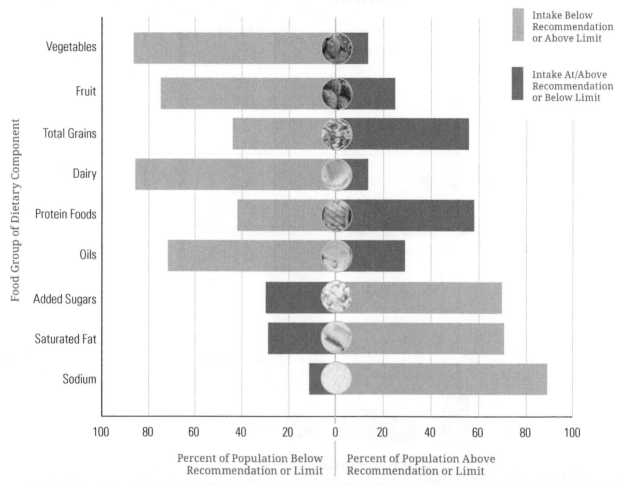

NOTE: The center (0) line is the goal or limit. For most, those represented by the orange sections of the bars, shifting toward the center line will improve their eating pattern.

DATA SOURCES: What We Eat in America, NHANES 2007-2010 for average intakes by age-sex group. Healthy U.S.-Style Food Patterns, which vary based on age, sex, and activity level, for recommended intakes and limits.

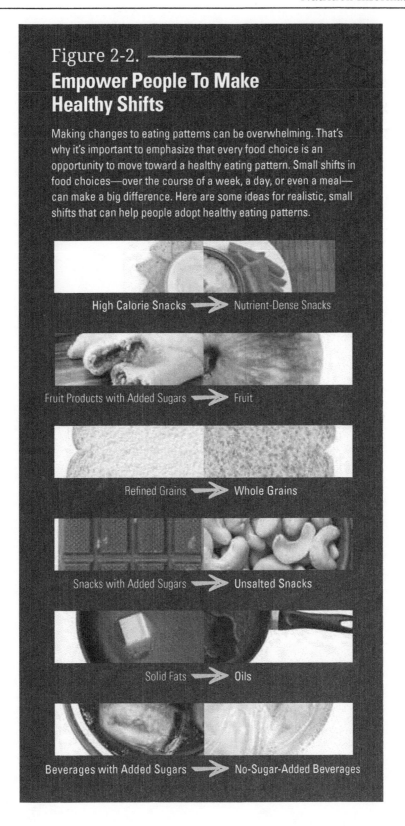

Figure 2-2.

Empower People To Make Healthy Shifts

Making changes to eating patterns can be overwhelming. That's why it's important to emphasize that every food choice is an opportunity to move toward a healthy eating pattern. Small shifts in food choices—over the course of a week, a day, or even a meal—can make a big difference. Here are some ideas for realistic, small shifts that can help people adopt healthy eating patterns.

High Calorie Snacks ➡ Nutrient-Dense Snacks

Fruit Products with Added Sugars ➡ Fruit

Refined Grains ➡ Whole Grains

Snacks with Added Sugars ➡ Unsalted Snacks

Solid Fats ➡ Oils

Beverages with Added Sugars ➡ No-Sugar-Added Beverages

Figure 2-3.

Average Daily Food Group Intakes by Age-Sex Groups, Compared to Ranges of Recommended Intake

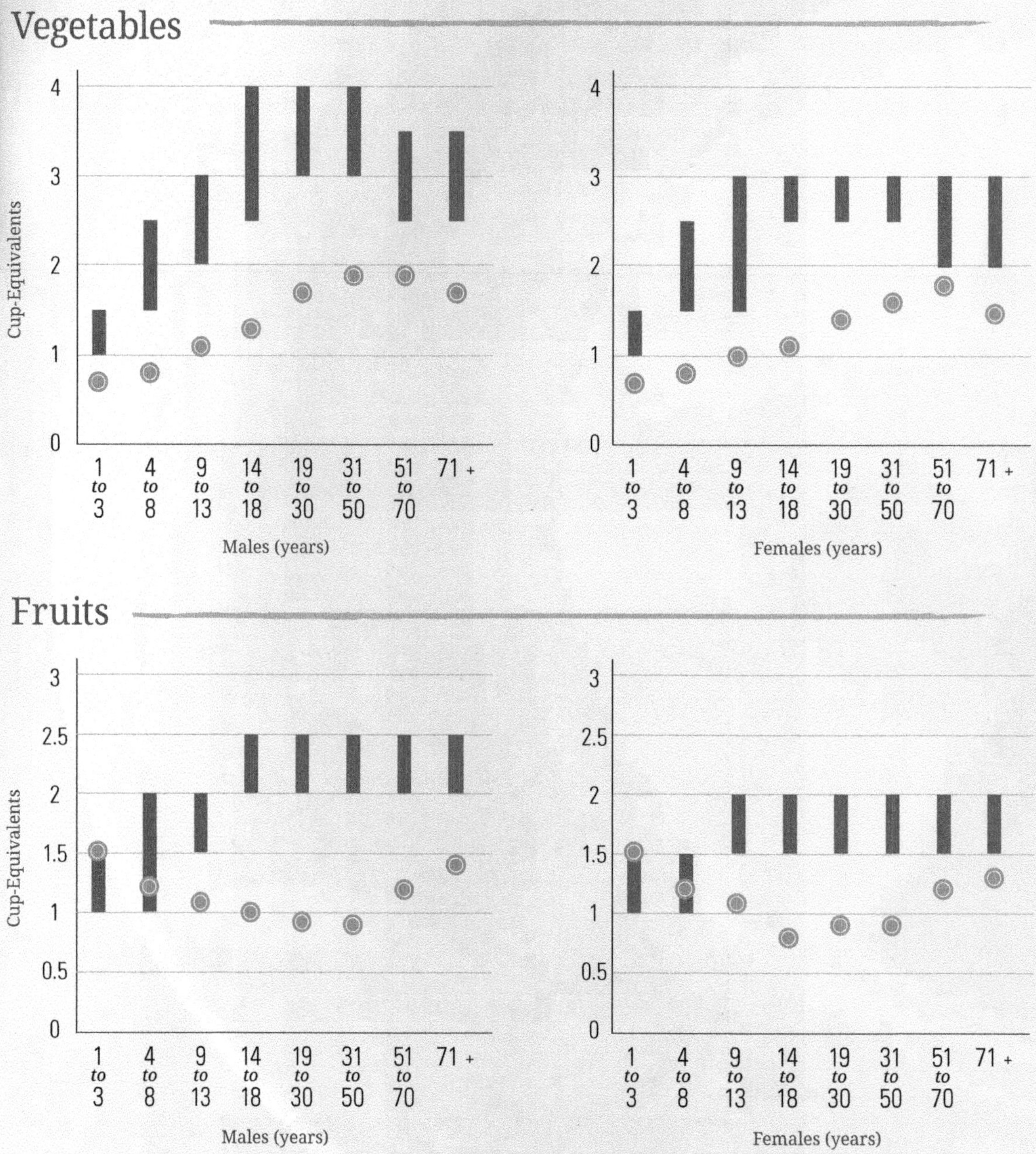

■ Recommended Intake Ranges
◉ Average Intake

Vegetables

Males (years)

Females (years)

Fruits

Males (years)

Females (years)

■ Recommended Intake Ranges   ◉ Average Intake

Total Grains

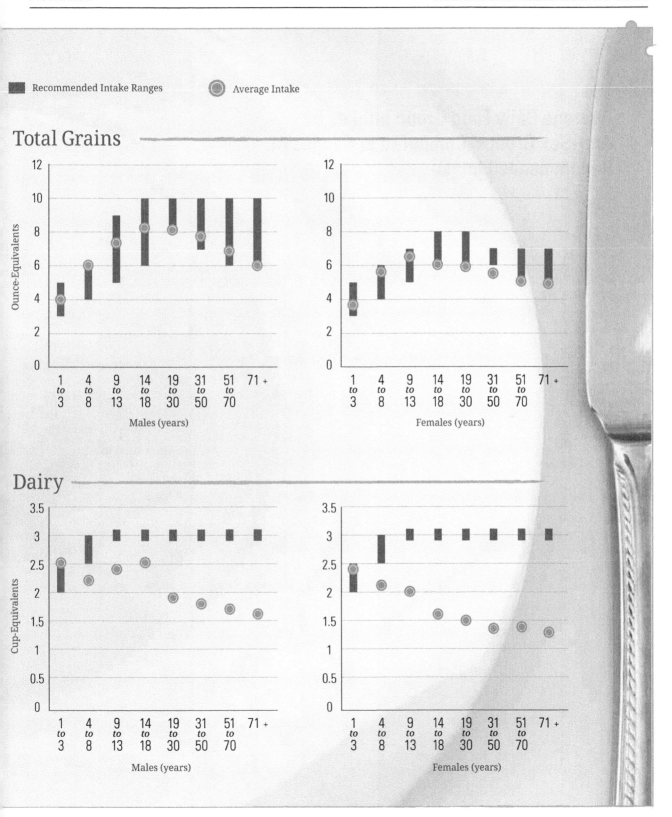

Dairy

Figure 2-3. *(continued...)*

Average Daily Food Group Intakes by Age-Sex Groups, Compared to Ranges of Recommended Intake

■ Recommended Intake Ranges

⬤ Average Intake

Protein Foods

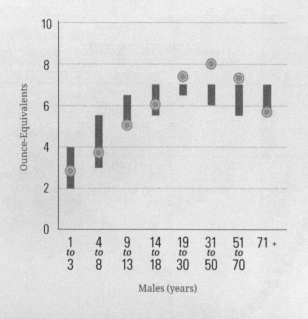

Males (years)

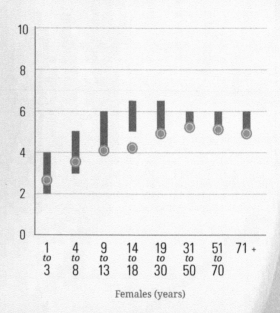

Females (years)

DATA SOURCES: What We Eat in America, NHANES 2007-2010 for average intakes by age-sex group. Healthy U.S.-Style Food Patterns, which vary based on age, sex, and activity level, for recommended intake ranges.

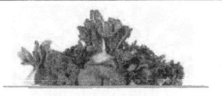

Figure 2-4.

Average Vegetable Subgroup Intakes in Cup-Equivalents per Week by Age-Sex Groups, Compared to Ranges of Recommended Intakes per Week

Dark Green Vegetables

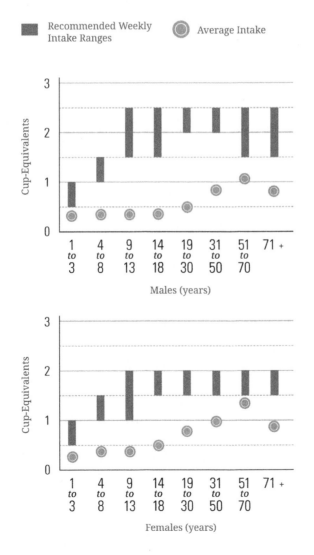

Figure 2-4. *(continued...)*

Average Vegetable Subgroup Intakes in Cup-Equivalents per Week by Age-Sex Groups, Compared to Ranges of Recommended Intakes per Week

■ Recommended Intake Ranges

◉ Average Intake

Red & Orange Vegetables

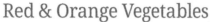

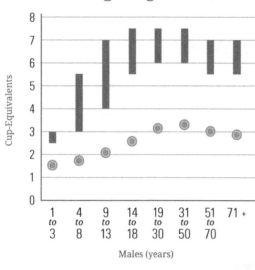

Males (years)

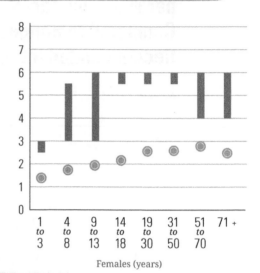

Females (years)

Legumes (Beans & Peas)

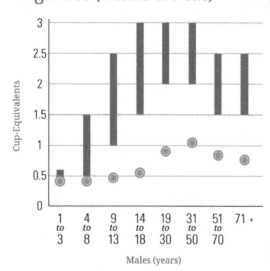

Males (years)

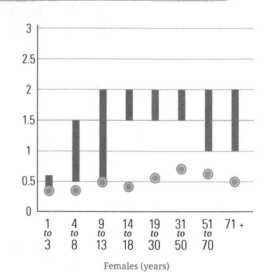

Females (years)

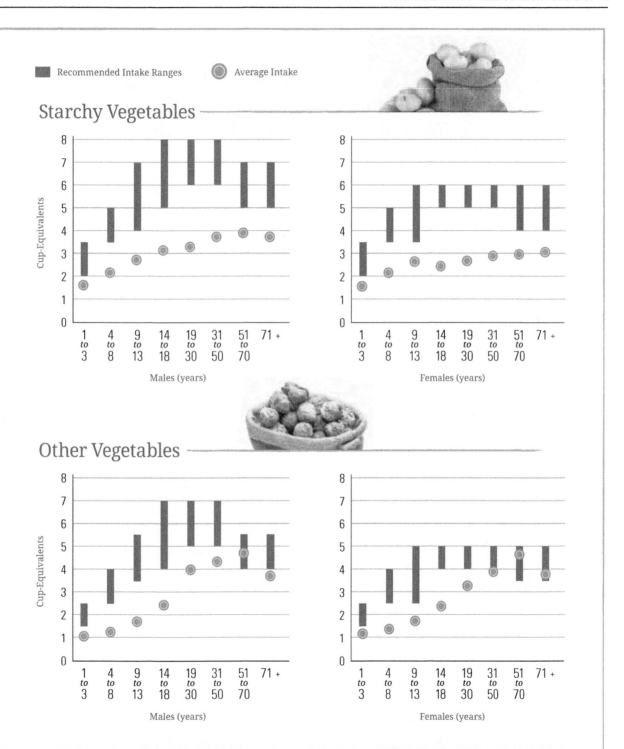

Recommended Intake Ranges   **Average Intake**

Starchy Vegetables

Males (years)

Females (years)

Other Vegetables

Males (years)

Females (years)

DATA SOURCES: What We Eat in America, NHANES 2007-2010 for average intakes by age-sex group. Healthy U.S.-Style Food Patterns, which vary based on age, sex, and activity level, for recommended intake ranges.

Figure 2-5.

Average Whole & Refined Grain Intakes in Ounce-Equivalents per Day by Age-Sex Groups, Compared to Ranges of Recommended Daily Intake for Whole Grains & Limits for Refined Grains*

■ Range of Recommended Intake for Whole Grains/Limits for Refined Grains Intake

● Average Refined Grains Intake

◆ Average Whole Grains Intake

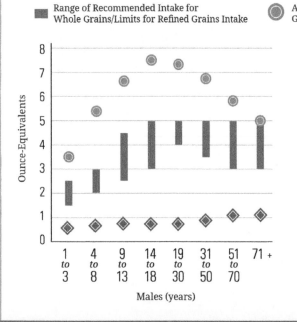

Males (years)

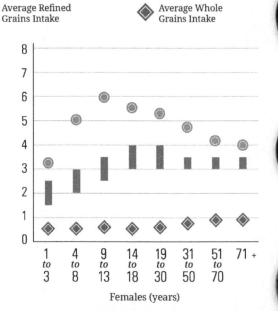

Females (years)

*NOTE: Recommended daily intake of whole grains is to be at least half of total grain consumption, and the limit for refined grains is to be no more than half of total grain consumption. The blue vertical bars on this graph represent one half of the total grain recommendations for each age-sex group, and therefore indicate recommendations for the minimum amounts to consume of whole grains or maximum amounts of refined grains. To meet recommendations, whole grain intake should be within or above the blue bars and refined grain intake within or below the bars.

DATA SOURCES: What We Eat in America, NHANES 2007-2010 for average intakes by age-sex group. Healthy U.S.-Style Food Patterns, which vary based on age, sex, and activity level, for recommended intake ranges.

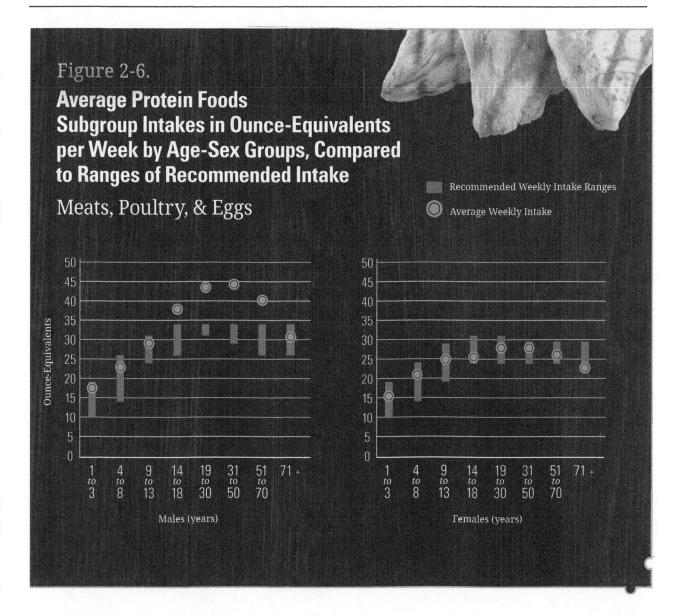

Figure 2-6.

Average Protein Foods Subgroup Intakes in Ounce-Equivalents per Week by Age-Sex Groups, Compared to Ranges of Recommended Intake

Meats, Poultry, & Eggs

Recommended Weekly Intake Ranges

Average Weekly Intake

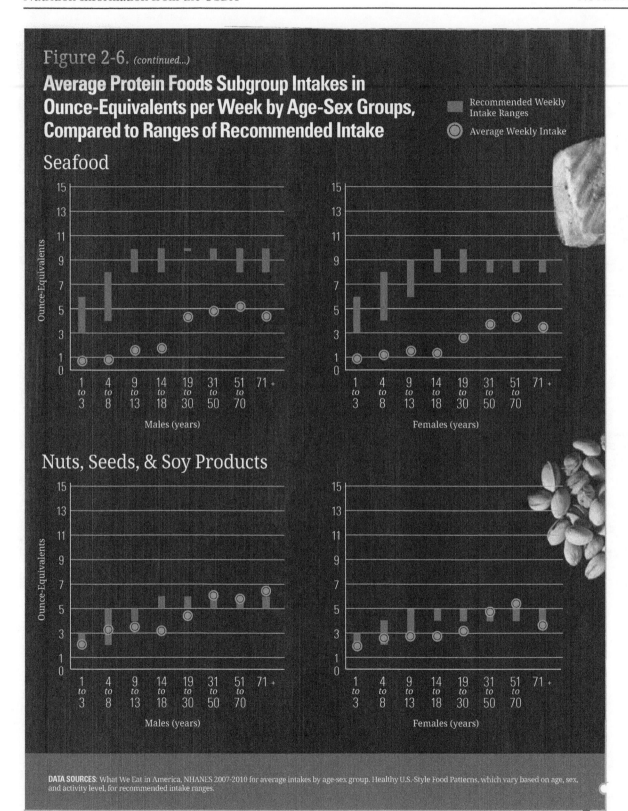

Figure 2-6. *(continued...)*

Average Protein Foods Subgroup Intakes in Ounce-Equivalents per Week by Age-Sex Groups, Compared to Ranges of Recommended Intake

■ Recommended Weekly Intake Ranges

◎ Average Weekly Intake

Seafood

Males (years)

Females (years)

Nuts, Seeds, & Soy Products

Males (years)

Females (years)

DATA SOURCES: What We Eat in America, NHANES 2007-2010 for average intakes by age-sex group. Healthy U.S.-Style Food Patterns, which vary based on age, sex, and activity level, for recommended intake ranges.

Figure 2-7.

Average Intakes of Oils & Solid Fats in Grams per Day by Age-Sex Group, in Comparison to Ranges of Recommended Intake for Oils

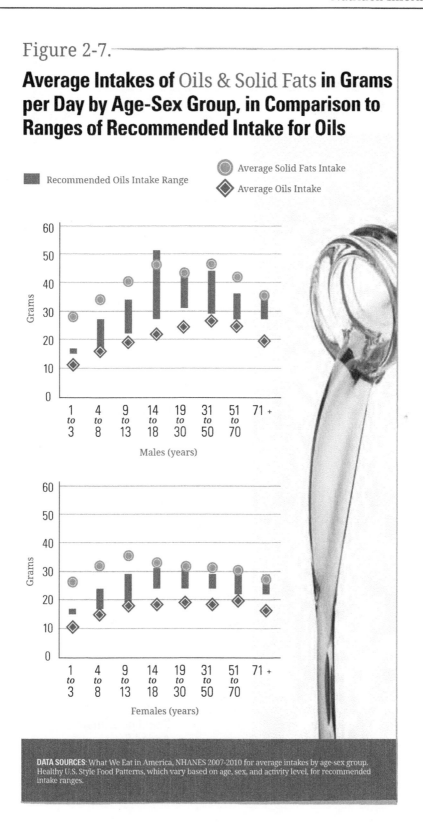

DATA SOURCES: What We Eat in America, NHANES 2007-2010 for average intakes by age-sex group. Healthy U.S. Style Food Patterns, which vary based on age, sex, and activity level, for recommended intake ranges.

281

Figure 2-8.
Typical Versus Nutrient-Dense Foods & Beverages

Achieving a healthy eating pattern means shifting typical food choices to more nutrient-dense options—that is, foods with important nutrients that aren't packed with extra calories or sodium. Nutrient-dense foods and beverages are naturally lean or low in solid fats and have little or no **added** solid fats, sugars, refined starches, or sodium.

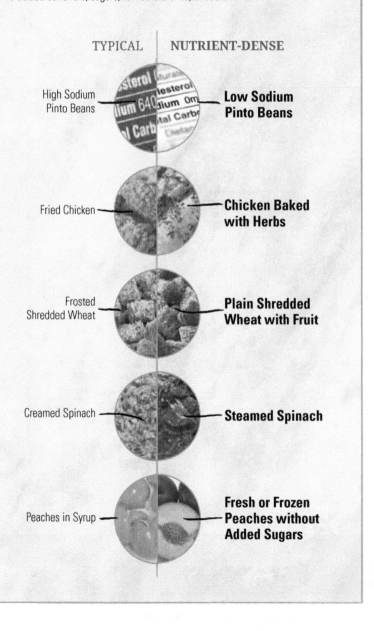

TYPICAL | NUTRIENT-DENSE

High Sodium Pinto Beans — **Low Sodium Pinto Beans**

Fried Chicken — **Chicken Baked with Herbs**

Frosted Shredded Wheat — **Plain Shredded Wheat with Fruit**

Creamed Spinach — **Steamed Spinach**

Peaches in Syrup — **Fresh or Frozen Peaches without Added Sugars**

Figure 2-9.

Average Intakes of Added Sugars as a Percent of Calories per Day by Age-Sex Group, in Comparison to the *Dietary Guidelines* Maximum Limit of Less than 10 Percent of Calories

■ Recommended Maximum Limit   ● Average Intake

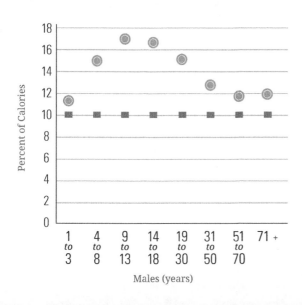

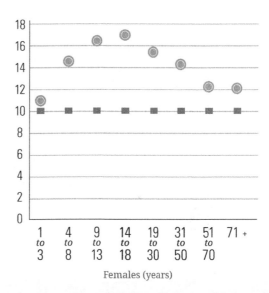

NOTE: The maximum amount of added sugars allowable in a Healthy U.S.-Style Eating Pattern at the 1,200-to-1,800 calorie levels is less than the *Dietary Guidelines* limit of 10 percent of calories. Patterns at these calorie levels are appropriate for many children and older women who are not physically active.

DATA SOURCE: What We Eat in America, NHANES 2007-2010 for average intakes by age-sex group.

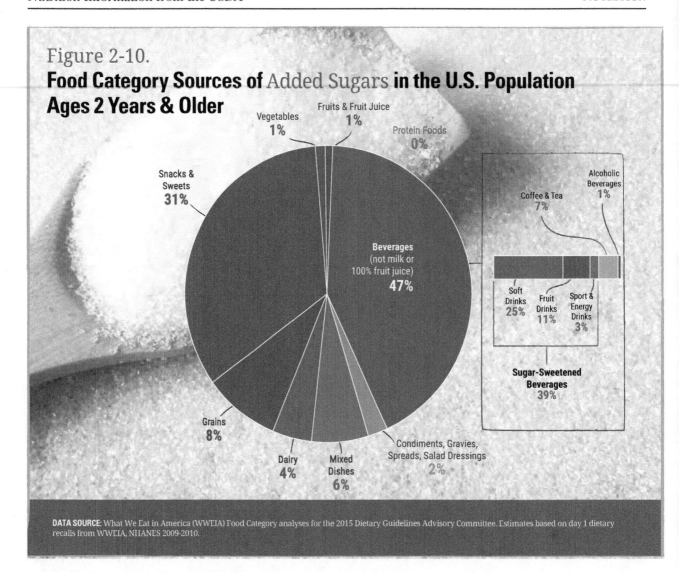

Figure 2-10.

Food Category Sources of Added Sugars in the U.S. Population Ages 2 Years & Older

Vegetables 1%

Fruits & Fruit Juice 1%

Protein Foods 0%

Snacks & Sweets 31%

Beverages (not milk or 100% fruit juice) 47%

Grains 8%

Dairy 4%

Mixed Dishes 6%

Condiments, Gravies, Spreads, Salad Dressings 2%

Coffee & Tea 7%

Alcoholic Beverages 1%

Soft Drinks 25%

Fruit Drinks 11%

Sport & Energy Drinks 3%

Sugar-Sweetened Beverages 39%

DATA SOURCE: What We Eat in America (WWEIA) Food Category analyses for the 2015 Dietary Guidelines Advisory Committee. Estimates based on day 1 dietary recalls from WWEIA, NHANES 2009-2010.

Figure 2-11.

Average Intakes of Saturated Fats as a Percent of Calories per Day by Age-Sex Groups, in Comparison to the *Dietary Guidelines* Maximum Limit of Less Than 10 Percent of Calories

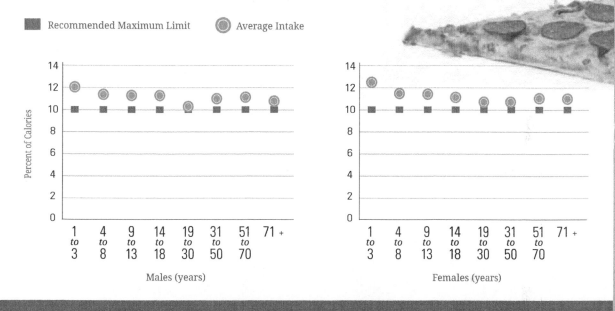

■ Recommended Maximum Limit   ◉ Average Intake

Males (years)

Females (years)

DATA SOURCE: What We Eat in America, NHANES 2007-2010 for average intakes by age-sex group.

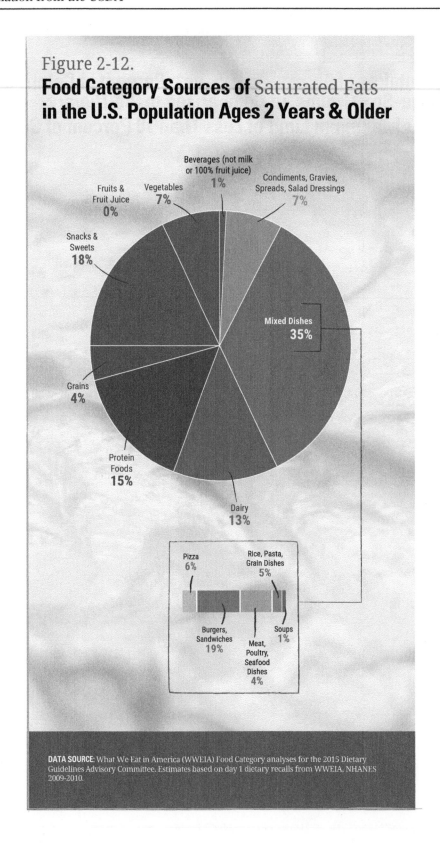

Figure 2-12.
Food Category Sources of Saturated Fats in the U.S. Population Ages 2 Years & Older

Beverages (not milk or 100% fruit juice)
1%

Condiments, Gravies, Spreads, Salad Dressings
7%

Fruits & Fruit Juice
0%

Vegetables
7%

Snacks & Sweets
18%

Mixed Dishes
35%

Grains
4%

Protein Foods
15%

Dairy
13%

Pizza
6%

Rice, Pasta, Grain Dishes
5%

Burgers, Sandwiches
19%

Meat, Poultry, Seafood Dishes
4%

Soups
1%

DATA SOURCE: What We Eat in America (WWEIA) Food Category analyses for the 2015 Dietary Guidelines Advisory Committee. Estimates based on day 1 dietary recalls from WWEIA, NHANES 2009-2010.

Figure 2-13.

Average Intake of Sodium in Milligrams per Day by Age-Sex Groups, Compared to Tolerable Upper Intake Levels (UL)

■ Recommended Maximum Limit (UL)   ◉ Average Intake

Males (years)

Females (years)

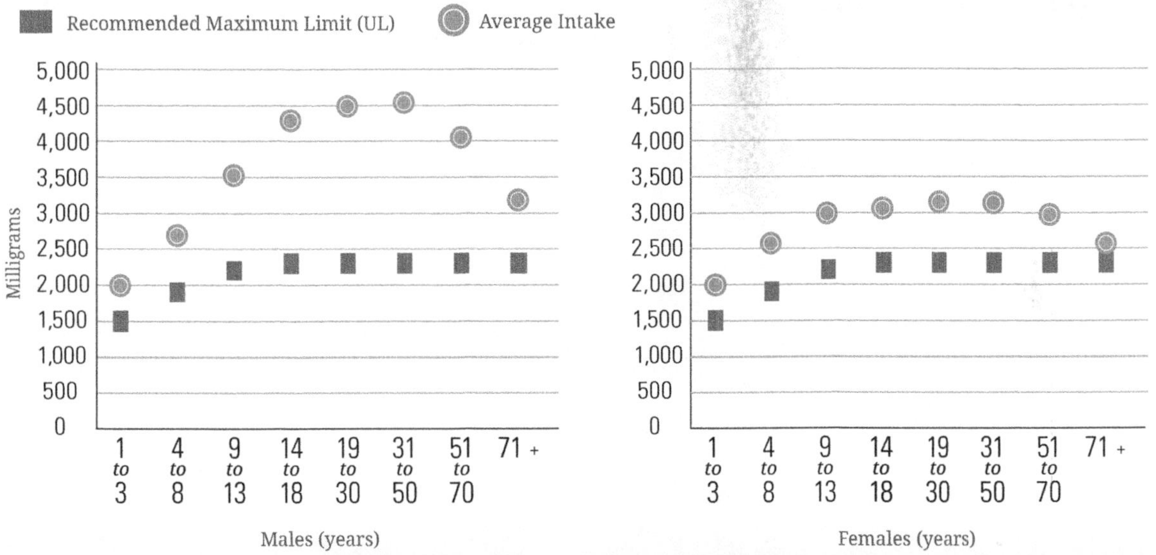

DATA SOURCES: What We Eat in America, NHANES 2007-2010 for average intakes by age-sex group. Institute of Medicine Dietary Reference Intakes for Tolerable Upper Intake Levels (UL).

Figure 2-14.
Food Category Sources of Sodium in the U.S. Population Ages 2 Years & Older

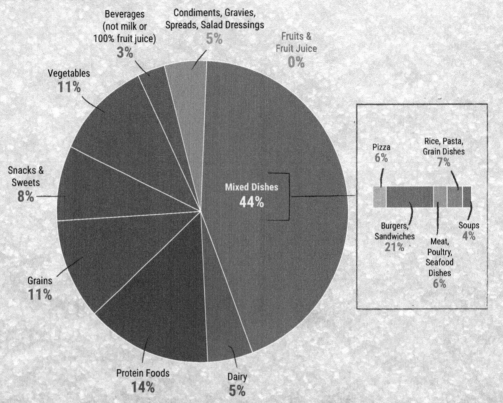

Beverages (not milk or 100% fruit juice) 3%

Condiments, Gravies, Spreads, Salad Dressings 5%

Fruits & Fruit Juice 0%

Vegetables 11%

Snacks & Sweets 8%

Mixed Dishes 44%

Pizza 6%

Rice, Pasta, Grain Dishes 7%

Burgers, Sandwiches 21%

Meat, Poultry, Seafood Dishes 6%

Soups 4%

Grains 11%

Protein Foods 14%

Dairy 5%

DATA SOURCE: What We Eat in America (WWEIA) Food Category analyses for the 2015 Dietary Guidelines Advisory Committee. Estimates based on day 1 dietary recalls from WWEIA, NHANES 2009-2010.

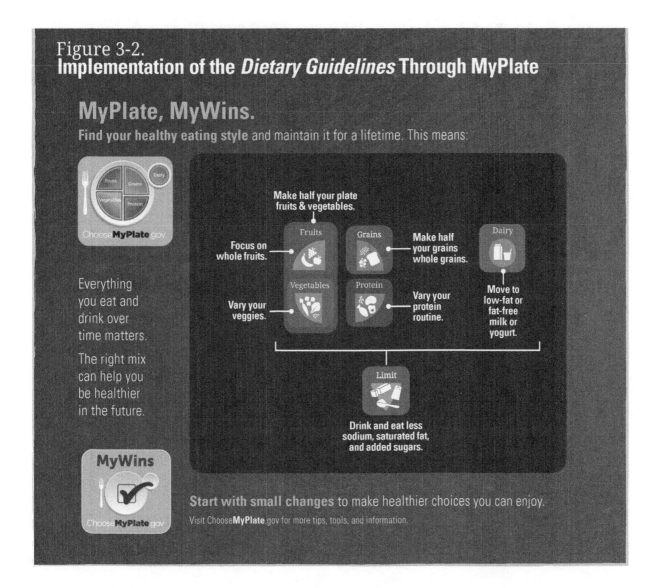

Figure 3-2.
Implementation of the *Dietary Guidelines* Through MyPlate

Figure 3-3.

Strategies To Align Settings With the *2015-2020 Dietary Guidelines*

Americans make food and beverage choices in a variety of settings at home, at work, and at play. Aligning these settings with the *2015-2020 Dietary Guidelines* will not only influence individual choices—it can also have broader population level impact when multiple sectors commit to make changes together.

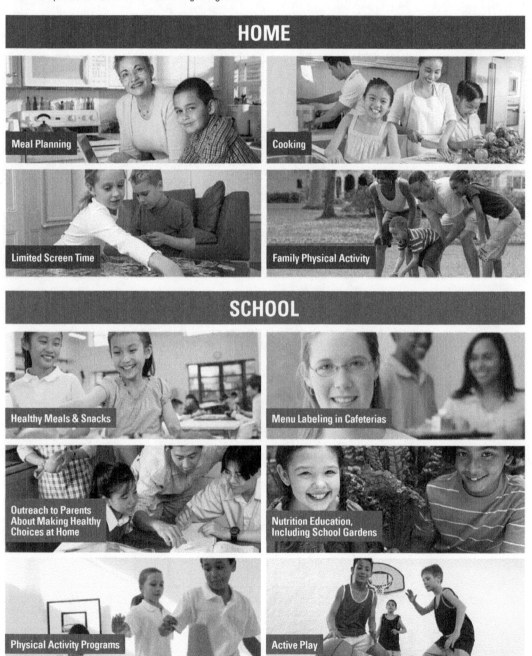

Figure 3-3. *(continued...)*

Strategies To Align Settings With the *2015-2020 Dietary Guidelines*

Americans make food and beverage choices in a variety of settings at home, at work, and at play. Aligning these settings with the *2015-2020 Dietary Guidelines* will not only influence individual choices—it can also have broader population level impact when multiple sectors commit to make changes together.

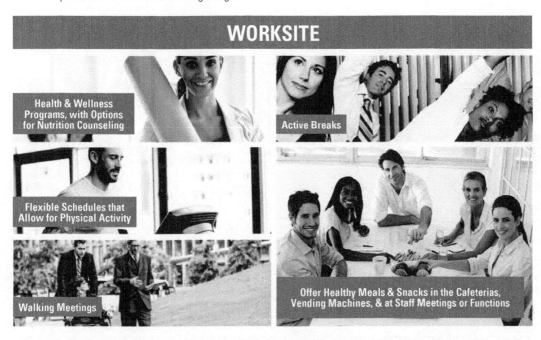

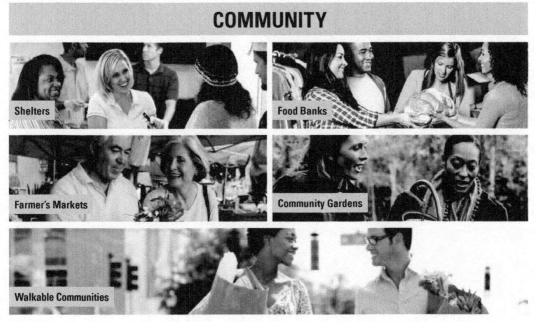

FOOD RETAIL

Outreach to Consumers About Making Healthy Changes

Access to Healthy Food Options

PRODUCE

Access to Healthy Food Choices

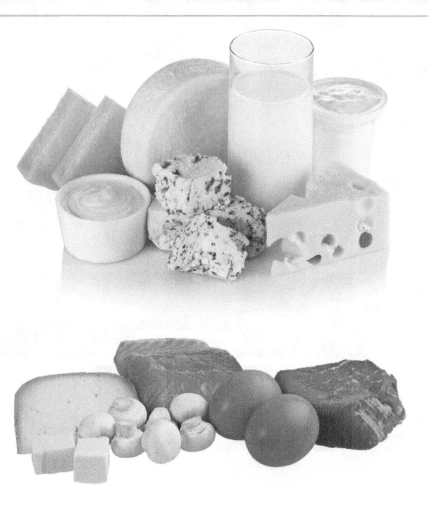

Table A2-1.

Estimated Calorie Needs per Day, by Age, Sex, & Physical Activity Level

Males

Age	Sedentary[a]	Moderately Active[b]	Active[c]
2	1,000	1,000	1,000
3	1,000	1,400	1,400
4	1,200	1,400	1,600
5	1,200	1,400	1,600
6	1,400	1,600	1,800
7	1,400	1,600	1,800
8	1,400	1,600	2,000

Females[d]

Age	Sedentary[a]	Moderately Active[b]	Active[c]
2	1,000	1,000	1,000
3	1,000	1,200	1,400
4	1,200	1,400	1,400
5	1,200	1,400	1,600
6	1,200	1,400	1,600
7	1,200	1,600	1,800
8	1,400	1,600	1,800

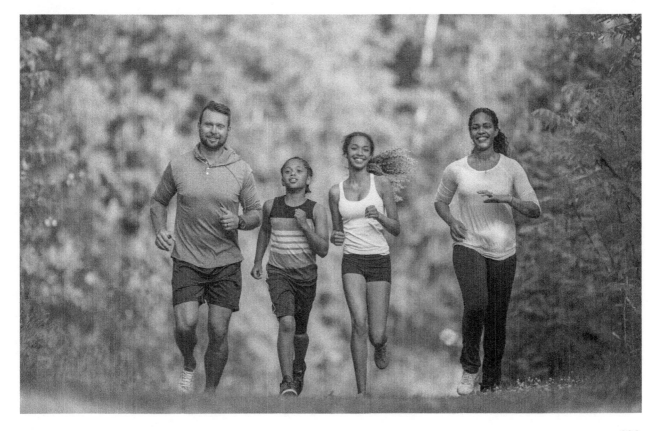

Males

Age	Sedentary[a]	Moderately Active[b]	Active[c]
9	1,600	1,800	2,000
10	1,600	1,800	2,200
11	1,800	2,000	2,200
12	1,800	2,200	2,400
13	2,000	2,200	2,600
14	2,000	2,400	2,800
15	2,200	2,600	3,000
16	2,400	2,800	3,200
17	2,400	2,800	3,200
18	2,400	2,800	3,200
19-20	2,600	2,800	3,000
21-25	2,400	2,800	3,000
26-30	2,400	2,600	3,000
31-35	2,400	2,600	3,000
36-40	2,400	2,600	2,800
41-45	2,200	2,600	2,800
46-50	2,200	2,400	2,800
51-55	2,200	2,400	2,800
56-60	2,200	2,400	2,600
61-65	2,000	2,400	2,600
66-70	2,000	2,200	2,600
71-75	2,000	2,200	2,600
76 & Up	2,000	2,200	2,400

Females[d]

Age	Sedentary[a]	Moderately Active[b]	Active[c]
9	1,400	1,600	1,800
10	1,400	1,800	2,000
11	1,600	1,800	2,000
12	1,600	2,000	2,200
13	1,600	2,000	2,200
14	1,800	2,000	2,400
15	1,800	2,000	2,400
16	1,800	2,000	2,400
17	1,800	2,000	2,400
18	1,800	2,000	2,400
19-20	2,000	2,200	2,400
21-25	2,000	2,200	2,400
26-30	1,800	2,000	2,400
31-35	1,800	2,000	2,200
36-40	1,800	2,000	2,200
41-45	1,800	2,000	2,200
46-50	1,800	2,000	2,200
51-55	1,600	1,800	2,200
56-60	1,600	1,800	2,200
61-65	1,600	1,800	2,000
66-70	1,600	1,800	2,000
71-75	1,600	1,800	2,000
76 & Up	1,600	1,800	2,000

[a] Sedentary means a lifestyle that includes only the physical activity of independent living.

[b] Moderately Active means a lifestyle that includes physical activity equivalent to walking about 1.5 to 3 miles per day at 3 to 4 miles per hour, in addition to the activities of independent living.

[c] Active means a lifestyle that includes physical activity equivalent to walking more than 3 miles per day at 3 to 4 miles per hour, in addition to the activities of independent living.

[d] Estimates for females do not include women who are pregnant or breastfeeding.

SOURCE: Institute of Medicine. Dietary Reference Intakes for Energy, Carbohydrate, Fiber, Fat, Fatty Acids, Cholesterol, Protein, and Amino Acids. Washington (DC): The National Academies Press; 2002.

Table A3-1.

Healthy U.S.-Style Eating Pattern: Recommended Amounts of Food From Each Food Group at 12 Calorie Levels

Calorie Level of Pattern[a]	1,000	1,200	1,400	1,600	1,800	2,000	2,200	2,400	2,600	2,800	3,000	3,200
Food Group[b]	Daily Amount[c] of Food From Each Group (vegetable and protein foods subgroup amounts are per week)											
Vegetables	1 c-eq	1½ c-eq	1½ c-eq	2 c-eq	2½ c-eq	2½ c-eq	3 c-eq	3 c-eq	3½ c-eq	3½ c-eq	4 c-eq	4 c-eq
Dark-Green Vegetables (c-eq/wk)	½	1	1	1½	1½	1½	2	2	2½	2½	2½	2½
Red & Orange Vegetables (c-eq/wk)	2½	3	3	4	5½	5½	6	6	7	7	7½	7½
Legumes (Beans & Peas) (c-eq/wk)	½	½	½	1	1½	1½	2	2	2½	2½	3	3
Starchy Vegetables (c-eq/wk)	2	3½	3½	4	5	5	6	6	7	7	8	8
Other Vegetables (c-eq/wk)	1½	2½	2½	3½	4	4	5	5	5½	5½	7	7
Fruits	1 c-eq	1 c-eq	1½ c-eq	1½ c-eq	1½ c-eq	2 c-eq	2 c-eq	2 c-eq	2 c-eq	2½ c-eq	2½ c-eq	2½ c-eq
Grains	3 oz-eq	4 oz-eq	5 oz-eq	5 oz-eq	6 oz-eq	6 oz-eq	7 oz-eq	8 oz-eq	9 oz-eq	10 oz-eq	10 oz-eq	10 oz-eq
Whole Grains[d] (oz-eq/day)	1½	2	2½	3	3	3	3½	4	4½	5	5	5
Refined Grains (oz-eq/day)	1½	2	2½	2	3	3	3½	4	4½	5	5	5

Table A3-1. (continued...)
Healthy U.S.-Style Eating Pattern: Recommended Amounts of Food From Each Food Group at 12 Calorie Levels

Calorie Level of Pattern[a]	1,000	1,200	1,400	1,600	1,800	2,000	2,200	2,400	2,600	2,800	3,000	3,200
Food Group[b]	Daily Amount[c] of Food From Each Group (vegetable and protein foods subgroup amounts are per week)											
Dairy	2 c-eq	2½ c-eq	2½ c-eq	3 c-eq	3 c-eq	3 c-eq	3 c-eq	3 c-eq	3 c-eq	3 c-eq	3 c-eq	3 c-eq
Protein Foods	2 oz-eq	3 oz-eq	4 oz-eq	5 oz-eq	5 oz-eq	5½ oz-eq	6 oz-eq	6½ oz-eq	6½ oz-eq	7 oz-eq	7 oz-eq	7 oz-eq
Seafood (oz-eq/wk)	3	4	6	8	8	8	9	10	10	10	10	10
Meats, Poultry, Eggs (oz-eq/wk)	10	14	19	23	23	26	28	31	31	33	33	33
Nuts Seeds, Soy Products (oz-eq/wk)	2	2	3	4	4	5	5	5	5	6	6	6
Oils	15 g	17 g	17 g	22 g	24 g	27 g	29 g	31 g	34 g	36 g	44 g	51 g
Limit on Calories for Other Uses, Calories (% of Calories)[e,f]	150 (15%)	100 (8%)	110 (8%)	130 (8%)	170 (9%)	270 (14%)	280 (13%)	350 (15%)	380 (15%)	400 (14%)	470 (16%)	610 (19%)

[a] Food intake patterns at 1,000, 1,200, and 1,400 calories are designed to meet the nutritional needs of 2- to 8-year-old children. Patterns from 1,600 to 3,200 calories are designed to meet the nutritional needs of children 9 years and older and adults. If a child 4 to 8 years of age needs more calories and, therefore, is following a pattern at 1,600 calories or more, his/her recommended amount from the dairy group should be 2.5 cups per day. Children 9 years and older and adults should not use the 1,000-, 1,200-, or 1,400-calorie patterns.

[b] Foods in each group and subgroup are:

• Vegetables

  • Dark-green vegetables: All fresh, frozen, and canned dark-green leafy vegetables and broccoli, cooked or raw: for example, broccoli; spinach; romaine; kale; collard, turnip, and mustard greens.

  • Red and orange vegetables: All fresh, frozen, and canned red and orange vegetables or juice, cooked or raw: for example, tomatoes, tomato juice, red peppers, carrots, sweet potatoes, winter squash, and pumpkin.

  • Legumes (beans and peas): All cooked from dry or canned beans and peas: for example, kidney beans, white beans, black beans, lentils, chickpeas, pinto beans, split peas, and edamame (green soybeans). Does not include green beans or green peas.

- • Starchy vegetables: All fresh, frozen, and canned starchy vegetables: for example, white potatoes, corn, green peas, green lima beans, plantains, and cassava.
- • Other vegetables: All other fresh, frozen, and canned vegetables, cooked or raw: for example, iceberg lettuce, green beans, onions, cucumbers, cabbage, celery, zucchini, mushrooms, and green peppers.
- • Fruits
  - • All fresh, frozen, canned, and dried fruits and fruit juices: for example, oranges and orange juice, apples and apple juice, bananas, grapes, melons, berries, and raisins.
- • Grains
  - • Whole grains: All whole-grain products and whole grains used as ingredients: for example, whole-wheat bread, whole-grain cereals and crackers, oatmeal, quinoa, popcorn, and brown rice.
  - • Refined grains: All refined-grain products and refined grains used as ingredients: for example, white breads, refined grain cereals and crackers, pasta, and white rice. Refined grain choices should be enriched.
- • Dairy
  - • All milk, including lactose-free and lactose-reduced products and fortified soy beverages (soymilk), yogurt, frozen yogurt, dairy desserts, and cheeses. Most choices should be fat-free or low-fat. Cream, sour cream, and cream cheese are not included due to their low calcium content.
- • Protein Foods
  - • All seafood, meats, poultry, eggs, soy products, nuts, and seeds. Meats and poultry should be lean or low-fat and nuts should be unsalted. Legumes (beans and peas) can be considered part of this group as well as the vegetable group, but should be counted in one group only.

[c] Food group amounts shown in cup-(c) or ounce-equivalents (oz-eq). Oils are shown in grams (g). Quantity equivalents for each food group are:

- • Vegetables and fruits, 1 cup-equivalent is: 1 cup raw or cooked vegetable or fruit, 1 cup vegetable or fruit juice, 2 cups leafy salad greens, ½ cup dried fruit or vegetable.
- • Grains, 1 ounce-equivalent is: ½ cup cooked rice, pasta, or cereal; 1 ounce dry pasta or rice; 1 medium (1 ounce) slice bread; 1 ounce of ready-to-eat cereal (about 1 cup of flaked cereal).
- • Dairy, 1 cup-equivalent is: 1 cup milk, yogurt, or fortified soymilk; 1½ ounces natural cheese such as cheddar cheese or 2 ounces of processed cheese.
- • Protein Foods, 1 ounce-equivalent is: 1 ounce lean meat, poultry, or seafood; 1 egg; ¼ cup cooked beans or tofu; 1 Tbsp peanut butter; ½ ounce nuts or seeds.

[d] Amounts of whole grains in the Patterns for children are less than the minimum of 3 oz-eq in all Patterns recommended for adults.

[e] All foods are assumed to be in nutrient-dense forms, lean or low-fat and prepared without added fats, sugars, refined starches, or salt. If all food choices to meet food group recommendations are in nutrient-dense forms, a small number of calories remain within the overall calorie limit of the Pattern (i.e., limit on calories for other uses). The number of these calories depends on the overall calorie limit in the Pattern and the amounts of food from each food group required to meet nutritional goals. Nutritional goals are higher for the 1,200- to 1,600-calorie Patterns than for the 1,000-calorie Pattern, so the limit on calories for other uses is lower in the 1,200- to 1,600-calorie Patterns. Calories up to the specified limit can be used for added sugars, added refined starches, solid fats, alcohol, or to eat more than the recommended amount of food in a food group. The overall eating Pattern also should not exceed the limits of less than 10 percent of calories from added sugars and less than 10 percent of calories from saturated fats. At most calorie levels, amounts that can be accommodated are less than these limits. For adults of legal drinking age who choose to drink alcohol, a limit of up to 1 drink per day for women and up to 2 drinks per day for men within limits on calories for other uses applies (see Appendix 9. Alcohol for additional guidance); and calories from protein, carbohydrate, and total fats should be within the Acceptable Macronutrient Distribution Ranges (AMDRs).

[f] Values are rounded.

Table A4-1.
Healthy Mediterranean-Style Eating Pattern: Recommended Amounts of Food From Each Food Group at 12 Calorie Levels

Calorie Level of Pattern[a]	1,000	1,200	1,400	1,600	1,800	2,000	2,200	2,400	2,600	2,800	3,000	3,200
Food Group[b]	Daily Amount[c] of Food From Each Group (vegetable and protein foods subgroup amounts are per week)											
Vegetables	1 c-eq	1½ c-eq	1½ c-eq	2 c-eq	2½ c-eq	2½ c-eq	3 c-eq	3 c-eq	3½ c-eq	3½ c-eq	4 c-eq	4 c-eq
Dark-Green Vegetables (c-eq/wk)	½	1	1	1½	1½	1½	2	2	2½	2½	2½	2½
Red & Orange Vegetables (c-eq/wk)	2½	3	3	4	5½	5½	6	6	7	7	7½	7½
Legumes (Beans & Peas) (c-eq/wk)	½	½	½	1	1½	1½	2	2	2½	2½	3	3
Starchy Vegetables (c-eq/wk)	2	3½	3½	4	5	5	6	6	7	7	8	8
Other Vegetables (c-eq/wk)	1½	2½	2½	3½	4	4	5	5	5½	5½	7	7
Fruits	1 c-eq	1 c-eq	1½ c-eq	2 c-eq	2 c-eq	2½ c-eq	2½ c-eq	2½ c-eq	2½ c-eq	3 c-eq	3 c-eq	3 c-eq
Grains	3 oz-eq	4 oz-eq	5 oz-eq	5 oz-eq	6 oz-eq	6 oz-eq	7 oz-eq	8 oz-eq	9 oz-eq	10 oz-eq	10 oz-eq	10 oz-eq
Whole Grains[d] (oz-eq/day)	1½	2	2½	3	3	3	3½	4	4½	5	5	5
Refined Grains (oz-eq/day)	1½	2	2½	2	3	3	3½	4	4½	5	5	5

Table A4-1. *(continued...)*
Healthy Mediterranean-Style Eating Pattern: Recommended Amounts of Food From Each Food Group at 12 Calorie Levels

Calorie Level of Pattern[a]	1,000	1,200	1,400	1,600	1,800	2,000	2,200	2,400	2,600	2,800	3,000	3,200
Food Group[b]	Daily Amount[c] of Food From Each Group (vegetable and protein foods subgroup amounts are per week)											
Dairy[e]	2 c-eq	2½ c-eq	2½ c-eq	2 c-eq	2 c-eq	2 c-eq	2 c-eq	2½ c-eq	2½ c-eq	2½ c-eq	2½ c-eq	2½ c-eq
Protein Foods	2 oz-eq	3 oz-eq	4 oz-eq	5½ oz-eq	6 oz-eq	6½ oz-eq	7 oz-eq	7½ oz-eq	7½ oz-eq	8 oz-eq	8 oz-eq	8 oz-eq
Seafood (oz-eq/wk)[f]	3	4	6	11	15	15	16	16	17	17	17	17
Meats, Poultry, Eggs (oz-eq/wk)	10	14	19	23	23	26	28	31	31	33	33	33
Nuts Seeds, Soy Products (oz-eq/wk)	2	2	3	4	4	5	5	5	5	6	6	6
Oils	15 g	17 g	17 g	22 g	24 g	27 g	29 g	31 g	34 g	36 g	44 g	51 g
Limit on Calories for Other Uses, Calories (% of Calories)[g,h]	150 (15%)	100 (8%)	110 (8%)	140 (9%)	160 (9%)	260 (13%)	270 (12%)	300 (13%)	330 (13%)	350 (13%)	430 (14%)	570 (18%)

[a, b, c, d] See Appendix 3. USDA Food Patterns: Healthy U.S.-Style Eating Pattern, notes a through d.

[e] Amounts of dairy recommended for children and adolescents are as follows, regardless of the calorie level of the Pattern: For 2 year-olds, 2 cup-eq per day; for 3 to 8 year-olds, 2 ½ cup-eq per day; for 9 to 18 year-olds, 3 cup-eq per day.

[f] The U.S. Food and Drug Administration (FDA) and the U.S. Environmental Protection Agency (EPA) provide joint guidance regarding seafood consumption for women who are pregnant or breastfeeding and young children. For more information, see the FDA or EPA websites www.FDA.gov/fishadvice; www.EPA.gov/fishadvice.

[g,h] See Appendix 3, notes e through f.

Table A5-1.

Healthy Vegetarian Eating Pattern: Recommended Amounts of Food From Each Food Group at 12 Calorie Levels

Calorie Level of Pattern[a]	1,000	1,200	1,400	1,600	1,800	2,000	2,200	2,400	2,600	2,800	3,000	3,200
Food Group[b]	Daily Amount[c] of Food From Each Group (vegetable and protein foods subgroup amounts are per week)											
Vegetables	1 c-eq	1½ c-eq	1½ c-eq	2 c-eq	2½ c-eq	2½ c-eq	3 c-eq	3 c-eq	3½ c-eq	3½ c-eq	4 c-eq	4 c-eq
Dark-Green Vegetables (c-eq/wk)	½	1	1	1½	1½	1½	2	2	2½	2½	2½	2½
Red & Orange Vegetables (c-eq/wk)	2½	3	3	4	5½	5½	6	6	7	7	7½	7½
Legumes (Beans & Peas) (c-eq/wk)[d]	½	½	½	1	1½	1½	2	2	2½	2½	3	3
Starchy Vegetables (c-eq/wk)	2	3½	3½	4	5	5	6	6	7	7	8	8
Other Vegetables (c-eq/wk)	1½	2½	2½	3½	4	4	5	5	5½	5½	7	7
Fruits	1 c-eq	1 c-eq	1½ c-eq	1½ c-eq	1½ c-eq	2 c-eq	2 c-eq	2 c-eq	2 c-eq	2½ c-eq	2½ c-eq	2½ c-eq
Grains	3 oz-eq	4 oz-eq	5 oz-eq	5½ oz-eq	6½ oz-eq	6½ oz-eq	7½ oz-eq	8½ oz-eq	9½ oz-eq	10½ oz-eq	10½ oz-eq	10½ oz-eq
Whole Grains[e] (oz-eq/day)	1½	2	2½	3	3½	3½	4	4½	5	5½	5½	5½
Refined Grains (oz-eq/day)	1½	2	2½	2½	3	3	3 ½	4	4 ½	5	5	5
Dairy	2 c-eq	2.5 c-eq	2.5 c-eq	3 c-eq	3 c-eq	3 c-eq	3 c-eq	3 c-eq	3 c-eq	3 c-eq	3 c-eq	3 c-eq

Calorie Level of Pattern[a]	1,000	1,200	1,400	1,600	1,800	2,000	2,200	2,400	2,600	2,800	3,000	3,200
Food Group[b]	**Daily Amount**[e] of Food From Each Group (vegetable and protein foods subgroup amounts are per week)											
Protein Foods	1 oz-eq	1½ oz-eq	2 oz-eq	2½ oz-eq	3 oz-eq	3½ oz-eq	3½ oz-eq	4 oz-eq	4½ oz-eq	5 oz-eq	5½ oz-eq	6 oz-eq
Eggs (oz-eq/wk)	2	3	3	3	3	3	3	3	3	4	4	4
Legumes (Beans & Peas) (oz-eq/wk)[d]	1	2	4	4	6	6	6	8	9	10	11	12
Soy Products (oz-eq/wk)	2	3	4	6	6	8	8	9	10	11	12	13
Nuts & Seeds (oz-eq/wk)	2	2	3	5	6	7	7	8	9	10	12	13
Oils	15 g	17 g	17 g	22 g	24 g	27 g	29 g	31 g	34 g	36 g	44 g	51 g
Limit on Calories for Other Uses, Calories (% of Calories)[f,g]	190 (19%)	170 (14%)	190 (14%)	180 (11%)	190 (11%)	290 (15%)	330 (15%)	390 (16%)	390 (15%)	400 (14%)	440 (15%)	550 (17%)

[a, b, c] See Appendix 3, USDA Food Patterns: Healthy U.S.-Style Eating Pattern, notes a through c.

[d] About half of total legumes are shown as vegetables, in cup-eq, and half as protein foods, in oz-eq. Total legumes in the Patterns, in cup-eq, is the amount in the vegetable group plus the amount in protein foods group (in oz-eq) divided by 4.

Calorie Level of Pattern[a]	1,000	1,200	1,400	1,600	1,800	2,000	2,200	2,400	2,600	2,800	3,000	3,200
Total Legumes (Beans & Peas) (c-eq/wk)	1	1	1½	2	3	3	3½	4	5	5	6	6

[e, f, g] See Appendix 3, notes d through f.

Glossary of Terms

A

Acculturation—The process by which individuals who immigrate into a new country adopt the attitudes, values, customs, beliefs, and behaviors of the new culture. Acculturation is the gradual exchange between the original attitudes and behaviors associated with the originating country and those of the host culture.

Added Refined Starch—The starch constituent (see Carbohydrates) of a grain, such as corn, or of a vegetable, such as potato, used as an ingredient in another food. Starches have been refined to remove other components of the food, such as fiber, protein, and minerals. Refined starches can be added to foods as a thickener, a stabilizer, a bulking agent, or an anti-caking agent. While refined starches are made from grains or vegetables, they contain little or none of the many other components of these foods that together create a nutrient-dense food. They are a source of calories but few or no other nutrients.

Added Sugars—Syrups and other caloric sweeteners used as a sweetener in other food products. Naturally occurring sugars such as those in fruit or milk are not added sugars. Specific examples of added sugars that can be listed as an ingredient include brown sugar, corn sweetener, corn syrup, dextrose, fructose, glucose, high-fructose corn syrup, honey, invert sugar, lactose, malt syrup, maltose, molasses, raw sugar, sucrose, trehalose, and turbinado sugar. (See Carbohydrates, Sugars.)

B

Body Mass Index (BMI)—A measure of weight in kilograms (kg) relative to height in meters squared (m²). BMI is considered a reasonably reliable indicator of total body fat, which is related to the risk of disease and death. BMI status categories include underweight, healthy weight, overweight, and obese (**Table A6-1**). Overweight and obese describe ranges of weight that are greater than what is considered healthy

Table A6-1.

Body Mass Index (BMI) & Corresponding Body Weight Categories for Children & Adults

Body Weight Category	Children & Adolescents (Ages 2 to 19 Years) (BMI-for-Age Percentile Range)	Adults (BMI)
Underweight	Less than the 5th percentile	Less than 18.5 kg/m²
Normal Weight	5th percentile to less than the 85th percentile	18.5 to 24.9 kg/m²
Overweight	85th to less than the 95th percentile	25.0 to 29.9 kg/m²
Obese	Equal to or greater than the 95th percentile	30.0 kg/m² & greater

for a given height, while underweight describes a weight that is lower than what is considered healthy. Because children and adolescents are growing, their BMI is plotted on growth charts for sex and age. The percentile indicates the relative position of the child's BMI among children of the same sex and age.

C

Calorie Balance—The balance between calories consumed through eating and drinking and calories expended through physical activity and metabolic processes.

- **Calorie**—A unit commonly used to measure energy content of foods and beverages as well as energy use (expenditure) by the body. A kilocalorie is equal to the amount of energy (heat) required to raise the temperature of 1 kilogram of water 1 degree centigrade. Energy is required to sustain the body's various functions, including metabolic processes and physical activity. Carbohydrate, fat, protein, and alcohol provide all of the energy supplied by foods and beverages. If not specified explicitly, references to "calories" refer to "kilocalories."

Carbohydrates—One of the macronutrients and a source of energy. They include sugars, starches, and fiber:

- **Fiber**—Total fiber is the sum of *dietary fiber* and *functional fiber*. Dietary fiber consists of nondigestible carbohydrates and lignin that are intrinsic and intact in plants (i.e., the fiber naturally occurring in foods). Functional fiber consists of isolated, nondigestible carbohydrates that have beneficial physiological effects in humans. Functional fibers are either extracted from natural sources or are synthetically manufactured and added to foods, beverages, and supplements.

- **Starches**—Many glucose units linked together into long chains. Examples of foods containing starch include vegetables (e.g., potatoes, carrots), grains (e.g., brown rice, oats, wheat, barley, corn), and legumes (beans and peas; e.g., kidney beans, garbanzo beans, lentils, split peas).

- **Sugars**—Composed of one unit (a monosaccharide, such as glucose or fructose) or two joined units (a disaccharide, such as lactose or sucrose). Sugars include those occurring naturally in foods and beverages, those added to foods and beverages during processing and preparation, and those consumed separately. (See Added Sugars.)

Cardiovascular Disease (CVD)—Heart disease as well as diseases of the blood vessel system (arteries, capillaries, veins) that can lead to heart attack, chest pain (angina), or stroke.

Cholesterol—A natural sterol present in all animal tissues. Free cholesterol is a component of cell membranes and serves as a precursor for steroid hormones (estrogen, testosterone, aldosterone), and for bile acids. Humans are able to synthesize sufficient cholesterol to meet biologic requirements, and there is no evidence for a dietary requirement for cholesterol.

- **Blood Cholesterol**—Cholesterol that travels in the serum of the blood as distinct particles containing both lipids and proteins (lipoproteins). Also referred to as serum cholesterol. Two kinds of lipoproteins are:

  - **High-Density Lipoprotein (HDL-cholesterol)**—Blood cholesterol often called "good" cholesterol; carries cholesterol from tissues to the liver, which removes it from the body.

  - **Low-Density Lipoprotein (LDL-Cholesterol)**—Blood cholesterol often called "bad" cholesterol; carries cholesterol to arteries and tissues. A high LDL-cholesterol level in the blood leads to a buildup of cholesterol in arteries.

- **Dietary Cholesterol**—Cholesterol found in foods of animal origin, including meat, seafood, poultry, eggs, and dairy products. Plant foods, such as grains, vegetables, fruits, and oils do not contain dietary cholesterol.

Cup-Equivalent (cup-eq or c-eq)—The amount of a food or beverage product that is considered equal to 1 cup from the vegetables, fruits, or dairy food groups. A cup-eq for some foods or beverages may differ from a measured cup in volume because the foods have been concentrated (such as raisins or tomato paste), the foods are airy in their raw form and do not compress well into a cup (such as salad greens), or the foods are measured in a different form (such as cheese).

D

DASH Eating Plan—The DASH (Dietary Approaches to Stop Hypertension) Eating Plan exemplifies healthy eating. It was designed to increase intake of foods expected to lower blood pressure while being heart healthy and meeting Institute of Medicine (IOM) nutrient recommendations. It is available at specific calorie levels. It was adapted from the dietary pattern developed for the Dietary Approaches to Stop Hypertension (DASH) research trials. In the trials, the DASH dietary pattern lowered blood pressure and LDL-cholesterol levels, resulting in reduced cardiovascular disease risk. The DASH Eating Plan is low in saturated fats and rich in potassium, calcium, and magnesium, as well as fiber and protein. It also is lower in sodium than the typical American diet, and includes menus with two levels of sodium, 2,300 and 1,500 mg per day. It meets the Dietary Reference Intakes for all essential nutrients and stays within limits for overconsumed nutrients, while allowing adaptable food choices based on food preferences, cost, and availability.

Diabetes—A disorder of metabolism—the way the body uses digested food (specifically carbohydrate) for growth and energy. In diabetes, the pancreas either produces little or no insulin (a hormone that helps glucose, the body's main source of fuel, get into cells), or the cells do not respond appropriately to the insulin that is produced, which causes too much glucose to be released in the blood. The three main types of diabetes are type 1, type 2, and gestational diabetes. If not controlled, diabetes can lead to serious complications.

Dietary Reference Intakes (DRIs)—A set of nutrient-based reference values that are quantitative estimates of nutrient intakes to be used for planning and assessing diets for healthy people. DRIs expand on the periodic reports called Recommended Dietary Allowances (RDAs), which were first published by the Institute of Medicine in 1941.

- **Acceptable Macronutrient Distribution Ranges (AMDR)**—Range of intake for a particular energy source (i.e., carbohydrate, fat, and protein) that is associated with reduced risk of chronic disease while providing intakes of essential nutrients. If an individual's intake is outside of the AMDR, there is a potential of increasing the risk of chronic diseases and/or insufficient intakes of essential nutrients.

- **Adequate Intakes (AI)**—A recommended average daily nutrient intake level based on observed or experimentally determined approximations or estimates of mean nutrient intake by a group (or groups) of apparently healthy people. An AI is used when the Recommended Dietary Allowance cannot be determined.

- **Estimated Average Requirements (EAR)**—The average daily nutrient intake level estimated to meet the requirement of half the healthy individuals in a particular life stage and sex group.

- **Recommended Dietary Allowances (RDA)**—The average daily dietary intake level that is sufficient to meet the nutrient requirement of nearly all (97 to 98%) healthy individuals in a particular life stage and sex group.

- **Tolerable Upper Intake Levels (UL)**—The highest average daily nutrient intake level likely to pose no risk of adverse health effects for nearly all individuals in a particular life stage and sex group. As intake increases above the UL, the potential risk of adverse health effects increases.

E

Eating Behaviors—Individual behaviors that affect food and beverage choices and intake patterns, such as what, where, when, why, and how much people eat.

Eating Pattern (also called "dietary pattern")—The combination of foods and beverages that constitute an individual's complete dietary intake over time. This may be a description of a customary way of eating or a description of a combination of foods recommended for consumption. Specific examples include USDA Food Patterns and the Dietary Approaches to Stop Hypertension (DASH) Eating Plan. (See USDA Food Patterns and DASH Eating Plan.)

Energy Drink—A beverage that contains caffeine as an ingredient, along with other ingredients, such as taurine, herbal supplements, vitamins, and added sugars. It is usually marketed as a product that can improve perceived energy, stamina, athletic performance, or concentration.

Enrichment—The addition of specific nutrients (i.e., iron, thiamin, riboflavin, and niacin) to refined grain products in order to replace losses of the nutrients that occur during processing. Enrichment of refined grains is not mandatory; however, those that are labeled as enriched (e.g., enriched flour) must meet the standard of identity for enrichment set by the FDA. When cereal grains are labeled as enriched, it is mandatory that they be fortified with folic acid. (The addition of specific nutrients to whole-grain products is referred to as fortification; see Fortification.)

Essential Nutrient—A vitamin, mineral, fatty acid, or amino acid required for normal body functioning that either cannot be synthesized by the body at all, or cannot be synthesized in amounts adequate for good health, and thus must be obtained from a dietary source. Other food components, such as dietary fiber, while not essential, also are considered to be nutrients.

Existing Report—An existing systematic review, meta-analysis, or report by a Federal agency or leading scientific organization examined by the 2015 Dietary Guidelines Advisory Committee in its review of the scientific evidence. A systematic process was used by the Advisory Committee to assess the quality and comprehensiveness of the review for addressing the question of interest. (See Nutrition Evidence Library (NEL) systematic review.)

F

Fats—One of the macronutrients and a source of energy. (See Solid Fats and Oils.)

- **Monounsaturated Fatty Acids (MUFAs)**—Fatty acids that have one double bond and are usually liquid at room temperature. Plant sources rich in MUFAs include vegetable oils (e.g., canola, olive, high oleic safflower and sunflower), as well as nuts.

- **Polyunsaturated Fatty Acids (PUFAs)**—Fatty acids that have two or more double bonds and are usually liquid at room temperature. Primary sources are vegetable oils and some nuts and seeds. PUFAs provide essential fats such as n-3 and n-6 fatty acids.

- **n-3 PUFAs**—A carboxylic acid with an 18-carbon chain and three cis double bonds, Alpha-linolenic acid (ALA) is an n-3 fatty acid that is essential in the diet because it cannot be synthesized by humans. Primary sources include soybean oil, canola oil, walnuts, and flaxseed. Eicosapentaenoic acid (EPA) and docosahexaenoic acid (DHA) are very long chain n-3 fatty acids that are contained in fish and shellfish. Also called omega-3 fatty acids.

- **n-6 PUFAs**—A carboxylic acid with an 18-carbon chain and two cis double bonds, Linoleic acid (LA), one of the n-6 fatty acids, is essential in the diet because it cannot be synthesized by humans. Primary sources are nuts and liquid vegetable oils, including soybean oil, corn oil, and safflower oil. Also called omega-6 fatty acids.

- **Saturated Fatty Acids**—Fatty acids that have no double bonds. Fats high in saturated fatty acids are usually solid at room temperature. Major sources include animal products such as meats and dairy products, and tropical oils such as coconut or palm oils.

- *Trans* **Fatty Acids**—Unsaturated fatty acids that are structurally different from the unsaturated fatty acids that occur naturally in plant foods. Sources of *trans* fatty acids include partially hydrogenated vegetable oils used in processed foods such as desserts, microwave popcorn, frozen pizza, some margarines, and coffee creamer. *Trans* fatty acids also are present naturally in foods that come from ruminant animals (e.g., cattle and sheep), such as dairy products, beef, and lamb.

Food Access—Ability to obtain and maintain levels of sufficient amounts of healthy, safe, and affordable food for all family members in various settings including where they live, learn, work and play. Food access is often measured by distance to a store or the number of stores in an area; individual-level resources such as family income or vehicle availability; and neighborhood-level indicators of resources, such as average income of the neighborhood and the availability of public transportation.

Food Categories—A method of grouping similar foods in their as-consumed forms, for descriptive purposes. The USDA's Agricultural Research Service (ARS) has created 150 mutually exclusive food categories to account for each food or beverage item reported in What We Eat in America (WWEIA), the food intake survey component of the National Health and Nutrition Examination Survey (for more information, visit: http://seprl.ars.usda.gov/Services/docs.htm?docid=23429). Examples of WWEIA Food Categories include soups, nachos, and yeast breads. In contrast to food groups, items are not disaggregated into their component parts for assignment to food categories. For example, all pizzas are put into the pizza category.

Food Hub—A community space anchored by a food store with adjacent social and financial services where businesses or organizations can actively manage the aggregation, distribution, and marketing of source-identified food products to strengthen their ability to satisfy wholesale, retail, and institutional demand.

Food Groups—A method of grouping similar foods for descriptive and guidance purposes. Food groups in the USDA Food Patterns are defined as vegetables, fruits, grains, dairy, and protein foods. Some of these groups are divided into subgroups, such as dark-green vegetables or whole grains, which may have intake goals or limits. Foods are grouped within food groups based on their similarity in nutritional composition and other dietary benefits. For assignment to food groups, mixed dishes are disaggregated into their major component parts.

Food Pattern Modeling—The process of developing and adjusting daily intake amounts from food categories or groups to meet specific criteria, such as meeting nutrient intake goals, limiting nutrients or other food components, or varying proportions or amounts of specific food categories or groups. This methodology includes using current food consumption data to determine the mix and proportions of foods to include in each group, using current food composition data to select a nutrient-dense representative for each food, calculating nutrient profiles for each food group using these nutrient-dense representative foods, and modeling various combinations of foods and amounts to meet specific criteria. (See USDA Food Patterns.)

Food & Nutrition Policies—Regulations, laws, policymaking actions, or formal or informal rules established by formal organizations or government units. Food and nutrition policies are those that influence food settings and/or eating behaviors to improve food and/or nutrition choices, and potentially, health outcomes (e.g., body weight).

Fortification—As defined by the U.S. Food and Drug Administration (FDA), the deliberate addition of one or more essential nutrients to a food, whether or not it is normally contained in the food. Fortification may be used to prevent or correct a demonstrated deficiency in the population or specific population groups; restore naturally occurring nutrients lost during processing, storage, or handling; or to add a nutrient to a food at the level found in a comparable traditional food. When cereal grains are labeled as enriched, it is mandatory that they be fortified with folic acid.

H

Health—A state of complete physical, mental, and social well-being and not merely the absence of disease or infirmity.

Healthy Eating Index (HEI)—A measure of diet quality that assesses adherence to the *Dietary Guidelines*. The HEI is used to monitor diet quality in the United States and to examine relationships between diet and health-related outcomes. The HEI is a scoring metric that can be applied to any defined set of foods, such as previously collected dietary data, a defined menu, or a market basket. Thus, the HEI can be used to assess the quality of food assistance packages, menus, and the U.S. food supply.

High-Intensity Sweeteners—Ingredients commonly used as sugar substitutes or sugar alternatives to sweeten and enhance the flavor of foods and beverages. People may choose these sweeteners in place of sugar for a number of reasons, including that they contribute few or no calories to the diet. Because high-intensity sweeteners are many times sweeter than table sugar (sucrose), smaller amounts

of high-intensity sweeteners are needed to achieve the same level of sweetness as sugar in food and beverages. (Other terms commonly used to refer to sugar substitutes or alternatives include non-caloric, low-calorie, no-calorie, and artificial sweeteners, which may have different definitions and applications. A high-intensity sweetener may or may not be non-caloric, low-calorie, no-calorie, or artificial sweeteners.)

Household Food Insecurity— Circumstances in which the availability of nutritionally adequate and safe food, or the ability to acquire acceptable foods in socially acceptable ways, is limited or uncertain.

Hypertension—A condition, also known as high blood pressure, in which blood pressure remains elevated over time. Hypertension makes the heart work too hard, and the high force of the blood flow can harm arteries and organs, such as the heart, kidneys, brain, and eyes. Uncontrolled hypertension can lead to heart attacks, heart failure, kidney disease, stroke, and blindness. Prehypertension is defined as blood pressure that is higher than normal but not high enough to be defined as hypertension.

M

Macronutrient—A dietary component that provides energy. Macronutrients include protein, fats, carbohydrates, and alcohol.

Meats & Poultry—Foods that come from the flesh of land animals and birds. In the USDA Food Patterns, organs (such as liver) are also considered to be meat or poultry.

- **Meat** (also known as "red meat")—All forms of beef, pork, lamb, veal, goat, and non-bird game (e.g., venison, bison, elk).

- **Poultry**—All forms of chicken, turkey, duck, geese, guineas, and game birds (e.g., quail, pheasant).

- **Lean Meat & Lean Poultry**—Any meat or poultry that contains less than 10 g of fat, 4.5 g or less of saturated fats, and less than 95 mg of cholesterol per 100 g and per labeled serving size, based on USDA definitions for food label use. Examples include 95% lean cooked ground beef, beef top round steak or roast, beef tenderloin, pork top loin chop or roast, pork tenderloin, ham or turkey deli slices, skinless chicken breast, and skinless turkey breast.

- **Processed Meat & Processed Poultry**—All meat or poultry products preserved by smoking, curing, salting, and/or the addition of chemical preservatives. Processed meats and poultry include all types of meat or poultry sausages (bologna, frankfurters, luncheon meats and loaves, sandwich spreads, viennas, chorizos, kielbasa, pepperoni, salami, and summer sausages), bacon, smoked or cured ham or pork shoulder, corned beef, pastrami, pig's feet, beef jerky, marinated chicken breasts, and smoked turkey products.

Mixed Dishes—Savory food items eaten as a single entity that include foods from more than one food group. These foods often are mixtures of grains, protein foods, vegetables, and/or dairy. Examples of mixed dishes include burgers, sandwiches, tacos, burritos, pizzas, macaroni and cheese, stir-fries, spaghetti and meatballs, casseroles, soups, egg rolls, and Caesar salad.

Moderate Alcohol Consumption—Up to one drink per day for women and up to two drinks per day for men. One drink-equivalent is described using the reference beverages of 12 fl oz of regular beer (5% alcohol), 5 fl oz of wine (12% alcohol), or 1.5 fl oz of 80 proof (40%) distilled spirits. One drink-equivalent is described as containing 14 g (0.6 fl oz) of pure alcohol.[1]

Multi-Component Intervention—Interventions that use a combination of strategies to promote behavior change. These strategies can be employed across or within different settings or levels of influence.

Multi-Level Intervention—Interventions are those that target change at the individual level as well as additional levels, such as in the community (e.g., public health campaigns), schools (e.g., education), and food service (e.g., menu modification).

N

Nutrient Dense—A characteristic of foods and beverages that provide vitamins, minerals, and other substances that contribute to adequate nutrient intakes or may have positive health effects, with little or no solid fats and added sugars, refined starches, and sodium. Ideally, these foods and beverages also are in forms that retain naturally occurring components, such as dietary fiber. All vegetables, fruits, whole grains, seafood, eggs, beans and peas, unsalted nuts and seeds, fat-free and low-fat dairy products, and lean meats and poultry—when prepared with little or no added solid fats, sugars, refined starches, and sodium—are nutrient-dense foods. These foods contribute to meeting food group recommendations within calorie and sodium limits. The term "nutrient dense" indicates the nutrients and other beneficial substances in a food have not been "diluted" by the addition of calories from added solid fats, sugars, or refined starches, or by the

solid fats naturally present in the food.

Nutrient of Concern—Nutrients that are overconsumed or underconsumed and current intakes may pose a substantial public health concern. Data on nutrient intake, corroborated with biochemical markers of nutritional status where available, and association with health outcomes are all used to establish a nutrient as a nutrient of concern. Underconsumed nutrients, or "shortfall nutrients," are those with a high prevalence of inadequate intake either across the U.S. population or in specific groups, relative to IOM-based standards, such as the Estimated Average Requirement (EAR) or the Adequate Intake (AI). Overconsumed nutrients are those with a high prevalence of excess intake either across the population or in specific groups, related to IOM-based standards such as the Tolerable Upper Intake Level (UL) or other expert group standards.

Nutrition Evidence Library (NEL) Systematic Review—A process that uses state-of-the-art methods to identify, evaluate, and synthesize research to provide timely answers to important food and nutrition-related questions to inform U.S. Federal nutrition policies, programs, and recommendations. This rigorous, protocol-driven methodology is designed to minimize bias, maximize transparency, and ensure the use of all available relevant and high-quality research. The NEL is a program within the USDA Center for Nutrition Policy and Promotion. For more detailed information, visit: www.NEL.gov.

O

Oils—Fats that are liquid at room temperature. Oils come from many different plants and some fish. Some common oils include canola, corn, olive, peanut, safflower, soybean, and sunflower oils.

A number of foods are naturally high in oils such as nuts, olives, some fish, and avocados. Foods that are mainly made up of oil include mayonnaise, certain salad dressings, and soft (tub or squeeze) margarine with no *trans* fats. Oils are high in monounsaturated or polyunsaturated fats, and lower in saturated fats than solid fats. A few plant oils, termed tropical oils, including coconut oil, palm oil and palm kernel oil, are high in saturated fats and for nutritional purposes should be considered as solid fats. Partially hydrogenated oils that contain *trans* fats should also be considered as solid fats for nutritional purposes. (See Fats.)

Ounce-Equivalent (oz-eq)—The amount of a food product that is considered equal to 1 ounce from the grain or protein foods food group. An oz-eq for some foods may be less than a measured ounce in weight if the food is concentrated or low in water content (nuts, peanut butter, dried meats, flour) or more than a measured ounce in weight if the food contains a large amount of water (tofu, cooked beans, cooked rice or pasta).

P

Physical Activity—Any bodily movement produced by the contraction of skeletal muscle that increases energy expenditure above a basal level; generally refers to the subset of physical activity that enhances health.

Point-of-Purchase—A place where sales are made. Various intervention strategies have been proposed to affect individuals' purchasing decisions at the point of purchase, such as board or menu labeling with various amounts of nutrition information or shelf tags in grocery stores.

Portion Size—The amount of a food served or consumed in one eating

[1] Drink-equivalents are not intended to serve as a standard drink definition for regulatory purposes.

occasion. A portion is not a standardized amount, and the amount considered to be a portion is subjective and varies.

Prehypertension—See Hypertension.

Protein—One of the macronutrients; a major functional and structural component of every animal cell. Proteins are composed of amino acids, nine of which are indispensable (essential), meaning they cannot be synthesized by humans and therefore must be obtained from the diet. The quality of dietary protein is determined by its amino acid profile relative to human requirements as determined by the body's requirements for growth, maintenance, and repair. Protein quality is determined by two factors: digestibility and amino acid composition.

R

Refined Grains—Grains and grain products with the bran and germ removed; any grain product that is not a whole-grain product. Many refined grains are low in fiber but enriched with thiamin, riboflavin, niacin, and iron, and fortified with folic acid.

S

Screen Time—Time spent in front of a computer, television, video or computer game system, smart phone or tablet, or related device.

Seafood—Marine animals that live in the sea and in freshwater lakes and rivers. Seafood includes fish (e.g., salmon, tuna, trout, and tilapia) and shellfish (e.g., shrimp, crab, and oysters).

Sedentary Behavior—Any waking activity predominantly done while in a sitting or reclining posture. A behavior that expends energy at or minimally

above a person's resting level (between 1.0 and 1.5 metabolic equivalents) is considered sedentary behavior.

Serving Size—A standardized amount of a food, such as a cup or an ounce, used in providing information about a food within a food group, such as in dietary guidance. Serving size on the Nutrition Facts label is determined based on the Reference Amounts Customarily Consumed (RACC) for foods that have similar dietary usage, product characteristics, and customarily consumed amounts for consumers to make "like product" comparisons. (See Portion Size.)

Shortfall Nutrient—
See Nutrient of Concern.

Social-Ecological Model—
A framework developed to illustrate how sectors, settings, social and cultural norms, and individual factors converge to influence individual food and physical activity choices.

Solid Fats—Fats that are usually not liquid at room temperature. Solid fats are found in animal foods, except for seafood, and can be made from vegetable oils through hydrogenation. Some tropical oil plants, such as coconut and palm, are considered as solid fats due to their fatty acid composition. The fat component of milk and cream (butter) is solid at room temperature. Solid fats contain more saturated fats and/or *trans* fats than liquid oils (e.g., soybean, canola, and corn oils), with lower amounts of monounsaturated or polyunsaturated fatty acids. Common fats considered to be solid fats include: butter, beef fat (tallow), chicken fat, pork fat (lard), shortening, coconut oil, palm oil and palm kernel oil. Foods high in solid fats include: full-fat (regular) cheeses, creams, whole milk, ice cream, marbled cuts of meats, regular ground beef, bacon, sausages, poultry skin, and many baked

goods made with solid fats (such as cookies, crackers, doughnuts, pastries, and croissants). (See Fats and Nutrient Dense)

Sugar-Sweetened Beverages—
Liquids that are sweetened with various forms of added sugars. These beverages include, but are not limited to, soda (regular, not sugar-free), fruitades, sports drinks, energy drinks, sweetened waters, and coffee and tea beverages with added sugars. Also called calorically sweetened beverages. (See Added Sugars and Carbohydrates: Sugars.)

U

USDA Food Patterns—A set of eating patterns that exemplify healthy eating, which all include recommended intakes for the five food groups (vegetables, fruits, grains, dairy, and protein foods) and for subgroups within the vegetables, grains, and protein foods groups. They also recommend an allowance for intake of oils. Patterns are provided at 12 calorie levels from 1,000 to 3,200 calories to meet varied calorie needs. The Healthy U.S.-Style Pattern is the base USDA Food Pattern.

- **Healthy U.S.-Style Eating Pattern**—A pattern that exemplifies healthy eating based on the types and proportions of foods Americans typically consume, but in nutrient-dense forms and appropriate amounts, designed to meet nutrient needs while not exceeding calorie requirements. It is substantially unchanged from the primary USDA Food Patterns of the *2010 Dietary Guidelines*. This pattern is evaluated in comparison to meeting Dietary Reference Intakes for essential nutrients and staying within limits set by the IOM or *Dietary Guidelines* for overconsumed food components. It aligns closely with the Dietary Approaches to Stop Hypertension

(DASH) Eating Plan, a guide for healthy eating based on the DASH diet which was tested in clinical trials. (See Nutrient Dense and DASH Eating Plan.)

- **Healthy Mediterranean-Style Eating Pattern**—A pattern that exemplifies healthy eating, designed by modifying the Healthy U.S.-Style Pattern to more closely reflect eating patterns that have been associated with positive health outcomes in studies of Mediterranean-Style diets. This pattern is evaluated based on its similarity to food group intakes of groups with positive health outcomes in these studies rather than on meeting specified nutrient standards. It differs from the Healthy U.S.-Style Pattern in that it includes more fruits and seafood and less dairy.

- **Healthy Vegetarian Eating Pattern**—A pattern that exemplifies healthy eating, designed by modifying the Healthy U.S.-Style Pattern to more closely reflect eating patterns reported by self-identified vegetarians. This pattern is evaluated in comparison to meeting Dietary Reference Intakes for essential nutrients and staying within limits set by the IOM or *Dietary Guidelines* for overconsumed food components. It differs from the Healthy U.S.-Style Pattern in that it includes more legumes, soy products, nuts and seeds, and whole grains, and no meat, poultry, or seafood.

V

Variety—A diverse assortment of foods and beverages across and within all food groups and subgroups selected to fulfill the recommended amounts without exceeding the limits for calories and other dietary components. For example, in the vegetables food group, selecting a variety of foods could be accomplished over the course of a week by choosing from all subgroups, including dark green, red and orange, legumes (beans and peas), starchy, and other vegetables.

W

Whole Fruits—All fresh, frozen, canned, and dried fruit but not fruit juice.

Whole Grains—Grains and grain products made from the entire grain seed, usually called the kernel, which consists of the bran, germ, and endosperm. If the kernel has been cracked, crushed, or flaked, it must retain the same relative proportions of bran, germ, and endosperm as the original grain in order to be called whole grain. Many, but not all, whole grains are also sources of dietary fiber.

Table A10-1.
Potassium: Food Sources Ranked by Amounts of Potassium & Energy per Standard Food Portions & per 100 Grams of Foods

Food	Standard Portion Size	Calories in Standard Portion[a]	Potassium in Standard Portion (mg)[a]	Calories per 100 grams[a]	Potassium per 100 grams (mg)[a]
Potato, Baked, Flesh & Skin	1 medium	163	941	94	544
Prune Juice, Canned	1 cup	182	707	71	276
Carrot Juice, Canned	1 cup	94	689	40	292
Passion-Fruit Juice, Yellow or Purple	1 cup	126-148	687	51-60	278
Tomato Paste, Canned	¼ cup	54	669	82	1,014
Beet Greens, Cooked from Fresh	½ cup	19	654	27	909
Adzuki Beans, Cooked	½ cup	147	612	128	532
White Beans, Canned	½ cup	149	595	114	454
Plain Yogurt, Nonfat	1 cup	127	579	56	255
Tomato Puree	½ cup	48	549	38	439
Sweet Potato, Baked in Skin	1 medium	103	542	90	475
Salmon, Atlantic, Wild, Cooked	3 ounces	155	534	182	628

Table A10-1. *(continued...)*

Potassium: Food Sources Ranked by Amounts of Potassium & Energy per Standard Food Portions & per 100 Grams of Foods

Food	Standard Portion Size	Calories in Standard Portion[a]	Potassium in Standard Portion (mg)[a]	Calories per 100 grams[a]	Potassium per 100 grams (mg)[a]
Clams, Canned	3 ounces	121	534	142	628
Pomegranate Juice	1 cup	134	533	54	214
Plain Yogurt, Low-Fat	8 ounces	143	531	63	234
Tomato Juice, Canned	1 cup	41	527	17	217
Orange Juice, Fresh	1 cup	112	496	45	200
Soybeans, Green, Cooked	½ cup	127	485	141	539
Chard, Swiss, Cooked	½ cup	18	481	20	549
Lima Beans, Cooked	½ cup	108	478	115	508
Mackerel, Various Types, Cooked	3 ounces	114-171	443-474	134-201	521-558
Vegetable Juice, Canned	1 cup	48	468	19	185
Chili with Beans, Canned	½ cup	144	467	112	365
Great Northern Beans, Canned	½ cup	150	460	114	351
Yam, Cooked	½ cup	79	456	116	670
Halibut, Cooked	3 ounces	94	449	111	528
Tuna, Yellowfin, Cooked	3 ounces	111	448	130	527
Acorn Squash, Cooked	½ cup	58	448	56	437

Food	Standard Portion Size	Calories in Standard Portion[a]	Potassium in Standard Portion (mg)[a]	Calories per 100 grams[a]	Potassium per 100 grams (mg)[a]
Snapper, Cooked	3 ounces	109	444	128	522
Soybeans, Mature, Cooked	½ cup	149	443	173	515
Tangerine Juice, Fresh	1 cup	106	440	43	178
Pink Beans, Cooked	½ cup	126	430	149	508
Chocolate Milk (1%, 2% & Whole)	1 cup	178-208	418-425	71-83	167-170
Amaranth Leaves, Cooked	½ cup	14	423	21	641
Banana	1 medium	105	422	89	358
Spinach, Cooked from Fresh or Canned	½ cup	21-25	370-419	23	346-466
Black Turtle Beans, Cooked	½ cup	121	401	130	433
Peaches, Dried, Uncooked	¼ cup	96	399	239	996
Prunes, Stewed	½ cup	133	398	107	321
Rockfish, Pacific, Cooked	3 ounces	93	397	109	467
Rainbow Trout, Wild or Farmed, Cooked	3 ounces	128-143	381-383	150-168	448-450
Skim Milk (Nonfat)	1 cup	83	382	34	156
Refried Beans, Canned, Traditional	½ cup	106	380	89	319
Apricots, Dried, Uncooked	¼ cup	78	378	241	1162
Pinto Beans, Cooked	½ cup	123	373	143	436

Table A10-1. *(continued...)*
Potassium: Food Sources Ranked by Amounts of Potassium & Energy per Standard Food Portions & per 100 Grams of Foods

Food	Standard Portion Size	Calories in Standard Portion[a]	Potassium in Standard Portion (mg)[a]	Calories per 100 grams[a]	Potassium per 100 grams (mg)[a]
Lentils, Cooked	½ cup	115	365	116	369
Avocado	½ cup	120	364	160	485
Tomato Sauce, Canned	½ cup	30	364	24	297
Plantains, Slices, Cooked	½ cup	89	358	116	465
Kidney Beans, Cooked	½ cup	113	357	127	403
Navy Beans, Cooked	½ cup	128	354	140	389

[a] Source: U.S Department of Agriculture. Agricultural Research Service. Nutrient Data Laboratory. 2014. USDA National Nutrient Database for Standard Reference, Release 27. Available at: http://www.ars.usda.gov/nutrientdata.

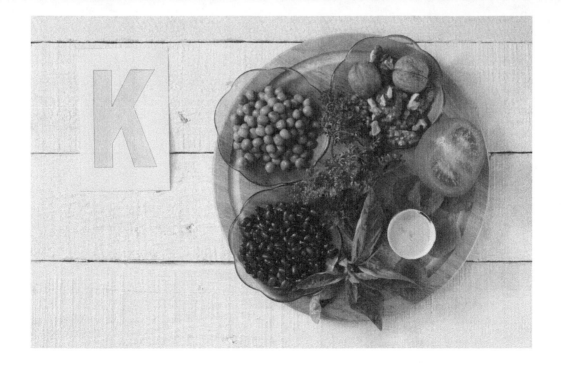

Table A11-1.
Calcium: Food Sources Ranked by Amounts of Calcium & Energy per Standard Food Portions & per 100 Grams of Foods

Food	Standard Portion Size	Calories in Standard Portion[a]	Calcium in Standard Portion (mg)[a]	Calories per 100 grams[a]	Calcium per 100 grams (mg)[a]
Fortified Ready-to-Eat Cereals (Various)[b]	¾-1¼ cup	70-197	137-1,000	234-394	455-3,333
Pasteurized Processed American Cheese	2 ounces	210	593	371	1,045
Parmesan Cheese, Hard	1.5 ounces	167	503	392	1,184
Plain Yogurt, Nonfat	8 ounces	127	452	56	199
Romano Cheese	1.5 ounces	165	452	387	1,064
Almond Milk (All Flavors)[b]	1 cup	91-120	451	38-50	188
Pasteurized Processed Swiss Cheese	2 ounces	189	438	334	772
Tofu, Raw, Regular, Prepared with Calcium Sulfate	½ cup	94	434	76	350
Gruyere Cheese	1.5 ounces	176	430	413	1,011
Plain Yogurt, Low-Fat	8 ounces	143	415	63	183
Vanilla Yogurt, Low-Fat	8 ounces	193	388	85	171

Table A11-1. *(continued...)*

Calcium: Food Sources Ranked by Amounts of Calcium & Energy per Standard Food Portions & per 100 Grams of Foods

Food	Standard Portion Size	Calories in Standard Portion[a]	Calcium in Standard Portion (mg)[a]	Calories per 100 grams[a]	Calcium per 100 grams (mg)[a]
Pasteurized Processed American Cheese Food	2 ounces	187	387	330	682
Fruit Yogurt, Low-Fat	8 ounces	238	383	105	169
Orange Juice, Calcium Fortified[b]	1 cup	117	349	47	140
Soymilk (All Flavors)[b]	1 cup	109	340	45	140
Ricotta Cheese, Part Skim	½ cup	171	337	138	272
Swiss Cheese	1.5 ounces	162	336	380	791
Evaporated Milk	½ cup	170	329	135	261
Sardines, Canned in Oil, Drained	3 ounces	177	325	208	382
Provolone Cheese	1.5 ounces	149	321	351	756
Monterey Cheese	1.5 ounces	159	317	373	746
Mustard Spinach (Tendergreen), Raw	1 cup	33	315	22	210
Muenster Cheese	1.5 ounces	156	305	368	717
Low-Fat Milk (1%)	1 cup	102	305	42	125
Mozzarella Cheese, Part-Skim	1.5 ounces	128	304	301	716

Food	Standard Portion Size	Calories in Standard Portion[a]	Calcium in Standard Portion (mg)[a]	Calories per 100 grams[a]	Calcium per 100 grams (mg)[a]
Skim Milk (Nonfat)	1 cup	83	299	34	122
Reduced Fat Milk (2%)	1 cup	122	293	50	120
Colby Cheese	1.5 ounces	167	291	394	685
Low-Fat Chocolate Milk (1%)	1 cup	178	290	71	116
Cheddar Cheese	1.5 ounces	173	287	406	675
Rice Drink[b]	1 cup	113	283	47	118
Whole Buttermilk	1 cup	152	282	62	115
Whole Chocolate Milk	1 cup	208	280	83	112
Whole Milk	1 cup	149	276	61	113
Reduced Fat Chocolate Milk (2%)	1 cup	190	273	76	109
Ricotta Cheese, Whole Milk	½ cup	216	257	174	207

[a] Source: U.S Department of Agriculture, Agricultural Research Service, Nutrient Data Laboratory. 2014. USDA National Nutrient Database for Standard Reference, Release 27. Available at: http://www.ars.usda.gov/nutrientdata.

[b] Calcium fortified.

Table A12-1.

Vitamin D: Food Sources Ranked by Amounts of Vitamin D & Energy per Standard Food Portions & per 100 Grams of Foods

Food	Standard Portion Size	Calories in Standard Portion[a]	Vitamin D in Standard Portion (µg)[a,b]	Calories per 100 grams[a]	Vitamin D per 100 grams (µg)[a,b]
Salmon, Sockeye, Canned	3 ounces	142	17.9	167	21.0
Trout, Rainbow, Farmed, Cooked	3 ounces	143	16.2	168	19.0
Salmon, Chinook, Smoked	3 ounces	99	14.5	117	17.1
Swordfish, Cooked	3 ounces	146	14.1	172	16.6
Sturgeon, Mixed Species, Smoked	3 ounces	147	13.7	173	16.1
Salmon, Pink, Canned	3 ounces	117	12.3	138	14.5
Fish Oil, Cod Liver	1 tsp	41	11.3	902	250
Cisco, Smoked	3 ounces	150	11.3	177	13.3
Salmon, Sockeye, Cooked	3 ounces	144	11.1	169	13.1
Salmon, Pink, Cooked	3 ounces	130	11.1	153	13.0
Sturgeon, Mixed Species, Cooked	3 ounces	115	11.0	135	12.9

Food	Standard Portion Size	Calories in Standard Portion[a]	Vitamin D in Standard Portion (µg)[a,b]	Calories per 100 grams[a]	Vitamin D per 100 grams (µg)[a,b]
Whitefish, Mixed Species, Smoked	3 ounces	92	10.9	108	12.8
Mackerel, Pacific & Jack, Cooked	3 ounces	171	9.7	201	11.4
Salmon, Coho, Wild, Cooked	3 ounces	118	9.6	139	11.3
Mushrooms, Portabella, Exposed to Ultraviolet Light, Grilled	½ cup	18	7.9	29	13.1
Tuna, Light, Canned in Oil, Drained	3 ounces	168	5.7	198	6.7
Halibut, Atlantic & Pacific, Cooked	3 ounces	94	4.9	111	5.8
Herring, Atlantic, Cooked	3 ounces	173	4.6	203	5.4
Sardine, Canned in Oil, Drained	3 ounces	177	4.1	208	4.8
Rockfish, Pacific, Mixed Species, Cooked	3 ounces	93	3.9	109	4.6
Whole Milk[c]	1 cup	149	3.2	61	1.3
Whole Chocolate Milk[c]	1 cup	208	3.2	83	1.3
Tilapia, Cooked	3 ounces	109	3.1	128	3.7
Flatfish (Flounder & Sole), Cooked	3 ounces	73	3.0	86	3.5
Reduced Fat Chocolate Milk (2%)[c]	1 cup	190	3.0	76	1.2

Table A12-1. *(continued...)*
Vitamin D: Food Sources Ranked by Amounts of Vitamin D & Energy per Standard Food Portions & per 100 Grams of Foods

Food	Standard Portion Size	Calories in Standard Portion[a]	Vitamin D in Standard Portion (µg)[a,b]	Calories per 100 grams[a]	Vitamin D per 100 grams (µg)[a,b]
Yogurt (Various Types & Flavors)[c]	8 ounces	98-254	2.0-3.0	43-112	0.9-1.3
Milk (Non-Fat, 1% & 2%)[c]	1 cup	83-122	2.9	34-50	1.2
Soymilk[c]	1 cup	109	2.9	45	1.2
Low-Fat Chocolate Milk (1%)[c]	1 cup	178	2.8	71	1.1
Fortified Ready-to-Eat Cereals (Various)[c]	⅓-1¼ cup	74-247	0.2-2.5	248-443	0.8-8.6
Orange Juice, Fortified[c]	1 cup	117	2.5	47	1.0
Almond Milk (All Flavors)[c]	1 cup	91-120	2.4	38-50	1.0
Rice Drink[c]	1 cup	113	2.4	47	1.0
Pork, Cooked (Various Cuts)	3 ounces	122-390	0.2-2.2	143-459	0.2-2.6
Mushrooms, Morel, Raw	½ cup	10	1.7	31	5.1
Margarine (Various)[c]	1 Tbsp	75-100	1.5	533-717	10.7
Mushrooms, Chanterelle, Raw	½ cup	10	1.4	38	5.3
Egg, Hard-Boiled	1 large	78	1.1	155	2.2

[a] Source: U.S Department of Agriculture, Agricultural Research Service, Nutrient Data Laboratory. 2014. USDA National Nutrient Database for Standard Reference, Release 27. Available at: http://www.ars.usda.gov/nutrientdata.

[b] 1 µg of vitamin D is equivalent to 40 IU.

[c] Vitamin D fortified.

Table A13-1.

Dietary Fiber: Food Sources Ranked by Amounts of Dietary Fiber & Energy per Standard Food Portions & per 100 Grams of Foods

Food	Standard Portion Size	Calories in Standard Portion[a]	Dietary Fiber in Standard Portion (g)[a]	Calories per 100 grams[a]	Dietary Fiber per 100 grams (g)[a]
High Fiber Bran Ready-to-Eat Cereal	½-¾ cup	60-81	9.1-14.3	200-260	29.3-47.5
Navy Beans, Cooked	½ cup	127	9.6	140	10.5
Small White Beans, Cooked	½ cup	127	9.3	142	10.4
Yellow Beans, Cooked	½ cup	127	9.2	144	10.4
Shredded Wheat Ready-to-Eat Cereal (Various)	1-1¼ cup	155-220	5.0-9.0	321-373	9.6-15.0
Cranberry (Roman) Beans, Cooked	½ cup	120	8.9	136	10.0
Adzuki Beans, Cooked	½ cup	147	8.4	128	7.3
French Beans, Cooked	½ cup	114	8.3	129	9.4
Split Peas, Cooked	½ cup	114	8.1	116	8.3
Chickpeas, Canned	½ cup	176	8.1	139	6.4
Lentils, Cooked	½ cup	115	7.8	116	7.9

Table A13-1. *(continued...)*

Dietary Fiber: Food Sources Ranked by Amounts of Dietary Fiber & Energy per Standard Food Portions & per 100 Grams of Foods

Food	Standard Portion Size	Calories in Standard Portion[a]	Dietary Fiber in Standard Portion (g)[a]	Calories per 100 grams[a]	Dietary Fiber per 100 grams (g)[a]
Pinto Beans, Cooked	½ cup	122	7.7	143	9.0
Black Turtle Beans, Cooked	½ cup	120	7.7	130	8.3
Mung Beans, Cooked	½ cup	106	7.7	105	7.6
Black Beans, Cooked	½ cup	114	7.5	132	8.7
Artichoke, Globe or French, Cooked	½ cup	45	7.2	53	8.6
Lima Beans, Cooked	½ cup	108	6.6	115	7.0
Great Northern Beans, Canned	½ cup	149	6.4	114	4.9
White Beans, Canned	½ cup	149	6.3	114	4.8
Kidney Beans, All Types, Cooked	½ cup	112	5.7	127	6.4
Pigeon Peas, Cooked	½ cup	102	5.6	121	6.7
Cowpeas, Cooked	½ cup	99	5.6	116	6.5
Wheat Bran Flakes Ready-to-Eat Cereal (Various)	¾ cup	90-98	4.9-5.5	310-328	16.9-18.3
Pear, Raw	1 medium	101	5.5	57	3.1
Pumpkin Seeds, Whole, Roasted	1 ounce	126	5.2	446	18.4

Food	Standard Portion Size	Calories in Standard Portion[a]	Dietary Fiber in Standard Portion (g)[a]	Calories per 100 grams[a]	Dietary Fiber per 100 grams (g)[a]
Baked Beans, Canned, Plain	½ cup	119	5.2	94	4.1
Soybeans, Cooked	½ cup	149	5.2	173	6.0
Plain Rye Wafer Crackers	2 wafers	73	5.0	334	22.9
Avocado	½ cup	120	5.0	160	6.7
Broadbeans (Fava Beans), Cooked	½ cup	94	4.6	110	5.4
Pink Beans, Cooked	½ cup	126	4.5	149	5.3
Apple, with Skin	1 medium	95	4.4	52	2.4
Green Peas, Cooked (Fresh, Frozen, Canned)	½ cup	59-67	3.5-4.4	69-84	4.1-5.5
Refried Beans, Canned	½ cup	107	4.4	90	3.7
Chia Seeds, Dried	1 Tbsp	58	4.1	486	34.4
Bulgur, Cooked	½ cup	76	4.1	83	4.5
Mixed Vegetables, Cooked from Frozen	½ cup	59	4.0	65	4.4
Raspberries	½ cup	32	4.0	52	6.5
Blackberries	½ cup	31	3.8	43	5.3
Collards, Cooked	½ cup	32	3.8	33	4.0
Soybeans, Green, Cooked	½ cup	127	3.8	141	4.2
Prunes, Stewed	½ cup	133	3.8	107	3.1

Table A13-1. *(continued...)*
Dietary Fiber: Food Sources Ranked by Amounts of Dietary Fiber & Energy per Standard Food Portions & per 100 Grams of Foods

Food	Standard Portion Size	Calories in Standard Portion[a]	Dietary Fiber in Standard Portion (g)[a]	Calories per 100 grams[a]	Dietary Fiber per 100 grams (g)[a]
Sweet Potato, Baked in Skin	1 medium	103	3.8	90	3.3
Figs, Dried	¼ cup	93	3.7	249	9.8
Pumpkin, Canned	½ cup	42	3.6	34	2.9
Potato, Baked, with Skin	1 medium	163	3.6	94	2.1
Popcorn, Air-Popped	3 cups	93	3.5	387	14.5
Almonds	1 ounce	164	3.5	579	12.5
Pears, Dried	¼ cup	118	3.4	262	7.5
Whole Wheat Spaghetti, Cooked	½ cup	87	3.2	124	4.5
Parsnips, Cooked	½ cup	55	3.1	71	4.0
Sunflower Seed Kernels, Dry Roasted	1 ounce	165	3.1	582	11.1
Orange	1 medium	69	3.1	49	2.2
Banana	1 medium	105	3.1	89	2.6
Guava	1 fruit	37	3.0	68	5.4
Oat Bran Muffin	1 small	178	3.0	270	4.6
Pearled Barley, Cooked	½ cup	97	3.0	123	3.8

Food	Standard Portion Size	Calories in Standard Portion[a]	Dietary Fiber in Standard Portion (g)[a]	Calories per 100 grams[a]	Dietary Fiber per 100 grams (g)[a]
Winter Squash, Cooked	½ cup	38	2.9	37	2.8
Dates	¼ cup	104	2.9	282	8.0
Pistachios, Dry Roasted	1 ounce	161	2.8	567	9.9
Pecans, Oil Roasted	1 ounce	203	2.7	715	9.5
Hazelnuts or Filberts	1 ounce	178	2.7	628	9.7
Peanuts, Oil Roasted	1 ounce	170	2.7	599	9.4
Whole Wheat Paratha Bread	1 ounce	92	2.7	326	9.6
Quinoa, Cooked	½ cup	111	2.6	120	2.8

[a] Source: U.S Department of Agriculture, Agricultural Research Service, Nutrient Data Laboratory. 2014. USDA National Nutrient Database for Standard Reference, Release 27. Available at: http://www.ars.usda.gov/nutrientdata.

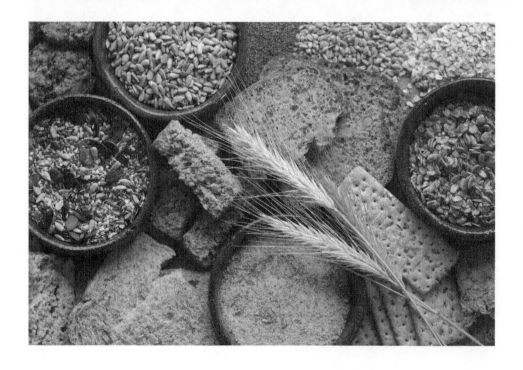

SIDE-BY-SIDE COMPARISON

Original Label

Nutrition Facts

Serving Size 2/3 cup (55g)
Servings Per Container About 8

Amount Per Serving

Calories 230	Calories from Fat 72
	% Daily Value*
Total Fat 8g	**12%**
Saturated Fat 1g	**5%**
Trans Fat 0g	
Cholesterol 0mg	**0%**
Sodium 160mg	**7%**
Total Carbohydrate 37g	**12%**
Dietary Fiber 4g	**16%**
Sugars 1g	
Protein 3g	
Vitamin A	10%
Vitamin C	8%
Calcium	20%
Iron	45%

* Percent Daily Values are based on a 2,000 calorie diet.
Your daily value may be higher or lower depending on
your calorie needs.

	Calories:	2,000	2,500
Total Fat	Less than	65g	80g
Sat Fat	Less than	20g	25g
Cholesterol	Less than	300mg	300mg
Sodium	Less than	2,400mg	2,400mg
Total Carbohydrate		300g	375g
Dietary Fiber		25g	30g

New Label

Nutrition Facts

8 servings per container
Serving size 2/3 cup (55g)

Amount per serving

Calories 230

	% Daily Value*
Total Fat 8g	**10%**
Saturated Fat 1g	**5%**
Trans Fat 0g	
Cholesterol 0mg	**0%**
Sodium 160mg	**7%**
Total Carbohydrate 37g	**13%**
Dietary Fiber 4g	**14%**
Total Sugars 12g	
Includes 10g Added Sugars	**20%**
Protein 3g	
Vitamin D 2mcg	10%
Calcium 260mg	20%
Iron 8mg	45%
Potassium 235mg	6%

* The % Daily Value (DV) tells you how much a nutrient in
a serving of food contributes to a daily diet. 2,000 calories
a day is used for general nutrition advice.

Note: The images above are meant for illustrative purposes to show how the new Nutrition Facts label might look compared to the old label. Both labels represent fictional products. When the original hypothetical label was developed in 2014 (the image on the left-hand side), added sugars was not yet proposed so the "original" label shows 1g of sugar as an example. The image created for the "new" label (shown on the right-hand side) lists 12g total sugar and 10g added sugar to give an example of how added sugars would be broken out with a % Daily Value.

NEW LABEL / WHAT'S DIFFERENT

Servings: larger, bolder type

Serving sizes updated

Calories: larger type

New: added sugars

Updated daily values

Change in nutrients required

Actual amounts declared

New footnote

Nutrition Facts

8 servings per container
Serving size   2/3 cup (55g)

Amount per serving
Calories   230

	% Daily Value*
Total Fat 8g	**10%**
Saturated Fat 1g	**5%**
Trans Fat 0g	
Cholesterol 0mg	**0%**
Sodium 160mg	**7%**
Total Carbohydrate 37g	**13%**
Dietary Fiber 4g	**14%**
Total Sugars 12g	
Includes 10g Added Sugars	**20%**
Protein 3g	

Vitamin D 2mcg	10%
Calcium 260mg	20%
Iron 8mg	45%
Potassium 235mg	6%

* The % Daily Value (DV) tells you how much a nutrient in a serving of food contributes to a daily diet. 2,000 calories a day is used for general nutrition advice.

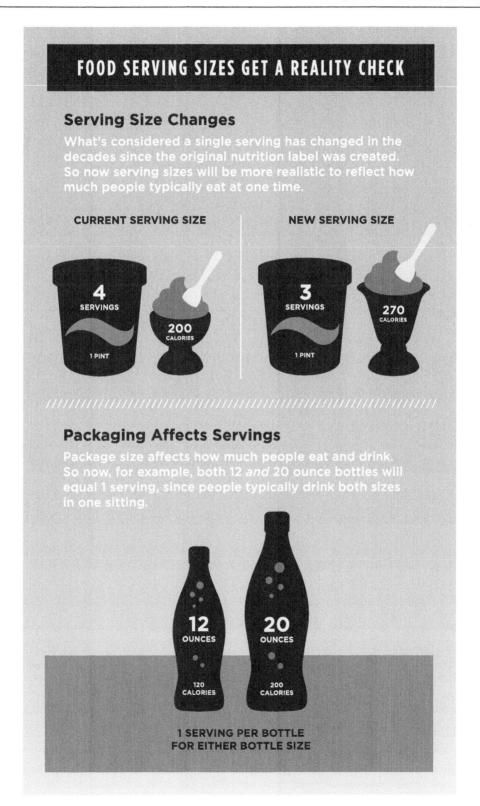

FOOD SERVING SIZES GET A REALITY CHECK

Serving Size Changes

What's considered a single serving has changed in the decades since the original nutrition label was created. So now serving sizes will be more realistic to reflect how much people typically eat at one time.

CURRENT SERVING SIZE

NEW SERVING SIZE

4 SERVINGS

1 PINT

200 CALORIES

3 SERVINGS

1 PINT

270 CALORIES

Packaging Affects Servings

Package size affects how much people eat and drink. So now, for example, both 12 *and* 20 ounce bottles will equal 1 serving, since people typically drink both sizes in one sitting.

12 OUNCES

120 CALORIES

20 OUNCES

200 CALORIES

1 SERVING PER BOTTLE FOR EITHER BOTTLE SIZE